Inguinal Hernia

advances or controversies?

Inguinal Hernia

advances or controversies?

Edited by
MAURICE E ARREGUI

Director of Fellowship in Laparoscopy, Endoscopy and Ultrasound,
St Vincent Hospital and Health Care Center, Indianapolis, Indiana, USA

and

ROBERT F NAGAN

Staff Surgeon, St Vincent Hospital and Health Care Center;
Assistant Clinical Professor, Indiana University, Indianapolis, Indiana, USA

Radcliffe Medical Press, Oxford • New York

15 Kings Meadow, Ferry Hinksey Road, Oxford OX2 0DP, UK

141 Fifth Avenue, Suite N, New York, NY 10010, USA

British Library Cataloguing in Publication Data

A catalogue record for this book is available from the British Library

Library of Congress Cataloging-in-Publication Data

Inguinal hernia : advances or controversies? / edited by Maurice E. Arregui and Robert Nagan.
p. cm.
Includes bibliographical references and index.
ISBN 1-85775-046-2 : $99.50
1. Inguinal hernia—Surgery. 2. Inguinal hernia. I. Arregui, Maurice E., 1951- . II. Nagan, Robert, 1921- .
[DNLM: 1. Hernia, Inguinal. WI 960 I55 1994]
RD621.I52 1994
617.5′59—dc20
DNLM/DLC
for Library of Congress 94-7987
CIP

ISBN 1 85775 046 2

Typset by AMA Graphics Ltd., Preston
Printed and bound in Great Britain by Biddles Ltd., Guildford and King's Lynn

Contents

Complications and controversies in open hernia repair

Part III: Laparoscopic hernia repairs

Techniques of laparoscopic hernia repairs

Laparoscopic ring closure techniques

Laparoscopic repair with intraperitoneal onlay mesh

Laparoscopic transabdominal preperitoneal approach to hernia repair

Laparoscopic extraperitoneal approach to hernia repair

Complications, recurrences and technical considerations in laparoscopic hernia repair

Part IV: Selected studies on hernia repair

Diagnosis of inguinal hernias

Classification of inguinal hernias

Open repair of inguinal hernias

Laparoscopic repair of inguinal hernias

Transabdominal preperitoneal repair of inguinal hernias

Transabdominal preperitoneal repair of recurrent hernias

Mesh considerations in hernia repairs

Repair of ventral hernias

Contributors

Toshio Akamatsu, Puget Sound Hospital, Tacoma, Washington, USA

Parviz K Amid, Lichtenstein Hernia Institute, Los Angeles, California, USA

Gabriel Angres, Department of Radiology, St Joseph Hospital, Elgin, Illinois, USA

Riccardo Annibali, Milan, Italy

Maurice E Arregui, St Vincent Hospital and Health Care Center, Indianapolis, Indiana, USA

Toshihisa Ashikawa, First Department of Surgery, Tokyo Medical and Dental School of Medicine, Tokyo, Japan

Mohammed Badruddoja, Department of General Surgery, Sherman Hospital, Elgin, Illinois, USA

Robert Bendavid, Shouldice Hospital, Thornhill, Ontario, Canada

Stanley D Berliner, Albert Einstein School of Medicine, New York, USA

M Bonenti, General Surgery Department, City Hospital, Belluno, Italy

William V Booth, Surgical Specialty Group Inc, Baton Rouge, Louisiana, USA

O Boudouris, Centre Hospitalier Universitaire, Amiens, France

Roderick B Brown, Glacial Ridge Hospital, Glenwood, Minnesota, USA

Armin Bruggemann, Department of Surgery, University of Goettingen, Goettingen, Germany

Jean A Bruyns, Saint Pierre Hospital, Brussels, Belgium

E Burgio, General Surgery Department, City Hospital, Belluno, Italy

Irving M Bush, Department of Urology and General Surgery, Chicago Medical School and Mount Sinai Medical Center, Chicago, Illinois, USA

Guy B Cadiere, Saint Pierre Hospital, Brussels, Belgium

Fábio G Campos, Mae de Deus Hospital, Sao Paulo, Brazil

Luis I Campos, Sacred Heart Hospital, Allentown, Pennsylvania, USA

José AV Carim, Samaritano Hospital, Sao Paulo, Brazil

Brendan J Carroll, Cedars-Sinai Medical Center, Los Angeles, California, USA

F Casa, CNR Ceriseie Ariel Center, Milan, Italy

Daniel Castro, Department of Surgery, St Vincent Hospital and Health Care Center, Indianapolis, Indiana, USA

Jamal Charara, Quebec Biomaterials Institute, St-Francois d'Assise Hospital, Quebec City, Canada

E Chiesara, Pharmacological Department, E Trabucchi, University of Medicine, Milan, Italy

Robert E Condon, The Medical College of Wisconsin, Milwaukee, Wisconsin, USA

John Corbitt Jr, JFK Medical Center, Atlantis, Florida, USA

Douglas Cornet, Department of Surgery, Creighton University School of Medicine, Omaha, Nebraska, USA

Frank T Crossland, M-J Insurance Inc, Indianapolis, Indiana, USA

A Da Rold, General Surgery Department, City Hospital, Belluno, Italy

Chad J Davis, Department of Surgery, St Vincent Hospital and Health Care Center, Indianapolis, Indiana, USA

Aureo L dePaula, Santa Rita Hospital, Sao Paulo, Brazil

L De Lazzer, General Surgery department, City Hospital, Belluno, Italy

Glenn A Deyo, Puget Sound Hospital, Tacoma, Washington, USA

Yves-Marie Dion, Department of Surgery, Laval University and Quebec Biomaterials Institute, St Francois de'Assise Hospital, Quebec City, Quebec, Canada

Tennison Dong, Department of Surgery, Valley Presbyterian Hospital, Van Nuys, California, USA

Jean L Dulucq, Hopital Bagatelle, Talance, France

Titus Duncan, George Baptist Medical Center, Atlanta, Georgia, USA

Francis A Dysarz, Department of Surgery, Staten Island University Hospital, New York, USA

Mitsuo Endo, First Department of Surgery, Tokyo Medical and Dental School of Medicine, Tokyo, Japan

W Steve Eubanks, Department of Surgery, Duke University Medical Center, Durham, North Carolina, USA

Moses J Fallas, Cedars-Sinai Medical Center, Los Angeles, California, USA

Franco Favretti, Divisione Chirurgia Generale, Presidio Ospedaliero, Belluno, Italy

Edward L Felix, Surgical Associates of Fresno Medical Clinic Inc., Fresno, California, USA

George S Ferzli, Department of Surgery, Staten Island University Hospital, New York, USA

Alberic GTW Fiennes, Department of Surgery, St George's Hospital Medical School, London, UK

Charles J Filipi, Department of Surgery, Creighton University School of Medicine, Omaha, Nebraska, USA

Robert J Fitzgibbons Jr, Department of Surgery, Creighton University School of Medicine, Omaha, Nebraska, USA

Morris E Franklin Jr, Health Science Center, University of Texas, San Antonio, Texas, USA

Arthur I Gilbert, Hernia Institute of Florida Inc, Florida, USA

PMNYH Go, Department of Surgery, University of Limberg, The Netherlands

Dalila Greco, Surgery Department, Hospital Niguarda, Ca' Granda, Milano, Italy

Lisa M Grininger, Kaiser Foundation Hospital, Honolulu, Hawaii

Jay L Grosfeld, Department of Surgery, Indiana University School of Medicine, Indianapolis, Indiana, USA

Robert Guidoin, Quebec Biomaterials Institute, St-Francois d'Assise Hospital, Quebec City, Canada

Joel C Hammond, Department of Surgery, St Vincent Hospital and Health Care Center, Indianapolis, Indiana, USA

William Harrop-Griffiths, St Mary's Hospital, London, UK

Kiyoshi Hashiba, Mae de Deus Hospital, Sao Paulo, Brazil

Abdelkader Hawasli, Eastside Surgical Specialists PC, St Clair Shores, Michigan, USA

Jacques M Himpens, Saint Pierre Hospital, Brussels, Belgium

Shing-Moo Huang, Department of Surgery, Veterans General Hospital, Taipei, Taiwan

Mark T Izawa, Kaiser Foundation Hospital, Honolulu, Hawaii

Rama Jager, Hernia Center Plus, Indianapolis, Indiana, USA

Namir Katkhouda, University of Southern California School of Medicine, Department of Surgery, Los Angeles, California, USA

Toru Kawamura, First Department of Surgery, Tokyo Medical and Dental School of Medicine, Tokyo, Japan

Maciej J Kieturakis, Sequioia Hospital, Redwood City, California, USA

Karl A LeBlanc, Surgical Specialty Group Inc, Baton Rouge, Louisiana, USA

PW Leopold, Department of Surgery, St George's Hospital, London, UK

Irving L Lichtenstein, Department of Surgery, Cedars-Sinai Medical Center, Harbor-UCLA Research and Education Institute, Los Angeles, California, USA

Paula J Lindahl, Kaiser Foundation Hospital, Honolulu, Hawaii

Bradley Litke, Department of Surgery, Creighton University School of Medicine, Omaha, Nebraska, USA

Demetrius Litwin, Mount Sinai Hospital, Toronto, Canada

A Loh, Department of Surgery, St George's Hospital, London, UK

George W Lucas, Georgia Baptist Medical Center, Atlanta, Georgia, USA

Wing-Yiu Lui, Department of Surgery, Veterans General Hospital, Taipei, Taiwan

Bruce V MacFadyen Jr, Department of Surgery, The University of Texas Medical School, Houston, Texas, USA

L Marabini, Pharmacological Department, E Trabucchi, University of Medicine, Milan, Italy

Edward Mason, George Baptist Medical Center, Atlanta, Georgia, USA

J Barry McKernan, Department of Surgery, Metropolitan and West Paces Ferry Hospital, Atlanta, Georgia, USA

Pablo Miguel, Samaritano Hospital, Sao Paulo, Brazil

John A Morrison, Department of Surgery, James Paton Memorial Hospital, Gander, Newfoundland, Canada

Takeshi Nagahama, Department of Surgery, Tokyo Metropolitan Komagome General Hospital, Tokyo, Japan

Robert F Nagan, Department of Surgery, St Vincent Hospital and Health Care Center, Indianapolis, Indiana, USA

Akira Nakashima, Department of Surgery, Nissan Kouseikai Tamagawa Hospital, Tokyo, Japan

Jorge Navarrete, Department of Surgery, St Vincent Hospital and Health Care Center, Indianapolis, Indiana, USA

Thomas Neufang, Department of Surgery, Georg-August University, Göttingen, Germany

Lucian Newman Jr III, George Baptist Medical Center, Atlanta, Georgia, USA

Lloyd M Nyhus, Department of Surgery, College of Medicine, University of Illinois, Chicago, California, USA

Howard A Olgin, Department of Surgery, Valley Presbyterian Hospital, Van Nuys, California, USA

Satoru Ootawa, Department of Surgery, Nissan Kouseikai Tamagawa Hospital, Tokyo, Japan

G Ortisi, Granda Milano Microbiological Department, H Niguarda CA', Milan, Italy

John H Payne Jr, Kaiser Foundation Hospital, Honolulu, Hawaii

Joseph A Perkins, M-J Insurance Inc, Indianapolis, Indiana, USA

Edward H Phillips, Cedars-Sinai Medical Towers, Los Angeles, California, USA

Joseph Pietrafita, Abbott Northwestern Hospital, Minneapolis, Minnesota, USA

Eileen F Podoll, Kaiser Foundation Hospital, Honolulu, Hawaii

Thomas Quinn, Division of Anatomy, Creighton University School of Medicine, Omaha, Nebraska, USA

Prasanta Raj, Department of Surgery, Fairview General Hospital, Cleveland, Ohio, USA

Raymond C Read, John L McClellan Memorial Veterans Hospital, Little Rock, Arkansas, USA

Stephen G ReMine, Department of Surgery, Fairview General Hospital, Cleveland, Ohio, USA

Luis Reyes, Department of Surgery, Fairview General Hospital, Cleveland, Ohio, USA

Jack K Riner, Hernia Center Plus, Indianapolis, Indiana, USA

Ronald N Riner, Department of Medical Affairs, Daughters of Charity National Health System, St Louis, Missouri, USA

Sérgio Roll, Santa Rita Hospital, Sao Paulo, Brazil

R David Rosin, St Mary's Hospital, London, UK

Ira M Rutkow, The Hernia Center, Freehold, New Jersey, USA

Robb H Rutledge, Harris Methodist Fort Worth Hospital, Fort Worth, Texas, USA

Yasushi Sato, Department of Surgery, Nissan Kouseikai Tamagawa Hospital, Tokyo, Japan

Leonard S Schultz, Laser Technologies Group Inc., Minneapolis, Minnesota, USA

Michael P Schwartz, Department of Radiology, St Joseph Hospital, Elgin, Illinois, USA

Arnold S Seid, Saint John's Hospital and Health Center, Santa Monica, California, USA

Chester J Semel, Cedars-Sinai Medical Center, Los Angeles, California, USA

Robert W Sewell, Harris Methodist – HEB, Bedford, Texas, USA

Alex G Shulman, Department of Surgery, Cedars-Sinai Medical Center, Harbor-UCLA Research and Education Institute, Los Angeles, California, USA

John E Skandalakis, Centers for Surgical Anatomy and Technique, Emory University School of Medicine, Atlanta, Georgia, USA

Leif Spangen, Central Hospital, Karlstad, Sweden

Albert T Spaw, HCA Center for Research and Education, Nashville, Tennessee, USA

James R Starling, Department of Surgery, University of Wisconsin-Madison Medical School, Madison, Wisconsin, USA

René E Stoppa, Hopital Nord, Amiens, France

Norihide Sugano, First Department of Surgery, Tokyo Medical and Dental School of Medicine, Tokyo, Japan

Kenneth P Sullivan, Department of Radiology, St Joseph Hospital, Elgin, Illinois, USA

Robert S Taylor, Department of Surgery, St George's Hospital London, UK

Cihat Tetik, Department of Surgery, St Vincent Hospital and Health Care Center, Indianapolis, Indiana, USA

C Tosi, Granda Physical Department, H Niguarda CA', Milan, Italy

Frederick K Toy, Department of Surgery, Nanticoke Memorial Hospital, Seaford, Delaware, USA

S Valletta, General Surgery Department, City Hospital, Belluno, Italy

H van Mameren, Department of Anatomy and Embryology, University of Limburg, Maastricht, The Netherlands

Cornelis J van Steensel, Reiner de Graaf Hospital, Delft, The Netherlands

Robert L Waddell, Harris Methodist-HEB, Bedford, Texas, USA

George E Wantz, The New York Hospital-Cornell Medical Center, New York, USA

Wibo F Weidema, Reiner de Graaf Hospital, Delft, The Netherlands

Also: John N Graber, David F Hickok, G Lepsien, F-E Ludtke,
Robert L McKnight Jr and Constantine A Michas

Publisher's Note

The last manuscript to reach us arrived on 21st March, leaving only 10 weeks in which to complete publication. This timescale, and the difficulty of communicating with 126 contributors from around the world, (some of whom do not use English as their first language), forced us to accept some inconsistencies of presentation. We are rather sensitive about this matter but we believe that only the most vigilant of our readers will notice where we have had to compromise on the high standards of production normally associated with our publications.

Radcliffe Medical Press
April 1994

Preface

Never before has interest in inguinal herniorrhaphy been so intense. This is due to the current enthusiasm for the laparoscopic approach. Approximately 700 000 hernias are repaired annually, 500 000 of which are inguinal hernias. Hernia operations have generally been considered as simple and not of great importance to many surgeons. During residency training, there is little enthusiasm by the senior staff and senior residents for the 'lowly' inguinal hernia, and it is often the junior residents who perform this anatomically complicated procedure. As a result, most surgeons complete their training in general surgery with only a minimal understanding of inguinal herniorrhaphy and a very vague concept of the related anatomy. When asked to explain which tissues are approximated, the reply is often 'stuff to stuff'. This is why recurrence rates in the 'real' world are so high.

As a result of the remarkable success of laparoscopic cholecystectomy—the most common procedure performed by the general surgeon—many have applied this approach to inguinal herniorrhaphy—the second most common procedure they perform. This book brings together several pioneers in the field of laparoscopic inguinal hernia repair, who present not only their experience but also the combined experience of numerous investigators internationally. Initial experiences are analysed and modifications suggested. Complications are honestly presented, and a detailed anatomy as seen from the laparoscopic perspective is introduced.

As the title suggests, laparoscopic inguinal herniorrhaphy may indeed be an advance. However, many also feel that it is controversial, in that inguinal herniorrhaphy may just as easily be accomplished by contemporary anterior approaches with less risk, less cost and confer the same advantages of rapid recovery and minimal pain claimed by the proponents of the laparoscopic approach. This book tries to temper the enthusiasm for laparoscopic inguinal herniorrhaphy by presenting the work of renowned experienced surgeons who are expert at open preperitoneal and anterior inguinal hernia repair. Their excellent results make us question whether inguinal herniorrhaphy is indeed an advance or a break-away from minimally invasive surgery to more invasive surgery.

This book is based on Hernias '93: Advances or Controversies, an international conference held May 24–27, 1993 in Indianapolis, Indiana. Speakers included major investigators in open as well as laparoscopic inguinal herniorrhaphy. The book is divided into four sections; the first part dealing with the basics including: anatomy, biology and classification of hernias. It also deals with biomaterials and the economics of hernia repair. Part Two deals with the various classical and contemporary open hernia repairs. Part Three presents techniques of laparoscopic repair as well as the complications and technical considerations, and Part Four is based on the numerous Free Paper presentations presented during the conference.

Because of the intense interest in inguinal herniorrhaphy, a concerted effort has been made to produce this book in a short period of time. The material presented is both current and practical as it addresses many of the contemporary questions asked by surgeons in practice. The Editors hope that it will stimulate further interest in the proper understanding of inguinal herniorrhaphy – which has finally received the attention that it has long deserved.

The Editors wish to thank Karl Storz Inc, Ethicon Inc, Cook Inc and WL Gore Inc, who have provided generous grants making possible the publication of this very timely book.

Maurice E Arregui
Robert F Nagan
May 1994

We dedicate this work to our wonderful wives, Pam and Dete, for their great love, support and encouragement. We deeply appreciate the sacrifices they make to accommodate the many scheduled and unscheduled hours we spend away from the warm homes they have made for us. Knowing that their welcoming arms await us at the end of each day means everything to us.

The Editors and Publishers of this book would like to acknowledge the considerable help provided by the following Sponsors, without which publication may not have been possible.

Cook Inc

Ethicon Inc

W. L. Gore Inc

Karl Storz Inc

Part I: General Considerations

History, embryology and anatomy
Biology of hernia formation
Diagnosis, classification and anaesthesia
Biomaterials in hernia repairs
Economics of hernia repair

1

History of Inguinal Herniorrhaphy

RAYMOND C READ

Of all the studies by which man acquires citizenship of the intellectual commonwealth, no single one is so indispensable as the study of the past. Bertrand Russell

The development of techniques for the repair of inguinal herniation is best divided into ancient and modern by the decade 1884–94 when Bassini introduced the first radical operation[1]. Halsted, just before his death, pointed out that Bassini unquestionably has the priority. 'I've not seen a single paper since Bassini's which contributed anything new. Prior to Bassini's publications inguinal hernia had rarely been cured'[2]. Willis Andrews in 1905 pointed out that the 'most original important step in the Bassini method was reconstructing a posterior wall of the canal up to and including the inguinal ring which was narrowed by suturing the conjoint tendon and transversalis fascia firmly to Poupart's ligament'[3]. William B. Coley in 1936, after a long surgical career, said that 'Bassini's method was original and not a modification of any of the earlier techniques'[4].

Ancient

The ancient era was largely taken up with understanding of surface anatomy[5]. The Romans in particular were very interested in the human body, taking baths and enjoying statuary. Celsus in AD 25 described, in his encyclopaedia, taxis and the difference between a hydrocele and an inguinal hernia. Heliodorus a hundred years later twisted the sac of the hernia to avoid castration. Paul of Aegina, AD 700, distinguished incomplete herniation into the canal itself (bubonocele) from complete herniation, which descended into the scrotum. He also, for causation, championed stretching of the peritoneum rather than its rupture as described by Galen. Roland of Parma in 1383 introduced the Trendelenburg manoeuvre to enhance reduction by taxis. Franco of Berne in 1556 made an important advance, describing a director that could be inserted into the canal and allow incision of inguinal rings in those patients resistant to taxis. Heister in 1724 resected strangulated bowel and performed a bowel diversion.

The ancient era before Bassini culminated in the golden age of anatomy, 1770–1840. Camper, Cloquet, Cooper, de Gimbernat, Hesselbach, Hunter, Morton, Scarpa and Thompson all contributed to a detailed understanding of the inguinal canal and its components. Because dissection was limited by the absence of both anaesthesia and antisepsis, all operations documented prior to Bassini were conducted beneath or through the external ring, including Marcy's first attempts[6]. Occasional incisors performed laparotomy, starting in India in 800 BC, in cases of strangulated bowel. The big argument was over the need for castration, which was avoided by dissecting the peritoneal sac, at the top of the scrotum, from the testicle. However, wounds were left open and sutures hanging, causing sepsis from which the testicle frequently sloughed anyway. As Zimmerman commented in 1937 at the 50th year commemoration of Bassini's world-shaking contribution, 'Edoardo Bassini found hernial surgery in the same stage of development it had reached during the Dark Ages and left it where it stands today'[7].

Bassini's era

Bassini was born in Pavia in northern Italy near Milan in 1844. He graduated from the medical school there in 1866 and fought with Garibaldi in the struggle for Italian independence. Interestingly enough, he was bayoneted in the groin and developed a faecal fistula which required dressings for over a year. He travelled widely, visited Lister and returned to introduce antisepsis to Italy. He became the Chairman of Surgery at Padua, and died, 80 years old, at Verona in 1924. His contributions included:

- complete division of the external oblique aponeurosis to expose the canal
- excision of the cremaster
- complete division of the transversalis fascial floor
- dissection and isolation of the spermatic cord
- ligature of the processus vaginalis flush with the peritoneum in the iliac fossa
- use of the preperitoneal plane
- construction of a new floor for the inguinal canal mediolaterally, including transversalis fascia with the conjoint tendon, his 'triple layer'.

The cord was transplanted anterolaterally, restoring obliquity to the inguinal canal. He explanted the cord laterally to within 2.5 cm (1 inch) of the anterior superior iliac spine, constructing a new internal abdominal ring. He used the rectus sheath in repair, and fixed it with interrupted deep silk sutures. He allowed the patient to wake from anaesthesia to test the repair intraoperatively. His infection rate was only 4% and he rarely used drains. He shortened hospitalization to a couple of weeks, and insisted on early ambulation. After operation the patient was not given a truss.

Modern era

Bassini's follow up, reported in the German literature[8], was over 90% for up to four and a half years in a large series of 262 patients, including children and adults, men and women, indirect and direct herniation. He published extensively on his work but, although he remained as Chairman for another 25 years, his last discussion of inguinal herniorrhaphy was in 1894, and he didn't participate in the arguments regarding the many modifications that were soon introduced. These were designed to decrease the risk to the femoral vein, the bladder and the blood supply to the testicle, and consisted frequently of suturing the internal oblique muscle down to the inguinal ligament as initiated by Bull and Coley in 1890[9,10]. Berger described the use of the cremasteric muscle in the repair in 1902[11], whereas Ferguson (1899)[12] and later Halsted II[13] described bringing the internal oblique muscle over the cord, which was undisturbed, and suturing it to the inguinal ligament. This was a particularly pernicious technique because the processus vaginalis was ligated in the canal rather than above the internal abdominal ring. Russell in 1912[14] championed simple ligation of the processus vaginalis without closure of the ring in indirect herniation, particularly in children. This idea was taken up between the World Wars because it preserved the shutter mechanism, particularly important in young recruits.

Wolfler in 1892[15] introduced the rectus sheath relaxing incision. Marcy in 1895[16] described the posterior repair of the internal inguinal ring, and Narath in 1896[17] is credited with the first use of a prosthesis made of silver filigree. Later modifications included in 1896 Lotheissen's[18] using the Cooper's ligament rather than inguinal ligament for fixation, later popularized by McVay. McArthur[19] described suturing of the pedicled external oblique aponeurotic graft. Kirschner in 1910[20] introduced fascia lata for this purpose, and Usher in 1958[21] described Marlex, the most successful of the plastic prostheses.

These various modifications, along with an increase in the incidence of direct hernia from ageing and cigarette smoking, resulted in the 1920s and 30s in bad results. The Bassini operation fell into disrepute, largely because it was not done properly. The difficulty with recurrence after repair of direct herniation prompted the wide use of fascial grafts, championed by Gallie of Canada, and the further development of artificial prostheses to reinforce the repair. It also prompted a return to the original Bassini operation, which was the origin of the Shouldice procedure which over the last 30 years has dominated inguinal herniorrhaphy without prosthetic replacement. Harrison in 1922, while working in Saudi Arabia, made an important contribution. He pointed out that 'the natural conclusion regarding the cause of an indirect and direct hernia is the failure of the transversalis fascia'[22]. This concept stimulated exposures of this layer by other avenues, in particular the posterior or abdominal approach.

With the explosion of abdominal surgery that followed the introduction of anaesthesia by Morton in 1846[23] and antisepsis by Lister 20 years later[24], repair of inguinal herniation by transabdominal section was widely discussed in Europe and Great Britain in the late nineteenth century. This transperitoneal method persisted up until the Second World War. It was modified by LaRoque of Richmond, Virginia, in the early part of this century, to be combined with the classic anterior repair. However, Cheatle in 1920[25] at Kings College Hospital in London was the first to use the preperitoneal space in the inguinal hernia repair. His contribution was ignored and it had to be rediscovered in 1936 by Henry[26]. This technique has been exploited with excellent results by Stoppa in France during the last 25 years. McEvedy in England (1950)[27] made a significant contribution by describing a unilateral preperitoneal exposure through the rectus sheath, retracting the rectus muscle medially rather than laterally. This technique was popularized and extended by Nyhus and his associates ten years later[28] at the suggestion of Professor Bruce of Edinburgh. It is important to point out that, whereas the Cheatle–Henry incision allows the repair to be conducted internal to the inferior epigastric vessels which are retracted laterally with the rectus muscles, the McEvedy approach comes down on these structures and the fissile bloodless plane has to be reached beneath them by incising the posterior lamina of the transversalis fascia, originally described by Astley Cooper. Wantz[29] has successfully employed unilateral prosthetic repair through this incision whereas Rives[30], a colleague of Stoppa (his work being carried on recently by Flament at Rheims), entered the preperitoneal plane from the groin for prosthetic placement. Stoppa made another important contribution in pointing out that the cord could be dissected and separated back into its contributions from the vas deferens and the spermatic vessels, so that it could be parietalized onto the iliopsoas muscle[31]. Prostheses can then be placed internal to these extraperitoneal structures, thus essentially explanting the internal abdominal ring up retroperitoneally so that a separate incision in the prosthesis is not necessary for passage of the cord.

An important contribution to inguinal herniorrhaphy was made by Mahorner and Goss in 1962[32], operating on two patients with large recurrences following multiple operations. They were faced with a repair without either inguinal or Astley Cooper's ligament remaining. They constructed an angle iron dermal graft sutured retroperitoneally and anteriorly over the peritoneum, beneath the abdominal wall where it was widely sutured. This principle has been used in Stoppa and Wantz' work with the posterior approach and has influenced Rives and certainly myself in performing prosthetic preperitoneal placement from the classic anterior incision.

Conclusion

The advent of laparoscopic herniorrhaphy has led to a re-examination of where we have been and where we are going with the fundamentals of inguinal herniation and which structures are important for repair regardless of the approach used to expose them.

References

1. Bassini E. Sulla cura radicale dell'ernia inguinale. *Arch Soc Ital Chir* 1887; **4**: 380.
2. Halsted WS. The cure of the more difficult as well as the simpler inguinal ruptures. *Johns Hopkins Hosp Bull* 1903; **14**: 208.
3. Andrews EW. Imbrication or lap joint method: a plastik operation for hernia. *Chicago Med Rec* 1895; **9**: 67.
4. Coley WB. Review of the radical cure of hernia during the last half of the century. (editorial) *Am J Surg* 1936; **31**: 397–402.
5. Read RC. The development of inguinal herniorrhaphy. *Surg Clin North Am* 1984; **64**: 185.
6. Marcy HO. A new use for catabolized catgut sutures. *Boston Med Surg J* 1871; **85**: 315.
7. Zimmerman LM, Heller RE. Edoardo Bassini and his role in the development of hernial surgery. In: Fasiani GM, Catterina A, eds. Scritti di Chirurgia Erniaria per Commemorare il Cinquantenario della Operazion di Bassini, 2 vols. Padova, Italy: Universita di Padova, 1937: 606–13.
8. Bassini E. Ueber de Behandlung des Leistenbruches. *Arch Klin Chir* 1890; **40**: 429.
9. Bull WT. Notes on cases of hernia which have relapsed after various operations for radical cure. *NY Med J* 1891; **53**: 615.
10. Coley WB. The operative treatment of hernia with a report of 200 cases. *Ann Surg* 1895; **21**: 389.
11. Berger P. La hernie inguino-interstitielle et son traitment par la cure radicale. *Rev Chir Paris* 1902; **25**: 1.
12. Ferguson AH. Oblique inguinal hernia: typical operation for its radical cure. *JAMA* 1899; **33**: 6.
13. Halsted WS. The radical cure of hernia. *Johns Hopkins Hosp Bull* 1889; **1**: 12.
14. Russell RH. The saccular theory of hernia and the radical operation. *Lancet* 1906; **2**: 1197.
15. Wolfler A. Zur Radikaloperation des Freien Leistenbruches. *Beitr Chir* (Festchrift Geuidmet Theodor Billroth). Stuttgart, 1892: 552.
16. Marcy HO. The surgical treatment of inguinal hernia. *Med News* 1895; **66**: 35.
17. Read RC. Historical survey of the treatment of hernia. In: Nyhus LM, Condon RE, eds. *Hernia*, 3rd ed. Philadelphia JB Lippincott, 1989: 3–17.
18. Lotheissen G. Zur Radicaloperation des Schenkelhernien. *Zentralbl Chir* 1898; **25**: 548.
19. McArthur LL. Autoplastic suture in hernia and other diastases; preliminary report. *JAMA* 1901; **37**: 1162.
20. Kirschner M. Die praktischen Ergebnisse der freien Fascien-Transplantation. *Arch Klin Chir* 1910; **92**: 888.
21. Usher FC, Oschner, J, Tuttle Jr LL. Use of Marlex mesh in the repair of incisional hernias. *Am Surg* 1958; **24**: 969.
22. Harrison PW. Inguinal hernia: a study of the principles involved in surgical treatment. *Arch Surg* 1922; **4**: 680.
23. Fulton JF. The vision and daring of youth. *Yale J Biol Med* 1946; **19**: 207.

24. Ellis H. Lord Lister and the compound fracture. *Contemp Surg* 1979; **15**: 67.

25. Cheatle GL. An operation for the radical cure of inguinal and femoral hernia. *BMJ* 1920; **2**: 68.

26. Henry AK. Operation for femoral hernia by a midline extraperitoneal approach: with a preliminary note on the use of this route for reducible inguinal hernia. *Lancet* 1936; **1**: 531.

27. McEvedy PG. Femoral hernia. *Ann R Coll Surg Engl* 1950; **7**: 484.

28. Nyhus LM, Condon RE, Harkins HN. Clinical experiences with preperitoneal hernial repair for all types of hernia of the groin. *Am J Surg* 1960; **100**: 234.

29. Wantz GE. Giant prosthetic reinforcement of the visceral sac. *Surg Gynecol Obstet* 1989; **169**: 408–17.

30. Rives J. Surgical treatment of the inguinal hernia with Dacron patch. *Int Surg* 1967; **47**: 360–1.

31. Stoppa RE, Warlaumont CR, Verhaegthe PJ, *et al.* Prosthetic repair in the treatment of groin hernias. *Int Surg* 1986; **71**: 154.

32. Mahorner H, Goss CM. Herniation following destruction of Poupart's and Cooper's ligaments: a method of repair. *Ann Surg* 1962; **155**: 741.

2

The Anatomy of the Groin: the Basis for Anatomical Repair of Groin Hernias

ROBERT E CONDON

Groin anatomy

The tissues of the groin are layered:

1 skin

2 subcutaneous fat (Scarpa's)

3 external oblique

4 internal oblique

5 TRANSVERSUS ABDOMINIS

6 preperitoneal fat

7 peritoneum

A groin hernia is the result of a *defect in the integrity of the transversus abdominis lamina* of the body wall, permitting protrusion of the peritoneum and its contents into or through the more superficial layers of the abdominal wall. Anatomical groin hernia repair is a surgical exercise in applied anatomy directed to restoration or replacement of tissue continuity in the transversus abdominis lamina.

Knowledge of groin anatomy has for years been confused by inaccurate descriptions based on observations made in embalmed cadavers. Groin anatomy is best learned using fresh material for dissection, and thus is best learned in the operating room or in the autopsy suite. Publications based on dissections of fresh material[1–4] provide a base of accurate description on which to build a three-dimensional conception of normal anatomy. Furthermore, dissection of fresh material leads to an understanding of the range of alterations associated with groin hernia, thus allowing more effective repair.

The transversus abdominis lamina of the groin, the layer in which the primary musculoaponeurotic defect occurs in a groin hernia, is muscular laterally and aponeurotic (fascial tendinous) medially. The line of transition connects the deep inguinal ring and the costoxiphoid angle. The transversus abdominis muscle and aponeurosis are lined internally by a thin investing layer of tissue, the transversalis fascia. *The transversalis fascia is of no use in hernia repair.* Misconceptions regarding the transversalis fascia are a major source of confusion and error in discussions of groin hernia repair.

The medial aponeurotic portion of the transversus abdominis layer is, for the most part, a continuous tendinous sheet passing posterior to the rectus abdominis muscle to insert into the linea alba. However, below the semicircular line – located several centimetres below the umbilicus – the transversus abdominis aponeurosis passes anterior to the belly of the rectus abdominis muscle. In this area it is joined at the lateral border of the rectus, and is thus reinforced by the aponeurosis of the internal oblique.

In the most inferior portion of the groin, however, the continuity of the transversus abdominis lamina is lost. The inferior border of the continuous superior portion is the transversus abdominis arch; this structure is easily identified by palpation. It arches across the groin from the iliopsoas fascia, laterally, passing *above* the deep inguinal ring, to insert medially into the most inferior portion of the rectus sheath and into, but usually not beyond, the pubic tubercle. It is relatively uncommon (11%) for this insertion to go beyond the pubic tubercle, but when it does insert into the medial part of the superior pubic ramus then a true conjoined tendon (falx inguinalis) is present. *Remember: a true conjoined tendon is present in only a small minority of patients.*

At the most inferior portion of the transversus abdominis lamina, another band of connective tissue is found, the iliopubic tract. This structure, like the transversus abdominis arch, is attached laterally to the iliopsoas fascia. But, in crossing the groin, it passes *below* the deep inguinal ring, forming the upper margin of the femoral sheath and then recurves inferiorly to define the medial margin of the femoral canal; it finally inserts broadly into the superior pubic ramus. The inguinal ligament, the inferior margin of the external oblique lamina, lies immediately external to and parallel with the iliopubic tract, but is not so firmly attached to the femoral sheath and does not recurve but goes directly to its insertion between the pubic tubercles. *Thus, it is the iliopubic tract rather than the inguinal ligament that defines the femoral canal and forms the so-called lacunar ligament.*

The medial area of the groin between the iliopubic tract and the transversus abdominis arch forms the posterior wall of the inguinal canal. In this area, the reinforcement of transversalis fascia by aponeurotic fibres is very variable. This is the area in which a direct hernia occurs. The vertical extent of the posterior wall of the inguinal canal is variable and is related to the steepness of the pelvis. Women have a broad, flat pelvis with a very short gap between the iliopubic tract and transversus abdominis arch, which accounts for the fact that women rarely develop a direct inguinal hernia. Men, in contrast, have a variably steep, funnel-like pelvic skeleton and, associated with this, a relatively more extensive gap between the iliopubic tract and transversus abdominis arch, thus leading to the liability in men to develop a direct hernia.

Direct hernias

Direct hernias occur through the posterior wall of the inguinal canal and may be repaired, if small, by using a relaxing incision to create a bipedicled sliding tissue flap, permitting suture approximation of the transversus abdominis arch to the iliopubic tract. This restores the continuity of the transversus abdominis lamina. More often, however, even the use of a relaxing incision will not permit primary tissue approximation without tension. Tissue replacement with a prosthesis is frequently required in the repair of a typical medium to large direct inguinal hernia.

Indirect hernias

Indirect hernias occur through the superior aspect of the deep inguinal ring, between the transversus abdominis arch above, and the iliopubic tract below. Plastic repair of small to moderate sized indirect inguinal hernias is accomplished by suturing the transversus abdominis arch to the iliopubic tract about the cord to reconstitute an intact deep inguinal ring. A prosthesis is not usually needed in the repair of a typical indirect inguinal hernia. In some cases, indirect hernias enlarge medially into the posterior wall of the inguinal canal. These large indirect (complete) hernias are repaired by reconstruction of the deep ring together with tissue replacement or primary repair as for a direct hernia.

Femoral hernias

Femoral hernias progress down the femoral canal and are repaired by suturing the iliopubic tract above, to Cooper's ligament and pectineus fascia below. Prosthetic repair is not needed in the treatment of femoral hernias.

Hernia repair

The principles of anatomical repair of a groin hernia are:

1 the approach (anterior through the inguinal canal or posterior through the preperitoneal space) does not alter the structures nor the technique used in hernia repairs

2 the margins of the hernia defect are cleared of transversalis fascia and any other attenuated tissues to define the true fascial margins of the hernia defect

3 determine if the margins of the hernia defect can be approximated without tension (more than three pounds pull)

4 if tissues can be approximated without tension, conduct primary repair with sutures, testing each suture bite to make sure it will hold

5 if the anatomical margins cannot be approximated without tension, replace the missing tissue by inserting a prosthesis; test each suture holding the prosthesis about the defect to ensure that it will hold in the body wall.

References

1. Condon RE. Surgical anatomy of the transversus abdominis and transversalis fascia. *Ann Surg* 1971; **173**: 105.

2. Condon RE. 1989 The anatomy of the inguinal region and its relation to groin hernia. In: Nyhus LM, Condon RE, eds. *Hernia*, 3rd ed. Philadelphia: JB Lippincott, 1989: 18–60.

3. Nyhus LM, Condon RE, Harkins HN. Clinical experiences with preperitoneal hernial repair for all types of hernia of the groin; with particular reference to the importance of transversalis fascia analogues. *Am J Surg* 1960; **100**: 234–44.

4. Gilroy AM, Marks Jr SC, Lei Q, Page DW. Anatomical characteristics of the iliopubic tract: implications for repair of inguinal hernias. *Clin Anat* 1992; **5**: 255–63.

3

Gonadal Descent and the Surgical Anatomy of the Inguinal Canal

JOHN E SKANDALAKIS

Embryology

Differentiation of the gonads between male and female takes place at the seventh week of development. There are three embryological entities responsible for the genesis of the gonads:

- the mesodermal epithelium (mesothelium)
- the underlying mesenchyme
- the primordial germ cells.

The mesothelium and the mesenchyme produce the gonads, which are located between the mesonephros and the mesentery of the hindgut. This production is the genital ridge.

This primordial germ cells can be seen around the third week in the wall of the yolk sac, very close to the allantois, among endodermal cells. These peculiar cells migrate along the mesentery of the hindgut, invade the genital ridge around the sixth week, and later, by stimulation of the Y chromosome, differentiate in testicular tissue.

Prior to the differentiation in testicular tissue, the formation of primitive sex cords takes place. Later, during differentiation to the testis and ovary, these sex cords become the medullary cords. In time, the tunica albuginea is formed.

With the absence of the Y chromosome, the gonad differentiates into the ovary which, characteristically, does not have a tunica albuginea but rather a surface epithelium. Anatomists are currently debating if this epithelium is peritoneum. (I do not believe that the ovary is covered by peritoneum.)

The differentiation of the sex to ovary does not depend on hormones, and differentiation takes place even if the ovaries are absent. If the germ cells do not reach the indifferent gonad, the gonad remains indifferent or absent. The Leydig cells are of mesenchymal origin and, at about the eighth week of gestation, they start producing testosterone. The cells of Sertoli, a product of differentiation of the germ cells, are responsible for the production of sperm at puberty.

As to the ovary, the germ cells develop into oögonia and the surface epithelium forms the follicular cells[1].

Embryology of the groin

The embryology of the inguinal canal is peculiar. In a highly synergistic way, the skin above, the parietal peritoneum below and the embryological and anatomical entities between produce the future pathway for the testicles. They also, on occasion, provide a home for several congenital anomalies.

The skin forms the scrotum in the male and the labia in the female. The parietal peritoneum produces the processus vaginalis, a diverticulum that is present initially in all fetuses. It is, however, more important to the male because it permits the descent of the testicles. The embryological entities between the skin and peritoneum permit the processus vaginalis to penetrate them and to form the inguinal canal. Later, the inguinal canal will allow the downward journey of the testicle to the scrotum but will prevent the descent of the ovary outside of the peritoneal cavity.

The descent of the gonads

At the end of the second month or at the beginning of the third month, the testis is attached to the retroperitoneal space by a mesentery, the caudal genital ligament. The distal part of this ligament is the gubernaculum, which grows toward the scrotal swelling, which appears around the third month.

Exactly when the journey starts is unknown but, around the 28th week, the testis approaches the inguinal canal and, three days later, is posterior to the processus vaginalis (which has already formed)[2]. The processus vaginalis is still communicating with the peritoneal cavity in newborn infants and usually obliterates after the baby is born. Many times, however, it is quite open and a congenital indirect hernia may form.

When the testis travels downward, the kidney ascends, and the adrenal gland, which is developed *in situ*, is waiting to welcome the kidney. Factors responsible for testicular descent are perhaps:

- *Gubernaculum* – Backhouse and Butler[3] concluded that final descent results from invasion of the remaining gubernaculum by the growing cauda epididymis.
- *Androgens* – Androgens and the fetal testicle are stimulated by maternal gonadotrophin or chorionic gonadotrophin[4].
- *Intra-abdominal pressure* – The testicle does not like the warm environment of the abdominal cavity, because spermatogenesis requires a cool climate (as provided in the scrotum). Normal body temperature, which is abnormal for the undescended testicle, arrests spermatogenesis and enables only the Sertoli cells to survive.

Surgical anatomy

This section is divided into four parts: posterior inguinal wall; blood supply of the lower abdomen, testicles and scrotum; fossae and spaces; and the 'good stuff'.

Posterior inguinal wall

It is accepted that the posterior inguinal wall is formed by the fusion of the transversus abdominis aponeurosis and the transversalis fasciae. However, part of the posterior wall (perhaps one-third or one-quarter) is not covered by the transversus abdominis aponeurosis. This part is located at the area just above the distal part of Cooper's ligament and iliopubic tract laterally to the Gimbernat's ligament, with upward extension to the arch. In that area, we see the formation of the direct and supravesicular hernias. The uncovered part is the weak area, at least anatomically, of the posterior inguinal wall.

With the patient in the supine position, and after the aponeurosis of the external oblique has been incised, the surgeon deals with the following anatomical areas and entities of the inguinal region that are incorporated into an elliptical area: the floor of the inguinal canal, a superior medial edge (above), an inferior lateral edge (below), a medial apex and a lateral apex[5] (Figure 3.1).

Fruchaud's approach to this area differs[6]. His work is discussed by Madden[7] and Wantz[8] while Chevrel[9] details the components of the fibromuscular frame.

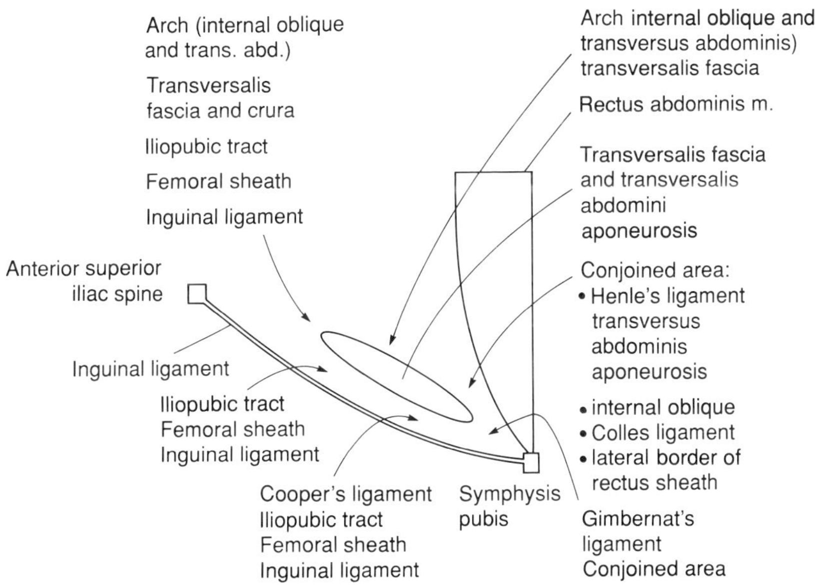

Figure 3.1: The surgical ellipse of the inguinal area. (From Skandalakis JE, Colborn GL, Gray SW, Skandalakis LJ, Pemberton LB. The surgical anatomy of the inguinal area. *Contemp Surg* 1991; **38** (1,2): 20–34.)

The 'pyriform fossa' of Fruchaud forms part of the posterior wall ('floor') of the inguinal canal. This potential structure is a semi-ovoid space filled with fibrofatty tissue located at the medial part of the floor. It is defined as having the iliopubic tract, which inserts into Cooper's ligament as its superior border, the shelving edge of the inguinal ligament as its inferior border, Gimbernat's ligament as its medial border and 'floor', and the medial wall of the femoral sheath as its lateral border[6].

Fruchaud believed that all groin hernias began in a single weak area within the groin, an area that he called the 'myopectineal orifice'[8]. The myopectineal orifice (Figure 3.2) is bounded superiorly by the arch of the internal oblique muscle and the transversus abdominis muscle, laterally by the iliopsoas muscle, medially by the lateral border of the rectus muscle and its anterior lamina, and inferiorly by the pubic pecten. The inguinal ligament spans and divides this framework. The area is transversed by the spermatic cord and femoral vessels, and is bridged on its inner surface by the transversalis fascia only.

The blood supply

The surgeon should be familiar with the blood supply of the lower abdominal wall, spermatic cord and scrotum.

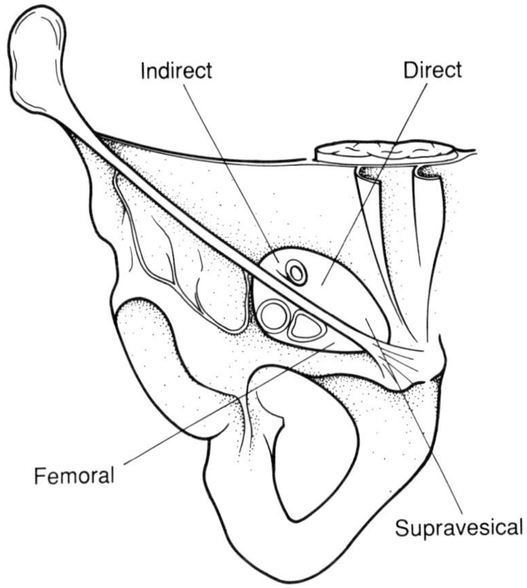

Figure 3.2: Posterior view of Fruchaud's myopectineal orifice. (Modified from Wantz GE. *Atlas of Hernia Surgery.* New York: Raven Press, 1991: 4.)

The arteries (Figure 3.3)

The arteries of the lower abdominal wall, related to the inguinal area, are:

- superficial epigastric artery from the femoral
- inferior epigastric artery from the external iliac
- superficial iliac circumflex from the femoral
- superficial external pudendal from the femoral.

Those of the spermatic cord are:

- testicular from the aorta
- differential from the inferior epigastric
- cremasteric from the inferior epigastric.

Those to the scrotum are:

- superficial external pudendal from the femoral
- deep external pudendal from the femoral
- internal pudendal from the internal iliac.

Characteristically, the superficial external pudendal gives the anterior scrotal, and the internal pudendal gives the posterior scrotal artery. The inferior epigastric forms the lateral superior border of the triangle of Hesselbach and, at the lateral border of the rectus sheath, penetrates the border and travels upward between the muscle and the posterior lamina, to anastomose with the superior epigastric artery. The cremasteric artery is a branch of the inferior epigastric artery. Occasionally (one in ten times), the obturator artery is a branch of the inferior epigastric artery and not of the internal iliac.

The enemy below is the aberrant obturator artery, just beneath the lacunar ligament, which connects the pubic branch of the obturator artery with the pubic branch of the inferior epigastric artery.

The vessels of the spermatic cord anastomose directly or indirectly with the vessels of the scrotum.

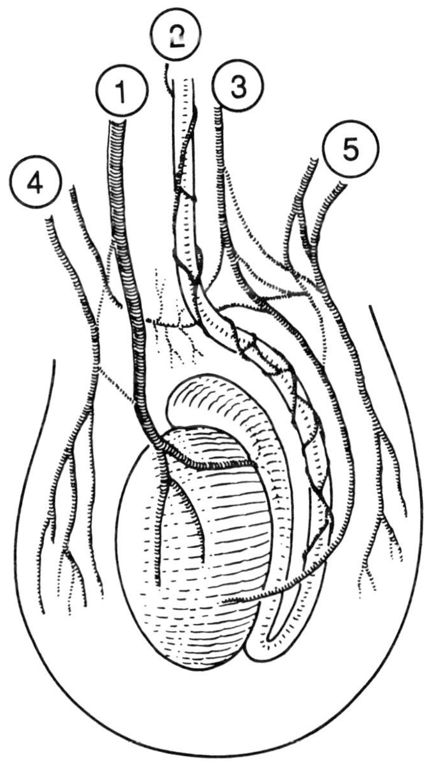

Figure 3.3: The arterial supply of the testis and epididymis. The testicular artery is the chief source of blood to the testis, but four other arteries anastomose with the testicular artery and each other to form a collateral circulation. 1, Testicular artery; 2, deferential artery; 3, cremaster artery; 4, posterior scrotal artery; 5, anterior artery. (From Skandalakis JE, Gray SW, Rowe Jr JS. Hernias. In *Anatomical Complications in General Surgery*. New York: McGraw-Hill, 1983: 252–81.)

The testicular arteries arise from the aorta. They descend in front of the ureter and lower part of the external iliac artery, to enter the internal inguinal ring and spermatic cord. The artery provides branches to the ureter, the cremaster muscle and the epididymis. The testicular artery divides at the upper end of the posterior border of the testis into medial and lateral branches. They pierce the capsule and form a tunica vasculosa beneath it.

The deferential artery arising from a vesical artery supplies the ductus deferens. Anastomoses exist between the testicular and deferential vessels.

Additional anastomoses seem to exist between the testicular, cremasteric and scrotal vessels[10]. Neuhof and Mencher[11] found that section of the spermatic cord resulted in testicular atrophy, but not gangrene, in 19 of their 24 patients. This indicates the presence of a real but inadequate collateral circulation in about two-thirds of patients[12]. In a larger study population, Burdick and Higginbotham[13] found gangrene in 2%.

Remember – the undescended testes do not have collateral circulation from the following arteries: posterior scrotal, external pudendal and the cremasteric. Therefore, preservation of their present blood supply is required.

The veins

Familiarity with the venous circulation of the testicle is necessary because we occasionally have to operate on a varicocele. Jordan[12] divides the testicular veins into two groups: deep and superficial. The deep is composed chiefly of one vein, the internal spermatic vein, which is the upward continuation, as a single unit, of the pampiniform plexus.

The pampiniform plexus is formed by three groups of veins:

- anterior group, around the testicular artery

- posterior group, from the epididymis
- middle group, around the vas

However, the middle group is often associated with the anterior or posterior groups and therefore is absent.

The superficial system consists of the superfical and deep inferior epigastric veins, the superficial internal circumflex and scrotal tributaries of the superficial and deep external and internal pudendal veins.

Fossae and spaces

The fossae of the anterior abdominal wall and their relation to possible inguinofemoral hernias may be appreciated in Figure 3.4.

- *Superficial perineal pouch* – between the Scarpa's fascia and the urogenital diaphragm. For all practical purposes, this pouch corresponds to the scrotum or the labia majora.
- *Space of Bogros* – this is the lateral extension of the retropubic space of Retzius. It is located under the posterior lamina of transversalis fascia[14] (Figure 3.5).
- *Fossae of the anterior abdominal wall* (lateral, medial, supravesical and femoral) – these are interesting because of their relation to the external supravesical hernia. By definition, the external supravesical hernia leaves the peritoneal cavity through the supravesical fossa, which lies medial to the site of a direct hernia.

The 'good stuff'

The 'good stuff' for repair consists of the following: inguinal ligament, lacunar ligament, pectineal ligament, transversalis fascia and transversus abdominis aponeurosis, iliopubic tract, anterior femoral sheath, transversalis fascia crura, conjoined area, arch of internal oblique and transversus abdominis muscle, and prosthetic material.

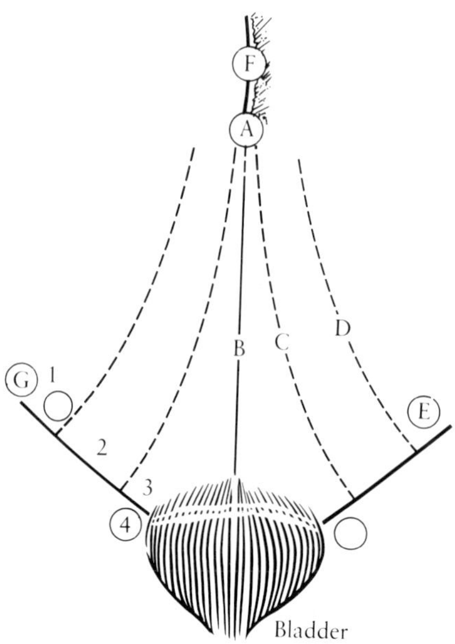

Figure 3.4: Diagram of the sites of groin hernias and their relationships to the bladder and the ligaments of the lower abdominal wall. **A**, umbilicus; **B**, urachus; **C**, lateral umbilical ligament (obliterated hypogastric artery); **D**, deep epigastric artery; **E**, internal inguinal ring; **F**, falciform ligament; **G**, inguinal ligament; **1**, lateral fossa (indirect inguinal hernia); **2**, medial fossa (direct inguinal hernia); **3**, supravesical fossa (paravesical hernia); **4**, femoral ring (femoral hernia). (Modified from Rowe JS Jr, Skandalakis FE, Gray SW. Multiple bilateral inguinal hernias. *Am Surg* 1973; **39**(5): 269–70.)

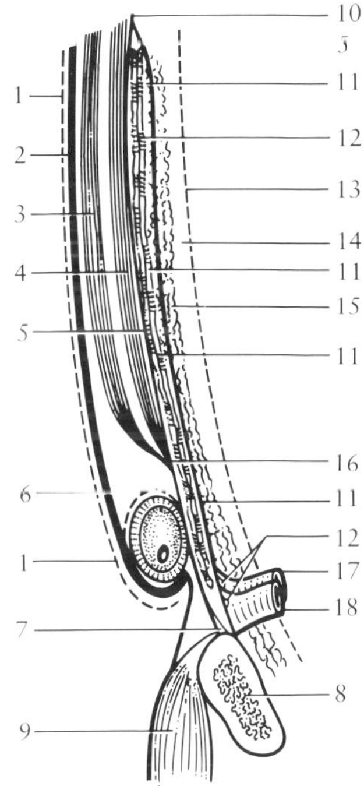

Figure 3.5: The space of Bogros.
1 = innominate; 2 = external oblique aponeurosis; 3 = internal oblique muscle; 4 = transversus abdominis muscle; 5 = transversalis fascia; 7 = Cooper's ligament; 8 = pubic bone; 9 = pectineus muscle; 10 = transversalis fascia; 11 = transversalis fascia posterior lamina; 12 = vessels; 13 - peritoneum; 14 - home (space) of the prosthesis space of Bogros; 15 = preperitoneal fat; 16 = transversus abdominis aponeurosis fascia; 17 = femoral artery; 18 = femoral vein. (*Drawn with* R. C. Read.) (From Skandalakis JE, Colborn GL, Androulakis JA, Skandalakis LJ, Pemberton LB. Embryologic and anatomic basis of inguinal herniorrhaphy. *Surg Clin North Am* 1993, **73**(4): 799–836)

The inguinal ligament

This is the lower edge of the external oblique aponeurosis from the anterior superior iliac spine to the pubic tubercle. No muscles enter or originate in the inguinal ligament. The inguinal ligament is responsible for the formation of the ligament of Gimbernat and the reflected inguinal ligament.

The lacunar ligament (Gimbernat's)

Gimbernat's ligament is a triangular extension of the inguinal ligament before its insertion to the pubic tubercle. It is inserted at the pecten pubis, and its lateral end meets the proximal end of Cooper's ligament. According to Condon, 'it never forms the medial border of the normal femoral canal'[15]. However, other investigators believe the opposite.

Remember the relationship of the aberrant accessory obturator artery to the lacunar ligament.

Cooper's ligament

Cooper first reported this 'ligament' nearly 200 years ago. Authors[7,15–20] since have described it in different ways. It is my opinion that this ligament is composed of:

- periosteum
- aponeurosis of pectineus muscle
- iliopubic tract
- distal end of Gimbernat's ligament.

The iliopubic tract

The iliopubic tract is an aponeurotic band extending from the iliopectineal arch to the superior ramus of the pubis. It creates the inferior margin of the deep musculoaponeurotic layer, which is composed of the transversus abdominis muscle and aponeurosis and the transversalis fascia.

Laterally, the tract is attached to the iliacus and psoas fascia and continues to the anterior superior spine of the ilium. This continuation is not surgically important.

Medially, it forms the lower border of the internal inguinal ring, crossing the femoral vessels to form the anterior margin of the femoral sheath and composing part of the transversalis fascia.

In reality, these anatomical entities perhaps all originate from the transversalis fascia.

The tract curves around the medial surface of the femoral sheath to attach to the pectineal ligament. Condon[21] found the iliopubic tract present in 98% of dissections. He noted that it is frequently confused with the inguinal ligament, which, although nearby, belongs to the anterior lamina (superficial musculoaponeurotic layer), and that the iliopubic tract is part of the deep layer (posterior lamina structures). In other words, the iliopubic tract is the inferior segment of the posterior wall of the inguinal canal of Madden[7].

The femoral canal and the femoral sheath

Between the inguinal ligament and the linea terminalis (iliopectineal line), which is that part of the pelvic brim extending from the ala of the sacrum to the pubic tubercle, is a space organized into three compartments. The most lateral of these is the neuromuscular compartment. This area contains the iliopsoas muscle, the femoral nerve and the lateral femoral cutaneous nerve. Medial to this, the vascular compartment contains the femoral artery and vein. Still more medial is the compartment of the femoral canal.

The femoral sheath, an extension of the transversalis fascia, envelops the femoral artery, vein and femoral canal. The femoral canal is the most medial of the three compartments of the sheath and is where a femoral hernia may pass. This canal is conical, approximately 1.25–2 cm in length.

The fossa ovalis, the opening for the great saphenous vein, is at its apex. Thus, a femoral hernia may present as a bulge of the skin over the fossa ovalis.

The femoral ring is inflexible. The transverse diameter ranges from 8 to 27 mm, and the anteroposterior diameter ranges from 9 to 19 mm; however, in 70% of patients these diameters are 10–14 mm and 12–16 mm, respectively[19].

The boundaries are:

- lateral: the femoral vein and connective tissue
- posterior: the pectineal Cooper's ligament
- anterior: the iliopubic tract or the inguinal ligament, or both
- medial: the transversalis fascia, aponeurotic insertion of the transversus abdominis muscle and the lacunar ligament.

McVay[19] located the lacunar ligament at the medial margin of the femoral ring in only eight of 362 subjects. He suggested that the aponeurosis of transversus abdominis is the usual boundary. Condon[15] proposed that either the aponeurosis or the recurved iliopubic tract may form the medial boundary.

Where is the site of obstruction in an incarcerated or strangulated femoral hernia? The femoral ring or a point 1.5 cm below the ring? Lytle[22] maintained that it is the latter and advised partial transection of the ligament of Gimbernat. I prefer partial transection of the inguinal ligament, for two reasons: (1) to avoid injury to an aberrant obturator artery passing medial to the hernial sac; and (2) it is the easy way to transect partially the inguinal ligament.

The exit of the femoral canal is:

- anterior = fascia lata
- posterior = pectineal fascia
- lateral = femoral sheath
- medial = iliopubic tract and, occasionally, the lacunar ligament.

To me, the formation of a femoral hernia is an enigma.

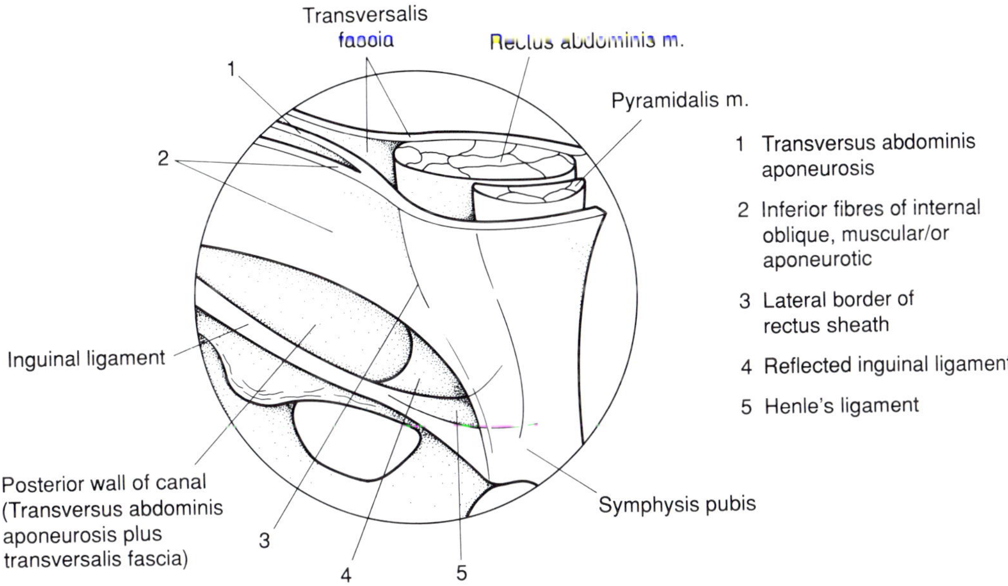

Figure 3.6: The 'conjoined area'. (From Skandalakis JE, Colborn GL, Androulakis JA, Skandalakis LJ, Pemberton LB. Embryologic and Anatomic Basis of Inguinal Herniorrhaphy. *Surg Clin North Am* 1993; **73**: 799–836

Femoral sheath

'The femoral artery, vein, and some lymph vessels are wrapped up in a prolongation of the extraperitoneal areolar tissue that envelops the external iliac vessels in the abdomen. This wrapping is the femoral sheath[23].

It is formed by the transversalis fascia and the fascia of the iliacus muscle[24].

'The iliopubic tract arches over the psoas and the femoral vessels where it forms an integral part of the anterior femoral sheath'[25].

The transversalis fascia crura

The transversalis fascia forms a sling around the internal ring, an incomplete ring that consists of a thickening forming two crura: a long anterior crus and a short posterior crus. Characteristically, the anterior crus is fixed to the transversus abdominis muscle or aponeurosis above and to the internal ring medially. The posterior crus is fixed to, or inserts on, the iliopubic tract. This arrangement forms an inverted U-shaped sling. By contraction of the transversus abdominis muscle, the sling closes the internal ring under the muscular edge of the internal oblique muscle.

Do not suture the transversalis fascia to the shelving edge of the inguinal ligament. Such a suture will not permit sphincteric action of the transversus abdominis muscle.

The conjoined area (Figure 3.6)

The conjoined tendon is the fusion of lower fibres of the internal oblique aponeurosis with similar fibres from the aponeurosis of the transversus abdominis just as they insert on the pubic tubercle and superior ramus of the pubis. This anatomical configuration, however, is rare. Hollinshead[17] considered it to exist in only 5% of subjects, Condon[21] allowed 3%, and McVay[26] believed it to be only an artefact of dissection.

Because the word 'conjoined' is universally accepted and as the conjoined tendon practically does not exist, we named this topography the 'conjoined area'. This area is formed by the following anatomical entities:

- transversus abdominis aponeurosis
- inferior fibres of internal oblique, muscular/or aponeurotic
- lateral border of rectus sheath
- reflected inguinal ligament
- Henle's ligament.

An inguinal hernia is repaired using the transversus abdominis aponeurosis, the transversalis fascia and the lateral edge of the rectus sheath. On occasion, the internal oblique muscle, the internal oblique aponeurosis, the ligament of Henle (falx inguinalis), the ligamentum interfoveolar or the reflected inguinal ligament may also be used in the repair. Although none of these is really conjoined, there is a tendency among surgeons to use the term for any mass of fascia or aponeurosis from the internal oblique or the transversus abdominis muscles.

References

1. Sadler TW. *Langman's Medical Embryology*, 6th ed. Baltimore: Williams & Wilkins, 1990: 8.
2. Wyndam NR. A morphological study of testicular descent. *J Anat* 1943; **77**: 179.
3. Backhouse KM, Butler H. The gubernaculum testis of the pig (sus scropha). *J Anat* 1960; **94**: 107.
4. Wislocki GB. Observations on descent of testes in macaque and in chimpanzee. *Anat Rec* 1933; **57**: 133.
5. Skandalakis JE, Colborn GL, Gray SW, Skandalakis LJ, Pemberton LB. The surgical anatomy of the inguinal area. *Contemp Surg* 1991; **38**: 20–34.
6. Fruchaud H. *Anatomie chirurgicale des hernies de l'aine*. Paris: C Doin, 1956: 169.
7. Madden JL. *Abdominal Wall Hernias*. Philadelphia: WB Saunders, 1989.
8. Wantz GE. *Atlas of Hernia Surgery*. New York: Raven Press, 1991: 4, 5, 101, 104.
9. Chevrel JP. *Surgery of the Abdominal Wall*. Berlin: Springer Verlag, 1985: 17–18.
10. Hanley HG, Harrison RG. Nature and surgical treatment of varicocele. *Br J Surg* 1962; **50**: 64.
11. Neuhof H, Mencher WH. The viability of the testis following complete severance of the spermatic cord. *Surgery* 1940; **8**: 672.
12. Jordan Jr WP. Hydroceles and varicoceles. *Surg Clin North Am* 1965; **45**: 1535.
13. Burdick CG, Higinbotham NL. Division of the spermatic cord as an aid in operating on selected types of inguinal hernia. *Ann Surg* 1935; **102**: 863.
14. Bendavid R. The space of Bogros and the deep inguinal venous circulation. *Surg Gynecol Obstet* 1992; **174**: 355.
15. Condon RE. Surgical anatomy of the transversus abdominis and transversalis fascia. *Ann Surg* 1971; **173**: 1.
16. Ellis H. *Clinical Anatomy: A Revision and Applied Anatomy for Clinical Students*, 6th ed. Oxford: Blackwell Scientific, 1977.
17. Hollinshead WH. The abdominal wall and inguinal region. In: *Anatomy for Surgeons: The Thorax, Abdomen and Pelvis*, vol 2. New York: Paul B Hoeber, 1956: 216–68.
18. Jones FW. *Buchanan's Manual of Anatomy*, 8th ed. Baltimore: Williams & Wilkins, 1943: 750.
19. McVay CB. The anatomic basis for inguinal and femoral hernioplasty. *Surg Gynecol Obstet* 1974; **139**: 931.

20. Nyhus LM, Bombeck CT. Hernias. In: Sabiston DC, ed. *Textbook of Surgery*, 13th ed. Philadelphia: WB Saunders, 1986: 1232, 1321–52.

21. Condon RE. The anatomy of the inguinal region and its relationship to groin hernia. In: Nyhus LM, Condon RE, eds. *Hernia*, 2nd ed. Philadelphia: JB Lippincott, 1978: 14–78.

22. Lytle WJ. Femoral hernia. *Ann R Coll Surg Engl* 1957; **21**: 244–62.

23. Grant JCB, Basmajian JV. *Grant's Method of Anatomy*, 7th ed. Baltimore: Williams & Wilkins, 1965: 363.

24. Brantigan OC. *Clinical Anatomy*. New York: McGraw Hill, 1963: 141.

25. Nyhus LM. An anatomic reappraisal of the posterior inguinal wall: special consideration of the iliopubic tract and its relation to groin hernias. *Surg Clin North Am* 1964; **44**: 1305.

26. McVay CB. *Surgical Anatomy*, 6th ed. Philadelphia: WB Saunders, 1984: 484–584.

Portions of this chapter have appeared in the following: *Embryology for surgeons* by SW Gray, JE Skandalakis.[‡] Surgical anatomy of hernial rings by JE Skandalakis, SW Gray, JT Akin, *Surg Clin North Am* 1974; 54: 1227–47[§]. *Anatomical complications in general surgery* by JE Skandalakis, SW Gray, JS Rowe.[‡] Surgical anatomy of the inguinal area by JE Skandalakis, GL Colborn, SW Gray, LJ Skandalakis, LB Pemberton, *World Journal of Surgery* 1989; 13: 490–8[§]. Hernia: surgical anatomy and technique by JE Skandalakis, SW Gray, AR Mansberger, GL Colborn, LJ Skandalakis[‡]. 'Surgical anatomy of the inguinal area by JE Skandalakis, GL Colborn, SW Gray, LJ Skandalakis, LB Pemberton, *Contemp Surg* 1991; 38 (1,2)[§]. Atlas of surgical anatomy for general surgeons by SW Gray, JE SKandalakis, DA McClusky[‡]. Embryologic and anatomical basis of modern herniorrhaphy by LJ Skandalakis, GL Colborn, SW Gray, JE Skandalakis, LB Pemberton, *Emory Univ J Med* 1992; 6 (2,3,4)[§]. Embryologic and anatomic basis of inguinal herniorrhaphy *Surg Clin North Am* 1993; 73 (4).

[‡]Copyright owned by author

[§] Paraphrased or reproduced

4

Anatomy of the Peritoneum, Preperitoneal Fascia and Posterior Lamina of the Transversalis Fascia in the Inguinal Area

MAURICE E ARREGUI, DANIEL CASTRO AND ROBERT F NAGAN

Numerous publications exist on the anatomy of the groin. Most deal with the anterior anatomy of the inguinal area because this is the most common approach to inguinal herniorrhaphy used by surgeons throughout the world. Recently, preperitoneal techniques have become more widely used. These techniques have been popularized by Nyhus, Stoppa and Wantz[1–4]. Indeed, many articles deal with the anatomy of the anterior abdominal wall from a preperitoneal perspective[5–9]. The current literature on laparoscopy also describes the musculoaponeurotic, vascular and nervous

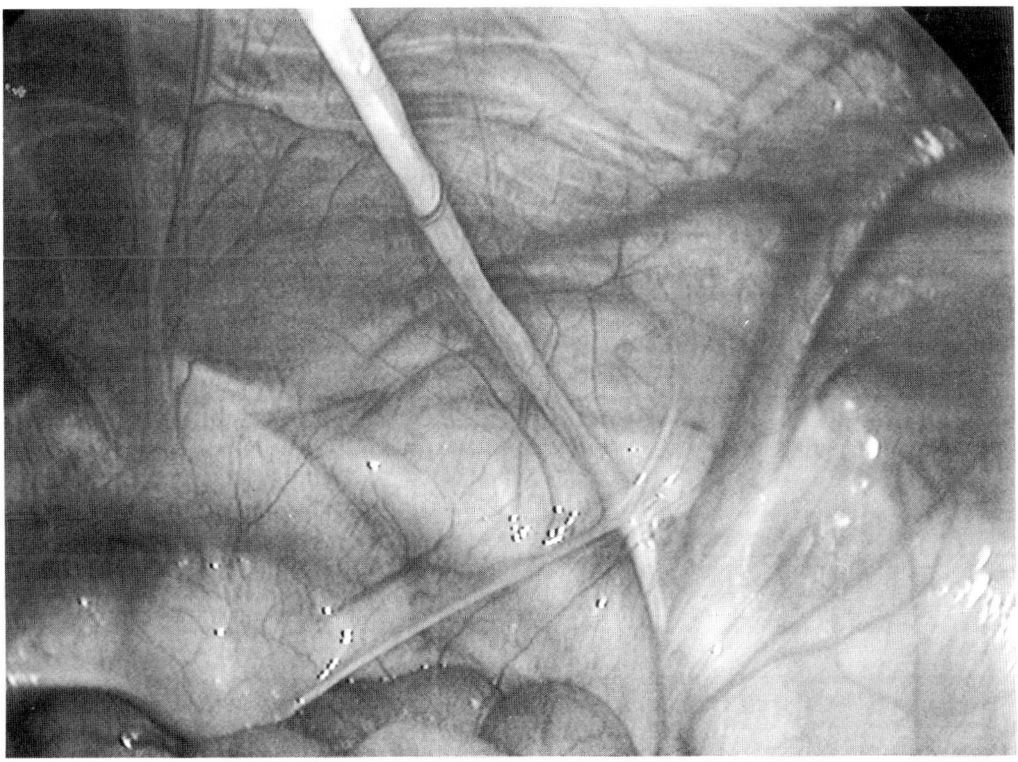

Figure 4.1: Median, medial and lateral umbilical ligaments create the umbilical fossa. The bladder is decompressed by a Foley catheter. The transverse vesicular fold extends from the bladder to the lateral pelvic wall. This patient, who was undergoing a laparoscopic cholecystectomy, did not have a clinical hernia.

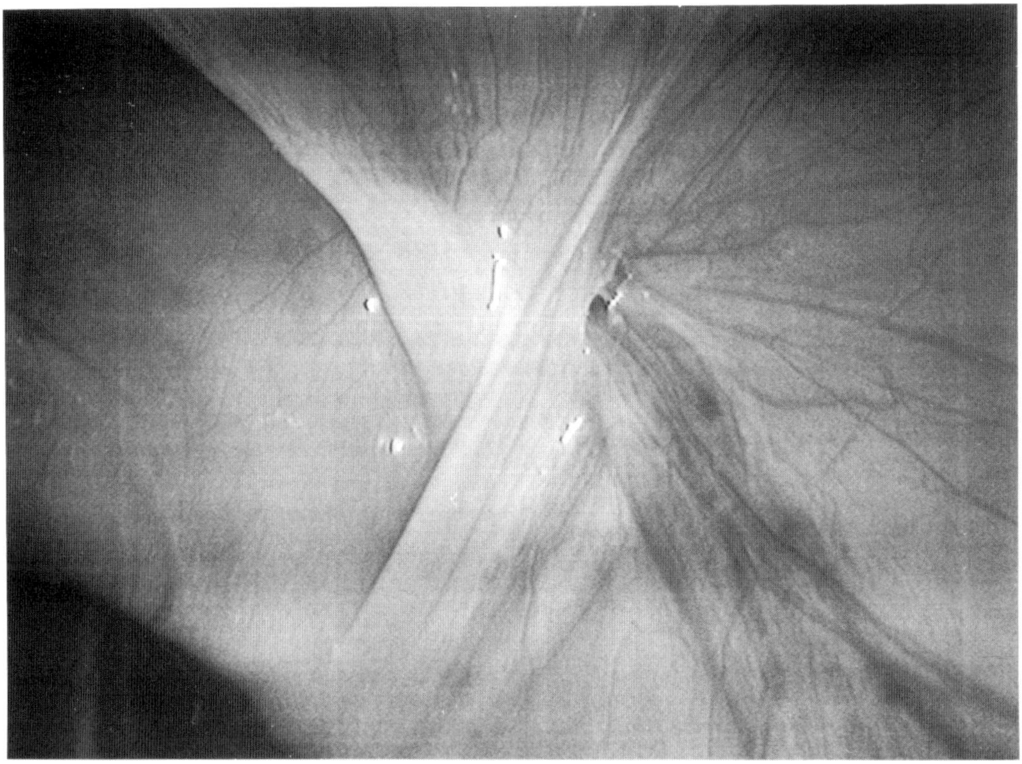

Figure 4.2: Patent processus vaginalis marks the entrance of the cord structures to the internal inguinal ring. Note the thickened lateral attachment of the transverse vesicular fold. (From Arregui ME, Dulucq JL, Teti C, *et al*: Laparoscopic Inguinal Hernia Repair with Preperitioneal Prosthetic Replacement. In 'Prostheses and Abdominal Wall Surgery, fig 1, Landes Medical Publishing, 1994, in press; with permission)

structures of the inguinal area[10]. In spite of all the anatomical literature available, there continues to exist significant confusion and disinterest regarding the transversalis fascia and the preperitoneal and peritoneal structures. In groin hernias, the transversalis fascia, peritoneum and preperitoneal fascias are involved. Especially with preperitoneal herniorrhaphy, the operating surgeon must possess a good knowledge of the anatomy of these structures to perform an accurate repair and to prevent injury.

The peritoneum and preperitoneal fascia probably play a very significant role in the aetiology and repair of indirect inguinal hernias of the congenital variety. These hernias in children originate from persistence of the processus vaginalis[11]. Knowledge of the failure of obliteration of the processus vaginalis may hold important clues for the selective repair of these very common hernias.

In spite of the agreement that groin hernias represent a defect in the transversalis fascia, there is significant disagreement as to its true definition. Stoppa has written '. . . the only area of resistance in this area (groin) is the transversalis fascia'[3]. Why, then, do we not understand this better?

The purpose of this chapter is to define better the peritoneum and the preperitoneal fascia and distinguish these layers from that of the posterior lamina of the transversalis fascia.

Inguinal anatomy

Our understanding of the anatomy of the preperitoneal fascia and spaces is derived from experience with repair of 202 hernias in 156 patients. Of these patients, 107 underwent repair with a

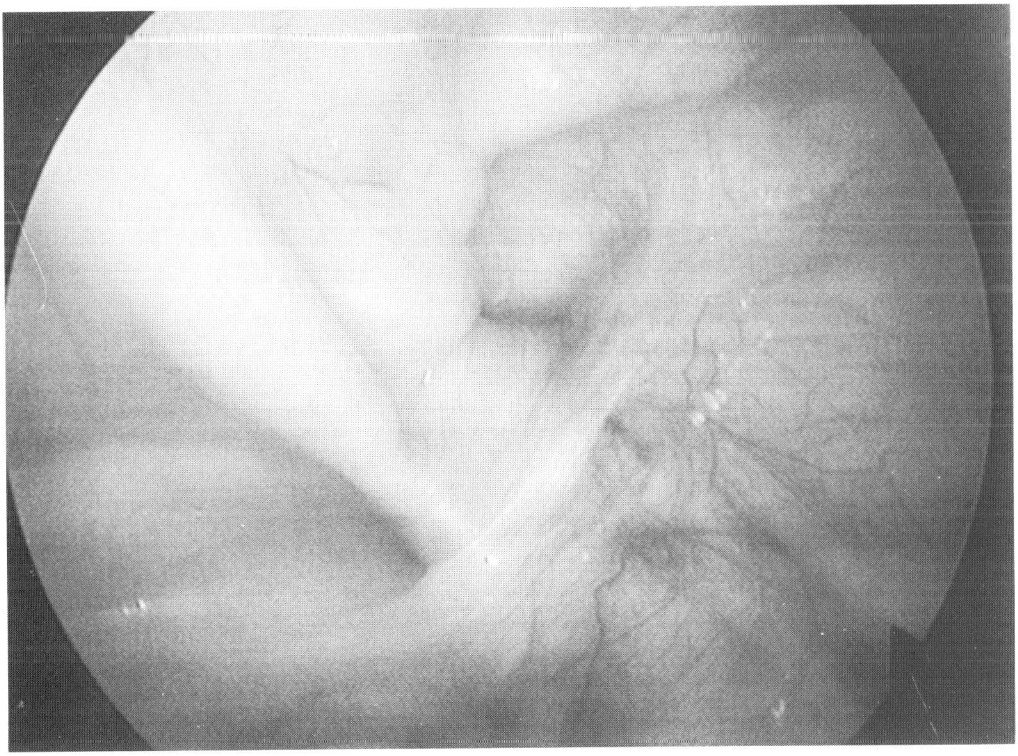

Figure 4.3: Acquired indirect inguinal hernia. This results from a weakness in the transversalis fascia lateral to the medial umbilical ligament but medial to the orifice of the internal ring. It does not result from a patent processus vaginalis. This type of defect is poorly appreciated from an anterior or totally preperitoneal approach.

transabdominal preperitoneal approach; 90 with the laparoscopic extraperitoneal approach; and five with ring closure technique. In addition to detailed laparoscopic dissection, we reviewed the literature, including anatomical textbooks and atlases. Attempts were made at cadaver dissections but these provided suboptimal conditions for intricate analysis of the various fascial planes of the preperitoneal space.

Peritoneum

The peritoneum is the largest serosal membrane. The other serosal membranes include the pleura and the pericardium. The surface of the peritoneum is equal to that of the skin. Its functions include absorption of fluids, storing fats, resisting or localizing infections, and minimizing friction. The innermost layer of the peritoneum includes mesothelial cells which are arranged as a single layer. Each cell has numerous microvilli to increase its absorptive surface. These cells have the capability of transforming into macrophages and fibroblasts. Supporting the mesothelial cells is the submesothelial connective tissue which has an increased number of macrophages and lymphocytes as well as, in certain areas including the omentum, increased numbers of fat cells[12]. This submesothelial connective tissue has a discrete blood supply and lymphatic drainage which in many areas, including the inguinal area, is separate from the anterior abdominal wall. There are two forms of innervation:

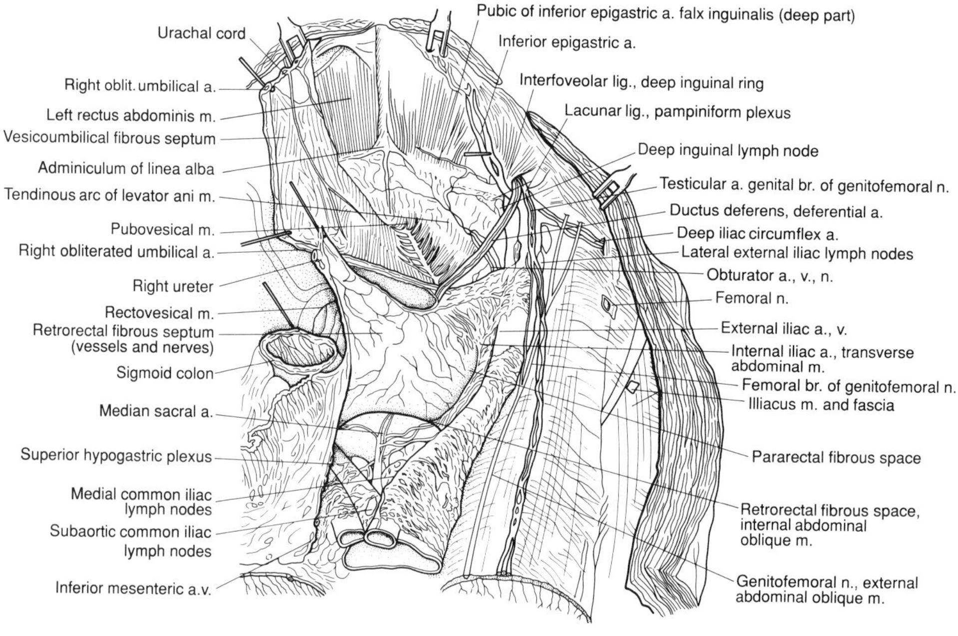

Figure 4.4: Excellent illustration of the umbilical prevesicular fascia containing the median and medial umbilical ligaments, bladder and their blood supply which is discrete from the anterior abdominal wall. The posterior lamina of the transversalis fascia is not well illustrated here. (From Platzer W: Atlas of Topographic and Applied Human Anatomy, fig. 263. In 'Pernkopf Anatomy', Urban & Schwarzenberg, 1987, vol II, 3rd ed; with permission.)

the *visceral innervation* comes from the sympathetic nerves which can perceive pain induced by tension and ischaemia; the *parietal innervation* comes from somatic nerves.

In the lower abdominal wall, the surface characteristics include the median umbilical ligament which represents the obliterated urachus connecting the bladder to the umbilicus, the medial umbilical ligament which represents the obliterated umbilical artery, and the lateral umbilical ligament which represents a prominence caused by the inferior epigastric vessels[9]. In addition, the transverse vesical folds can often be seen going from the bladder, following the vas deferens and attaching laterally and anterior to the internal inguinal ring. Between the median and medial umbilical ligaments lies the supravesical fossa which is the usual location for the infrequent suprapubic hernias. Between the medial umbilical fold and the lateral umbilical fold lies the medial inguinal fossa which marks the site of direct hernias (Figure 4.1). Lateral to the inferior epigastric vessels (lateral umbilical fold) lies the confluence of the blood supply and cord to the testicle lateral to the attachment of the transverse vesicular fold. This marks the site of indirect hernias (Figure 4.2). Occasionally, an indirect hernia arising lateral to the epigastric vessels but medial to the confluence of the vas deferens and spermatic vessels will be encountered. This represents weakness in the lateral aspect of the transversalis fascia and does not result from a patent processus vaginalis (Figure 4.3). In most, the preperitoneal tissue medial to the medial umbilical folds contains an increased amount of fat.

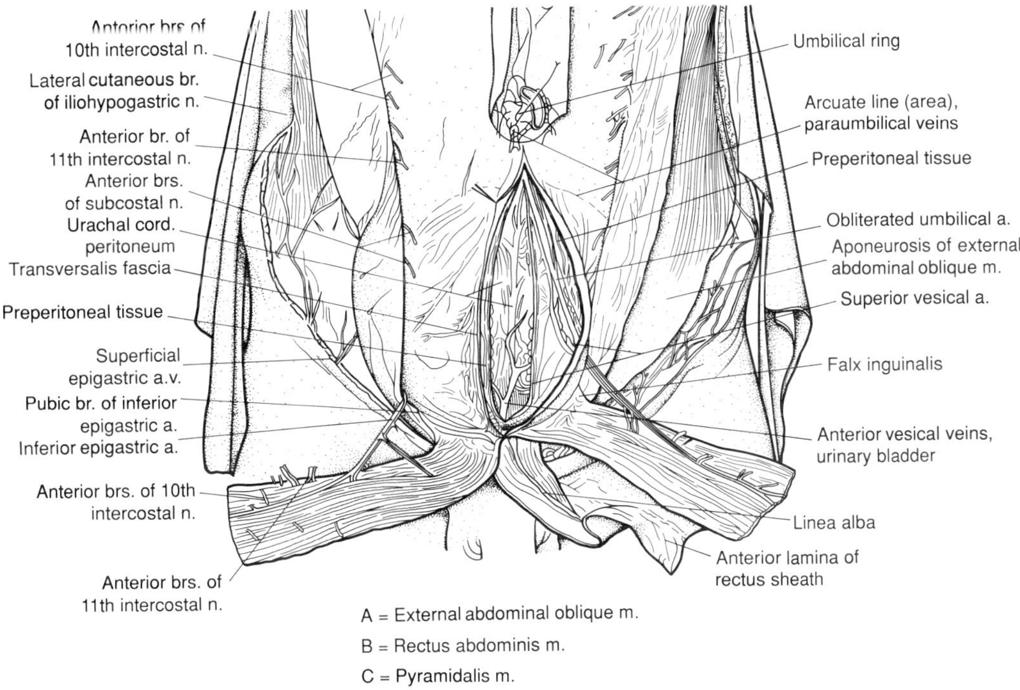

Figure 4.5: Excellent illustration showing the rectus muscle and inferior epigastric vessels separated from the posterior lamina of the transversalis fascia (labelled 'transversalis fascia'). Also illustrated here is a separate preperitoneal fascia (labelled 'preperitoneal tissue') separated by the preperitoneal space. The umbilical ligaments and bladder are deep to this. (From Platzer W: Atlas of Topographic and Applied Human Anatomy, fig. 178. In 'Pernkopf Anatomy', Urban & Schwarzenberg, 1987, vol II, 3rd ed; with permission.)

At the umbilicus, the umbilical ligaments will penetrate the transversalis fascia in the posterior rectus sheath to get to a more superficial position allowing exit at the umbilicus. Deep to the umbilicus this is seen as the umbilical fascia. When absent or attenuated, the umbilical area is relatively unsupported and this could predispose to an umbilical hernia[8].

Preperitoneal fascia

From the area of the umbilicus extending down to the inguinal area and pelvis, there are several layers of tissue planes. The deepest is the peritoneum. The next layer includes the preperitoneal fat which surrounds the median umbilical ligaments, bladder and blood supply. This area acts as a mesentery to the bladder and umbilical ligaments. The layer superficial to the bladder and umbilical ligaments is the prevesical umbilical fascia[13–16]. The blood supply, lymphatics and innervation to all of these tissues are separate from that of the anterior abdominal wall (Figures 4.4 and 4.5). The next plane is the true preperitoneal space which separates the prevesical umbilical fascia from the posterior lamina of the transversalis fascia. Medially this space is a well developed bloodless plane (Figure 4.6). Somewhat laterally, where there is little preperitoneal fat, the preperitoneal prevesicular fasica and the posterior lamina of the transversalis fascia are fused and more difficult to separate

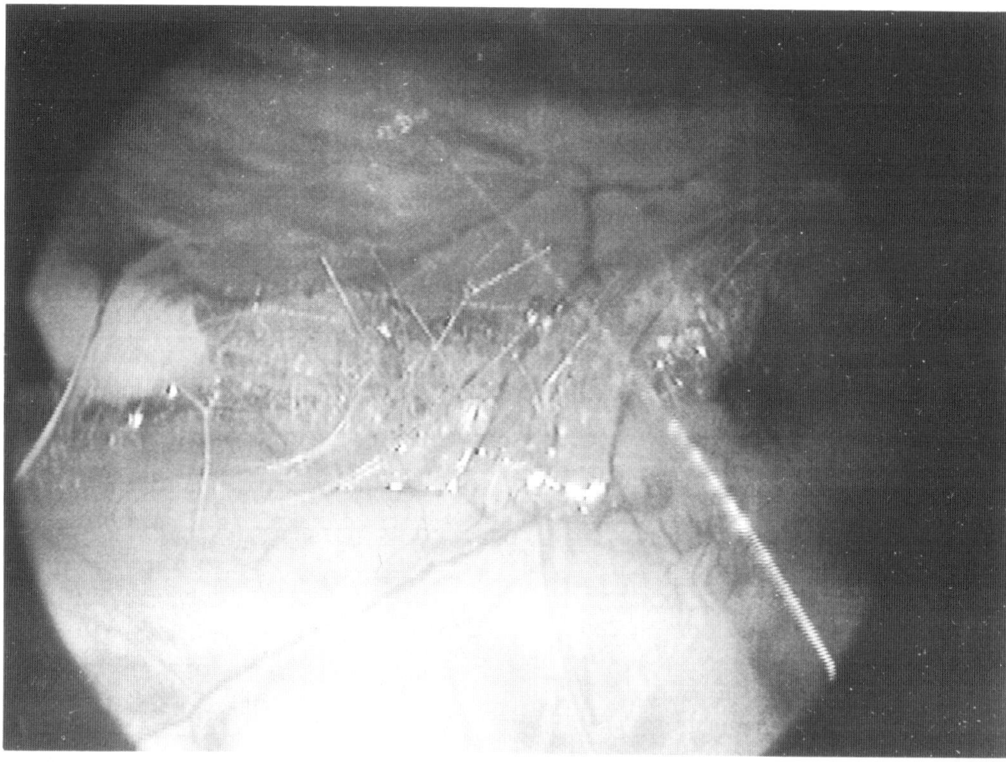

Figure 4.6: Laparoscopic view of the preperitoneal space. The umbilical prevesicular fascia is posterior and the posterior lamina of the transversalis fascia is anterior. Medially, the bloodless plane separates easily.

(Figure 4.7). Anterior to the posterior lamina of the transversalis fascia courses the inferior epigastric vessel with its branches and the rectus abdominis muscle (*see* Figure 4.5). The next layer is the anterior lamina of the transversalis fascia or the anterior rectus sheath composed of aponeurosis of the transverse muscles of the anterior abdominal wall. The inferior epigastric vessels provide the blood supply to the anterior abdominal wall. The true preperitoneal space is continuous with the space of Retzius which is superficial to the preperitoneal fascia and deep to the posterior lamina of the transversalis fascia.

At the level of the internal ring, the transversalis fascia forms a sling around the cord structures. Fowler described 'the deeper main membranous sheet of the preperitoneal fascia displays a circumferential arrangements of fibers surrounding the vas, spermatic vessels and any patent processus vaginalis when present, forming what is here called the secondary internal inguinal ring'[7]. Indeed, the preperitoneal fascia surrounding the cord structures is discrete from the transversalis fascia (Figure 4.8). Tobin recognized this and said, 'At the abdominal internal ring the ventral lamina, surrounding the spermatic vessels from kidney on and part of the intermediate stratum around the vas deferens, from bladder region, fuse with the dorsal lamina and continue as the innermost layer, internal spermatic fascia of the spermatic cord'[17]. Indeed, our dissections support the concept that the internal spermatic fascia is made up of the preperitoneal fascia rather than the transversalis fascia, as often reported in numerous textbooks and articles (Figure 4.9). During preperitoneal dissection, in order to get to the indirect hernia sac, the preperitoneal fascial fibres must be separated. The blood supply to the vas deferens and the preperitoneal fascia are derived from the internal iliac vessels. The spermatic vessels arise from the aorta or renal artery.

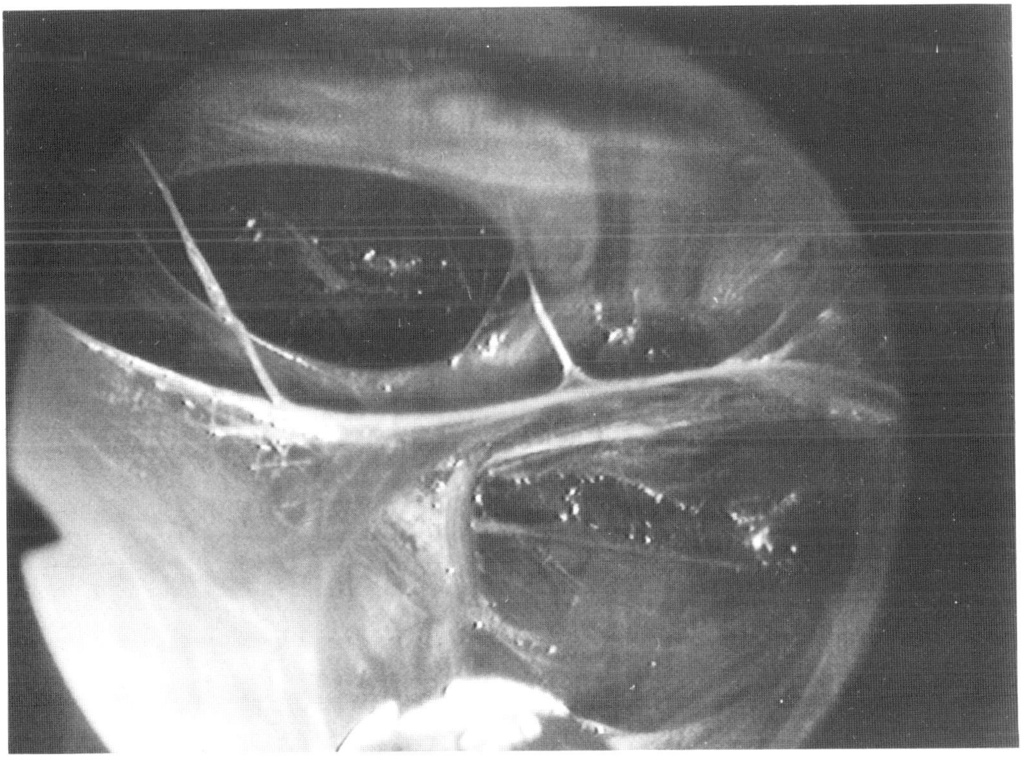

Figure 4.7: Lateral dissection in the preperitoneal space demonstrates the posterior lamina of the transversalis fascia. Here it is fused with the preperitoneal tissues. Note that the inferior epigastric vessels are located in the anterior compartment. This dissection is below the semicircular line of Douglas.

The significance of the preperitoneal fascia and the orifice of the indirect hernia lies in the failed obliteration of the processus vaginalis. In select type I indirect hernias, high ligation alone will repair the hernia defect. This is the same technique used in infants who undergo anterior repairs with high ligation alone without any attempt at reconstruction of the inguinal floor[11].

Although much confusion exists about the preperitoneal fascias, our studies indicate that this fascia is discrete from the posterior lamina of the transversalis fascia. During preperitoneal dissection, if the anatomy is not well understood, confusion can result which can lead to bleeding or injury to the structures contained within the preperitoneal fascia – notably the bladder.

Posterior lamina of the transversalis fascia

In spite of the fact that the transversalis fascia has been described as the layer of weakness resulting in inguinal hernia, there is much disagreement as to its exact definition. Cooper originally described it as being a bilaminar structure[19], and Read has recently attempted to clarify this[20]. Others, however, doubt its existence or describe it as the preperitoneal fascia[5,21]. The generally accepted view of the transversalis fascia is that covering of the transversus abdominis muscle which lies in between that muscle and the epigastric vessels[22].

It is often quite difficult to distinguish the preperitoneal fascia from the posterior lamina of the transversalis fascia because lateral to the medial umbilical folds, where there is very little fat between the peritoneum and the anterior abdominal wall, the peritoneum, preperitoneal fascia and posterior

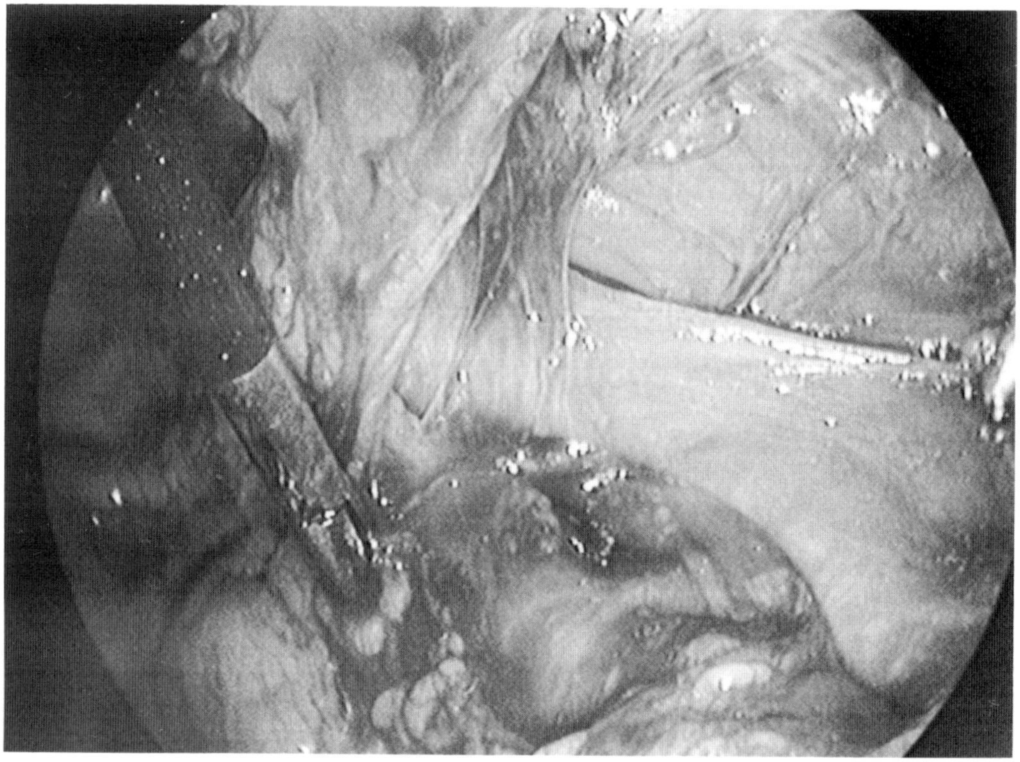

Figure 4.8: The preperitoneal fascia envelopes the cord structures as they enter the internal ring. This fascia is discrete from the transversalis fascia sling. (From Arregui ME, Dulucq JL, Tetic *et al*: Laparoscopic Inguinal Hernia Repair with Preperitoneal Prosthetic Replacement, fig 18. In 'Prostheses and Abdominal Wall Surgery', Landes Medical Publishing, 1994, in press; with permission.)

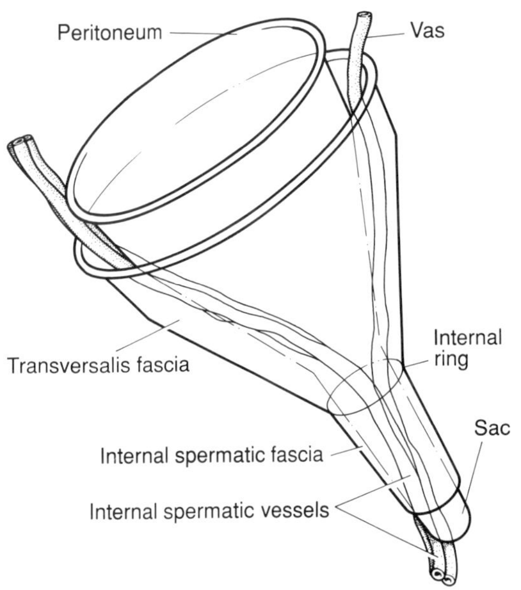

Figure 4.9: The common misconception that the internal spermatic fascia arises from the transversalis fascia rather than the preperitoneal fascia. (From Griffith CA: The Marcy Repair of Indirect Inguinal Hernia, fig 2. In 'Hernia', JB Lippincott Co., 178, 2nd ed; with permission.)

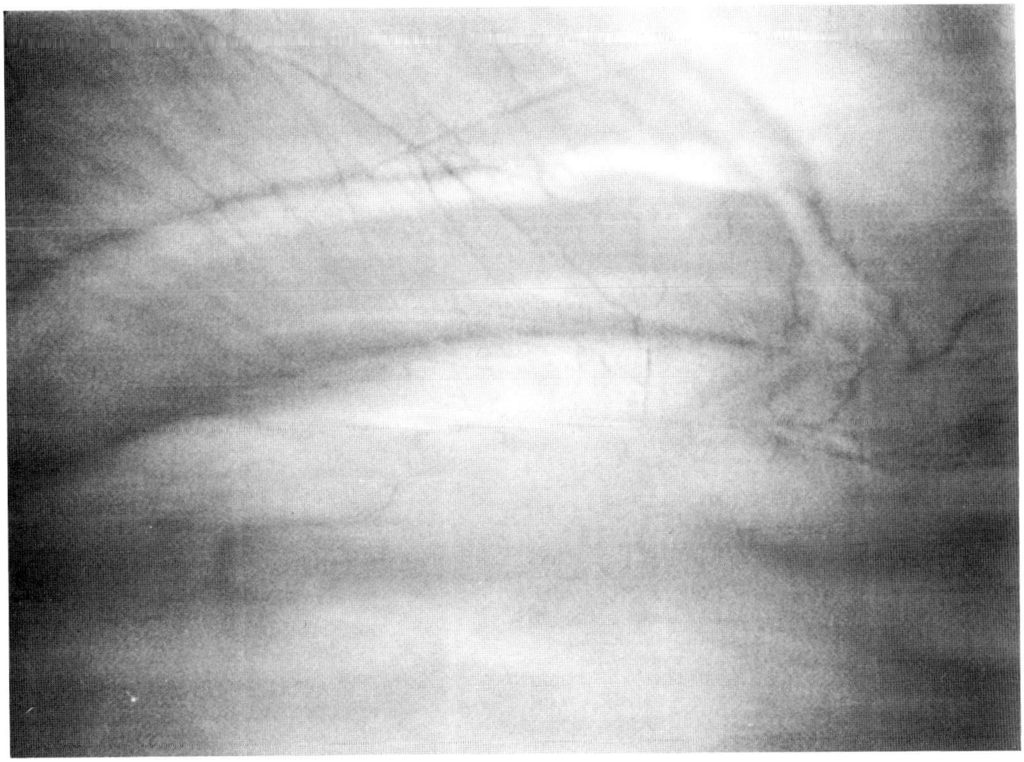

Figure 4.10: Laparoscopic transperitoneal view of the well delineated semicircular line of Douglas near the level of the umbilicus. The 45° view laparoscope is in the umbilicus.

lamina of the transversalis fascia are fused. This same confusion exists at the level of the umbilicus above the semicircular line of Douglas. However, above the semicircular line of Douglas, the posterior rectus sheath containing multiple thick fascial layers is very discrete (Figure 4.10). Below this it often thins out but continues. Anson, Morgan and McVay have described '. . . some of the fibers may pass posteriorly and thus form a relatively low linea-semicircularis in the upper area of the inguinal region. Frequently some of the lower aponeurotic fibers of the transversus may pass posterior to the rectus and gaining attachment to the caudal part of the linea alba and to the pubis.'[23] Indeed, in numerous laparoscopic views we have obtained of the anterior abdominal wall below the linea semicircularis, the posterior rectus sheath does not completely disappear but merely thins out (Figure 4.11). During preperitoneal dissection, this posterior rectus sheath often is composed of several layers, supporting the concept that this is a continuation of the posterior rectus sheath in an attenuated form. McKay described the posterior lamina of the transversalis fascia: 'the lower portion of the posterior aspect of the rectus sheath below the semilunar fold is composed not only of transversalis muscle but also of components of the internal oblique . . . proved by the occasional presence of muscular fibrous belonging to the internal oblique in the wall of the sheath below the level of the semilunar fold . . . The deep epigastric artery, immediately upon its origin from the external iliac, pierces the fascia transversalis . . .'[24] In fact, in our dissections we have seen the posterior rectus sheath extending and attaching to Cooper's ligament and enveloping the epigastric vessels posteriorly. The internal ring lies lateral to the separation of anterior and posterior lamina of the transversalis fascia or separation of the aponeurosis of the abdominal wall muscles which make up the anterior and posterior rectus sheath. Simply stated, the posterior rectus sheath does not stop

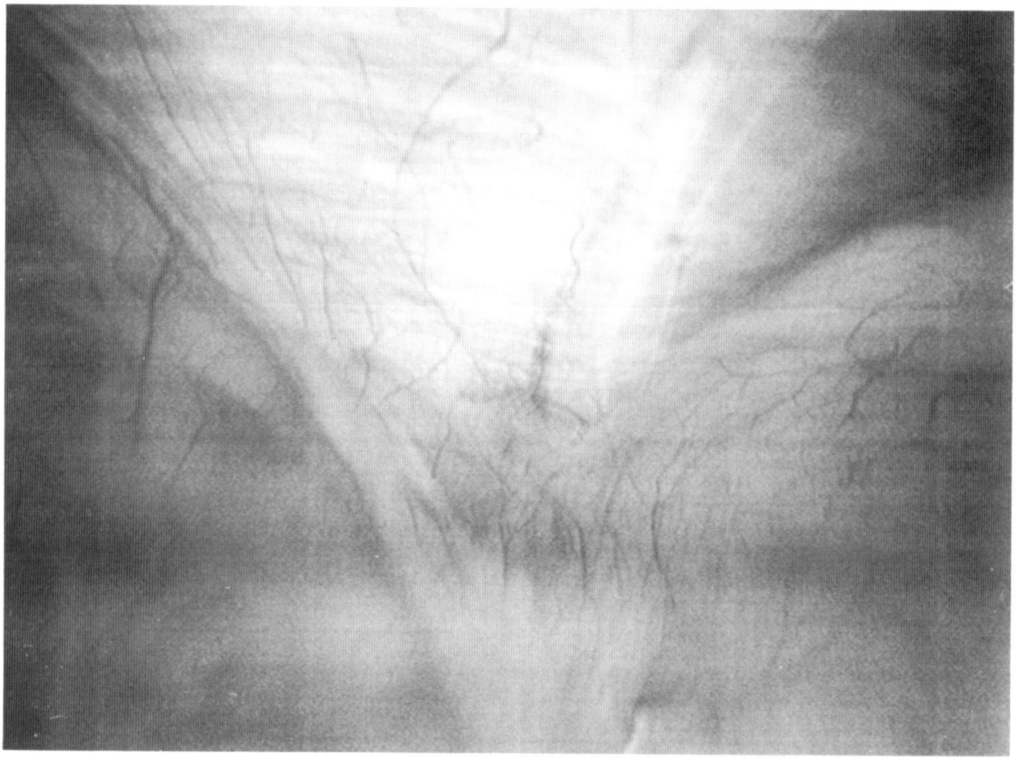

Figure 4.11: A lower view of the patient in Figure 4.10. Note the continuation of some transverse fibres below. These are deep to the inferior epigastric vessels. This represents the posterior lamina of the transversalis fascia or a continuation of an attenuated posterior rectus sheath.

at the semilunar fold of Douglas but continues on down to Cooper's ligament. It is usually multilayered, has a variable thickness, and often is very attenuated, thus leading to the confusion that it does not exist (Figure 4.12).

The posterior lamina of the transversalis fascia is posterior to the epigastric vessels. The blood supply is derived from the epigastric vessels. It represents the attenuated continuation of the posterior rectus sheath and is composed of multiple fascial layers. It lies anterior to the prevesicular umbilical fascia separated by the true preperitoneal space.

Conclusions

The transversalis fascia has been poorly described. This structure is critical in the formation of all groin hernias. The literature and our laparoscopic dissections support the concept of a bilaminar structure. Our observations show that it probably represents an attenuated continuation of the posterior rectus sheath. It derives its blood supply from the inferior epigastric vessels. Although in certain locations it is fused with the preperitoneal fascia, it remains a discrete structure. The blood supply for the preperitoneal fascias in the inguinal area is derived from the branches of the internal iliac vessels.

Preperitoneal inguinal herniorrhaphy not only requires a firm understanding of the musculoaponeurotic, vascular, bony and nervous structures but also demands a proper understanding of the

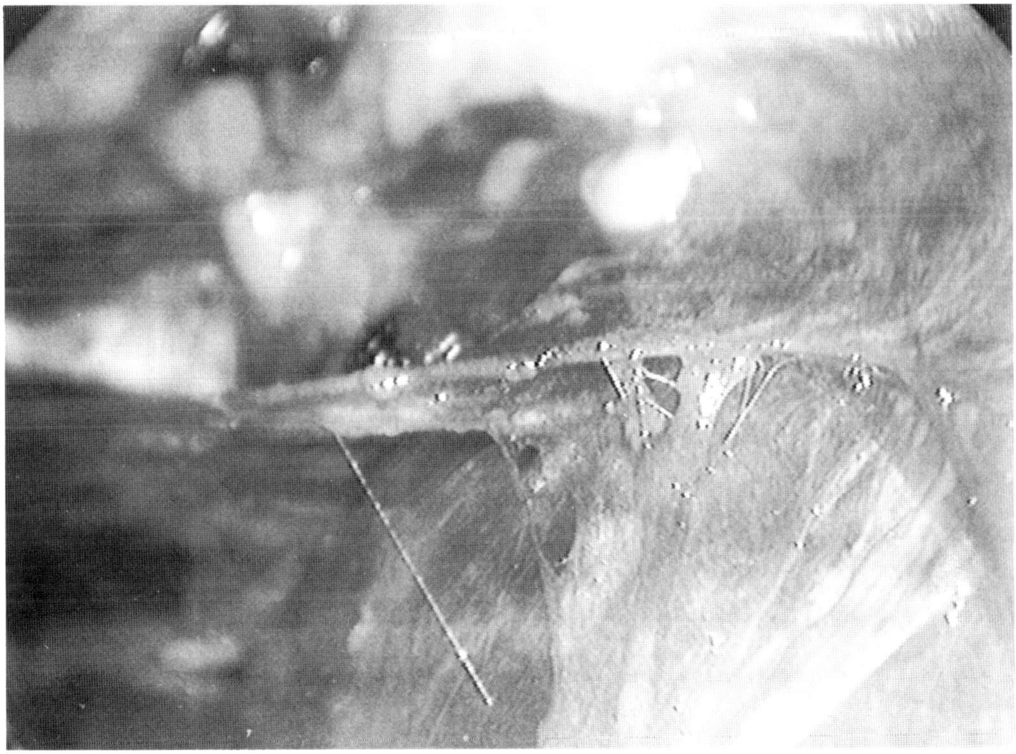

Figure 4.12: Preperitoneal dissection of the posterior lamina of the transversalis fascia. Multiple layers are clearly identified, supporting the view that this is an attenuated continuation of the posterior rectus sheath made up of the multiple layers of aponeurosis of the transverse muscles

peritoneum, preperitoneal fascia with contained structures, and the posterior lamina of the transversalis fascia.

References

1. Nyhus LM. The preperitoneal approach and ileopubic tract repair of inguinal hernia. In: Nyhus LM, Condon RE, eds. *Hernia*, 3rd ed. Philadelphia: JB Lippincott, 1989: 154–88.
2. Stoppa RE, Warlaumont CR. The preperitoneal approach and prosthetic repair of groin hernia. In: Nyhus LM, Condon RE, eds. *Hernia*, 3rd ed. Philadelphia: JB Lippincott, 1989: 199–255.
3. Stoppa R. Hernia of the abdominal wall. In: Chevrel JP, ed. *Surgery of the abdominal wall*. Berlin: Springer-Verlag, 1987: 156–224.
4. Wantz GE. Anatomy of hernias of the groin. In: Wantz GE. *Atlas of hernia surgery*. New York: Raven Press, 1991: 1–10.
5. Condon RE. Surgical anatomy of the transversus abdominis and transversalis fascia. *Ann Surg*, 1971; **173**: 1–5.
6. Condon RE. The anatomy of the inguinal region and its relation to groin hernia. In: Nyhus LM, Condon RE, eds. *Hernia*, 3rd ed. Philadelphia: JB Lippincott, 1989: 18–64.
7. Fowler R. The applied surgical anatomy of the peritoneal fascia of the groin and the 'secondary' internal inguinal ring. *Aust NZ J Surg* 1975; **45**: 8–14.

8. Skandalakis JE, Gray SW, Mansberger AR, Colborn GL, Skandalakis LJ. *Hernia: surgical anatomy and technique*. New York: McGraw-Hill, 1989.

9. Skandalakis JE, Gray SW, Skandalakis LJ, *et al.* Surgical anatomy of the inguinal area. *World J Surg* 1989; **13**: 490–8.

10. Spaw AT, Ennis BW, Spaw LP. Laparoscopic hernia repair: the anatomical basis. *J Laparoendosc Surg* 1991; **1**: 269–77.

11. Grosfeld JL. Groin hernia in infants and children. In: Nyhus LM, Condon RE eds. *Hernia*, 3rd ed. Philadelphia: JB Lippincott, 1989: 81–105.

12. di Zerega GS, Rodgers KE. *The peritoneum*. New York: Springer-Verlag, 1992: 2–22.

13. Pernkopf E. In: Platzer W, ed. *Pernkopf anatomy: atlas of topographic and applied human anatomy*, vol 2, 3rd ed. Munich: Urban & Schwarzenberg, 1989: Figures 178 and 263.

14. Netter FH. *Atlas of human anatomy*. Ciba-Geigy, Basle 1989: Plates 333 and 345.

15. Sobotta J. *Atlas of human anatomy*, Vol 2, *Thorax, abdomen, pelvis, lower limbs*. Staubesand J, ed. Munich: Urban & Schwarzenberg, 1990.

16. Hollingshead WH. *Textbook of Anatomy*, 2nd ed. Hagerstown, Maryland: Harper and Row, 1967: 683.

17. Tobin CE, Benjamin JA, Wells JC. Continuity of the fasciae lining the abdomen, pelvis, and spermatic cord. *Surg, Gynecol Obstet* 1946; **83**: 575–96.

18. Griffith CA. The Marcy repair revisited. *Surg Clin North Am* 1984; **64**: 215–27.

19. Cooper AP. *The anatomy and surgical treatment of inguinal and congenital hernia*. London: Longman, 1804.

20. Read RC. Cooper's posterior lamina of transversalis fascia. *Surg Gynecol Obstet* 1992; **174**: 426–34.

21. Brauss H. *Anatomie des menschen*, band I. Berlin: Julius Springer, 1921.

22. Lampe EW. Special comment: transversalis fascia. In: Nyhus LM, Condon RE, eds. *Hernia*, 2nd ed. Philadelphia: JB Lippincott, 1978: 60–4.

23. Anson BJ, Morgan EH, McVay CB. Surgical anatomy of the inguinal region based upon a study of 500 body-halves. *Surg Gynecol Obstet* 1960; **3**: 707–25.

24. Cleland J, Mackay JY, Young BJ. The relations of the aponeurosis of the transversalis and internal oblique muscles to the deep epigastric artery and to the inguinal canal. In: *Memoirs and memoranda in anatomy*, Vol I. London: Williams and Norgate, 1889.

5

Transversalis Fascia – a Reanalysis

RAYMOND C READ

Everything has been said before, but since nobody listens we have to keep going back and begin all over again. Andre Gide

No disease of the human body belonging to the province of the surgeon requires in its treatment a better combination of accurate anatomical knowledge with surgical skill than hernia in all its varieties. Astley Cooper[1]

History

Harrison in 1922[2] was the first to stress the importance of the fascia transversalis in the pathology and repair of inguinal hernias. Condon more recently has affirmed this relationship: 'the fundamental rupture, relaxation or discontinuity in the musculo-aponeurotic structure in cases of groin hernia occurs in the deeply placed transversus abdominis–transversalis fascial layer'[3].

We have all been taught that this layer envelops the peritoneum extending from the diaphragm to the pelvis, connecting the lumbar fascia to the linea alba. Thicker in the groin, it passes anterior to the recti and attaches inferiorly to the superior pubic ramus and femoral vessels. Condensations are referred to as internal spermatic fascia, iliopubic tract, Hesselbach's ligament, Henle's ligament, internal abdominal ring crura, and the rectus fascia of Anson and McVay. Condon's terminology, including the transversalis fascia in the transverse layer, harks back to Anson and McVay in 1938: 'the medially placed tendinous plate is in almost all descriptions correctly termed aponeurosis, but curiously enough the inferior continuation of the same structure is called a fascia, more specifically 'transversalis fascia'. That the two are merely areas of the same layer is clearly evident.[4] It is interesting that the epigastric vessels, although recognized as the line of dermarcation between direct and indirect defects, are rarely illustrated in hernial texts depicting hernias along with fascias. Condon has said:

> *This vasculature is contained within the preperitoneal space throughout their course in the groin, therefore they are deep or internal to the transversalis fascia, not superficial to it, and these vessels have no immediate connection with the musculo-aponeurotic abdominal wall in the groin. The branches of the inferior epigastric vessels usually do not pierce the transversalis fascia until they have crossed the lateral border of the rectus abdominis muscle. Between the iliac vessels and the border of the rectus muscle, the inferior epigastric vessels lie free in the preperitoneal space and have no intimate anatomical connection with the transversalis fascia. This fact is not enough appreciated*[3].

Gray's Textbook of Anatomy[5] shows the only structure behind the rectus abdominis muscles to be the preperitoneal fascia, a condensation of extraperitoneal fat. Anson and McVay stated that 'inferior to the linea semicircularis the rectus muscle is invested by its own layer of fascia'[4]. The preperitoneal connective tissue is known to have, as Lampe reported in an earlier edition of *Hernia* (Nyhus), 'a membrane-like condensation of the fibrous stroma of the preperitoneal fatty layer, mistaken by some as the transversalis fascia'[6].

Recent experience

My experience with the properitoneal approach to the repair of inguinal herniation in the 1960s demonstrated that the structure of the transversalis fascia is not, as we have been led to believe, this simple. Surprisingly, I found that the extrapreperitoneal covering makes up most of the internal spermatic fascia with . . . a small contribution from the transversalis fascia at the internal ring[7]. The preperitoneal fascia was strongly connected to the internal ring and funnelled the vas deferens and spermatic vessels from the extraperitoneal fat into this structure. Later, Fowler reported 'the preperitoneal fascia of the groin is distinct from the transversalis fascia, although often mistaken for it . . . special features include the preperitoneal fascia ring or secondary internal ring which appears to have been confused in the past with the transversalis fascial opening or internal ring proper[8]. Lytle, in Sheffield, had earlier (1945)[9] described the extraperitoneal covering making up most of the internal spermatic fascia and attaching strongly to the internal ring. He referred to another, deeper, inner internal ring. This confusion in terminology led me to examine the original description of the transversalis fascia made by Sir Astley Cooper in his classic texts on hernia in 1804[1] and 1807[10].

'When the tendons of the internal oblique and transversalis muscles are raised as they insert into the pubis, a layer of fascia is encountered lying between them and the peritoneum and an opening in it giving passage to the spermatic cord.'[1] In his second book, he said, 'This fascia should be called fascia transversalis. It lines an opening for the passage of the spermatic cord which I venture to name the internal abdominal ring.'[10] He went further:

> *The fascia transversalis may be divided into two portions, the one being placed a little before the other. Its outer portion is attached to the greater part of the posterior edge of the crural arch (Poupart's ligament). The inner portion is thinner than the former; it is also slightly attached to the crural arch (Poupart's ligament), but is more firmly affixed to the ligament of the pubis and is extended over the pubis into the cavity of the pelvis; it rises to the tendon of the transversalis muscle on the inner side of the spermatic cord and is firmly attached to the linea semilunaris. It appears that the internal ring is not a circumscribed aperture like the external abdominal ring, but is formed by the separation of two portions.*

One of his etchings illustrates these two layers.

He added in his second edition[11], 'the inner portion will be found to descend to form the anterior part of the sheath that envelops the femoral vessels'. Also, he commented bitterly in his second edition that 'Scarpa (as far as I can judge) seems to think that this name, Fascia transversalis Cooperi, is applied only to the outer portion'. Scarpa in 1814[12] had said that 'From below the umbilicus to the pubis the rectus muscle has no aponeurotic sheath and lies immediately upon the peritoneum'. This denial of Cooper's posterior lamina has persisted from Scarpa's time to the present. However, one anatomist, Mackay of Edinburgh, was able to confirm Cooper's observations in 1889[13], stating:

> *Different to what I find by careful dissection of many cadavers, the standard text of anatomy shows the transversalis fascia below the*

> *linea semicircularis passing entirely in front of the rectus muscle – below the linea semicircularis the transversalis and internal oblique muscles contribute a posterior sheath, while distinct and easily separated from transversalis fascia behind, it is comparatively thin.*

Thus, Mackay pointed out that there is an investing sheath of transversalis fascia for the rectus muscles, later confirmed by Anson and McVay (1938)[4]. Added to that, he reported that what we have been taught to call the 'preperitoneal membrane', lying between the rectus muscles with their investing fascia and the peritoneum, is part of transversalis fascia. Furthermore, Mackay reported that 'the inferior epigastric artery immediately upon its origin from the external iliac pierces the transversalis fascia'. Thus Mackay vindicated Cooper's description of a bilaminar transversalis fascia, different from Condon who considers the bilaminar appearance to be an artefact of dissection:

> *This apparent bilaminar nature of the transversalis fascia is brought about by the redundancy of the transversalis fascia as it forms the transversalis fascia sling. A dissection similar to Cooper's is produced if transversalis fascia is dissected from its attachment to the spermatic cord, the cord excised and the redundant transversalis fascia smoothed into flat surfaces.*[3]

Discussion

Thus, my observation that the extraperitoneal covering makes up most of the internal spermatic fascia with a small contribution from the transversalis fascia at the internal ring is explained by the fact that people have mistaken the posterior lamina of Cooper's transversalis fascia for a separate preperitoneal fascia layer, when it is actually just a deeper component of the one transversalis fascia. If, using the classic anterior approach to the groin, the floor of the inguinal canal is transected and fat is encountered; it is not possible to pass a finger freely down into the pelvis up to the umbilicus or laterally to the iliopsoas musculature – which one would expect if the floor of the canal were the transversalis fascial envelope of the abdomen continuous from the diaphragm to the pelvis and covering the peritoneum. The inferior epigastric vessels and beneath them another layer, translucent but surprisingly tough, intervene.

This has been considered by the establishment in surgical anatomy (Lampe, Lytle, Fowler and, as I mentioned earlier, myself) to be the preperitoneal fascia, a condensation of the extraperitoneal fat similar to Scarpa's fascia in the subcutaneous layer. However, examination reveals that it inserts inferiorly into the spermatic cord at the internal ring and the iliopectineal ligament lying on the superior pubic ramus. Medially, it passes behind the rectus muscles to the linea semicircularis above and the linea alba medially. It does not descend smoothly into the pelvis as has been described by Lampe and would be predicted if it were just simply a condensation of extraperitoneal fat.

Interestingly enough, McVay and Anson in 1940[14] pointed out that the linea semicircularis may be almost as high as the umbilicus, or so close to the pubic crest that the aponeurotic defect resembles an enlarged foramen for transmission of the inferior epigastric vessels. Their finding of this considerable variation in humans is best explained by saying that normally there is a posterior lamina of transversalis fascia passing behind the rectus muscles. In some people this is much thicker and better reinforced with aponeurotic fibres. The foramen remaining for passage of the inferior epigastric vessels is consistent with Mackay's observation that these vascular structures, soon after their origin, pierce the posterior lamina of transversalis fascia.

Thus, I believe that the epigastric vessels run between the two laminae of Cooper's transversalis fascia, which can therefore be considered as a vascular envelope. These arterial and venous plexi, including the accessory obturator vessels, rectusial branches to the muscle and pubic bone blood supply have recently been documented by Bendavid[15] and confirmed by me, from both the preperitoneal approach and the classic anterior incision. Bendavid considers them to lie in the space of Bogros (extraperitoneal) whereas I believe they lie within the transversalis layers.

It is important to realize that, when the Cheatle–Henry incision is used for preperitoneal exposure and repair of inguinal herniation, the posterior lamina of transversalis fascia is divided in the linea alba. One enters the preperitoneal plane immediately with lateral retraction of both the epigastric vasculature and the posterior lamina of transversalis fascia with the rectus muscles. This is different from when the McEvedy–Nyhus–Wantz unilateral approach is employed, since here one enters between the anterior and posterior lamina of transversalis fascia and comes down on the epigastric vessels. It is important that any prosthesis be placed deep to the epigastric vessels and the posterior lamina transversalis fascia, but superficial to the vas deferens and parietalized spermatic vessels lying in the extraperitoneal fat.

In the Lotheissen–McVay repair, to get to Cooper's ligament lying along the iliopectineal line on the pubic bone, it is necessary to divide the posterior lamina of the transversalis fascia and loosen up the inferior epigastric vessels. Similarly, with the Rives placement of prostheses in the extraperitoneal plane from the groin, the inferior epigastric vessels have to be mobilized so that the buttress can be placed in its proper anatomical plane. Otherwise, there is a potential problem of interstitial recurrent inguinal herniation because the prosthesis may be lifted up off more superficial layers such as the inguinal ligament and the internal oblique muscle. As Usher said in 1958, 'When you fix a leak in a tire you place the boot on the inside'[16]. Or, put another way, 'the bath plug is inserted from within the bath'[17]. If the goal of inguinal hernia repair, with or without a prosthesis, is to do so between the viscera and the abdominal wall, the operation has to be performed 'a la Bassini and Halsted I – ie in the preperitoneal plane internal to the inferior epigastric vasculature coursing between the two layers of the transversalis fascia, the deepest component of the abdominal wall.

References

1. Cooper AP. *The Anatomy and Surgical Treatment of Inguinal and Congenital Hernia*. London: Longman, 1804.
2. Harrison PW. Inguinal hernia: a study of the principles involved in surgical treatment. *Arch Surg* 1922; **4**: 680.
3. Condon RE. The anatomy of the inguinal region and its relationship to groin hernias. In: Nyhus LM, Condon KE, eds. *Hernia*, 3rd ed. Philadelphia: JB Lippincott, 1989: 19–64.
4. Anson BJ, McVay CB. Inguinal hernia. I. The anatomy of the region. *Surg Gynecol Obstet* 1938; **66**: 186–91.
5. Clemente C, ed. *Gray's Anatomy*, 30th Am. ed. Philadelphia: Lea & Febiger, 1985; 494.
6. Lampe EW. Special comment: Transversalis fascia. In: Nyhus LM, Condon RE, eds. *Hernia*, 2nd ed. Philadelphia: JB Lippincott, 1978: 60–4.
7. McVay CB, Read RC, Ravitch MM. Inguinal hernia. *Curr Probl Surg* 1967; Oct, 1–50.
8. Fowler R. The applied surgical anatomy of the peritoneal fascia of the groin and the 'secondary' internal inguinal ring. *Aust NZ J Surg* 1975; **45**: 8–14.
9. Lytle WJ. Internal inguinal ring. *Br J Surg* 1945; **32**: 441–6.
10. Cooper AP. *The Anatomy and Surgical Treatment of Crural and Umbilical Hernia*. London: Longman, 1807: 3–4.
11. Cooper AP. *The Anatomy of Surgical Treatment of Abdominal Hernia*, 2nd ed. Am. ed. Key CA, ed. Philadelphia: Lea & Febiger, 1844: vol 7, 27–8.
12. Scarpa A. *et al. A Treatise on Hernia*, trans. John Henry Wishart. Edinburgh: Longman, Hurst, Rees *et al.*, 1814.

13. Cleland J, Mackay JY, Young BJ. The relations of the aponeurosis of the transversalis and internal oblique muscles to the deep epigastric artery and to the inguinal canal. In: *Memoirs and Memoranda in Anatomy*, vol 1. London: Williams & Norgate, 1889: 142–5.

14. McVay CB, Anson BJ. Composition of the rectus sheath. *Anat Rec* 1940; **77**: 213–25.

15. Bendavid R. The space of Bogros and the deep inguinal venous circulation. *Surg Gynecol Obstet* 1992; **174**: 355–8.

16. Usher FC, Oschner J, Tuttle Jr LL. Use of Marlex mesh in the repair of incisional hernias. *Am Surg* 1958; **24**: 969.

17. Estrin J, Lipton S, Block IR. The posterior approach to inguinal and femoral hernias. *Surg Gynecol Obstet* 1963; **116**: 547.

6

Avoiding Nerve Injury during Laparoscopic Hernia Repair: Critical Areas for Staple Placement

RICCARDO ANNIBALI, THOMAS QUINN AND ROBERT J FITZGIBBONS Jr

Following the excellent results obtained with laparoscopic cholecystectomy, laparoscopic hernia repair is gaining rapid acceptance by general surgeons. Some important controversies remain: the conventional operation is frequently performed under local anaesthesia on an outpatient basis, while general anaesthesia is generally recommended for the laparoscopic approach; most conventional herniorrhaphies do not require entry into the peritoneal cavity, thus avoiding the possible risks and consequences that are inherent to laparoscopy. Nevertheless, the economic impact of the operation in terms of an earlier return to work represents an attractive feature of this operation. Other goals to be achieved with laparoscopic hernia repair are a lower recurrence rate, decreased postoperative pain, minimal postoperative morbidity and improved cosmesis, at a reasonable cost on an outpatient basis[1].

The introduction of laparoscopy, however, has involved a different perspective for the surgeon used to the conventional anterior approach. In 1969, Ravitch stated that the 'operations for the cure of hernia would seem to be established and well known beyond the possible need for further discussion and demonstration'[2]. Actually, before the introduction of laparoscopic surgery, it seemed that 'hernia' was quite well defined, the term indicating the protrusion of a viscus from the abdominal cavity that needed to be repositioned and kept in place. The only variable was the type of repair preferred. The recent introduction of laparoscopic surgical techniques has challenged the general surgeon with a totally new approach to the 'problem hernia': through a laparoscope, the hernia itself is no longer viewed as a protrusion from the abdominal wall, but rather the extrusion of a viscus from the peritoneal cavity. The layers that constitute the inguinal region and the lower anterior abdominal wall are seen from an opposite viewpoint and dissected according to a reversed order. Most anatomical and surgical textbooks describe the critical layers in sequence as a dissection would proceed from the superficial layers to the deep ones, reserving little consideration for the internal view of the abdominal wall. Indeed, in 1945, Lytle wrote: 'The operating surgeon knows little of the posterior wall of the inguinal canal, so well it is hidden from his view.'[3] For a safe approach to laparoscopic herniorrhaphy, it would seem appropriate to reverse the habitual order and visualize the anatomy from the inner layers, since laparoscopy provides an optimal panoramic view of the posterior surface of the abdominal wall.

The unusual anatomical perspective was not the only factor that persuaded us to start a thorough review of the anatomy of the inguinal region and the lower deep abdominal wall soon after we began our training with laparoscopic hernia repair at the Department of Surgery of Creighton University. Early in our experience, we registered in the postoperative period an unsuspectingly high incidence not only of groin and testicular pain but also of meralgia paraesthetica (pain in the thigh). This finding was confirmed by the results of a multicentre international clinical trial on laparoscopic hernia repair co-ordinated by our group, including 636 repairs in 816 patients, which demonstrated that the cumulative incidence of neuralgia in the groin and testicular areas, combined with meralgia paraesthetica, represented by far the most frequently reported complication in almost all the surveys considered. We defined the pain 'temporary', when it resolved spontaneously within two months; otherwise it was considered as 'permanent'. Transient groin, testicular and thigh pain were observed in, respectively, 6.25%, 0.98% and 3.18% of patients considered, whereas permanent groin, testicular and thigh pain were reported in 1.84%, 0.49% and 0.98%. As a consequence, it became obvious that laparoscopic hernia repair might interfere with the innervation of the lower abdominal wall, genital region and thigh in a different, and probably more serious, way compared with conventional herniorrhaphy. On the basis of these results, we felt that we needed to go back to cadaver dissections and re-examine the anatomy of the inguinal region as well as that of the major nerves derived from the lumbar plexus. We preferred to begin our dissections with an enlarged bilateral subcostal incision instead of a midline incision, to preserve the anterior abdominal wall intact as a whole big flap.

Innervation

After removal of the peritoneum covering the lower portion of the posterior abdominal wall, five major nerves responsible for the innervation of the lower abdominal wall, the inguinal and genital region, the thigh and the leg are found in the extra-peritoneal space: the ilio-inguinal, the iliohypogastric, the genitofemoral, the femoral and the lateral femoral cutaneous (Figures 6.1 and 6.2). These nerves originate from the lumbar plexus (T1, L1–L4).

The *iliohypogastric nerve* (Figure 6.1) appears at the lateral margin of the psoas muscle and crosses obliquely on the quadratus lumborum, passes beneath the inferior pole of the kidney to pierce the transversus abdominis muscle, and then divides into two branches. The most important one is the hypogastric. The hypogastric nerve lies between the external and the internal oblique muscle at the level of the anterior superior iliac spine and reaches the suprapubic skin by piercing either the external oblique aponeurosis or the anterior rectus sheath. It innervates the skin of the anterior abdominal wall above the pubis (Figure 6.3).

The *ilioinguinal nerve* (*see* Figures 6.1 and 6.2) follows a course similar to that of the iliohypogastric, but more inferior. It crosses the quadratus lumborum and the iliacus muscles before piercing the transversus abdominis just above the anterior portion of the iliac crest. After piercing the internal oblique, it runs along the inguinal canal, over the cremasteric muscle, and finally exits through the external inguinal ring to innervate the skin of the superomedial portion of the thigh, the root of penis, the pubic region and the scrotum or labium majus (Figure 6.3).

The *genitofemoral nerve* (*see* Figures 6.1 and 6.2) emerges from the fibres of the psoas muscle at the level of the third or fourth lumbar vertebra, and crosses behind the ureter to divide into the genital and femoral branches at a variable distance from the iliopubic tract. The *genital branch* is medial, traverses the iliac vessels to reach the internal inguinal ring and runs along the inguinal canal together with the spermatic cord. The genital branch of the genitofemoral nerve provides motor innervation to the cremaster muscle and sensory innervation to the skin of the penis and scrotum (Figure 6.3). The *femoral branch* lies usually on the lateral edge of the psoas muscle, beneath the psoas fascia. It is not constantly a single trunk, and may bifurcate before crossing the deep circumflex iliac artery to pass under the iliopubic tract just lateral to the testicular vessels. In the femoral sheath, it lies lateral to the femoral artery. After piercing the anterior wall of the femoral sheath and the fascia lata, it reaches the superior portion of the femoral triangle in the thigh and supplies innervation to the femoral triangle and proximal part of the anterior thigh. It provides sensory innervation to the anteromedial surface of the upper thigh (Figure 6.3).

The *lateral femoral cutaneous nerve* emerges from the lateral margin of the psoas muscle, deep to the peritoneum and iliac fascia, through which it can often be seen (*see* Figures 6.1 and 6.2). It crosses the iliacus muscle obliquely towards the anterior superior iliac spine. Medial to the anterior superior iliac spine, it passes below the iliopubic tract to reach the thigh and divides into two branches. The anterior branch becomes superficial at a variable distance below the anterior superior

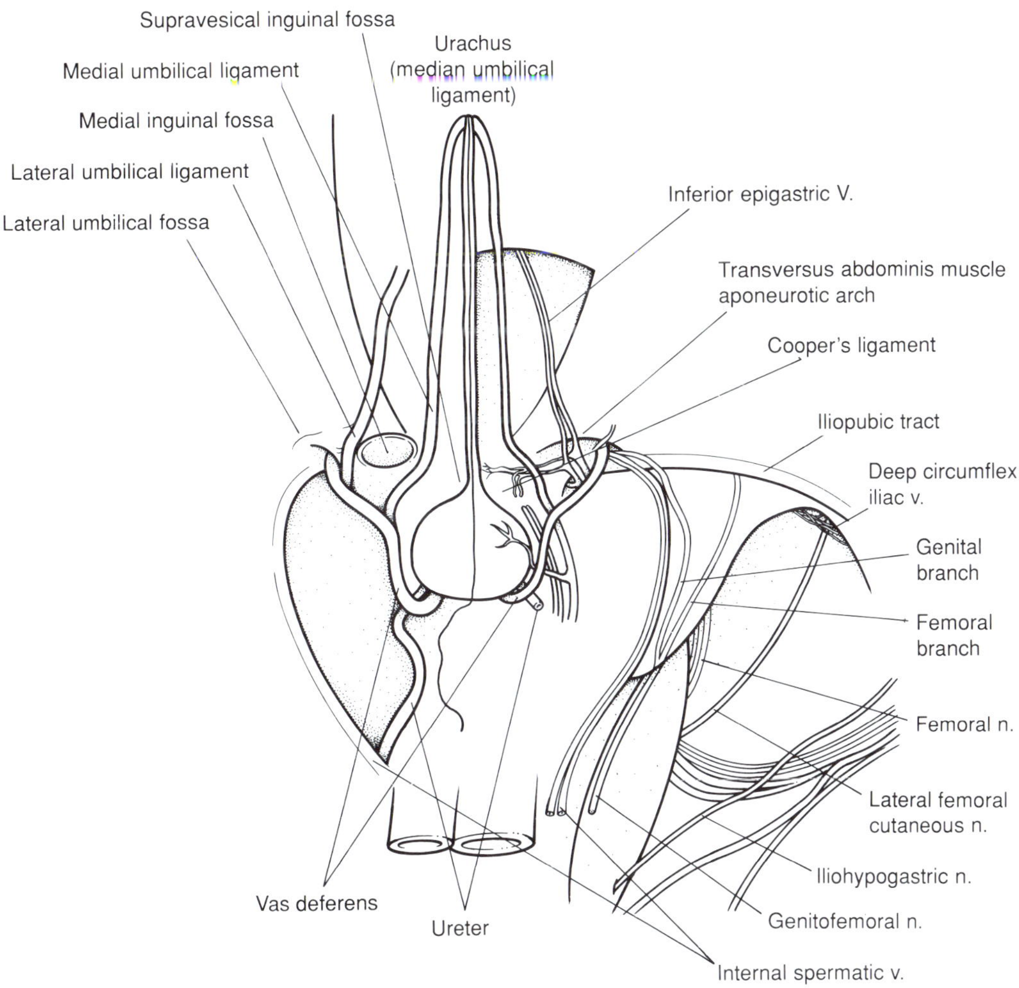

Figure 6.1: The anatomy of the internal surface of the lower abdominal wall, inguinal region and lower trunk.

iliac spine and innervates the skin of the anterior and lateral surfaces of the upper thigh as far as the knee (Figure 6.3). The posterior branch pierces the fascia lata at a higher level and then runs posterior to reach the skin of the lateral aspect of the thigh. The innervated area extends from the greater trocanter to the midcalf level.

The *femoral nerve* is the largest nerve originating from the lumbar plexus (Figure 6.3). It emerges from the inferior aspect of the psoas muscle, passes along the lateral border, and then runs between the iliacus and pectineus muscles, covered by a layer of fascia. It passes below the iliopubic tract, reaches the femoral triangle within the lacuna musculorum, and finally divides into anterior and posterior branches. The *anterior branch* originates approximately 8 cm distal to the inguinal ligament and provides the *intermediate femoral cutaneous* and the *medial femoral cutaneous* nerves, to innervate the skin of the lower anteromedial thigh. The *saphenous nerve* is the largest sensory branch of the femoral nerve, and continues to the leg to innervate the medial aspect of the leg and the great toe (Figure 6.3). The posterior branch contains the muscular branches, that provide motor innervation to the pectineus, sartorius and quadriceps.

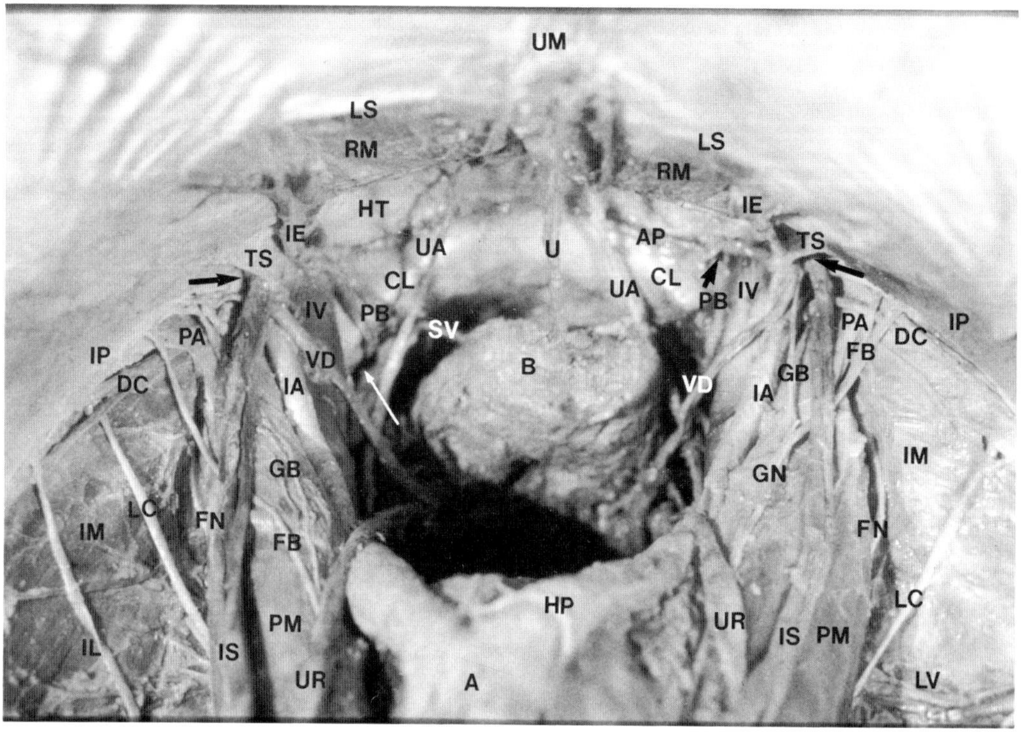

Figure 6.2: Panoramic view of the internal surface of the anterior lower abdominal wall, inguinal regions, lower trunk and pelvis in a cadaver dissection. A, abdominal aorta; AP, anterior pubic branch and iliopubic vein; CL, Cooper's ligament; DC, deep circumflex iliac vessels; FB, femoral branch of the genitofemoral nerve; FN, femoral nerve; GB, genital branch of the genitofemoral nerve; GN, genitofemoral nerve; HT, inguinal (Hesselbach's triangle); IA, external iliac artery; IE, inferior epigastric vessels; IL, ilioinguinal nerve; IM, iliacus muscle; IP, iliopubic tract; IS, internal spermatic (testicular) vessels; IV, external iliac vein; LC, lateral femoral cutaneous nerve; LS, linea semicircularies; LV, iliolumbal vessels; Thick black arrow, deep inguinal ring; white arrow, obturator forament; short arrow, femoral ring; PA, iliopectineal arch; PB, anastomotic pubic branches; PM, psoas major muscle; RM, rectus abdominis muscle; SV, superior vesical artery; TS, transversalis fascia sling; U, urachus; UA, umbilical artery; UM, umbilicus; UR, ureter; VD, vas deferens.

Anatomical areas critical for laparoscopic hernia repair

The term 'triangle of doom', first introduced by Spaw, indicates the triangular area between the vas deferens medially and spermatic vessels laterally[4] (Figures 6.4 and 6.5). Its importance is related to the fact that the external iliac vessels lie in its floor, usually hidden by the peritoneum and the transversalis fascia. To prevent injury to these important structures, it is strongly recommended that suturing or stapling be done only medial to the vas deferens or lateral to the spermatic vessels[4]. In our opinion, however, this statement could lead to the false belief that all major dangers involved in laparoscopic herniorrhaphy are located in that triangular area. As a consequence, this could lead

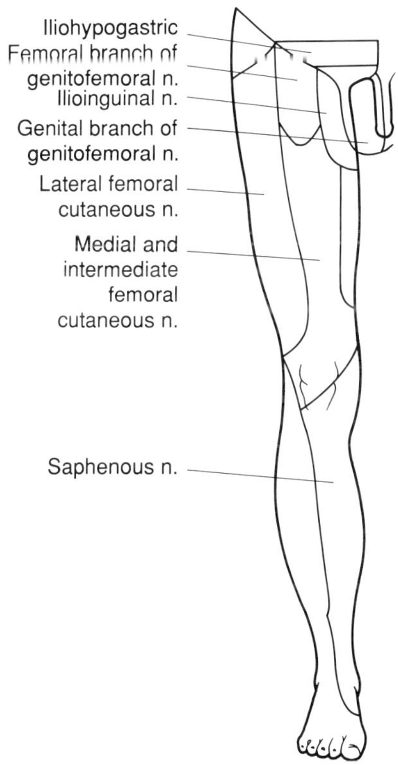

Figure 6.3: Areas of sensory innervation in the lower limb of relevant interest for the laparoscopic herniorraphist.

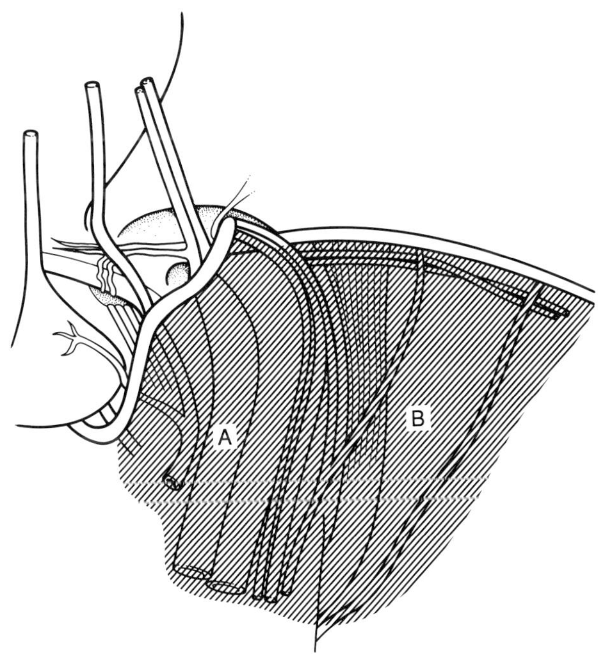

Figure 6.4: A indicates the area known as 'triangle of doom'. B is the triangular area area where staples placed inadvertently may cause nerve injury with an entrapment mechanism ('triangle of pain').

the inexperienced laparoscopic surgeon to a false sense of confidence when placing staples needed to hold the prosthetic mesh in place. Actually, we believe that the borders of the 'dangerous area' should be extended.

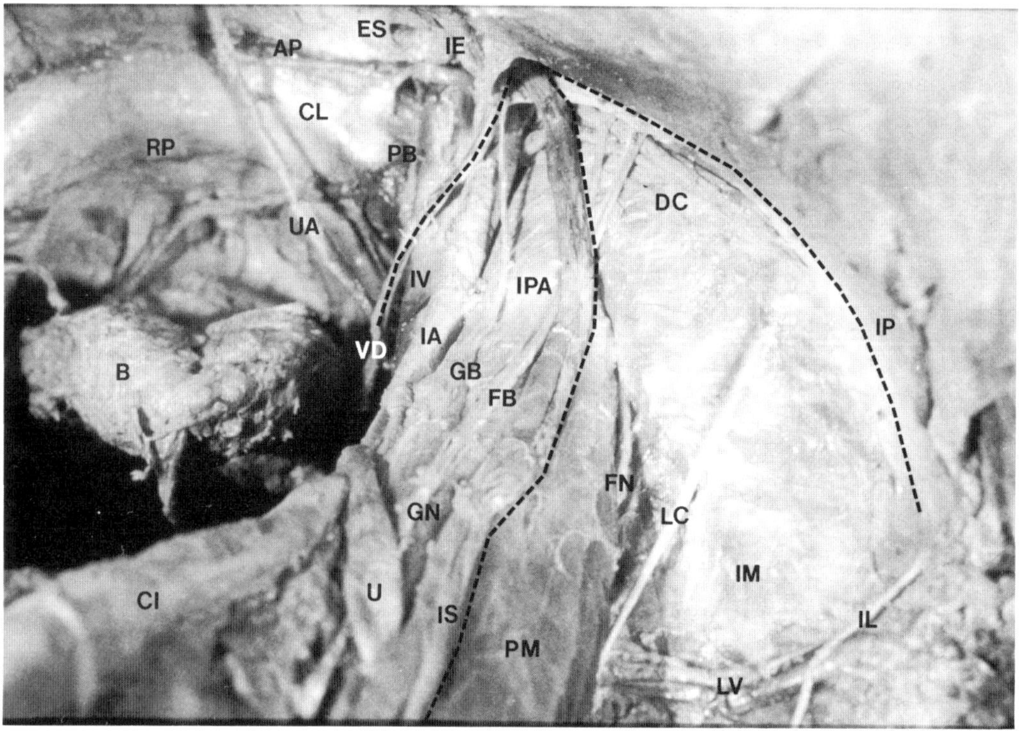

Figure 6.5: Cadaver preparation (right side) that shows the structures included within the 'triangle of doom' (medial triangle) and the dangerous area beside it, bordered by the internal spermatic (testicular) vessels inferomedially and the iliopubic tract superolaterally (lateral triangle), where no staples or sutures should be placed. AP, anterior pubic branch and iliopubic vein; B, bladder (reflected posteriorly); CI, common iliac artery; CL, Cooper's pectineal ligament; DC, deep circumflex iliac vessels' ES, external spermatic (cremasteric) vessels; FB, femoral branch of the genitofemoral nerve; FN, femoral nerve; GB, genital branch of the genitofemoral nerve; GN, genitofemoral nerve; IA, external iliac artery; IE, inferior epigastric vessels; IL, ilioinguinal nerve; IM, iliac muscle; IP, iliopubic tract; IPA, iliopectineal arch; IS, internal spermatic (testicular) vessels; IV, external iliac vein; LC, lateral femoral cutaneous nerve; LV, iliolumbal vessels; PB, anastomotic pubic branch; PM, psoas major muscle; RP, retropubic vein; U, ureter; UA, umbilical artery; VD, vas deferens.

For laparoscopic inguinal herniorrhaphy, the iliopubic tract is another extremely important landmark to observe if staples are to be applied safely[5,6]. In fact, lateral to the spermatic vessels and immediately below (or, in some instances, directly through) the fibres of the iliopubic tract are the genital and femoral branches of the genitofemoral nerve, the femoral nerve and the lateral femoral cutaneous nerve. Consequently, staples placed posterior to the iliopubic tract and lateral to the femoral vessels can result in transient or permanent neuralgia involving one or more of the above-mentioned nerves or branches (*see* Figure 6.6).

Pain in the groin or lower abdomen is noted if the *ilioinguinal* or the *iliohypogastric nerve* is injured, whereas pain along the cord and scrotum occurs if the genital branch of the genitofemoral nerve has been damaged[7,8]. Injury of the iliohypogastric and ilioinguinal nerves, however, is much less frequent during laparoscopic hernia repair than with conventional anterior inguinal herniorraphy, because they lie in a plane superficial to the preperitoneal space. On occasion, however, they can be compromised when staples are placed deeply, especially if a vigorous bimanual technique is used.

The importance of damaging the *genital branch of the genitofemoral nerve* during conventional hernia repair, and its relationship with subsequent development of neuralgia in the innervated district, has been largely debated[9,10,11]. Lichtenstein recommended the accurate preservation of the nerve fibres during sac dissection[12]. Obney, of the Shouldice Hospital, reported that this nerve is routinely

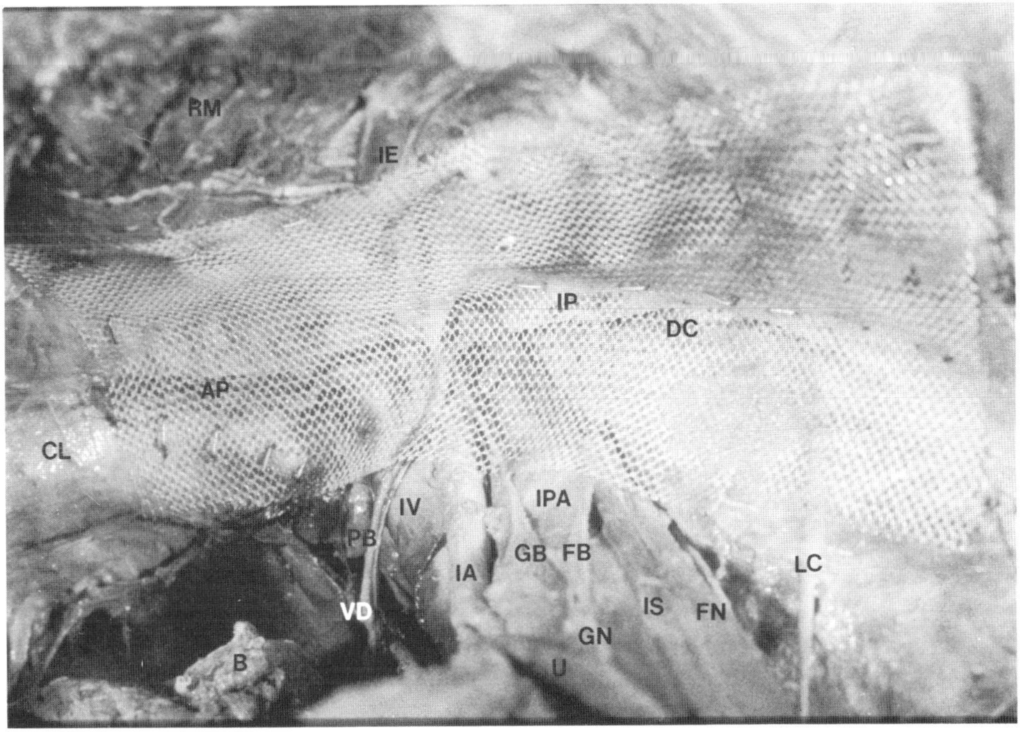

Figure 6.6: Mesh correctly positioned and tacked with staples to cover the three weak areas corresponding to the deep inguinal ring, the inguinal triangle and the femoral ring. AP, anterior pubic branch and iliopubic vein; B, bladder (reflected posteriorly); CL, Cooper's pectineal ligament; DC, deep circumflex iliac vessels; FB, femoral branch of the genitofemoral nerve; FN, femoral nerve; GB, genital branch of the genitofemoral nerve; GN, genitofemoral nerve; IA, external iliac artery; IE, inferior epigastric vessels; IM, iliacus muscle; IP, iliopubic tract; IPA, iliopectineal arch; IS, internal spermatic (testicular) vessels; IV, external iliac vein; LC, lateral femoral cutaneous nerve; PE, anastomotic pubic branch; PM, psoas major muscle; RM, rectus abdominis muscle; TM, transversus abdominis muscle; U, ureter; VD, vas deferens.

divided at that institution and they do not observe any significant postoperative discomfort[13]. The genital branch of the genitofemoral nerve is not encountered commonly in the area in which staples are applied. It might be damaged, however, by the manoeuvres used to reduce the sac of an indirect hernia, even if this event is probably rare. In addition, it is not unusual to observe the genital branch passing below the iliopubic tract in the vicinity of the deep inguinal ring, to enter the inguinal canal from below. This anatomical variation may occasionally lead to damage of the genital branch. The genital branch of the genitofemoral nerve is probably somehow involved in the painful sensation known as 'dysejaculation': this is a rare complication, described in 17 patients subjected to conventional anterior herniorrhaphy, and reported as a painful, burning or searing sensation during ejaculation. The onset of the condition is noted at variable times after surgery, and may be triggered by distention of the vas deferens by the ejaculate[14].

The *femoral branch of the genitofemoral nerve* and the *lateral femoral cutaneous nerve* are those at higher risk of being injured, because they are more superficial (they lie on the anterior surface of the psoas and iliacus muscles respectively) along the course where staples are usually applied to tack the inferior border and the outer corner of the mesh (Figures 6.6 and 6.7).

The *femoral nerve* (*see* Figures 6.1 and 6.2) is medial and in a relatively deeper position. Although less vulnerable, it may be injured by staples placed medially and close to the iliopectineal arch, with possible sensory (usually pain in the anteromedial region of the thigh) and/or functional consequences (inability to extend the leg, quadriceps atrophy).

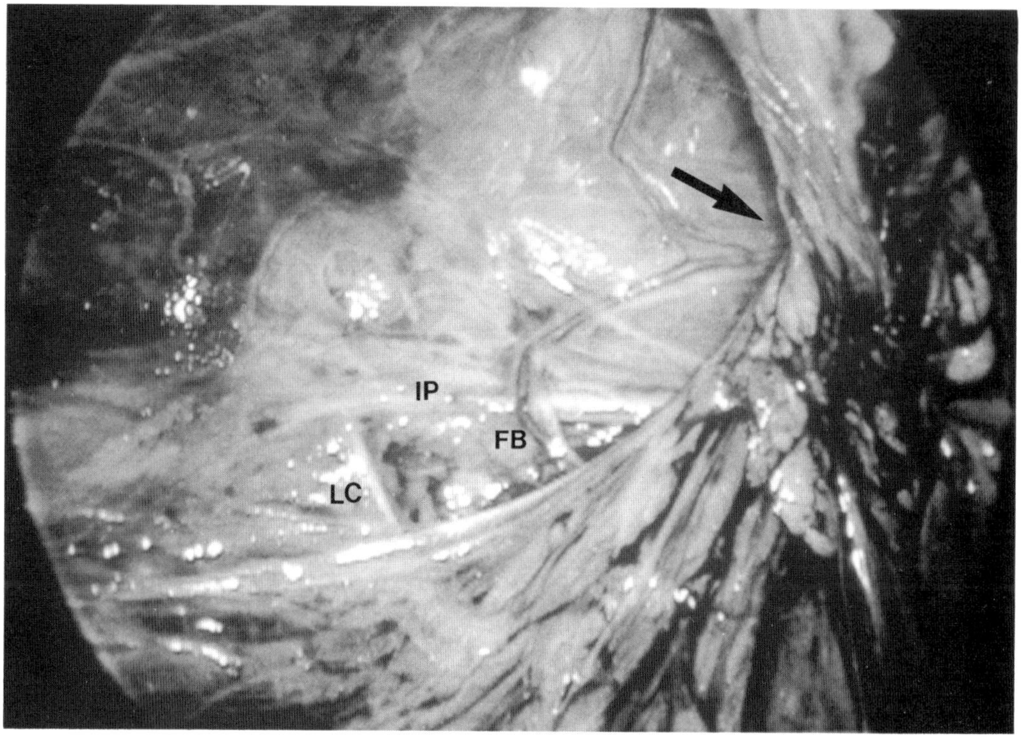

Figure 6.7: After an accurate surgical dissection, the femoral branch of the genitofemoral nerve and the lateral femoral cutaneous nerve have been identified during a laparoscopic hernia repair as they approach and pass below the iliopubic tract. FB, femoral branch of the genitofemoral nerve; IP, iliopubic tract; LC, lateral femoral cutaneous nerve; The arrow indicates the enlarged deep inguinal ring, through which an indirect inguinal hernia found its outlet.

To prevent damage to the nerves, as well as to the external iliac and deep circumflex iliac vessels, we recommend that, lateral to the vas deferens, staples should be placed only above and parallel to the iliopubic tract (*see* Figures 6.4–6.6).

In view of the dangers associated with improper placement of staples during herniorrhaphy, it seems appropriate to introduce a new triangular area in addition to the 'triangle of doom'. The boundaries of this second dangerous zone include the testicular vessels inferomedially and the iliopubic tract superolaterally (*see* Figures 6.4 and 6.5). We recommend that no staples or sutures be applied in this triangle.

Medial to the vas deferens, care should also be taken when tacking the inferomedial corner of the mesh. Staples should be applied on Cooper's pectineal ligament only, because staples placed too close to the deep inguinal ring and transversalis fascia sling could damage the terminal portion of the external iliac vein before it passes below the iliopubic tract (*see* Figure 6.5). Finally, when stapling the mesh to Cooper's ligament, it is important to avoid the anastomotic pubic branch, which usually lies on the lateral portion of the pectineal ligament (*see* Figures 6.1, 6.2, 6.5 and 6.6).

Conclusions

Laparoscopic hernia repair is a new, interesting surgical operation, and can be accomplished as a straightforward outpatient procedure. The incidence of groin and thigh pain, however, was disturbingly high in the early experience. We believe that a thorough knowledge of the anatomy of the inguinal region and lower abdominal wall from the unique perspective of laparoscopy, and with particular attention to the innervation, is essential if an operation that is safe, has a lower recurrence rate and a short operative time is expected and also if disturbing complications are to be prevented.

References

1. Filipi CJ, Fitzgibbons RJ, Salerno GM, Hart RO. Laparoscopic herniorraphy, *Surg Clin North Am* 1992; **72**: 1109–24.
2. Ravitch MM. *Repair of hernias*. Chicago: Year Book Medical Publishers, 1969: 9.
3. Lytle W. The internal inguinal ring. *Br J Surg* 1945; **32**: 441–6.
4. Spaw AT, Ennis BW, Spaw LP. Laparoscopic hernia repair: the anatomic basis. *J Laparoendosc Surg* 1991; **1**: 269–77.
5. Lichtenstein IL, Amid PK, Shulman AG. The iliopubic tract. The key to inguinal herniorraphy? *Int Surg* 1990; **75**: 244–6.
6. Lichtenstein IL, Amid PK, Shulman AG. The iliopubic tract. Is it important in groin herniorraphy? *Contemp Surg* 1992; **40**: 22–4.
7. Gaster J. *Hernia: one day repair*. Darien Conn: Hafner Publishing, 1970: 5–54.
8. Mandelkow H, Loeweneck H. The iliohypogastric and ilioinguinal nerves. Distribution in the abdominal walls, danger areas in surgical incisions in the inguinal and pubic regions and reflected visceral pain in their dermatomes. *Surg Radiol Anat* 1988; **10**: 145–9.
9. Starling JR, Harms BA, Schroeder ME, Eichman PL. Diagnosis and treatment of genitofemoral and ilioinguinal entrapment neuropathies. *Surgery* 1987; **102**: 581–6.
10. Starling JR, Harms BA. Diagnosis and treatment of genitofemoral and ilioinguinal neuralgia. *World J Surg* 1989; **13**: 586–91.
11. Magee RK. Genitofemoral causalgia. *Can Med Assoc J* 1942; **46**: 326–9.
12. Lichtenstein IL, Shulman AG, Amid P, Montilor M. The cause and prevention of postherniorraphy neuralgia. Proposed protocol for treatment. *Am J Surg* 1988; **155**: 786–90.
13. Obney N. Application of Shouldice technique in large scrotal hernias and sliding hernias. *Contemp Surg* 1984; **24**: 11–16.
14. Bendavid R. 'Dysejaculation': an unusual complication. *Postgrad Gen Surg* 1992; **4**: 139–41.

7

Inguinal Hernia in Infants and Children

JAY L GROSFELD

Aetiology

Inguinal hernia is one of the most common conditions in infants that requires operative repair. The aetiology of congenital indirect hernia is related to the descent of the testis and the fate of the primitive processus vaginalis. The testis arises in the retroperitoneal space near the developing kidney.

In the first phase of testicular descent (the abdominal phase) the testis follows the downward course of the migrating gubernaculum testis which, under the effect of hormonal influences, enlarges and leads the gonad through the internal inguinal ring into the groin. As it passes through the internal ring, a portion of the peritoneal lining known as the processus vaginalis is pulled along into the inguinal canal. Abdominal descent is blocked by oestrogens.

The second phase of testicular descent (the inguinoscrotal phase) is under the influence of androgenic stimulation that may be mediated by the genitofemoral nerve. Recent data suggest that, if the genitofemoral nerve is cut, testicular descent will not occur. It is theorized that the genitofemoral nerve releases calcitonin-related gene peptide (CRGP), which acts as secondary messenger for androgen receptors on the gubernaculum or testis. CRGP causes rhythmic contractions of the gubernaculum, and there are CRGP receptors identified in the developing cremasteric muscle.

The processus vaginalis subsequently follows the testis into a scrotal position by the seventh intrauterine month, and is attached to the anteromedial surface of the testis.

Failure of obliteration of the patent processus vaginalis results in the development of a number of inguinoscrotal anomalies, including scrotal hernia, distal obliteration with a patent proximal hernia sac, communicating hydrocele (a misnomer for an inguinal hernia with a narrow patent connection to the peritoneal cavity at the internal inguinal ring), hydrocele of the cord (in boys) or of the canal of Nuck (in girls) and, finally, an isolated hydrocele of the tunica vaginalis.

All except the last-named finding are indications for prompt surgical repair. Hydrocele of the tunica that persists beyond one year of age also requires operative management.

Incidence

Inguinal hernia is more common in boys than in girls (3–8:1), and occurs on the right side in 60% of cases, on the left side in 30% and bilaterally in 10% of cases. The incidence of inguinal hernia in infants varies significantly with gestational age and is 3–5% in full-term infants but may be as high as 35% in preterm babies of less than 28 weeks' gestation.

There is often a family history of inguinal hernia although the actual familial incidence is unknown. There is an increased risk of inguinal hernia in babies that are born prematurely, infants with increased intra-abdominal pressure due to ascites related to hydrops or from liver or renal disease, following the performance of ventriculoperitoneal shunts for hydrocephalus (VP shunts), and after placement of a Tenckhoff catheter for continuous ambulatory peritoneal dialysis (CAPD) in infants with renal failure.

An increased incidence of inguinal hernia has also been observed in babies with

- intersex problems (testicular feminization syndrome, male pseuodohermaphrodites, mixed gonadal dysgenesis, etc.)
- undescended testes
- exstrophy of the bladder or cloaca
- abdominal wall defects
- connective tissue disorders (Ehlers–Danlos syndrome, Marfan's syndrome, Hunter–Hurler syndrome)
- hypospadias
- epispadias

and in children with cystic fibrosis and occasionally other respiratory conditions associated with chronic straining due to excessive cough.

Diagnosis

The diagnosis of inguinal hernia is usually made by the parent, who notices a bulge in the groin when the infant cries or strains, or recognizes a fluctuation in the size of the infant's testis related to an exchange of fluid between the peritoneal cavity and a patent hernia sac in the scrotum. When the child is active the scrotum gets larger, when sleeping quietly it gets smaller. This observation is brought to the attention of the baby's paediatrician or family doctor, who verifies the presence of the hernia and refers the infant for repair. Occasionally, incarceration will be the presenting clinical manifestation of inguinal hernia in an infant in whom the diagnosis was never previously suspected.

Risks of inguinal hernia

The major risks associated with inguinal hernia are incarceration, strangulation obstruction and gonadal infarction. The risk of incarceration is 12–15% throughout childhood but is much higher in the first year of life (31%). Infants under six months of age have the greatest risk of bowel infarction. The gonad is at risk for infarction if hernia incarceration occurs in an infant with an undescended testis where the blood supply to the gonad is more vulnerable to compression at the level of the internal ring.

Treatment

The treatment of choice for inguinal hernias is prompt surgical repair. The risk from hernia repair is minimal and operation is associated with an extremely low cumulative complication rate in experienced hands (1–2%).

Complications include bleeding, wound infection, hernia recurrence, injury to the vas or spermatic vessels, and gonadal atrophy. However, the complication rate may be as high as 18–20% when operations are performed for instances of incarcerated hernia.

These observations suggest that incarcerated hernia in infants should be manually reduced when possible (successful in 80%), converting an emergency problem to an elective case. The technique of reducing an incarcerated hernia in infants includes the careful use of sedation, positioning (reversed Trendelenburg), the use of a cool-pack placed over a piece of petroleum jelly (Vaseline) gauze (to protect the skin), and gentle manual compression if the hernia doesn't reduce spontaneously. We admit the patient to the hospital and repair the hernia the next day. If the baby is sent home and scheduled electively, the incarceration will often recur. When attempted reduction of the incarcerated hernia is unsuccessful, an emergency procedure should be carried out.

These observations strongly suggest that early elective repair of inguinal hernia should be performed shortly after diagnosis to prevent such potentially life-threatening complications. Most cases can be managed in the outpatient setting; however, selective patients with a history of prematurity, previous ventilator support, episodes of apnoea or other co-morbid problems can be managed postoperatively in an extended observation facility for 12–23 hours.

Operation

Operative repair is carried out under carefully administered and well-monitored general tracheal anaesthesia, through a 2.5 cm transverse incision in the lowest inguinal crease. The infant's groin may contain a great deal of fatty tissue, and the planes of dissection may be more difficult to identify because of the presence of a very thickened well-defined Scarpa's fascial layer. Careful identification of the external oblique fibres and tracing the inguinal ligament inferiorly will allow accurate identification of the exact site of the external inguinal ring prior to making any fascial incisions.

The cremasteric muscle fibres can be teased open and the hernia sac located in an anteromedial position. The spermatic vessels and vas deferens are gently separated from the sac by careful blunt dissection of the areolar tissue attached to these structures to prevent injury or unnecessary bleeding. The vas itself should never be picked up directly by forceps, as this can result in injury to this important structure. It is unnecessary to mobilize the entire spermatic cord and place a Penrose drain around it prior to the dissection, as is commonplace in the performance of an adult inguinal herniorrhaphy. The floor of the inguinal canal should not be disturbed, to avoid damaging the transversalis fascia and the subsequent risk of a direct hernia. The sac should not be divided or cross-clamped until all the vital structures have been identified. The dissection of the sac is carried up to the internal ring, where identification of the retroperitoneal fat verifies that the dissection is high enough.

In most cases, simple high ligation of the sac at the internal inguinal ring with two separate non-absorbable suture ligatures (3/0 or 4/0 silk) is all that is necessary. In rare instances, an associated weakness of the floor may require repair, or an excessively enlarged internal ring may need a snugging suture inserted across the transversalis fascia inferior to the cord structures.

Contralateral groin exploration is most useful in infant boys less than two years of age, in girls less than four years of age, when the clinical hernia presents on the left side and in patients with increased abdominal pressure due to fluid in the abdomen (CAPD, VP shunts, etc.).

There is no indication for laparoscopic hernia repair in infants. The procedure may have a role in older children or in teenagers with recurrent hernia in whom a preperitoneal approach and the use of a prosthetic patch is anticipated.

Further reading

Cooney DR. Repair of inguinal hernia in children with ventriculoperitoneal shunts. In: Grosfeld JL, ed. *Current Problems in Pediatric Surgery*. Chicago: Year Book Medical Publ 1991: 17–28.

Fallat ME, Williams WPL, Farmer PG, Hutson JM. Histologic evaluation of inguinoscrotal migration of the gubernaculum in rodents during testicular descent and its relationship to the genitofemoral nerve. *Pediatr Surg Int* 1992; 7: 271

Grosfeld JL. Current concepts in inguinal hernia in infants and children. *World J Surg* 1989; **13**: 506–15.

Grosfeld JL, Minnick K, Shedd F, West KW, Rescorla FJ, Vane DW. Inguinal hernia in children: factors affecting recurrence in 62 cases. *J Pediatr Surg* 1991; **26**: 283–7.

Grosfeld JL. Inguinal hernia in the premature neonate. In: Grosfeld JL, ed. *Current Problems in Pediatric Surgery*. Chicago: Year Book Medical Publ, 1991: 3–8.

Kleinhaus S, Boley SJ. Recurrent inguinal hernia in children. In: Grosfeld JL, ed. *Current Problems in Pediatric Surgery*. Chicago: Year Book Medical Publ, 1991: 29–35.

Puri P, Guincy EJ, O'Donnell B. Inguinal hernia in infants: the fate of the testes following incarceration. *Pediatr Surg* 1984; **19**: 44.

Rescorla FJ, Grosfeld JL. Inguinal hernia repair in the perinatal period and early infancy: clinical considerations. *J Pediatr Surg* 1984; **19**: 832.

8

Shutter Mechanisms in the Inguinal Canal

LEIF SPANGEN

The shutter mechanisms in the groin and the role of their incompetence in the development of inguinal hernia are discussed in this chapter.

Inner shutter, closing mechanism and valve mechanism

The transversalis fascia in the groin is relatively thick and covers the inside of the musculature and aponeuroses. It is important to understand that the transversalis fascia is firmly attached to and inseparable from the transversus abdominis muscle and its aponeurosis. Functionally, the transversalis fascia and transversus abdominis muscle act as a single entity called the transversus abdominis layer.

Figure 8.1 is a schematic illustration showing the right groin seen from the inside. At the deep inguinal opening, the transversalis fascia merges with the funicle and continues within this as the internal cremasteric fascia, thereby forming the U-shaped inner inguinal ring. The margin is a duplication of the fascia, which is also greatly thickened here. This U-shaped margin of the inner inguinal ring is called the *transversalis fascia sling*. We see from the Figure that the two crura of the sling are attached to the posterior wall of the transversus abdominis muscle in fan-shaped fashion. The medial, superior, crus is attached to the aponeurosis part of the muscle and the lateral, inferior, crus is attached to the muscle belly. The curve of the U is normally situated at or just below the edge of the transversus abdominis arch so that the funicle can pass freely down to the inguinal canal. The largest part of the belly of the transversus abdominis and the internal oblique muscle are situated lateral to the inner inguinal opening. Because the aponeurosis medially is inelastic, contraction of the muscles occurs laterally to the inner inguinal opening. The crura of the sling are then stretched, and the ring and funicle will be lifted cranially and laterally up under the transversus abdominis

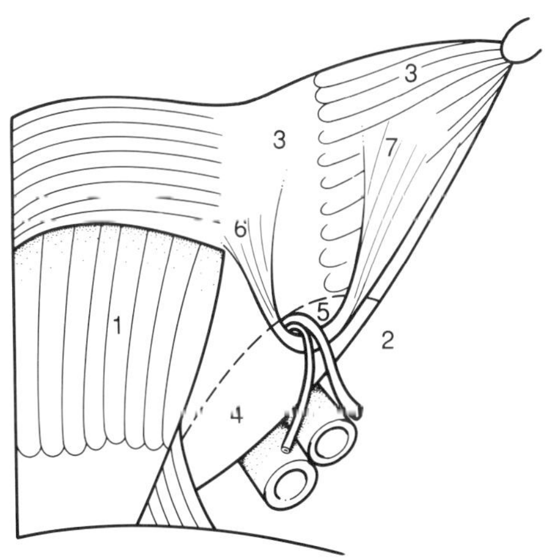

Figure 8.1: Posterior view of the lower part of the anterior abdominal wall. The peritoneum and preperitoneal fat have been removed. 1, rectus abdominis muscle; 2, inguinal ligament; 3, transversus abdominis muscle; 4, transversus abdominis arch; 5, inner inguinal ring; 6, superior crus and, 7, inferior crus of the transversalis fascia sling.

arch, at the same time that the arch is pulled towards the inguinal ligament. The movements in and between these structures may be compared to a curtain or a shutter, and are called the *inner shutter*.

The inner shutter, which is activated during a muscle contraction, contains two protective mechanisms against herniation. They are passive and secondary to the movement of the transversalis fascia sling. Figure 8.2 is a diagrammatic representation of the groin (a) at rest, and (b) during muscle contraction. With a competent inner shutter, the cords are pulled closer together in the sling, which also closes more tightly around the funicle when the inner inguinal opening is closed. This *Closing mechanism* functions because the transversus abdominis muscle and transversalis fascia are firmly attached to each other. Since the transversalis fascia sling is U-shaped, the closing mechanism has also been described as a semisphincter mechanism.

In situations of increased intra-abdominal pressure, the oblique course of the inguinal canal protects it against herniation. In the resting position the ceiling in the sling is formed by the transversus abdominis muscle except the part that lies caudally to the arch, where the dividing wall to the inguinal canal consists entirely of transversalis fascia (*see* Figure 8.2a). If the inner shutter is competent, the sling and funicle are pulled in the lateral and cranial direction up under the transversus abdominis arch as the opening in the transversalis fascia around the funicle is closed (*see* Figure 8.2b). When the intra-abdominal pressure increases, the transversalis fascia sling is pressed against the contracting transversus abdominis muscle, which, with a competent inner shutter, covers the entire ceiling of the sling and thereby offers a stable resistance or buttress. The lateralization of the transversalis fascia sling and funicle increases the oblique course of the inguinal canal, thereby creating an efficient pressure valve during increased intra-abdominal pressure. This protection is called the *pressure-valve mechanism.*

Activation of the abdominal muscles occurs voluntarily or via a reflex arch triggered by stretching or pressure on the muscle. If the intra-abdominal pressure increases or the transversalis fascia in the Hesselbach's triangle is pressed outwards, the pressure or tension on the transversus abdominis muscle increases, thereby causing a reflex increase of muscle tone. Thus, the higher the pressure in the abdomen, the greater the increase in muscle tone and the more efficient the protective mechanisms. A competent inner shutter can thus effectively protect the canal against the development of an indirect inguinal hernia.

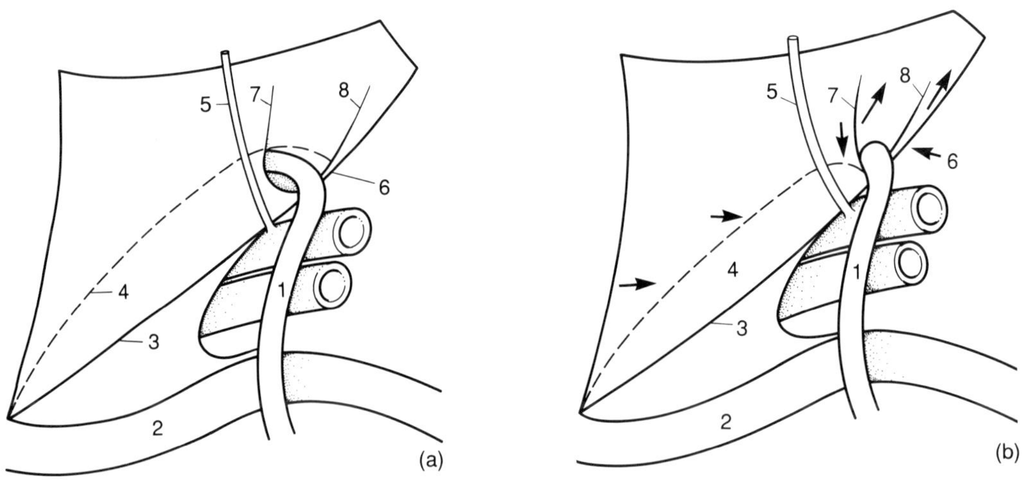

Figure 8.2: Diagrammatic posterior view of the right groin: (a) the abdominal muscles are in the relaxed position; (b) what happens when the internal oblique and transversus abdominis muscles contract. 1, Round ligament; 2, superior ramus of pubic bone; 3, inguinal ligament; 4, transversus abdominis arch; 5, inferior epigastric artery; 6, deep inguinal ring; 7, superior crus and, 8, inferior crus of the transversalis fascia sling. Arrows indicate the direction of contraction.

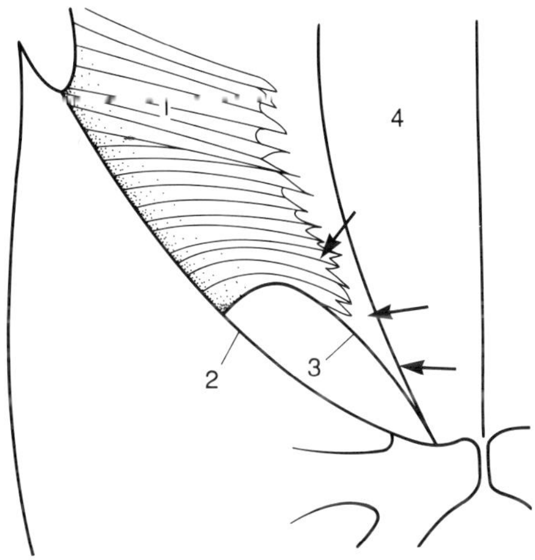

Figure 8.3: Diagrammatic anterior view of the right groin. The arrows show the main directions of movement of the transversus abdominis arch on muscle stimulation. 1, Internal oblique muscle; 2, inguinal ligament; 3, transversus abdominis arch; 4, anterior rectus sheath.

Shutter mechanisms related to the transversus abdominis arch

In order to describe the shutter mechanisms related to the transversus abdominis arch, it is easier to view the inguinal canal from the anterior side as in Figure 8.3.

The transversus abdominis arch forms the cranial boundary, or ceiling, of the inguinal canal. It consists mainly of the transversus abdominis muscle and its aponeurosis, and is strengthened ventrally by the internal oblique muscle. These two muscles are strongly adherent to each other and cannot be separated in distinct layers in the groin. They therefore function more or less as one muscle unit but with partly different contraction directions.

The transversus abdominis muscle has its origin in the most lateral part of the inguinal ligament, whereas the origin of the internal oblique muscle stretches from the superior anterior iliac spine to the level of the inner inguinal opening. From the inner inguinal opening to the attachment in the rectus sheath, the fibre direction and contraction direction in the two muscles are largely the same. Laterally, the transversus abdominis fibres have a lateral–cranial direction, whereas the fibres to the internal oblique muscle run in the lateral–caudal direction in front of the deep inguinal opening. During muscle activity, the lateral part of the arch is drawn further down over the internal inguinal opening so that the internal oblique muscle acts as a shutter. This is the *outer shutter*.

During muscle activity, the cremaster muscle lifts the funicle towards the inner ring – the so-called 'recoil action of the cremaster muscle'. The funicle can thereby be lifted with the transversalis fascia sling in the lateral–cranial direction without prolapsing down through the inner inguinal opening.

The transversus abdominis arch medial to the inner inguinal opening functions as a *partial shutter*. The arch cannot be actively or passively drawn completely down to the inguinal ligament without tension. The reason is that the aponeurotic tissue between the arch and the anterior rectus sheath is relatively immobile.

During muscle contraction, the medial part of the transversus abdominis arch is stretched laterally and partly towards the inguinal ligament. The contraction vectors are shown in Figure 8.3. The gap between the transversus abdominis arch and the inguinal ligament decreases somewhat but by no means disappears. The transversalis fascia is thereby also mobilized in the lateral direction within Hesselbach's triangle so that the U-shaped sling at the inner ring can move in the lateral–cranial direction during muscle activity. At the same time, the transversalis fascia is stretched in the triangle. If the transversalis fascia is already insufficient medially, the weak shutter effect of the arch will not be able to prevent the transversalis fascia from yielding and protruding. The different shutter mechanisms co-operate intimately with one another and normally prevent formation of an inguinal hernia. In my opinion, it is the inner shutter with its closing and pressure valve mechanisms that is most important. All factors that compromise its competence create the conditions for indirect herniation owing to a failing buttressing action of the transversus abdominis muscle at the deep inguinal ring.

Examples of factors that may contribute to the creation of an incompetent inner shutter are given in Table 8.1.

Table 8.1: Examples of factors that may contribute to creation of an incompetent inner shutter

Congenital anomalies (eg excessively wide inner inguinal ring)
Pathological connective tissue changes
Chronic cough
Chronically elevated intra-abdominal pressure (ascites, CAPD) – especially with a patent processus vaginalis
Neuromuscular injury (eg after appendectomy)

Table 8.2: Shutter mechanisms in the groin

1	Inner shutter mechanism	Closing mechanism Pressure-valve mechanism	
2	Outer shutter mechanism	Laterally	at the transversus abdominis arch
3	Partial shutter mechanism	Medially	at the transversus abdominis arch

How can the shutter mechanisms be studied?

The inner shutter and closing mechanism can readily be demonstrated during operation under local or epidural anaesthesia if the patient coughs or bears down. The inner inguinal ring, held under tension by an artery forceps or a finger, can then be seen to be displaced and pulled upwards and outwards behind the transversus abdominis arch if the shutter is competent[1,2].

Electromyographic studies can also be performed peroperatively. This is indicated particularly if a neuromuscular injury is suspected[3,4]. Herniographic examination gives little information as to the competence of the shutter mechanisms. The investigation merely shows the peritoneal surface of the groins, lined with larger or smaller amounts of preperitoneal fat which conceal the transversalis fascia sling and muscle contours. The techniques for demonstrating and studying the shutter mechanisms are otherwise unsatisfactory, and it should be noted that there is insufficient evidence that such a mechanism actually functions in this area.

Stabilization mechanisms (outer and inner guard)

In the groin, the external oblique muscle consists only of aponeurosis; it functions as a support for the deeper layers and stabilizes the inguinal canal. The external aponeurosis forms the *outer guard*. The aponeurosis does not contribute to the formation of the lateral margin of the rectus sheath in the inguinal region; it unites with the anterior rectus sheath more medially. During contraction of the external oblique muscle, the inguinal ligament is also stretched and may even be lifted ventrally 1–2 mm. During muscle activity, Hesselbach's triangle is therefore framed by the stable inguinal ligament, Cooper's ligament and transversus abdominis arch. This stable frame is called the *inner guard*. The gap within the frame is covered only by transversalis fascia and constitutes the weak area that is strengthened when mesh is used in hernia repair.

Conclusion

There are three different shutter mechanisms in the groin, and the inner shutter is the most important one (Table 8.2). As shown, the transversalis fascia sling is the basis of its function and is therefore an important structure in aetiology and repair of indirect inguinal hernias.

References

1. Lytle WJ. The internal inguinal ring. *Br J Surg* 1945; **32**: 441–6.
2. Lytle WJ. The deep inguinal ring, development, function and repair. *Br J Surg* 1970; **57**: 531–6.
3. Tobin GT, Scott Clark P, Peacock EE. A neuromuscular basis for development of indirect inguinal hernia. *Arch Surg* 1976; **111**: 464–6.
4. Arnbjörnsson E. A neuromuscular basis for the development of the right inguinal hernia after appendectomy. *Am J Surg* 1982; **143**: 367–9.

Brandon WJM. Inguinal hernia. The unpredictable result. *Br J Surg* 1946; **34**: 13–18.

Doran FSA. Inguinal herniography. *Lancet* 1955; **269**: 1307–10.

Keith A. On the origin and nature of hernia. *Br J Surg* 1924; **11**: 455–75.

Lytle WJ. Anatomy and function in hernia repair. *Proc Roy Soc Med* 1961; **54**: 967–70.

9

Collagen Synthesis and Direct Inguinal Herniation

RAYMOND C READ

History

Galen (AD 200), without dissecting the human body, stated that hernias were produced by rupture of the peritoneum. Paul of Aegina (AD 700), the last of the classical Greek writers, thought stretch rather than a break was involved. John Hunter in the mid eighteenth century was the first to document the congenital nature of certain indirect hernias, since the sac was continuous with the tunica vaginalis testis. His most famous pupil, Astley Cooper, considered the transversalis fascia, which he discovered, to be the main barrier to herniation through the inguinal canal. He listed factors that increase visceral pressure – cough, prostatism, constipation, pregnancy, obesity, ascites and heavy lifting – and those diminishing the strength of the abdominal wall – hereditary deficiency, debility, weight loss and ageing.

After Bassini introduced the modern operation to the world[1], surgical thought regarding causation became dominated by the saccular theory, 'rejects the view that hernia can ever be "acquired" in the pathological sense'[2]. This dogma was challenged in the 1920s when it became apparent that simple excision of the sac and closure of the defect gave disastrous results in direct inguinal herniation. Thus, Harrison[3] questioned why elderly men presented with herniation for the first time if it was congenital, and stated that the muscles appeared to be normal but the transversalis fascial floor of the canal was giving way. Keith[4] then stated that 'a pathological change in the connective tissues of the belly wall render certain individuals particularly liable to hernia'. He continued:

> *It is most important that surgeons should form a just and true opinion concerning the manner in which hernias arise. If they occur only in those who have hernial sacs already formed during fetal life, then we must either excise the sacs at birth or stand by and do nothing but trust to luck. If the occurrence of hernia is due to circumstances over which we have control then the prevention of hernia is a matter worthy of our serious study*[4].

Biochemical studies

In the 1960s, while repairing inguinal hernias through the posterior McEvedy approach, I noticed that the rectus sheath several centimetres away from the defects themselves appeared to be thinner than normal[5]. Samples of constant size weighed less than matched controls. Patients with bilateral or direct defects were more affected than those with unilateral indirect. Atrophy was unrelated to age or muscle mass. Hydroxyproline content, and therefore collagen which comprises 80% of dry weight in the rectus sheath, was strikingly decreased. Extraction of the remaining collagen revealed altered capacity for precipitation, with a reduced hydroxyproline/proline ratio suggesting impaired hydroxylation and lysyl oxidase activity. Synthesis of hydroxyproline, and therefore collagen, was inhibited. The diameter of the fibrils was variable, some remaining intracellular. Similar electron microscopic findings were present in pericardial and skin biopsies from the same patients. Because some of these findings had been described in emphysematous lung in association with cigarette smoking, we studied this relationship (metastatic emphysema). Circulating serum elastolytic activity was significantly greater than normal in patients with direct herniation who smoked ($p < 0.001$). Smokers with indirect defects had less change ($p < 0.01$)[6].

Confirmation was provided by Weitz *et al.*[7] who, using a specific fibrinopeptide cleavage product of fibrinogen, recovered the 'fingerprints' of free active unbound neutrophil elastase activity from the plasma of cigarette smokers. Furthermore, Bielecki *et al.*[8] then showed that smoking was significantly more common in adults with groin hernias, especially women. Similar findings have been found by us in veterans with aortic aneurysm[9]. This evidence of acquired damage to aponeurosis and fascia supports the use of prostheses in repair. Because attenuation is not restricted to the defect itself, large inserts should be used.

Discussion

These biochemical findings confirm Sir Arthur Keith's prescient observation that we are so apt to look on tendons' fascial structure in connective tissue as dead passive structures, when they are certainly alive, and the fact that hernia is so often multiple in middle-aged and old people leads one to suspect that a pathological change in the connective tissue of the stomach may render certain individuals particularly liable to hernia. It is interesting that the age distribution of herniation does not make this necessarily a senile phenomenon. The association with smoking was suggested by a considerable incidence of lung cancer and emphysema in these individuals, along with an increased white blood cell count. These cells contained large amounts of activated elastase enzyme. These are some of the same findings that occur in patients presenting with chronic obstructive lung disease from emphysema. Because the serum inhibitory capacity for proteolytic enzyme is fortunately much greater than any potential release of these substances, it is difficult to measure elastase directly. Most of our measurements were performed using the level of inhibitor that was remaining in the circulation, the activity presumably being reduced in those patients who were reacting against increased elastase levels.

Our observation[9] of an association between abdominal aortic aneurysm and inguinal herniation in cigarette smokers has been confirmed by Weitz *et al.*[10]. They conclude that 'our findings raised the possibility that other systemic complications to cigarette smoking, for example atherosclerotic disease, may be the result of uncontrolled neutrophil elastase activity'. It is these findings pointing out that the attenuation of fascia in inguinal herniation is not restricted to the defect itself that has discouraged the insertion of prostheses simply sutured to the outlines of the defect itself. As Usher recommended[11] and Stoppa has taught us all more recently[12], wide underlap to presumably more normal tissues is very important when prosthetic support is being provided in repair of inguinal herniation. A certain form rigidity of these plastic materials is also important, so that the prosthesis does not require fixation necessarily with a great number of sutures which may not hold. The widespread use of prostheses was dreamed of by Billroth[13], who stated 'if we could artificially produce tissue of the durability of the density and toughness of fascia and tendon, the secret to the radical cure of hernia would be known'.

Tension in the repair of inguinal herniation. It is fashionable today to have 'tension-free' or 'tensionless' repair of these defects. Yet our observation (reported in 1981[14]) is one of the few available where the actual force involved was measured directly at the operating room table. We studied a number of patients with direct or indirect inguinal herniation that was being repaired with or without a relaxing incision using either the Bassini or the McVay technique. We found that the maximal tension along the repair was medially just lateral to the pubis. This is in agreement with everyone's experience that the pubic angle is perhaps the commonest location of recurrence following repair of direct inguinal hernia. We also found that the McVay operation was associated with more suture tension after repair carried out during anaesthesia than the Bassini operation, but in both types of operation the relaxing incision reduced it significantly. This raises the question whether a relaxing incision should not be used more often in repair of inguinal herniation because it is innocuous. I have heard of only one case of an iatrogenic spigelian herniation at the lateral border of the rectus following this release. Certainly, the rectus fascia of Anson and McVay inserting at the lateral border prevents this, and therefore suture of the lateral relaxation is unnecessary. A muscle hernia may, however, occur.

Conclusion

Patients who present with inguinal herniation may have fascial deficiency elsewhere in the body. It is well known that they are more liable to incisional and ventral herniation and certainly other defects around the groin. These should be carefully looked for. The use of prostheses is encouraged. Fixation of these to hernial rings is to be discouraged. Wide underlapping is afforded. Prosthetic placement should be sutureless as much as possible and preferably placed right next to the peritoneum to reinforce this layer and provide a support for the viscera.

I finish here by quoting Sir Heneage Ogilvie: 'I know more than a hundred surgeons whom I would cheerfully allow to remove my gallbladder but only one to whom I should like to expose my inguinal canal'.

References

1. Bassini E. Nuovo metodo per la cura radicale dell'ernia inguinale. *Atti Congr Assoc Med Ital* 1887; **2**: 179.
2. Russell RH. The saccular theory of hernia and the radical operation. *Lancet*, 1906; **2**: 1197.
3. Harrison PW. Inguinal hernia: a study of the principles involved in surgical treatment. *Arch Surg* 1922; **4**: 680.
4. Keith A. On the origin and nature of hernia. *Br J Surg* 1924; **11**: 455.
5. Read RC. Attenuation of rectus sheath in inguinal herniation. *Am J Surg* 1970; **120**: 610.
6. Read RC. The role of protease-antiprotease in the pathogenesis of herniation and abdominal aortic aneurysm in certain smokers. *Postgrad Gen Surg* 1992; **14**: 161.
7. Weitz JI, Crowley KA, Landman SL, Lipman BI, Yu J. Increased neutrophil elastase activity in cigarette smokers. *Ann Intern Med* 1987; **107**: 68–2.
8. Bielecki K, Puawski R. Is cigarette smoking a causative factor in the development of inguinal hernia? *Pol Tyg Lek* 1988; **43**: 974–5.
9. Cannon DJ, Casteel L, Read RC. Abdominal aortic aneurysm, Leriche's syndrome, inguinal herniation, and smoking. *Arch Surg* 1984; **119**: 387.
10. Weitz JI, Landman SL, Crowley KA, Birken S, Morgan FJ. Development of an assay for *in vivo* human neutrophil elastase activity. Increased elastase activity in patients with alpha-1-proteinase inhibitor deficiency. *J Clin Invest* 1986; **78**: 155–62
11. Usher FC, Oschner J, Tuttle Jr IL. Use of Marlex mesh in the repair of incisional hernias. *Am Surg* 1958; **24**: 969

12. Stoppa RE, Warlaumont CR, Verhaegthe PJ *et al.* Prosthetic repair in the treatment of groin hernias. *Int Surg* 1986; **T1**: 154.

13. Wolfler A. Zur Radikaloperation des Freien Leistenbruches. *Beitr Chir* (Festchrift Geuidmet Theodor Billroth). Stuttgart, 1892: 552.

14. Read RC, McLeod MS Jr. Influence of a relaxing incision on suture tension in Bassini's and McVay's repairs. *Arch Surg* 1981; **116**: 440.

10

Groin Pain and the Occult Inguinal Hernia in Women

LEIF SPANGEN

A non-palpable inguinal hernia is often overlooked as the possible cause of inguinal pain in women. There are few reports on this type of hernia[1–5], but I believe that symptomatic, non-palpable inguinal hernia is relatively common in women but seldom diagnosed.

The patients

Over a period of 12 years, 180 inguinal explorations were performed in 168 women for suspected non-palpable inguinal hernia. Figure 10.1 shows that the majority of the patients were 20–50 years old (range 10–76 years). The mean age in this series was 32 years. A total of 172 inguinal hernias in 160 women were found; 117 were on the right and 55 on the left side.

Symptoms and findings at clinical examination (Tables 10.1 and 10.2)

All but two of the 168 patients had dull inguinal pain, which was usually aggravated by physical exertion. During periods of accentuated pain, three-quarters also reported neuralgia-like pain, often radiating towards the thigh, the flank or the lower abdomen on the same side. The neuralgia-like pain varied in intensity and occurred intermittently. In two-thirds of the patients there was pinprick hyperalgesia corresponding to the distribution of the ilioinguinal nerve (Figure 10.2). A tender point

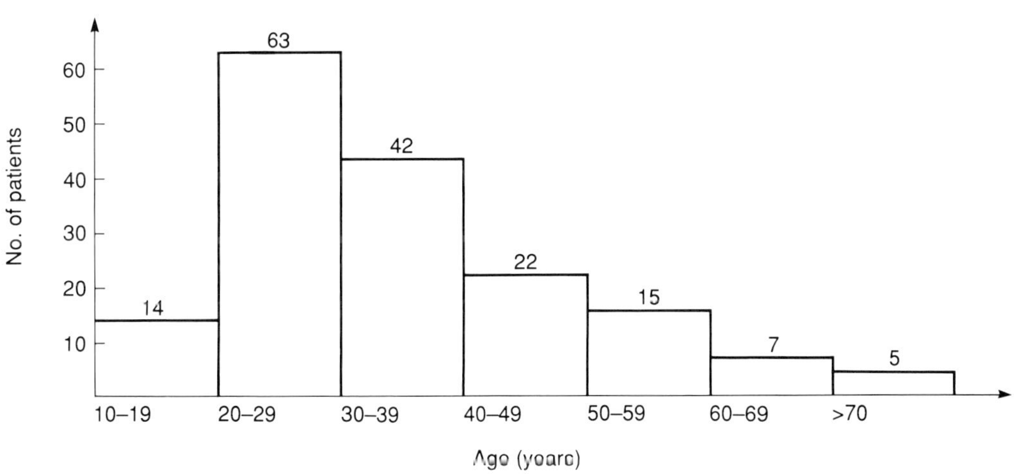

Figure 10.1: Age distribution of 168 patients with a history and clinical findings that prompted exploration for suspected occult inguinal hernia.

upon palpation corresponding to the deep inguinal ring during Valsalva's manoeuvre was a constant observation (Figure 10.3).

Table 10.1: Preoperative symptoms in 172 cases of occult inguinal hernia

	Number
Type of inguinal pain:	
Dull, drawing pain	170
Neuralgic pain only	2
Combined dull and neuralgia-like pain	126
Pain radiating from the groin to the ipsilateral:	
Thigh	96
Flank	61
Hypogastrium	28
Pain accentuated by:	
Physical exertion	161
Menstruation	18
Mental stress	3

Table 10.2: Preoperative clinical findings in 172 cases of occult inguinal hernia

	Number
Tenderness corresponding to the deep inguinal ring upon palpation during Valsalva's manoeuvre	172
Hyperalgesia of the skin corresponding to the distribution of the ilioinguinal nerve	109

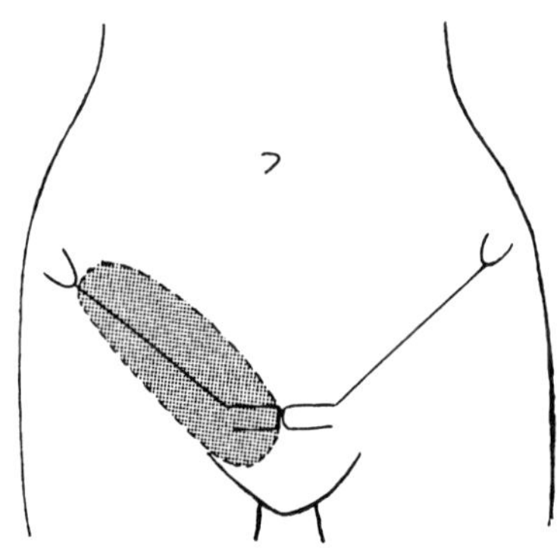

Figure 10.2: Distribution of skin innervation of the ilioinguinal nerve.

Differential diagnosis

There are many possible causes of inguinal pain and many different specialists are involved. For those diagnoses that are most relevant to me, I have prepared a check list which includes adductor-tendo-periostitis (ATP), different types of hernias and genuine neuralgia. Table 10.3 shows common symptoms of the different conditions. There is lack of neuralgic pain and pinprick hyperalgesia in patients with ATP and femoral hernia. In both indirect inguinal and obturator hernias there is initial, often intermittent neuralgic-like pain, combined with pinprick hyperalgesisa.

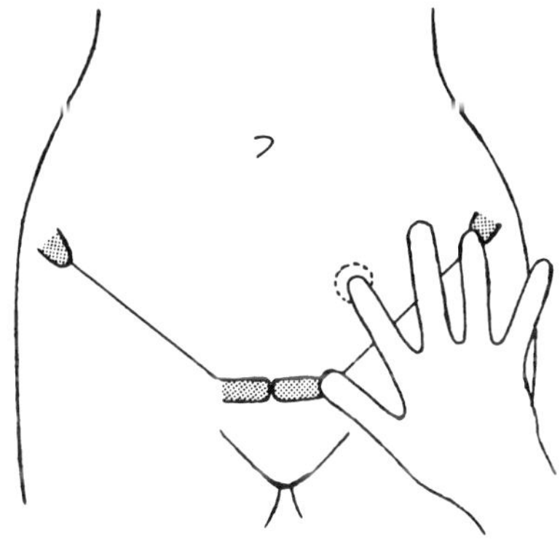

Figure 10.3: Location of the deep inguinal opening.

Table 10.3: Differential diagnosis of non-palpable inguinal hernia in women

		Hernia			*Genuine neuralgia*
Symptoms	*ATP*	*Femoral*	*Inguinal*	*Obturator*	
Pain:					
Neuralgic	—	—	+ 75% intermittent initially	+ 50–75% intermittent	++ Constant
Dull, drawing, spontaneous	++ even at night	+	+	+	—
Accentuated during physical exertion	++	+	+	+ (Howship–Romberg)	+
Radiating to the leg	++	+	+ (50%)	+	(+)
Tenderness on palpation	+	+(+)	++ Deep inguinal ring	(+) On palpation per vagina/ rectum	—
Pinprick hyperalgesia	—	—	+ 60–70% intermittent	+ 50–75%	++ Constant

++ = severe; (+) = moderate; ATP = addutor-tendo-periostitis

Operation and surgical findings

The inguinal canal was, with few exceptions, explored via an anterior approach, and all hernioplasties were performed with resorbable suture material (Dexon or Maxon 3–0).

The surgical findings are summarized in Table 10.4. All 172 inguinal hernias were indirect; 119 (70%) showed a hernial sac, varying in length between 1.5 and 5 cm, whereas in 51 cases (30%) the hernia consisted of a preperitoneal fat only. The deep inguinal ring, which was wider than normal in all cases, had a width of 2.5–4 cm. In addition to the inguinal hernias, a femoral hernia was found in four cases and a low spigelian hernia in Hesselbach's triangle in two cases. In one patient a femoral hernia was the only surgical finding, and in seven cases the exploration provided no explanation for the patient's complaints.

Patients with non-palpable inguinal hernia frequently have a secondary ATP, and vice versa. If a patient treated for an adductor-tendo-periostitis does not respond to conservative treatment, an

Table 10.4: Findings at operation in 180 inguinal explorations (in 168 patients) for suspected occult inguinal hernia

	Number
Indirect inguinal hernia consisting of:	
Hernial sac	119
Preperitoneal fat only	51
Sliding hernia	1
Combined indirect and direct hernia	1
Direct inguinal hernia	0
Femoral hernia only	1
Normal operation findings	7

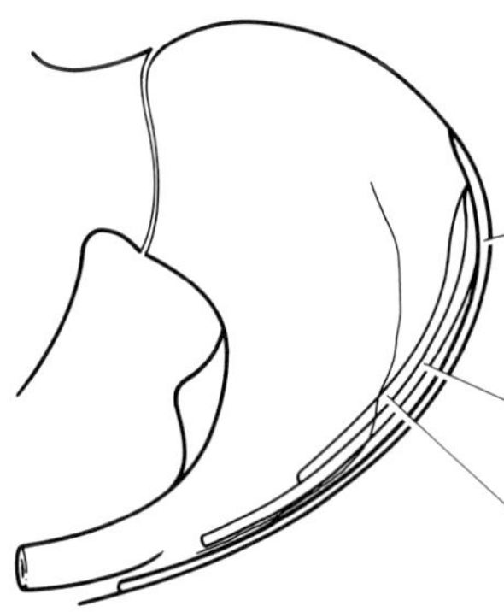

Figure 10.4: Topographic anatomy of the ilioinguinal nerve.

inguinal hernia should be suspected. Herniography is then strongly indicated at an early stage of the investigation[6,7].

Herniography has been found to be a sensitive and reliable diagnostic aid capable of demonstrating non-palpable hernial sacs in the groin with great accuracy[8–11]. One must remember, however, that in about one-third of non-palpable inguinal hernias in women, at least in my experience, the hernia consists entirely of preperitoneal fat, which represents a special case of indirect inguinal herniation. Characteristically, the lipoma is found within the internal cremasteric fascia. Herniography is not capable of demonstrating lipoma of the round ligament or the cord.

Since 1990 we have performed herniography in all patients with suspected non-palpable hernia, and the occurrence of a hernial sac at herniography and on operation agree closely. If the history and clinical findings in a woman suggest the presence of a hernia, we consider exploration. We do so despite a normal herniogram in the patient with no other explanation for her groin pain because we know that a hernia can consist of preperitoneal fat only.

Herniography is of great help in patients with postoperative pain and no palpable hernia but with clinical suspicion of recurrence[6,12]. Gullmo and his group report that non-palpable recurrent hernias are found in about 40% of symptomatic patients.

There may be tenderness to palpation several centimetres cranially to the inner inguinal opening, corresponding to the spigelian aponeurosis, in patients with indirect inguinal hernia. Many patients referred on suspicion of spigelian hernia below the interspinal plane have proved to have a non-palpable indirect inguinal hernia.

Follow up

During the first postoperative months, three cases of haematoma not requiring treatment and two cases of superficial wound infection were seen. No other serious early complications were observed. In about 20% of the cases, mild postoperative pain of neuralgic type was continued, but this pain usually disappeared after one to three months. Pinprick hyperalgesia could often be demonstrated days to weeks after the patients had been pain-free.

In all, 166 operated inguinal hernias were followed up, and the mean observation time was 20 months (range 3–60 months). At the latest examination, 92 of the 166 were symptomless and 54 were markedly improved, whereas 16 had unchanged and four aggravated symptoms. The procedure obtained good results in 87%.

The reason for persisting symptoms or deterioration are presented in Table 10.5. Neuralgia dominates, and recurrence of inguinal hernia was observed in two of the cases with postoperative neuralgia-like pain. In six cases the cause of the postoperative inguinal pain was not found.

Table 10.5: Causes of persisting or accentuated symptoms postoperatively in 20 of 166 operated cases of occult inguinal hernia

	Number
Postoperative neuralgia	6
Adductor-tendo-periostitis	5
Gynaecological disease	3
Recurrence of inguinal hernia	2
No known cause	6

Discussion

The dull pain is probably caused by stimulation of the pain fibres present in large numbers in both the preperitoneal fat and the peritoneum when these structures are forced through the deep inguinal ring. The pain is aggravated on palpation because the hernia is pressed against the hernial ring, which, during Valsalva's manoeuvre is well defined and firm. Pain is more common in the incipient stage than in palpable hernias, and neuralgia-like pain is the most common initial symptom produced by indirect inguinal hernia in both women and men[6,13].

To understand the patient's symptoms, it is important to be familiar with the topographic anatomy of the ilioinguinal nerve (Figure 10.4). This nerve runs from the retroperitoneal space and penetrates the transversus abdominis and internal oblique muscles stepwise somewhat cranially and laterally to the deep inguinal ring. The entrapment or trigger point is therefore located medial and somewhat caudally to the anterior superior iliac spine and there is also a distinct tenderness on palpation here in patients with neuralgia-like pain.

The hernia pain and the increased intra-abdominal pressure cause a local reflex increase of tone in the internal oblique and transversus abdominis muscles. As the nerve passes between the fibres of these muscles, it may be subject to mechanical pressure, thereby giving rise to neuralgia-like pain. This is a nerve entrapment. The increase in tone is only intermittent, which explains why the neuralgia-like pain and the pinprick hyperalgesia occur intermittently, too. On the other hand, the fact that the hyperalgesia can sometimes be demonstrated several days or weeks after the neuralgia-like pain has disappeared may be interpreted as an indication that the pressure can cause a nerve injury.

It is the pinprick hyperalgesia that is easiest to demonstrate in a patient with nerve entrapment. I use a safety-pin to test it. The hyperalgesia for touch and temperature is less pronounced. The pain in nerve entrapment is not as intense as in genuine or postoperative neuralgia, and typical features are that it is intermittent and varies in intensity. In genuine neuralgia the pain is constant and very intense, and accompanied by pronounced hyperalgesia for touch and temperature as well. In a patient with severe, continuous neuralgic pain, one must be very cautious and think the matter over very carefully before carrying out an inguinal exploration. The risk is that the cause of the pain is located in the central nervous system, in which case surgery should be avoided or be carefully planned. Four patients with severe postoperative neuralgia in my material proved, when re-evaluating the case history, to have had severe continuous neuralgia-like pain preoperatively and would therefore today have been treated differently. Two patients who developed postoperative neuralgia-like pain after a symptom-free period of four to six months had a non-palpable recurrent hernia, shown by herniography and verified at operation.

The deep inguinal ring in our patients with non-palpable inguinal hernias was open for one finger or more. The inner shutter is then incompetent and contraction of the muscles only reduces the width of the deep inguinal ring without being able to close it completely.

Conclusion

Non-palpable indirect inguinal hernia in a woman may be the cause of persistent pain in the groin and lower abdomen, and gives a typical clinical picture. It is important to keep this condition in mind, especially as the patients respond well to surgical treatment.

All patients experience distinct tenderness upon palpation over the deep inguinal ring during Valsalva's manoeuvre. Because of nerve entrapment the patient often complains of intermittent neuralgia-like pain, and pinprick hyperalgesia of the skin corresponding to the distribution of the ilioinguinal nerve can be demonstrated. Herniography is of great help in the investigation of these patients and is recommended, but is not capable of demonstrating the fatty inguinal hernias.

I would emphasize, however, that inguinal pain is a common symptom with multifactorial causes. The patient should therefore be thoroughly investigated for other possible or concomitant causes of pain before the decision is made to carry out an inguinal exploration.

References

1. Bondevik H. Inguinal prolaps of retroperitoneal fat. *Acta Chir Scand* 1966; **131**: 492–6.
2. Fodor PB, Webb WA. Indirect inguinal hernia in the female with no palpable sac. *South Med J* 1971; **64**: 15–16.
3. Herrington JK. Occult inguinal hernia in the female. *Ann Surg* 1975; **181**: 481–3.
4. Roos H, Smedberg S. Symptomatic non-palpable inguinal hernias. *Postgrad Gen Surg* 1992; **4**: 131–4.
5. Spangen L, Andersson R, Ohlsson L. Non-palpable inguinal hernia in the female. *Am Surgeon* 1988; **54**: 574–7.
6. Smedberg S. Herniography and Hernial Surgery. Bulletin 59 from the Department of Surgery, Lund University; 1986: 1–83.
7. Smedberg SGG, Broomé AEA, Elmèr O, Gullmo Å. Herniography in the diagnosis of obscure groin pain. *Acta Chir Scand* 1985; **151**: 663–7.
8. Ekberg O, Blomqvist P, Olsson S. Positive contrast herniography in adult patient with obscure groin pain. *Surgery* 1981; **89**: 532–5.
9. Gullmo Å. Herniography. *Acta Chir Scand Suppl* 1980; **361**.

10. Hall C, Hall PN, Wingate JP, Neoptolemos JP. Evaluation of herniography in the diagnosis of an occult abdominal wall hernia in symptomatic adults. *Br J Surg* 1990; **77**: 902–6.

11. Smedberg SGG, Broomé AEA, Elmèr O, Gullmo Å. Herniography in primary inguinal and femoral hernia: an analysis of 283 operated cases. *Contemp Surg* 1990; **36**: 48–51.

12. Ekberg O, Blomqvist P, Fritzdorf J. Herniography in patients with clinically suggested recurrence of inguinal hernia. *Acta Radiol Diagnosis* 1984; **25**: 225–9.

13. Ljungdahl I. Inguinal and femoral hernia. *Acta Chir Scand Suppl* 1973; **439**.

11

The Value of Ultrasound in the Diagnosis of Hernias

MAURICE E ARREGUI

Although most masses occurring on the anterior abdominal wall, including the inguinofemoral area, are easily diagnosed by palpation, the aetiology of some masses can be obscured by obesity, previous surgery, radiation or trauma[1]. There are patients in whom masses in the groin cannot be differentiated from an incarcerated hernia. Ultrasound can be helpful in these patients as well as in diagnosing non-palpable femoral hernias in patients with obscure groin pain[2,3,4,5]. The advantages of using ultrasonography for the evaluation of obscure masses or groin pain include: no preparation required; it is non-invasive; it does not use ionizing radiation; it is painless; and it is readily available.

With the use of modern real-time B mode imaging a dynamic picture can be obtained, allowing detailed evaluation of the inguinal area. Our preliminary experience has found ultrasonography of the inguinal area helpful in identifying occult femoral hernias and in evaluating postoperative groin

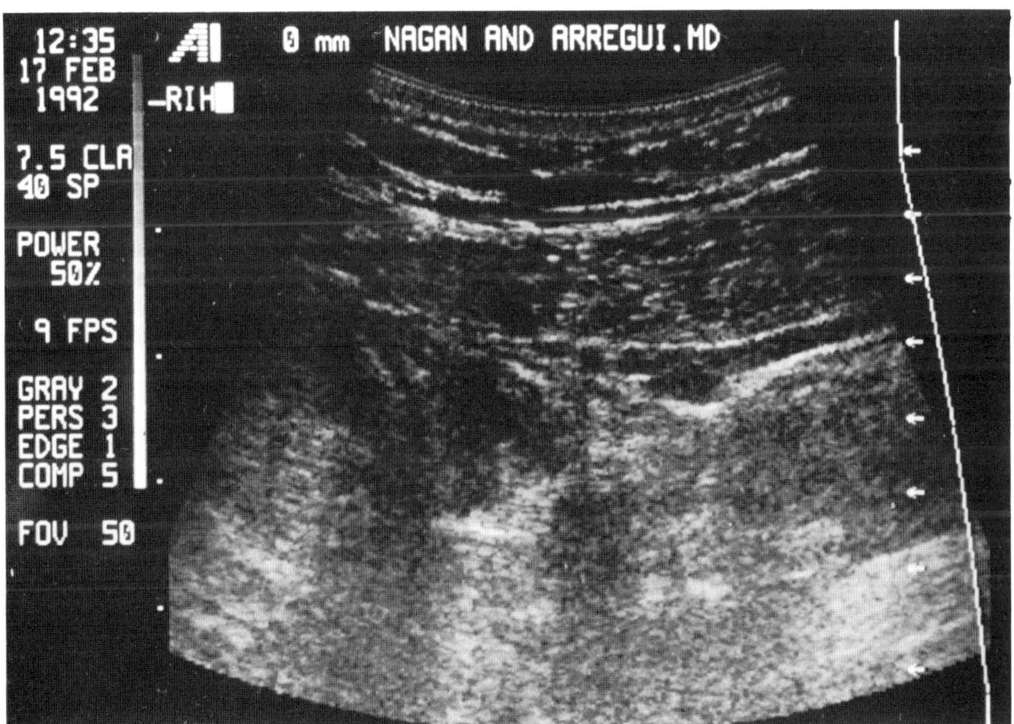

Figure 11.1: Transverse view of the right inguinal area using a 7.5 mHz linear transducer. Note the inferior epigastric vessels, seen just beneath the rectus abdominis muscle.

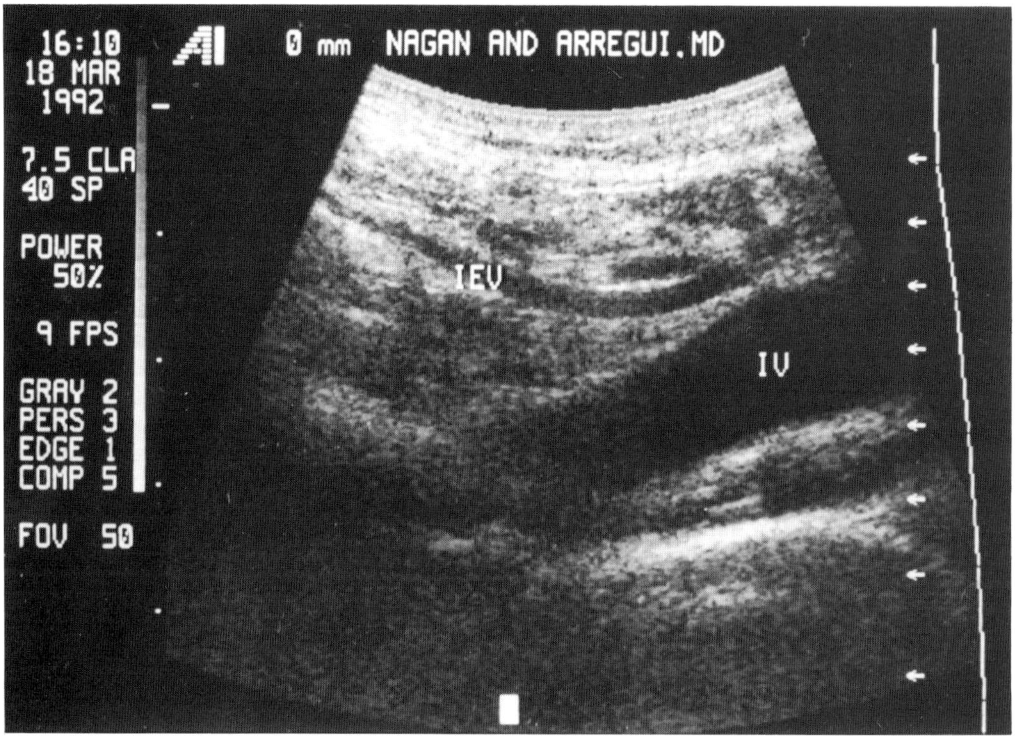

Figure 11.2: This oblique ultrasound view using a 7.5 mHz linear transducer gives an excellent view of the inferior epigastric vein (IEV) as it enters the external iliac vein (IV).

masses after laparoscopic hernia repair. We also report here a technique useful in differentiating indirect from direct hernias.

Technique

Patients are evaluated pre- and postoperatively with a 7½ mHz linear transducer linked to an AI 5200 unit (Acoustic Imaging Tech. Inc., Phoenix AZ). Examination is carried out with the patient in the supine position. Identifiable landmarks include: the rectus abdominis muscle, the inferior epigastric vessels, the femoral vessels, and the cord structures within the inguinal canal (Figures 11.1 and 11.2). Once the inferior epigastric vessels relative to the inguinal canal are identified, the patient is asked to perform the Valsalva manoeuvre – to create a protrusion of the hernia sac. Once the sac is identified, the patient is then asked to relax. The epigastric vessels are again identified. With careful observation of the patient performing the Valsalva manoeuvre, one can determine whether the sac is encroaching upon the epigastric vessels from a lateral position (Figures 11.3–11.5). If this is the case, it is an indirect hernia. In patients who are suspected of having a femoral hernia, the transducer is placed transversely over the femoral artery and vein. If a femoral hernia is present, a mass will be seen to enter into the femoral canal medial to the femoral vein during the Valsalva manoeuvre. In patients with suspected recurrent hernias in the early postoperative period, a 7½ mHz transducer is placed over the mass to determine whether the mass is a haematoma, a seroma or a recurrent hernia. In the early postoperative period, especially if preperitoneal fluid is present, the mesh can often be identified.

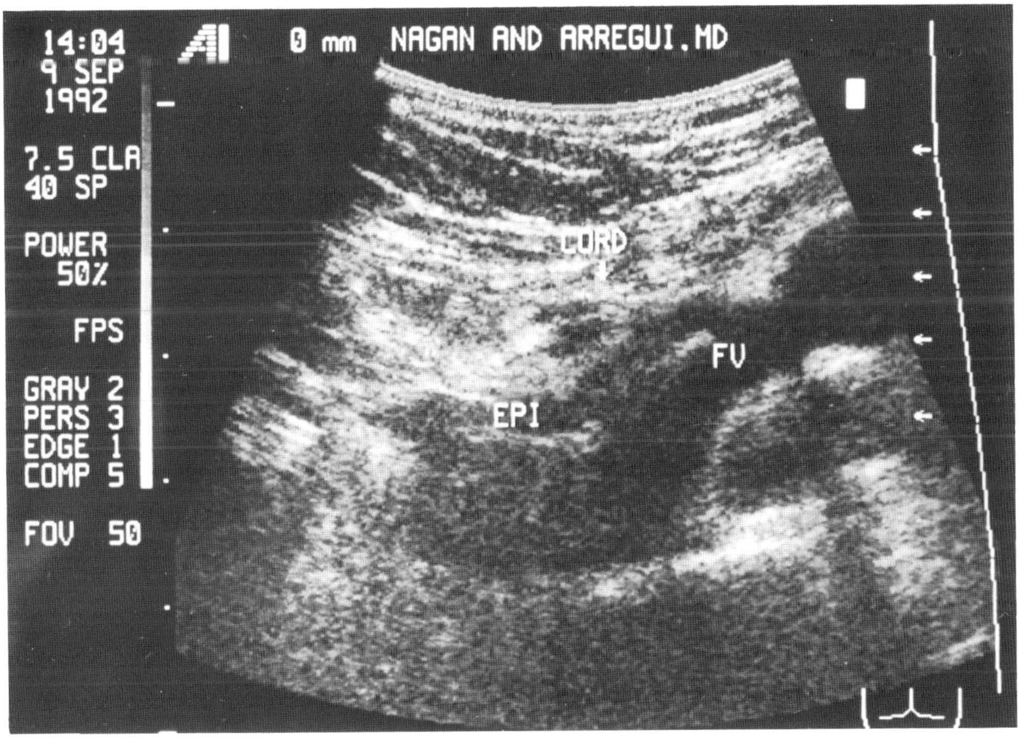

Figure 11.3: Ultrasound identification of indirect inguinal hernia. Prior to Valsalva manoeuvre. Note cord structures (Cord), inferior epigastric vessels (EPI), and femoral vein (FV).

Results

Our preliminary experience supports findings reported in the literature. We have diagnosed the femoral hernias in four patients preoperatively. These patients were being evaluated for obscure pain in the groin, and three of them had femoral hernias confirmed at surgery. The fourth had no femoral hernia; the femoral canal had only fat and lymph nodes.

We have evaluated three patients with palpable hernias preoperatively using ultrasound. Two were determined to have direct hernias and one was determined to have an indirect hernia; the preoperative diagnosis was confirmed at surgery in all three cases. With preoperative ultrasound evaluation, one obese patient with obscure pain in the right groin was suspected of having fat incarcerated in a groin hernia. This was not identified at surgery, and was therefore a false positive. In the postoperative period, we have been able to diagnose haematomas or seromas in several patients presenting with early inguinal masses, thus excluding the diagnosis of recurrence after laparoscopic hernia repair (Figure 11.6).

Conclusions

Abdominal wall masses are usually easily diagnosed by physical examination but occasionally difficulty is encountered. Lineaweaver used ultrasound to evaluate 23 obscure abdominal wall masses. He found a 91% accuracy in diagnosis, 39% (9) of these patients had findings that were unsuspected by the referring physician. Five of these, thought to be hernias, had a different diagnosis with ultrasonographic evaluation. The two failures in his series included two cases of adenopathy with abscess which were misdiagnosed as hernias[1].

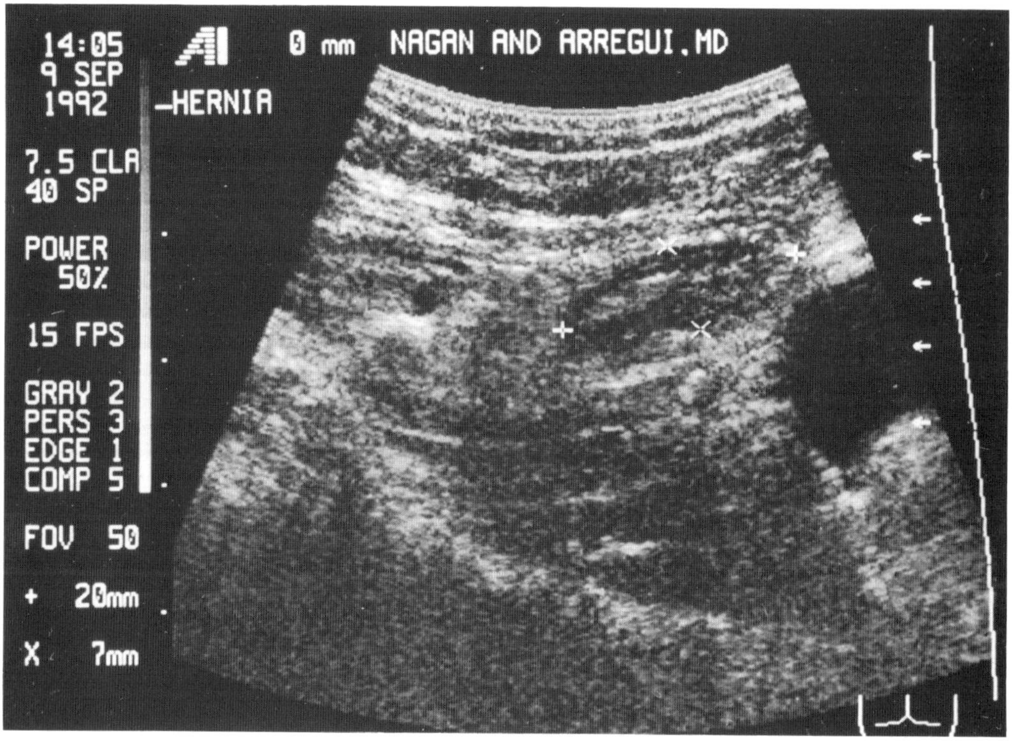

Figure 11.4: Ultrasound identification of indirect inguinal hernia. With early Valsalva manoeuvre the hernia sac and contents (marked with + and x) are entering the inguinal canal. During real-time B mode imaging, the dynamic view allows the ultrasonographer to see the hernia sac starting to protrude from lateral to the inferior epigastric vessels, thus establishing the diagnosis of an indirect inguinal hernia.

Yeh described the ultrasound characteristics of abdominal wall hernias, which include: a defect in the abdominal wall muscle, bowel located within the lesion and exaggeration of the mass with straining. He warned, however, about pitfalls in making the diagnosis. These included herniated loops of bowel that are not quite echogenic and could mimic a subcutaneous mass, a fluid-filled hernia sac which could mimic a cyst, a gas-containing hernia could be mistaken for an abscess, and an abscess due to an enteric fistula creating a muscular defect could be misdiagnosed as an incarcerated hernia[6].

Deitch reported 95 patients who underwent ultrasonographic evaluation of the inguinofemoral region: 70 of these patients subsequently had surgery; 68 of them had a correct diagnosis. This included 51 inguinal hernias, five femoral hernias, six sarcomas, five lymph nodes, two seromas and one femoral aneurysm. There were two false negatives; both were intermittently palpable hernias. With the patient in the supine position, the hernia could not be identified with ultrasonography[2].

Subramanyam identified the characteristics of a scrotal hernia which include: identifying loops of bowel within the scrotum, exclusion of testicular pathology by the demonstration of normal testicular elements, and the presence of the hernia sac in the inguinal region containing bowel and/or omentum. Using these criteria, he examined 65 patients with a clinical diagnosis of a primary scrotal mass. Ultrasound diagnosis revealed a scrotal hernia in six; five of these patients were found to have a hernia at the time of surgery. The false positive was due to an inguinoscrotal abscess. He also felt that in his experience a direct could not be distinguished from an indirect hernia[7]. With his technique, a 5 mHz short focus transducer was used. Longitudinal sonograms were obtained at 5 mm increments in transverse longitudinal sections.

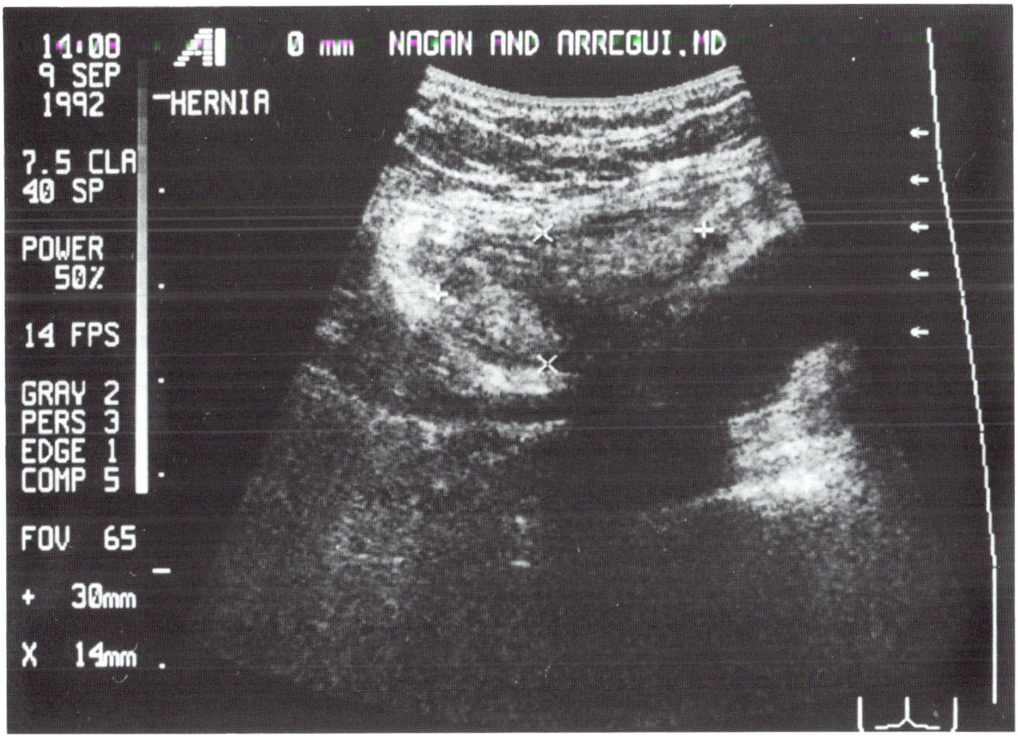

Figure 11.5: Ultrasound identification of indirect inguinal hernia. Sustained Valsalva manoeuvre further distends the hernia (marked with + and x). In this view the inferior epigastric vessels are displaced inferiorly.

With our technique, using a real-time 7½ mHz B mode transducer, we are able to visualize the epigastric vessels clearly. With modern high resolution dynamic real-time ultrasonography the anatomical layers and landmarks are better characterized, thus allowing the diagnosis to be made.

We have also found, as have others, that the diagnosis of occult femoral hernias can be aided by the use of ultrasonography. Deitch performed 45 ultrasound examinations using a 5 mHz gray scale scanner over the femoral area. With patients in the supine position, four hernias were found which were non-palpable on physical examination; three were for symptomatic groin pain; and one was asymptomatic. This fourth patient had a palpable left femoral hernia and a contralateral femoral hernia was found during the ultrasound examination[3]. Ponka reported a 25–55% incidence of strangulation and up to 33% mortality in patients with femoral hernias. He pointed out that, of 216 patients with femoral hernias, 24% had missed diagnoses. These misdiagnoses included inguinal hernias, lipomas, lymph nodes, hydroceles and saphenous varices. He also pointed out that in elderly or obese patients, nonpalpable Richter's femoral hernias can be encountered[5]. Deitch recommended that femoral sonography be performed in:

- patients with undiagnosed groin pain without palpable masses
- patients with questionable or clinically ambiguous femoral masses
- patients, especially if elderly or obese, with serious abdominal complaints of uncertain aetiology even in the absence of groin pain or palpable mass[3].

Machan has pointed out that 70% of non-obstructed femoral hernias are misdiagnosed by referring non-surgical medical practitioners. Even when symptoms are severe enough to warrant surgical intervention, 20–25% of femoral hernias are not diagnosed preoperatively by surgical staff[4].

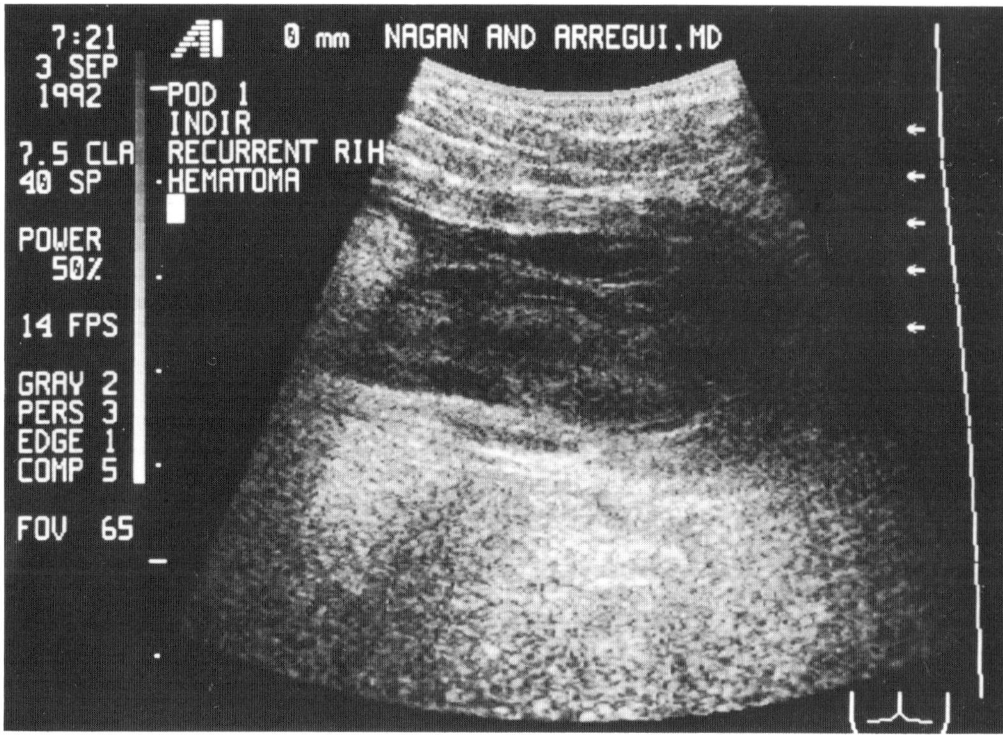

Figure 11.6: Postoperatively, this patient presented with a groin mass. Ultrasound evaluation shows an unequivocable haematoma, thus ruling out an early recurrence. The patient and surgeon are both reassured.

Preoperative evaluation of abdominal wall hernias is quite accurate. Spangen reported 94% accuracy with spigelian hernias[8]. Engel reported 93% accuracy with abdominal wall and scrotal masses[9]. Deitch reported 97% accuracy in surgically treated groin hernias[2]. Lineaweaver reported 91% accuracy with abdominal wall and groin hernias[1].

In the postoperative period, local complication rates can be as high as 8.7% with open inguinal hernia repairs[10]. Tetik and Arregui have recently reported a 4.7% incidence of postoperative haematoma or seroma following 1514 hernias repaired laparoscopically[11]. Archer defined the characteristics of postoperative haematoma. Early haematomas are hyperechoic. At 48–72 hours, liquefaction of the haematoma changes the characteristic to hypoechoic. Chronic haematomas show thickening, calcification or septation within the tunica vaginalis[12]. Rankin also found ultrasonography useful in differentiating abdominal wall haematomas from incisional hernias in six patients evaluated one and one-half to six months postoperatively[13]. We have, likewise, found the use of ultrasonography to be very helpful in confirming early postoperative haematomas versus recurrence after laparoscopic inguinal herniorrhaphy (*see* Figure 11.6).

Summary

Our early experience with perioperative use of ultrasonography in the evaluation of groin hernias and groin pain supports evidence reported in the literature. Ultrasonography is a safe, readily available technique that can add valuable information: distinguishing indirect from direct hernias, identifying obscure hernias in obese patients, diagnosing non-palpable femoral hernias, clarifying the diagnosis of palpable groin masses of uncertain nature, and evaluation of postoperative haematomas.

References

1. Lineaweaver W, Vlasak M, Muyshondt E. Ultrasonic evaluation of abdominal wall and groin masses. *South Med J* 1983; **76**: 590–2.
2. Deitch EA, Soncrant MC. Ultrasonic diagnosis of surgical disease of the inguinal–femoral region. *Surg Gynecol Obstet* 1981; **152**: 319–22.
3. Deitch EA, Soncrant MC. The value of ultrasound in the diagnosis of nonpalpable femoral hernias. *Surgery* 1981; **116**: 185–7.
4. Machan J, Cooperberg PL. A femoral hernia diagnosed by ultrasonography and fine-needle aspiration biopsy. *J Ultrasound Med* 1984; **3**: 379–80.
5. Ponka JL, Brush BE. Problem of femoral hernia. *Arch Surg* **102**: 417–23.
6. Yeh H-C, Lehr-Janus C, Cohen BA, *et al.* Ultrasonography and CT of abdominal and inguinal hernias. *J Clin Ultrasound* 1984; **12**: 479–86.
7. Subramanyam BR, Balthazar EJ, Raghavendra BN, *et al.* Sonographic diagnosis of scrotal hernia. *AJR* 1982; **139**: 535–8.
8. Spangen L. Spigelian hernia. *Acta Chir Scand Supp* 1976; **462**: 28–32.
9. Engel JM, Deitch EA. Sonography of the anterior abdominal wall. *AJR* 1981; **137**: 73–7.
10. Rydell W, Hanover WH. Inguinal and femoral hernias. *Arch Surg* 1963; **87**: 150–7.
11. Tetik C, Arregui ME, Castro D, *et al.* Complications and recurrences associated with laparoscopic repair of groin hernias: a multi-institutional retrospective analysis. Presented at Hernia 93: Advances or Controversies – An International Perspective. Symposium held Indianapolis, IN, USA, 23–27 May.
12. Archer A, Choyke PL, O'Brien W, *et al.* Scrotal enlargement following inguinal herniorrhaphy: ultrasound evaluation. *Urol Radiol* 1988; **9**: 249–52.
13. Rankin RN, Hutton L, Grace DM. Postoperative abdominal wall hematomas have a distinctive appearance on ultrasonography. *Can J Surg* 1985; **28**: 84–5.

12

General, Regional and Local Anaesthesia for Hernia Repair

WILLIAM HARROP-GRIFFITHS

This chapter discusses the advantages and disadvantages of general, regional and local anaesthesia for open hernia repair in the adult patient. The physiological challenges associated with laparoscopic repair are described and a case is put forward for the use of general anaesthesia for these procedures.

General anaesthesia

Advantages

General anaesthesia enjoys a higher overall success rate than locoregional anaesthesia and can provide the surgeon with optimal operating conditions in terms of patient immobility and muscular relaxation. General anaesthesia allows the surgeon to perform any procedure that is necessary. For instance, large or incarcerated hernias can be operated on without concern that the surgery may overwhelm the local or regional anaesthetic provided. In addition, the patient can be assured a pain-free and anxiety-free period during the operation.

Disadvantages

Recovery from the central hypnotic effects of general anaesthesia can be prolonged and therefore it may not lend itself ideally to day-care surgery. General anaesthesia incurs added costs which include anaesthesiologists, drugs, disposables and post-anaesthesia recovery facilities, and as a result it may not be able to compete with local anaesthesia in fiscal terms. In addition, there are a number of well-recognized complications of general anaesthesia, many of which are accentuated by age-related pathological changes.

Airway complications

Airway complications range from sore throat, a minor but often distressing complication, to life-threatening conditions such as hypoxaemia (due to difficulty in establishing or maintaining a clear airway) and the aspiration of stomach contents.

Respiratory complications

Respiratory complications include atelectasis, an increased incidence of respiratory tract infection and the possibility that patients with severe chronic pulmonary disease may become ventilator-dependent postoperatively.

Cardiovascular complications

The vast majority of general anaesthetics are cardiovascular depressants, and general anaesthesia may therefore pose a risk to some groups of patients with cardiovascular pathology.

Gastrointestinal complications

Gastrointestinal complications, in the form of nausea and vomiting, are distressing and common sequelae of general anaesthesia.

Urinary complications

In the elderly male population, urinary retention after general anaesthesia for hernia repair is common. This produces a high incidence of the need for catheterization, which carries with it the risk of urinary tract infections.

Regional anaesthesia

Advantages

Regional anaesthesia for hernia repair can be provided by either spinal (subarachnoid) or epidural (peridural) techniques. The use of regional anaesthesia avoids many of the airway, respiratory and gastrointestinal complications of general anaesthesia. Regional anaesthetic techniques provide good intraoperative and postoperative analgesia, and can provide the patient with awareness during the procedure if this is desired.

Disadvantages

The sympathectomy associated with regional anaesthesia can cause significant hypotension which may require treatment with intravenous fluids and vasoconstrictor agents. Sympathectomy can provide considerable risk to patients with heart valve stenosis, whilst substantial fluid administration can precipitate heart failure in susceptible patients after the offset of the sympathectomy. The injudicious use of vasoconstrictors may pose a threat to patients with coronary artery disease.

The motor blockade that accompanies regional anaesthesia may make rapid postoperative mobilization difficult. Indeed, the return of the patient to a 'street-fit' state may take longer than after general anaesthesia, for this reason. Postoperative urinary retention is even more common after regional anaesthesia than after general anaesthesia[1].

Local anaesthesia

Techniques

Local anaesthesia for open hernia repair can be achieved by literally a 'local anaesthetic' technique in which the surgeon is armed with syringes of local anaesthetic and infiltrates tissues before incising them. Alternatively, a technique that includes blockade of the nerves supplying the inguinal region may be used. These are often termed 'field blocks'. Several descriptions of the technique are available; they include those of Eriksson[2], Ponka[3] and Atkinson, Rushman and Lee[4]. They have at their basis the blockade of the ilioinguinal and iliohypogastric nerves as they pass approximately one finger's breadth medial to the anterior superior iliac spine lying either above the internal oblique muscle (iliohypogastric nerve) or below it (ilioinguinal nerve). To the blockade of these nerves may be added an attempt at blocking the genital branch of the genitofemoral nerve. It is stressed in each technique that complete skin analgesia should be achieved with a subcutaneous infiltration in addition to these nerve blocks, as fibres may cross from the other side of the body to supply the skin of the inguinal region. Further local anaesthetic infiltration is often needed during the operation, particularly for the hernial sac and into the pubic tubercle and inguinal ligament if these are to be used as a site for sutures.

Drugs for local anaesthesia

The most commonly used local anaesthetic drugs are bupivacaine and lignocaine. Large volumes (up to 100 ml) of local anaesthetic may be needed to provide high-quality anaesthesia, and care must therefore be taken to keep dose levels within the maximum amounts recommended. The Physicians' Desk Reference (an annotated American version of the Data Sheet Compendium) suggests a maximum of 175 mg of bupivacaine if given without adrenaline (epinephrine) or 225 mg if given in conjunction with adrenaline for an adult of average size. As 225 mg is contained in 45 ml of bupivacaine 0.5% or 90 ml of bupivacaine 0.25%, it is recommended that the 0.25% solution is used for local anaesthesia for hernia repair. A total of 500 mg of lignocaine should be considered the maximum dose when given with adrenaline. This amount is contained in 100 ml of 0.5% solution, and this is therefore a recommended solution.

Most commercial preparations of local anaesthetic already mixed with adrenaline consist of a 1 in 200 000 solution, ie a concentration of 5 μg/ml. If 100 ml of this solution is given, the total dose of adrenaline will be 500 μg. This high a dose may be associated with cardiovascular side-effects. In a recent study[5], 0.5% lignocaine with 1:200 000 adrenaline was used for local anaesthesia for inguinal hernia repair. Adrenaline doses ranged from 3.8 to 4.9 μg/kg, ie up to 1 ml/kg of the local anaesthetic solution. The mean increase in plasma adrenaline was 326%. Of the study group of 12, one patient developed multifocal ventricular ectopics and one patient suffered a supraventricular tachycardia which required treatment with intravenous verapamil. It is interesting to note that plasma noradrenaline (norepinephrine) levels were also significantly elevated in spite of sedation with midazolam. This would tend to indicate that patient anxiety caused a high degree of endogenous catecholamine release in addition to the administration of exogenous epinephrine.

Drugs for sedation

The administration of a local anaesthetic for inguinal hernia repair is not free from discomfort. This fact, allied to the anxiety that most patients feel in anticipation and in experiencing an operation without general anaesthesia, creates a requirement for sedation in many patients. Physicians often have their own favourite drugs that they find work well for them; however, a few general points can be made:

Opioids (narcotic analgesics) are a popular but potentially illogical choice. Although providing analgesia for the insertion of the block, opioid drugs are more likely, in the absence of a painful stimulus, to reveal their side-effects. Respiratory depression, nausea and vomiting may therefore be noted in this situation.

Benzodiazepines, and in particular the water-soluble agent midazolam, are popular in this context. The advantages of benzodiazepines include a low incidence of nausea and vomiting, a high therapeutic ratio and the ready availability of a specific antagonist (flumazenil). A disadvantage of midazolam is that its half-life, though much shorter than other readily available benzodiazepines such as diazepam (half-life 20–50 hours[6]), is nevertheless in the range of 1.7–2.6 hours[6] and recovery from heavy midazolam sedation can be prolonged.

Anaesthetic agents used in subanaesthetic doses can be excellent sedatives and have the advantage that half-lives tend to be short, that recovery is therefore rapid and that the level of sedation is easily titrated. The author's preference is for a low-dose propofol infusion supplemented by the administration of an oxygen/nitrous oxide mixture by mask. It should be pointed out that propofol in large doses may cause apnoea, and its administration by personnel inexperienced in airway management should be avoided.

Advantages

It is generally agreed that local anaesthesia for inguinal hernia repair in competent hands is a safe technique. Although there is a paucity of large-scale randomized, controlled trials comparing general, regional and local anaesthesia, the experience of such institutions as the Shouldice Clinic in performing very large numbers of inguinal hernia repairs with minimal morbidity and mortality is difficult to argue against. In addition to this, there is evidence[7] that locoregional anaesthesia has safety advantages for infraumbilical surgical procedures in general.

The administration of local anaesthesia for hernia repair is technically easy but requires practice and scrupulous attention to detail to produce the very high proportion of successful blocks that can be achieved.

Local anaesthesia for hernia repair avoids the vast majority of complications associated with general anaesthesia, and this fact must be looked on as a major advantage of its use. Added to this is another significant advantage, which is that the technique is ideally suited to day-care treatment as the drugs used have little direct central effect and motor blockade is not produced. Analgesia, as has been stated above, is excellent and can last up to 24 hours after the use of bupivacaine.

Disadvantages

Surgical conditions are not always ideal during local anaesthesia and the surgeon must be prepared for the occasional patient movement. The block can be painful to establish and the patient may complain if unblocked areas become apparent during surgery. As a result, sedation is often necessary and, if administered in an over-generous fashion, can occasionally approximate to general anaesthesia.

Some patients may prove to be unsuitable for local anaesthesia for hernia repair. These include the very young, the obese and those with large or incarcerated hernias.

General versus local anaesthesia

Evidence from studies

A study published in 1987[8] reported the results of a retrospective comparison of general, spinal and local anaesthesia. Patient satisfaction was found to be equal in all three groups. The general anaesthesia group suffered a higher incidence of sore throat than the other two groups, the spinal group suffered the highest incidence of urinary complications and the local anaesthesia group reported the greatest pain experienced during the operation. The overall advantages accrued by the local anaesthesia group were found to be greater if the patients were stratified into below and above 65 years old. Worthy of note is the fact that 2% of local anaesthesia patients required conversion to general anaesthesia and that 38% of the spinal anaesthetics were inadequate as judged by the need for the addition of local anaesthesia or conversion to a general anaesthetic.

A prospective randomized study compared general versus local anaesthesia for hernia repair[9]. No significant differences in cardiac output, mean arterial pressure, total peripheral resistance or heart rate between the two groups were identified at any point in the study period. Significant results included those that the local anaesthetic group required no postoperative pain medication whereas all the general anaesthesia group did, and that no member of the local anaesthetic group suffered nausea or vomiting postoperatively. The study identified a cost benefit of between $888 and $1341 per patient.

A verdict

In the hands of an enthusiastic and experienced medical and nursing team, local anaesthesia for hernia repair is safe and cost-effective while providing good overall patient satisfaction and acceptable surgical conditions. In saying this, I do not intend to indicate that general or regional anaesthesia is not safe and cannot be made cost-effective. Each individual institution must find a modus operandi that suits both its patients and those providing anaesthetic, surgical and nursing care. The author hails from a culture that is very resistant to the performance of surgical procedures on the awake patient. My own personal preference in this situation is to administer a general anaesthetic with agents that have a relatively short half-life and then to perform a field block with bupivacaine to provide both intraoperative and prolonged postoperative analgesia.

Laparoscopic hernia repair

In order to perform any operation, the surgeon must operate in a suitable transparent, fluid medium. The traditional medium used in open hernia repair is room air. Room air has certain advantages: it is freely available, has little physiological activity and exists at atmospheric pressure. The same cannot be said for the carbon dioxide (CO_2) introduced into the peritoneum for the performance of laparoscopic hernia repair. The CO_2 pneumoperitoneum extends the physiological impact of hernia surgery beyond the inguinal region. Problems may accrue as a result of the pressure effects of CO_2, the volume effects and its systemic absorption.

Pressure effects

Near-fatal gas embolism has been reported during laparoscopic cholecystectomy[10], as has a significant carbon dioxide pneumothorax[11], and these risks must be considered a possibility during laparoscopic hernia repair. External pressure on the stomach may increase the chance of the regurgitation and aspiration of stomach contents if the patient's stomach is not empty and the airway is not adequately protected by intact reflexes or a cuffed tracheal tube.

Pressure on vascular structures within the abdomen may give rise to cardiovascular physiological changes. Aortocaval compression similar to that seen in pregnancy may give rise to a reduction in venous return and cardiac output. Although young patients can often compensate for these effects, elderly patients may not have adequate cardiovascular reserve and may therefore become hypotensive. A study looking at the cardiovascular effects of laparoscopy in young fit women[12] showed that, although the commonly measured variables such as heart rate and blood pressure were maintained during the procedure, cardiac output and stroke index fell progressively. Normal heart rate and blood pressure were maintained only by intact cardiovascular responses.

Volume effects

The insufflation of carbon dioxide causes stretching of the peritoneum and is associated with bradyarrythmias[13], pain that is difficult to block with regional anaesthesia and impossible to block with local anaesthesia, and a high incidence of nausea and vomiting. It is usually assumed that these phenomena are vagally mediated, as they may still occur in the presence of extensive regional blockade.

A large pneumoperitoneum may splint the diaphragm, causing respiratory compromise. Functional residual capacity is decreased and limited diaphragmatic excursion may decrease overall lung and chest wall compliance[14].

Carbon dioxide absorption

The peritoneum is a highly effective absorptive layer, put into efficient use by the nephrologists in continuous ambulatory peritoneal dialysis. CO_2 is readily absorbed through the peritoneum into the systemic circulation and may effectively increase carbon dioxide production by up to 50%. However, the rate of absorption is very variable and it has been suggested that high pneumoperitoneum pressures may reduce CO_2 absorption by compressing vessels within the abdomen. There is evidence[15] that CO_2 absorption may be at its greatest after release of the peritoneum, as a result of the gas remaining within the peritoneum being absorbed by the now decompressed vessels. CO_2 excretion needs to be increased during laparoscopy if normal arterial gaseous homoeostasis is to be maintained and the acidosis associated with hypercapnia is to be prevented. An increase in minute volume will therefore be required. This can readily be achieved during general anaesthesia and controlled ventilation by increasing ventilatory frequency and/or tidal volume. In the spontaneously breathing patient, whether anaesthetized, sedated or awake, the mechanical effects of the pneumoperitoneum will make it more difficult to increase minute volume, and high arterial CO_2 levels may result.

General anaesthesia for laparoscopic hernia repair

Advantages

In placing a tracheal tube during general anaesthesia, the patient's airway can be safely and reliably protected from the aspiration of stomach contents. Even though the patient's airway is said to be well-protected during local or regional anaesthesia, the administration of substantial sedation may compromise the patient's ability to protect the airway, and it is therefore reasonable to assert that general anaesthesia with tracheal intubation will provide the patient with the most effective form of airway protection.

The muscular relaxation of the abdominal wall which can be provided by the use of neuromuscular blocking agents will decrease overall abdominal wall compliance and will therefore allow the insufflation of a given volume of CO_2 at a lower pressure, thereby reducing the pressure-related adverse effects of a pneumoperitoneum.

The presence of a tracheal tube allows the accurate measurement of end-tidal CO_2. This will assist the anaesthesiologist in ensuring that the patient's minute volume matches the need to excrete the increased CO_2 load. In addition, end-tidal CO_2 measurement will act as an effective monitor for gas embolism.

The placement of an oesophageal stethoscope is easy during general anaesthesia. This device is useful not only for the monitoring of heart and breath sounds but also can identify the millwheel murmur of ongoing gas embolism.

Disadvantages

The overall disadvantages of general anaesthesia have been discussed above. The main disadvantage of the use of general anaesthesia for hernia repair is that is constitutes a return to general anaesthesia for a procedure for which local anaesthesia has become increasingly popular! If laparoscopic hernia repair is to be expanded, many of the centres currently safely employing local anaesthesia for hernia repair will have to return to general anaesthesia and their patients may suffer complications as a result. As suggested above, elderly patients are more likely to suffer the complications of general anaesthesia and are less likely to have the cardiovascular and respiratory reserve necessary to overcome the physiological challenge of laparoscopy with a CO_2 pneumoperitoneum.

General versus local anaesthesia for laparoscopic surgery

A recently reported trial compared local and general anaesthesia for laparoscopic sterilization[16]. The reported results were that more than 90% of the patients undergoing sterilization under local anaesthesia found it 'highly acceptable'. The local anaesthetic group enjoyed a shorter operation time, a more rapid recovery, less abdominal pain and less sore throat. There was a significant cost reduction in providing local anaesthesia. It is interesting to note that overall heart rate and blood pressure were higher in the local anaesthesia group than in the general anaesthesia group, and that the local anaesthesia group (who were sedated) needed supplemental oxygen in order to prevent hypoxaemia.

Anaesthesia for laparoscopic hernia repair: conclusions

The general health of patients presenting for laparoscopic hernia repair is worse than in those who present for gynaecological laparoscopic procedures, the minimal access operations with which there is the most experience. Laparoscopic hernia repair poses respiratory and cardiovascular stresses upon the patient. Although young fit patients may be able to compensate for them, will these physiological stresses pose the greatest threat to those with the least respiratory and cardiac reserve? As it is these relatively unfit people who may benefit the most from minimally invasive techniques, are we posing the greatest threat to those who stand to benefit the most?

It is tempting to pursue local anaesthetic approaches to laparoscopic hernia repair, and many are already doing this. Purely preperitoneal surgical approaches to hernia repair may reduce the physiological impact of intraperitoneal CO_2 insufflation and may therefore assist in this development. However, only careful and honest audit will reveal the relative safety and efficacy of open and laparoscopic hernia repair. I believe that, if laparoscopic repair is to be adopted as the 'industry standard' for hernia repair, an approach that refines day-care general anaesthesia may be pragmatically preferable over the pursuit of local anaesthesia for what is no longer physiologically a 'local' procedure.

References

1. Finley RK, Miller SF, Jones LM. Elimination of urinary retention following inguinal herniorrhaphy. *Am Surg* 1991; **57**: 486–8.
2. Eriksson E. *Illustrated Handbook in Local Anaesthesia*, 2nd ed. London: Lloyd-Luke, 1979.
3. Ponka JL. Seven steps to local anaesthesia for inguinofemoral hernia repair. *Surg Gynecol Obstet* 1963; **117**: 115–20.
4. Atkinson RS, Rushman GB, Lee JA. Field block for repair of inguinal hernia. In: *A Synopsis of Anaesthesia*. London: Wright, 1982: 703–6.
5. Hayse-Gregson PB, Achola KJ, Smith G. Changes in haemodynamics and plasma catecholamine concentrations after field block for inguinal herniorrhaphy using lignocaine with adrenaline. *Anaesthesia* 1990; **45**: 7–10.
6. Reves JG. Benzodiazepines. In: Prys-Roberts C, Hugg CC, eds. *Pharmacokinetics of Anaesthesia*. Blackwell Scientific, Boston, 1984.
7. Scott NB, Kehlet H. Regional anaesthesia and surgical morbidity. *Br J Surg* 1988; **75**: 299–308.
8. Young DV. Comparison of local, spinal and general anesthesia for inguinal herniorrhaphy. *Am J Surg* 1987; **153**: 560–3.
9. Bethnia R, Hashemi F, Stryker SJ, Ujiki GT, Poticha SM. A comparison of general versus local anesthesia during inguinal herniorrhaphy. *Surg Gynecol Obstet* 1992; **174**: 277–80.
10. Au-Yeung P. Gas embolism during attempted laparoscopic vagotomy. *Anaesthesia* 1992; **47**: 817.
11. Gabbott DA, Dunkley AB, Roberts FL. Carbon dioxide pneumothorax occurring during laparoscopic cholecystectomy. *Anaesthesia* 1992; **47**: 587–8.
12. Johannsen G, Andersen M, Juhl B. The effect of general anaesthesia on the haemodynamic effects during laparoscopy with CO_2-insufflation. *Acta Anaesth Scand* 1989; **33**: 132–6.
13. Myles PS. Bradyarrhythmias and laparoscopy: a prospective study of heart rate changes with laparoscopy. Aust NZ J Obstet Gynaecol 1991; **31**: 171–3.
14. Bardoczky GI, Engelman E, Levarlet M, Simon P. Ventilatory effects of pneumoperitoneum monitored with continuous spirometry. *Anaesthesia* 1993; **48**: 309–11.
15. Lewis DG, Ryder W, Burn N, Wheldon JT, Tacchi D. Laparoscopy – an investigation during spontaneous ventilation with halothane. *Br J Anaesth* 1972; **44**: 685–91.
16. Bordahl PE, Raeder JC, Nordentoft J, Kirste U, Refsdal A. Laparoscopic sterilisation under local or general anaesthesia? A randomised study. *Obstet Gynecol* 1993; **81**: 137–41.

13

Regional Anaesthesia in Laparoscopic Hernia Repair

NAMIR KATKHOUDA

Groin hernia is the most frequent benign disease and the most common operation in the Western World. Indeed, more than 150 000 patients are operated on in France alone, and three times as many in the USA.

Laparoscopic hernia repair, although an effective and seducing approach, is not as widely accepted as it might be for three reasons.

- The paucity of scientific studies showing the advantages of laparoscopic hernia repair over conventional hernia repair. Several prospective randomized studies are under way, but the results are not yet available.
- The need for general anaesthesia when performing laparoscopic hernia repair. Indeed, the pneumoperitoneum can be established correctly only when the patient is under general anaesthesia: a carbon dioxide pneumoperitoneum under regional anaesthesia is not a recommended procedure, for reasons that are detailed below.
- The cost of the operation, particularly in terms of instrumentation.

The rationale behind regional anaesthesia is that this could allow an operation without pneumoperitoneum using a personal gasless suspension device. The advantage of regional anaesthesia is obvious: there is no loss of consciousness and therefore there is complete postoperative recovery, allowing the patient to resume work on the same day if he wishes to.

Definitions

Several types of anaesthesia are possible:

- local anaesthesia
- regional anaesthesia[1–3]. This can be an epidural anaesthetic given normally or a suspended epidural anaesthetic which consists of blocking only a few metamers.

  Spinal anaesthesia is performed by injecting the anaesthetic into the subarachnoidal space. A variation of this is continuous spinal anaesthesia, which involves the introduction of a catheter: this is usually reserved for older patients
- epidural anaesthesia plus narcosis. This is reserved for older high-risk patients and consists of light anaesthesia with good analgesia
- general anaesthesia. The patient is under mechanical ventilatory assistance.

Local anaesthesia

Local anaesthesia does not provide any general analgesia, and it is important to remember this if muscles, peritoneum or viscera are going to be dissected. It is therefore of no use in normal laparoscopic procedures involving traction or dissection or cutting of any intra-abdominal tissues. It could, however, be used for diagnostic laparoscopy using only one trocar with an operating scope where no intra-abdominal manoeuvres or dissection are planned.

Regional anaesthesia

Epidural anaesthesia is more comfortable than spinal anaesthesia. Indeed, it causes less vasoplegia, and therefore less lowering of blood pressure. There are no headaches, unless the subarachnoidal space is accidentally punctured, and it gives good postoperative analgesia. Prolonged anaesthesia may occur, which is limited when using spinal anaesthesia.

There are several contraindications to the use of regional anaesthesia.

- The major contraindication is the supraumbilical operation. The high puncture site required for these operations can induce blocking of respiratory muscles (at level T4) and require ventilatory control.

  Therefore, **laparoscopic cholecystectomy is not a good indication for regional anaesthesia** even if epidural anaesthesia is performed high up (at T_6–T_{10}). It could be considered as very risky anaesthesia with the possibility of respiratory failure and even cardiac problems.

- The second major contraindication for regional anaesthesia is coronary disease. The patient with coronary disease needs particularly good oxygenation and so is best controlled under general anaesthesia where they experience no fear or stress and oxygenation can be controlled well[4–9].

Other contraindications to epidural anaesthesia are[10–12]:

- unstabilized cardiac
- disorders in haemostasis
- local infection
- history of neurological disorder
- local anaesthetic agents contraindicated in the patient
- intellectual limitation
- no consent.

Epidural anaesthesia in laparoscopic hernia repair

This technique requires a skilled anaesthetic team, used not only for laparoscopic surgery, but also to the management of epidural anaesthesia. Our patients are given a preoperative anxiolytic, but not one which is hypnotic. The injection of 1–2 ml of lignocaine 2% plus BupiVacain 0.5% per blocked metamer (at L_4–L_5) is usually sufficient. Therefore, if six metamers are to be blocked, 12 ml is injected. If the patient should require a further injection during the procedure, it is important to avoid the Trendelenburg position as the drug can then take effect higher up leading to respiratory muscle blockage and the cardiac problems described above. In the postoperative period, the patient is placed in a supine position for a couple of hours, and can then leave hospital.

Possible complications of epidural anaesthesia[13–15]

During the operation, severe vasoplegia can occur, resulting in a drop in blood pressure and the risk of respiratory muscle blockage. This needs to be monitored very carefully by the anaesthetist.

In the postoperative period, apart from the usual complications, problems which may arise include urinary retention, infection and headaches if the arachnoidal space has been punctured.

Pneumoperitoneum with CO_2

It is of great importance to measure the expiratory fraction of CO_2 (FE CO_2 during the operation), and this is best done with tube capnography. The use of a tracheal tube requires the patient to be under general anaesthesia, so laparoscopic surgery using CO_2 pneumoperitoneum without general anaesthesia is hazardous and should be avoided.

Gasless surgery under regional anaesthesia (Figure 13.1)

A small incision is made in the umbilicus. The fascia is divided and the peritoneum opened under direct visual control as in open laparoscopy. The entire abdominal wall is lifted manually by the surgeon, and a blunt trocar is introduced through the incision with the scope. This allows limited but sufficient control of the intra-abdominal space. This exploration gives the surgeon the opportunity to see whether the operation is feasible. This manoeuvre can be carried out without insufflation.

A suspension device is then introduced near the trocar. This is done asymetrically so that the pelvic wall can be retracted and the laparoscopic hernia repair performed safely. The suspension device has a blunt end to prevent abdominal injuries. It is connected to a small chain and a metallic gallow is attached near the patient's leg. It is a simple, inexpensive device allowing efficient retraction of the abdominal wall for a patient under epidural anaesthesia.

Two trocars are then inserted in the normal positions, that is two fingers medially to the anterior iliac spines and one finger below this mark. Following penetration they are removed and simple grips or sleeves are left *in situ* as there is no risk of gas leakage. Theoretically gasless surgery is a more cost effective technique.

The procedure is performed using the transabdominal preperitoneal approach, with incision of a flap and the anatomical dissection of the area demonstrating the constant landmarks (Cooper's ligament) and where the pectineus muscle is attached, the rectus muscle above and laterally the psoas muscle. It is very important, once the peritoneal sac has been removed or dissected free, to parietalize the parts of the spermatic cord, that is to separate the vas and spermatic vessels, allowing them to be pushed laterally on to the pelvic wall and perfect placement of the mesh. The mesh must be large enough to cover the three hernia spaces (the indirect space, the direct space and the femoral space). The mesh in then stapled in place using only a few staples in Cooper's ligament, the rectus muscle and the psoas muscle laterally, taking care not to staple in the square of doom[6]. The square of doom is an extension of the triangle of doom, which comprises the vas and the spermatic arteries and veins, and where one can also find the iliac vessels. This triangle has now been extended to become the square of doom, limited by the iliopubic tract above and the vas medially.

In this square, running along the psoas muscle, is the genitofemoral nerve to which injury must be avoided. The lateral femorocutaneous nerve must also be avoided, but is much more lateral to the psoas muscle and is not usually reached in hernia surgery.

Finally, a very careful closure of the peritoneal flap is performed. This is best done using a running suture, appropriate needle holders and short threads or, if it needs to be stapled, then the closure should be performed in overlap fashion to avoid any windows being created which can lead to small bowel adhesion to the mesh or small bowel incarceration. One can use a Laparotie (Ethicon Endo-Surgery) to start and end the suture.

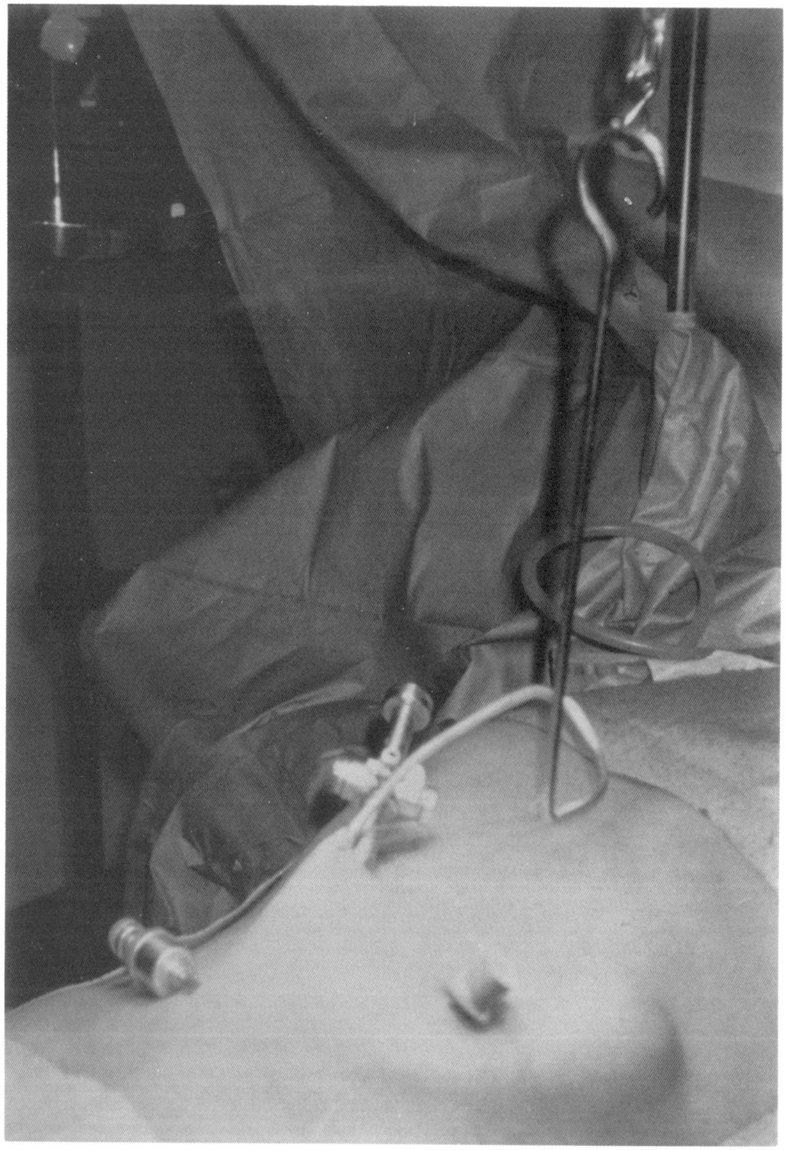

Figure 13.1:

Results

28 patients were operated on under regional anaesthesia using a gasless suspension device. The success rate was 85.7%. Four were converted to general anaesthesia: two due to operative dissection difficulties, one for failure of epidural anaesthesia and one due to a technical problem in a suspension device. A high percentage of patients were satisfied as they underwent a minimally invasive procedure without the risks associated with general anaesthesia.

Advantages of gasless laparoscopic surgery

No CO_2 means less risk. No general anaesthesia is used and there is no risk of retroperitoneal diffusion, inducing hypercarbia and cardiac arrythmias or more serious problems. A big advantage of gasless surgery is the reduction in costs as conventional trocars are not required.

There are, however, some drawbacks. It is technically more difficult to perform and requires experience. The introduction of the trocars must be done under strict visual control by the umbilical videoscope as there is no tension of the abdominal wall. We advise therefore, the use of open procedures to introduce the three trocars. A further disadvantage is the **absence of pneumodissection** with CO_2. This makes the dissection and the removal of tissues more difficult even when using sharp electrical scissors. In addition, the small bowel is not pushed away from the region when there is no CO_2, and so a steep Trendelenburg is needed; the dissection causes slightly more blood loss as CO_2 is absent and there is **no vascular compression**. Finally, a suspension device is needed, although our suspension device has shown to be efficient and of low cost.

In conclusion, gasless laparoscopic hernia repair under regional anaesthesia is a promising technique, although it needs more assessment which is being carried out by several teams at present. It answers two real problems in laparoscopic hernia repair: the use of general anaesthesia and the cost. It could represent a better procedure for performing laparoscopic hernia repair in the future.

Bibliography

1. Andrape P. A new interpretation of the origin of extradural space. *Br J Anaesth*, 1983; **55**: 85–8.
2. Bromage PR. Ageing and epidural dose requirements: segmental spread a predictability of epidural analgesia in youth and extreme age. *Br J Anaesth*, 1969; **4**: 1016–22.
3. Cousins MJ. Applied anatomy of epidural blockade. In: *Neural blockade in clinical anesthesia and management of pain*. Philadelphia: JB Lippincott, 1980, 194–195.
4. Fisher MD and Pennington JC. Allergy to local anaesthesia. *Br J Anaesth*, 1982; **54**: 893–4.
5. Domench RJ, Goich J. Effects of heart rate on regional coronary blood flow. *Cardiovasc Res*, 1976; **10**: 224–31.
6. Katkhouda N and Moviel J. Laparoscopic hernia repair: a personal approach. *Endo Surg New Tech*, 1993; **4**: 193–7
7. Klassen GA, Bramwell RS, Bromage PR *et al.* Effects of acute sympathectomy by epidural anesthesia of the canine coronary circulation. *Anesthes*, 1980; **52**: 8–15.
8. Lundt PC. Principles and practise of spinal anesthesia. Springfield Illinois: Charles C. Thomas Ed, 1971; 648.
9. Otton PC and Wilson EJ. The cardiocirculatory effects of upper thoracic epidural analgesia. *Canad Anaesth Soc J*, 1966; **13**: 541.
10. Ward RJ, Bonica JJ, Freund FG *et al.* Epidural and subarachnoidal anesthesia cardiovascular and respiratory effect. *JAMA*, 1965; **191**: 99–192.
11. Wells PH and Kaplan JA. Optimal management of patients with ischemic heart disease for non cardiac surgery by complementary anesthesiologist and cardiologist interaction. *Amer Heart J*, 1981; **102**: 1029–37.
12. Silver DJ, Dunsmore RH, Dickson CM. Spinal anesthesia for lumbar disc surgery: review of 576 operations. *Anesth Analg*, 1976; **55**: 550–4.
13. Swerdlow M. Complications of local anesthetic neural blockade. In: Cousins MJ, Bridenbaugh PO, Eds. *Neural blockade in clinical anesthesia and management of pain* Philadelphia: JB Lippincott 1980, 526–42.
14. Vandam LD. Complications of spinal and epidural anesthesic. In: Orkin FK, Copperman LH Eds. *Complications in anesthiology* Philadelphia. Lippincott JD, 1983, 75–105.
15. Vadam LD, Dripps RD. Long-term follow-up of patients who received 10 098 spinal anesthetics. III. Syndrome of decreased intracranial pressure (headache and ocular and auditory difficulties). *JAMA*, 1956; **161**: 586–91.

14

Laparoscopic Inguinal Herniorrhaphy Under Local Anaesthetic

GLENN A DEYO AND TOSHIO AKAMATSU

Introduction

A common complaint concerning laparoscopic herniorrhaphy has been the increased risk of changing a procedure commonly performed under local anaesthetic to one under general anaesthesia. A second problem has been some postoperative patients suffering from neuralgias — either genital femoral or even occasionally lateral femoral cutaneous. Both of these concerns could be addressed if laparoscopic hernias could routinely be performed using local anaesthetic with minimal sedation-analgesia. This chapter is an early report on the use of local anaesthesia for this purpose.

Materials and methods

It is important to note that this procedure is done as a 'local MAC'. This means that the patient has the advantage of having an anaesthetist present who provides intravenous sedation-analgesia and occasionally nitrous-oxygen as needed; and I have been fortunate to have access to an extremely competent anaesthetist who has taken an interest in this procedure. This procedure can be more work for the anaesthetist than if done under general or regional anaesthesia. The patient should always be given some form of an H-2 blocker the night prior, since they will not have their airway protected and will probably be in a Trendelenburg (head down) position. This should decrease the risk of complications from aspirations.

A Foley catheter is placed after lidocaine jelly had been inserted into the urethra and pentothal 50 mg IV has been administered. The procedure starts with an initial IV injection of 1 mg increments of Versed (midazolam HCL), Reglan 10 mg, Toradol 30 mg (ketorolac tromethamine) and Valium 10 mg followed by titrating doses of Versed and fentanyl during the initial insufflation. A local anaesthetic, Marcaine, 0.25% (bupivacaine hydrochloride), is used at the umbilicus. An open Hasson entry technique is used, which allows the anaesthetic to be placed in all layers under direct vision. The trocar is sutured in place with a figure of eight stitch (that is used to close the fascia at the end of the procedure).

Initial flow of CO_2 at 1.5 l/min is used until the maximum pressure of approximately 10 mmHg is obtained. Higher pressures tend to result in patient discomfort which will cause abdominal wall contraction. This can rapidly drive the pressure over 30 mmHg and completely collapse the field of view.

Full thickness infiltration of all levels of tissue is performed, using Marcaine, during placement of lateral ports. It is important to realize that the surgeon must limit the amount of abdominal wall compression during placement of these trocars to prevent an increased abdominal pressure. Therefore, the trocars must be sharp. Another method of tensionless entry that could be used is a deeper stab wound than usual down to the peritoneum. This is then followed by peritoneal puncture with the trocar.

The next step is irrigation of the abdominal cavity, which we are currently performing with 300–500 ml normal saline mixed with 20 ml 0.25% Marcaine/litre NACL. This grew out of a serendipitous finding that suggested that a portion of the discomfort patients feel with laparoscopy might be from desiccation. While passing a gauze sponge into the abdomen (to use for compression/haemostasis), it was accidentally dropped on the small bowel and the patient began to complain of pain. Since this was all that had occurred, the sponge was lifted from the bowel and the pain stopped. This was repeated several times with the same results. The abdomen was then flooded with normal saline and Marcaine. The patient stopped complaining. I now place this immediately after getting my first secondary port placed.

In the first group, Marcaine would be placed at the site of peritoneal incision over cutaneous nerve. Later, it was also found that the peritoneal incision did not seem to cause discomfort. Interestingly, the hernia sac can also be dissected free without local infiltration, therefore, it is unclear why a patient complains of such great discomfort when pulling up on the hernia sac during open herniorrhaphy under local anaesthetic.

Occasionally 1 cc of Marcaine at the pubic tubercle has been required if discomfort is noted during mesh attachment medially. It is very important that the patient is able to communicate with the surgeon as the mesh is being placed (either with sutures or staples) so that the patient can inform the surgeon of any paresthesias or pain. This has allowed careful placement of lateral staples (and sutures) to decrease the risks of lateral recurrences.

The surgeon should attempt to avoid the use of cautery since this could also result in accidental nerve conduction and injury. If bleeding near nerves cannot be controlled with pressure (gauze), then the use of Endoloops is a better alternative to cautery.

Originally, the peritoneum was closed using a running suture. Currently, a purse string stitch is being used (as recommended by Dr Maurice Arregui) to decrease the possible area of adhesion formation.

Results

Eight patients have been treated using this method and five procedures have been successfully completed. Three patients were converted to a general anaesthetic, one due to the patient's complaint of abdominal wall discomfort at the end of the procedure during closure of the peritoneum (an external traction device was being tested and was the cause of pain). The second was converted early in the procedure due to the patient's anxiety. The third patient was a much more complex patient who had a history of chronic right lower quadrant pain for several months, felt to be due to a small right inguinal hernia. This patient actually had his appendix abscessed into his indirect hernia sac and walled off with omentum and small bowel due to Crohn's disease. He did not require conversion until the devascularization of his appendix. This caused periumbilical pain, like one would see in early appendicitis. In retrospect, this could probably have been blocked with an injection of Marcaine in the mesoappendix. He had already undergone an extensive lysis of adhesions, partially using hydrodissection with the Marcaine/saline solution, as well as a suture ligation of his hernia sac prior to his appendectomy.

Our current technique, although still in evolution, has worked very well. It allows the patient to remain in an easily arousable state in which they can follow instructions and notify us of any paresthesias or pain due to nerve entrapment. Two patients warned us away from areas lateral and superior to the hernia defect.

In summary, salient points to remember for laparoscopic local procedures include:

- H-2 blockers night prior to surgery

- preoperative Reglan, Toradol (ketorolac tromethamine) and Valium
- urethral lubrication with lidocaine jelly and IV pentothal for Foley placement
- maintain low pressures of less than 10 mmHg
- low insufflator flow until pressures are reached, and then high flow used to maintain pressures
- limit desiccation with irrigation.

Conclusion

Laparoscopic herniorrhaphy using local anaesthesia appears to be a viable alternative to using a general anaesthetic. With continued investigation and experience, I believe that this can become a routine part of the procedure.

Bibliography

Hasson HM. Open laparoscopy: A report of 150 cases. *J. Reprod. Med.*, 1974; **12**: 234–8.

15

A Classification of Groin Hernia

LLOYD M NYHUS

The international conference on hernia held in Indianapolis, Indiana, 23–27 May 1993, highlighted the need for a simple, practical classification of hernia types. It is my premise that the rote use of one operation for the repair of all inguinal hernias, regardless of size or type, is tantamount to malfeasance. To subject a patient with a small fascial opening at the internal abdominal ring to any operative repair that opens an intact direct wall is incomprehensible. Similarly, there is no place for laparoscopic herniotomy in patients with minimal fascial defects. Why would one use general anaesthesia, as is required by laparosocpy, when local infiltration block of the regional nerves is all that is necessary for high ligation of the hernial sac and plastic repair of the internal abdominal ring? Furthermore, large, complex inguinal hernias, primary or recurrent, must be identified and typed preoperatively so that the best operative approach or technique can be selected from an array of proven procedures. This, then, is a plea for the study of each patient's specific problem, followed by selection of the operation best suited to cure the hernia.

The following classification (Table 15.1) is designed to aid the surgeon in individualizing each patient's problem and in matching it with appropriate therapy.

Classification of groin hernias (Table 15.1)

Type I

Type I comprises indirect inguinal hernias in which the internal abdominal ring is of normal size, configuration and structure. These usually occur in infants, children or young adults. The boundaries are well delineated and Hesselbach's triangle is normal. An indirect hernia sac extends variably from just distal to the internal abdominal ring to the middle of the inguinal canal.

Type II

Type II comprises the indirect inguinal hernias in which the internal ring is enlarged and distorted without impinging on the floor of the inguinal canal. Hesselbach's triangle (floor of the canal) is normal when palpated through the opened peritoneal sac. The hernial sac is not in the scrotum, but it may occupy the entire inguinal canal.

Type III

Type III hernias are of three subtypes: direct, indirect and femoral.

Type IIIA hernias are direct inguinal hernias in which the protrusion does not herniate through the internal abdominal (inguinal) ring. The weakened transversalis fascia (posterior inguinal wall medial to the inferior epigastric vessels) bulges outward in front of the hernial mass. All direct hernias, small or large, are type IIIA.

Table 15.1: Classification of groin hernias

Type I – Indirect inguinal hernia
  Internal inguinal ring normal (eg paediatric hernia)

Type II – Indirect inguinal hernia
  Internal inguinal ring dilated but posterior inguinal wall intact; inferior deep epigastric vessels not displaced

Type III – Posterior wall defects
  A Direct inguinal hernia
  B Indirect inguinal hernia
    Internal inguinal ring dilated, medially encroaching on or destroying the transversalis fascia of the Hesselbach triangle (eg massive scrotal, sliding or pantaloon hernias)
  C Femoral hernia

Type IV – Recurrent hernias
  A Direct
  B Indirect
  C Femoral
  D Combined

Type IIIB hernias are indirect hernias with a large dilated ring that has expanded medially and encroaches on the posterior inguinal wall (floor) to a greater or lesser degree. The hernial sac frequently is in the scrotum. Occasionally, the caecum on the right or the sigmoid colon on the left makes up a portion of the wall of the sac. These sliding hernias always destroy some of the inguinal floor. (The internal abdominal ring may be dilated without displacement of the inferior epigastric vessels. Direct and indirect components of the hernial sac may straddle those vessels to form a pantaloon hernia.)

Type IIIC hernias are femoral hernias, a specialized form of posterior wall defect.

Type IV

Recurrent hernias are type IV. They can be direct (type IVA), indirect (type IVB), femoral (type IVC) or a combination of these types (type IVD). These hernias cause intricate management problems and carry a higher morbidity than do other hernias.

Individualization of repair to type of hernia (Table 15.2)

Individualization of the approach to hernial repair should be based on a complete assessment of the internal inguinal ring, the condition of the posterior inguinal wall (floor), and inspection of the femoral ring to exlude an associated subclinical defect.

Digital exploration is the most effective way to evaluate the nature of the hernia. The exploration is performed by opening the hernial sac and inserting the index finger through the neck of the sac to draw up the internal ring. The finger inside the sac can feel the margin of the ring, test the strength of the posterior wall of the inguinal canal and detect a direct hernial weakness. This examination must be carried out before the sac is tied off.

Types I and II

Hernias (type I) need no fascial repair. High ligation of the hernial sac should suffice.

Table 15.2: Repair individualized to type of hernia

Type of hernia	*Repair*
Type I – Indirect with normal abdominal ring	High ligation of sac*; no repair: anterior approach
Type II – Indirect with internal abdominal ring dilated, posterior abdominal wall intact	High ligation of sac; transversalis fascia repair of internal abdominal ring: anterior approach
Type III – Posterior wall defects	
A Direct	Anterior approach – IPTR without mesh (Condon); Shouldice repair; Cooper ligament repair; *or*
B Large indirect	Posterior approach – IPTR with inlay buttress of polypropylene mesh; Stoppa GPRVS with Mersilene
C Femoral	Posterior approach – IPTR without mesh
Type IV – Recurrent	Posterior approach – IPTR with inlay buttress of polypropylene mesh

* Excision and ligation of hernial sac are performed for all indirect and femoral hernias. A direct sac is usually not opened, excised, or ligated.
GPRVS = giant prosthetic reinforcement of visceral sac; IPTR = iliopubic tract repair.

A small indirect hernia in which there is a slightly dilated internal ring but no weakening of the posterior inguinal wall (type II) is best treated from the anterior approach by high ligation of the sac and plastic closure of the transversalis fascia at the internal ring.

Hernias (type II) are for the most part overtreated; repair of the inguinal floor is unnecessary. In type I and II hernias, incision of a strong posterior layer (the first step in a Bassini, Shouldice or McVay repair) is inappropriate. An operation to repair type I or type II hernia is a simple procedure, and insertion of prosthetic mesh is not necessary.

Types III and IV

Direct inguinal (type IIIA) and large indirect (type IIIB) hernias are satisfactorily repaired by an anterior (Shouldice, Condon or Cooper ligament) or a posterior approach. The posterior approach and iliopubic tract repair of type IIIA or IIIB hernias should include an inlay buttress of mesh to support the anatomical repair.

I repair femoral (type IIIC) hernias by the posterior approach and close the defect by suturing the iliopubic tract to the Cooper ligament.

Recurrent hernias (type IV) are routinely treated by the posterior approach with iliopubic tract repair and an inlay buttress of prosthetic mesh. Extensive experience with this method has shown a re-recurrence rate of less than 2%.

Summary

The goal of successful operative procedures to repair common inguinal hernias is to duplicate the natural mechanisms (ie to close the sphincter or the shutter permanently. There is a natural system for guarding against indirect inguinal hernias (the sphincter mechanism of the internal abdominal ring) and direct inguinal hernias (the shutter mechanism of the transversus abdominis aponeurotic arch). If suture lines are placed to approximate the posterior inguinal wall to itself (ie transversus abdominis aponeurotic arch to iliopubic tract (shutter) and anterior transversalis fascia crus to posterior crus–iliopubic tract (sphincter)), a relatively tension-free repair results.

Prosthetic mesh is not necessary for routine hernia repairs. Mesh may be useful in patients with large direct or combined direct–indirect hernias.

To aid in surgical decision making, it is helpful to classify the types of inguinal hernias. Classifying hernias and matching the types of hernia with specific operations serve as a technical guide to hernia repair. This guide allows objective evaluation of treatment and verification of results.

16

Biomaterials in Hernia Surgery

STANLEY D BERLINER

Surgeons are scientists and artists. As scientists we must have a thorough knowledge of our field and a developed sense of technical proficiency; as artists we are required to utilize our creative and innovative skills. Since about 1983, defects of the abdominal wall have been corrected using a biomaterial with increasing frequency. The task of repairing this hernia can at times challenge both the scientific and the artistic talents of the most experienced surgeon.

Biomaterial

A biomaterial is any synthetic or non-pedicled natural substance that can be used for tissue replacement. Many substances have been employed, with varying degrees of success.

Autogenous fascia was used at the turn of the century. In 1910, Kirschner used non-pedicled fascial autografts as an onlay biomaterial in inguinal hernias. For incisional hernias, he used a double layer of fascia. One was positioned preperitoneally and the other placed as an onlay graft. Kirschner found that the graft site healed without reaction or sepsis, and correctly predicted that the graft would retain its original structure and remain viable[1].

In 1922, Harrison wrote of his dissatisfaction with the Bassini repair for direct hernias. Under local anaesthesia, Harrison incised and overlapped the posterior wall and reinforced this with a fascia lata onlay graft. Essentially, Harrison performed a prototype of the Shouldice hernioplasty and the Lichtenstein onlay graft. He did not report recurrences. Harrison operated on Bedouin tribesmen in the Middle East who would fold their tents and disappear into the night. It is not surprising that his major problem was wound infection[2].

Autogenous fascia has led an extensive clinical trial since 1910. It is the gold standard that serves as a model for the synthetics. Creating an ideal synthetic continues to be a challenge. The biomaterial should provide a non-antigenic framework that is gradually replaced by host fibroplasia so that a stable aponeurotic structure results. Many of the synthetics have not withstood the test of clinical trial. Pain, fragmentation, extrusion, early loss of tensile strength and low tolerance to infection have been major problems.

The use of absorbable biomaterials such as the glycolic acid polymers (Dexon and Vicryl) is limited. Studies demonstrate insufficient fibrous tissue incorporation into Vicryl mesh before hydrolysis occurred such that bursting strength at 12 weeks was much weaker than at three weeks. However, Vicryl and Dexon have proved successful as a buffer between exposed bowel and a non-absorbable synthetic. Dexon is also useful in temporary closure of large defects in the poor-risk patient. Vicryl appears to be less desirable because of more rapid hydrolysis.

In the 1940s a new world was opened to the surgeon with the introduction of non-absorbable synthetics. They avoid the necessity of the additional operation of a fascial autograft, and they eliminate the need for a homograft or heterograft bank. Pioneered by the investigative and clinical efforts of Usher in 1958, polypropylene mesh (Marlex, Prolene) has become the most commonly

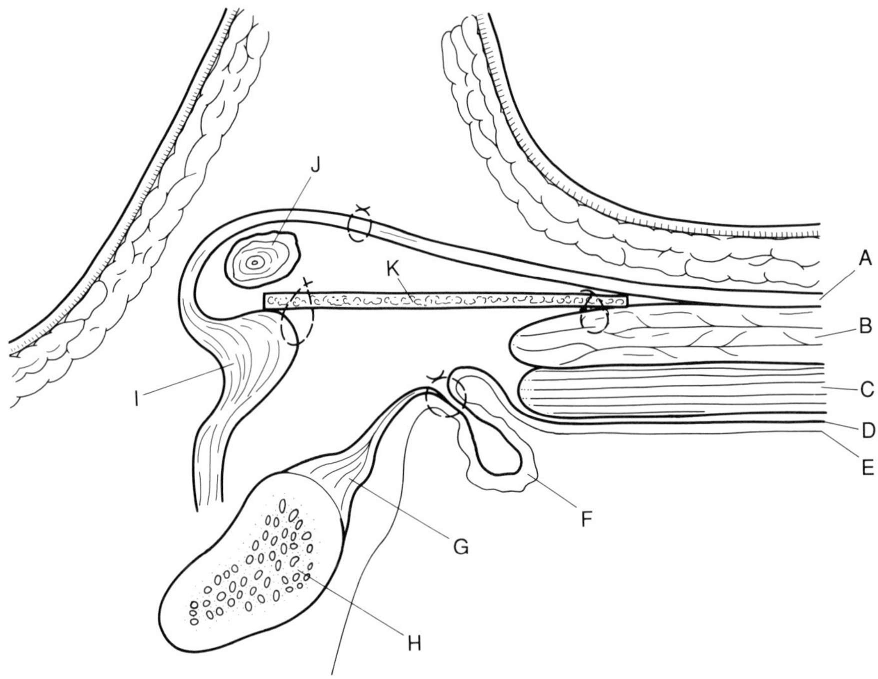

Figure 16.1 Sagittal view of the Lichtenstein onlay graft repair. The posterior wall defect has been corrected with a modified Bassini inversion of the direct sac (F). The mesh patch has been sutured to the inguinal ligament and to the internal oblique. This leaves a vulnerable area between inguinal ligament (I) and iliopubic tract (G). A, external oblique aponeurosis; B, internal oblique muscle; C, transversus aponeurosis; D, transversalis fascia; E, peritoneum; F, inverted direct sac; G, iliopubic tract insertion on Cooper's ligament; H, pubis; I, inguinal ligament; J, spermatic cord; K, mesh. (Reproduced, with permission, from *Am J Surg.* 1989; **157**: 192.)

used biomaterial for the repair of abdominal wall hernias. It serves as a durable framework for the ingrowth of collagen and has a high tolerance to infection, particularly the Prolene mesh which has a larger weave and has been used successfully in grossly contaminated situations.

Mersilene is a braided Dacron polyester, not a monofilament. Its lack of plastic memory allows it to conform to the preperitoneal structures it is encasing. It has had an extensive clinical trial in France, with good results.

Polytetrafluoroethylene (PTFE, Teflon) is an inert biomaterial. Early clinical experience with the porous weave mesh was not favourable because of infection and rejection. In 1975 a microporous expanded PTFE biomaterial was introduced by Gore and associates which has proven effective as a soft tissue patch for the repair of abdominal wall hernias. My personal experience with it has been excellent in selected groin hernias.

Carbon fibre is well tolerated in living tissues. Flexible filamentous carbon attracts fibroblastic ingrowth, and the result is a dense connective structure with the collagen bundles orientated along the lines of stress. It has been used successfully in orthopaedics as a tendon and ligament substitute. A composite polylactic acid and carbon cloth has been tried in incisional hernias in the laboratory and deserves more clinical trial.

Metals were used by German surgeons in the early 1900s. Whilst silver filigree is not practical for modern use, there is a ten-year study of 500 inguinal repairs in which the filigree was placed as an inlay graft, with only two known recurrences.

The synthetic is a foreign body and there is always the danger of wound infection. Fortunately, the incidence of infection has been low. Sinus tracts after Marlex repairs for incisional hernias can

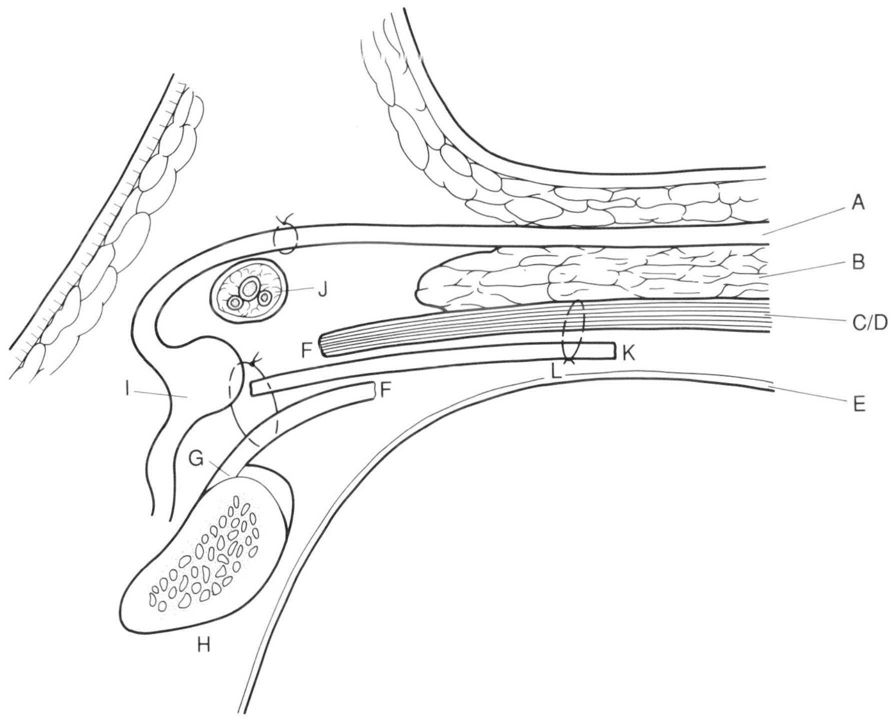

Figure 16.2 The inlay graft is sutured inferiorly to both inguinal ligament (I) and transversalis fascia (F), and superiorly to the white line of the transversus arch (L). Excess direct sac has been excised (F). A, inguinal ligament; B, internal oblique muscle; C and D. transversalis fascia (TF) and transversus abdominis aponeurosis (TAA) posterior wall; E, peritoneum; F, incised TF/TAA posterior wall, direct sac excised; G, iliopubic tract insertion on Cooper's ligament; H, pubis; I, inguinal ligament; J, spermatic cord; K, ePTFE soft tissue patch; L, graft sutured to transversus arch.

be managed conservatively. My experience with the larger weave Prolene mesh has been more favourable. It does better than Marlex in the face of gross contamination, and removes more easily than Marlex.

If infection does occur with the Dacron polyester, segments of the mersilene may require removal. Similarly, once bacteria lodge within the Gore-Tex soft tissue patch, it must be removed. There have been two infections in 600 inguinal repairs with the Gore-Tex soft tissue patch, which is an incidence of 0.3%. In one case, the hernia recurred four months after removal of the graft. The other patient developed a delayed sinus tract which was treated conservatively for nine months. The patch was then removed through the sinus tract, which rapidly closed. At the time of writing it two years later the hernia had not recurred.

Clinical material

During the 20-year period from January 1972 through December 1991, I repaired 6294 abdominal wall hernias in people over the age of 18: 96.6% were groin hernias and the remainder were ventral and incisional hernias. In males, 97.3% were inguinal and 2.7% femoral or inguinofemoral. In females, 74.5% were inguinal and 25.5% femoral or inguinofemoral.

Currently a biomaterial is employed in about 20% of inguinal hernias, 75% of femoral hernias, 100% of incisional hernias, 20% of epigastric hernias and 50% of umbilical hernias.

Groin hernias

I have yet to discover a single operation that fits all situations. My selection of the type of repair depends on the pathology encountered. In inguinal repairs where a major reconstruction of the posterior wall and deep ring is necessary, a Gore-Tex soft tissue patch is used as an inlay graft not as an onlay (Figures 16.1 and 16.2). Although this group represents more extensive pathology, the failure rate in 350 operations with a mean follow-up time of 4.5 years is 1.1%[3]. An expanded PTFE plug is used in about 75% of femoral hernias. The Gore-Tex glides more smoothly than the polypropylene materials as it is pulled alongside the femoral vein.

Incisional hernia

Incisional hernias require long-term follow up in order to evaluate the efficacy of the repair. During the ten-year period from 1970 through 1979, I performed 40 operations on 36 patients[4]. Three patients were lost to follow up. The mean follow-up time for 37 repairs was 74.4 months; 13 repairs had mesh inserted as an inlay graft and 27 repairs were by primary suture with a relaxing incision when necessary. There have been no recurrences in the biomaterial group; 12 of the 27 sutured repairs recurred, which is a failure rate of 44%. The recurrences developed between 7 and 98 months after operation, with an average recurrence time of 37.5 months.

Because of the high failure rate for sutured repairs, in 1980 primary approximation was limited to very small incisional hernias. During the four-year period from 1980 through 1983, 27 repairs were performed. Six operations were by primary suture, with two failures: one hernia recurred 13 months after surgery; the other recurred after nine years. In 21 cases a polypropylene material was used as an inlay graft, with one failure[4]. Because of the prohibitive failure rate for sutured repairs, every incisional hernia, regardless of size, is now repaired with a biomaterial.

References

1. Kirschner M. Die praktischen Ergebnisse der freien Fascien-Transplantation. *Arch Klin Chir* 1910; **92**: 888–912.

2. Harrison PW. Inguinal hernia: a study of the principles involved in the surgical treatment. *Arch Surg* 1922; **4**: 680–9.

3. Berliner SD. Clinical experience with an inlay expanded PTFE soft tissue patch as an adjunct in inguinal hernia repair. *Surg Gynecol Obstet* 1993; **176**: 323–6.

4. Berliner SD. Biomaterials in hernia repair. In: Nyhus LM, Condon RE, eds. *Hernia*, 3rd ed. Philadelphia: JB Lippincott, 1989: 541–54.

17

Biomaterials and Abdominal Wall Hernia Surgery

PARVIZ K AMID, ALEX G SHULMAN AND IRVING L LICHTENSTEIN

The importance of biomaterials in abdominal wall hernia surgery is increasingly appreciated. Improvement in the recurrence rate of incisional hernias from 46% and inguinal hernias from 10% to under 0.5% with the use of biomaterials has been reported[1,2]. Although decreasing, there exists and unjustified fear regarding the routine use of mesh in the repair of inguinal and incisional hernias. This is due to bad experiences in the past when a proper biomaterial was not available. When Francis Usher introduced Marlex mesh over two decades ago, proper suture material for fixation of the mesh in place was not available. This compounded the fear of mesh for the repair of abdominal wall hernias.

For the last 25 years, we have utilized Marlex mesh for the repair of more than 10 000 adult abdominal wall hernias. Its use together with a 'tension-free' technique of repair has been shown to be safe and effective[3]. More importantly, it reduces postoperative pain, disability period and the recurrence rate[2,4–7], thus making the management of abdominal wall hernias more cost-effective.

Materials and methods

The necessary qualities of synthetic biomaterials have been well described by Cumberland[8] and Scales[9]. Synthetic mesh should be physically unaltered by tissue fluids, be chemically inert, not cause foreign body reactions, be non-carcinogenic and non-allergenic, be capable of resisting mechanical strains and be capable of being sterilized.

Monofilamented polypropylene mesh (Figure 17.1) is the only biomaterial available today that fulfils all the requirements for a suitable mesh in general and the following critical characteristics in particular.

Inertness

All available biomaterials such as polypropylene mesh, expanded PTFE soft tissue patch, polyester mesh and Teflon mesh are well tolerated, without evidence of rejection; polypropylene mesh is the least reactive of plastic materials under test conditions[10,11]. Apparent instances of rejection are usually a misinterpreted infectious process or histiocytic reaction due to the microporosity of the materials used.

Permanence

A suitable mesh for hernia repair needs to be non-absorbable and permanent. Absorbable biomaterials are recommended only for temporary abdominal closure in contaminated cases. They are unsatisfactory materials for use in permanent abdominal wall replacement[12].

Experiments with the rat suggest possible benefit from implantation of polyglactin mesh in the groin for repair of inguinal hernias[13]. According to this study, the mesh becomes replaced by polarized collagen bundles orientated along the lines of stress. Morphologically, this implies that the newly

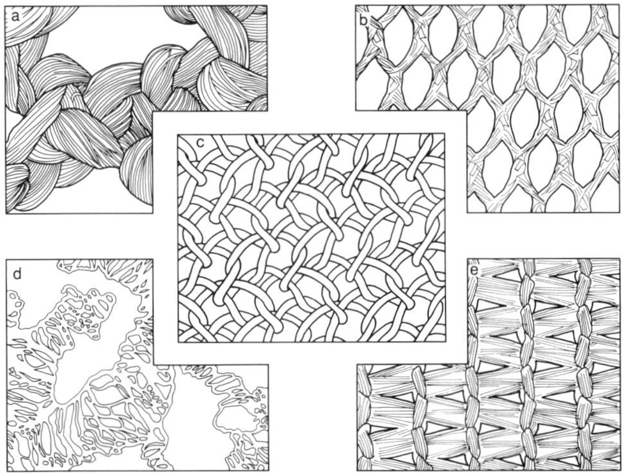

Figure 17.1: Scanning electron micrographs of frequently used biomaterials: (a) multifilamented PTFE mesh; (b) multifilamented polyester mesh; (c) monofilamented polypropylene mesh; (d) expanded PTFE soft tissue patch; and (e) multifilamented polypropylene mesh.

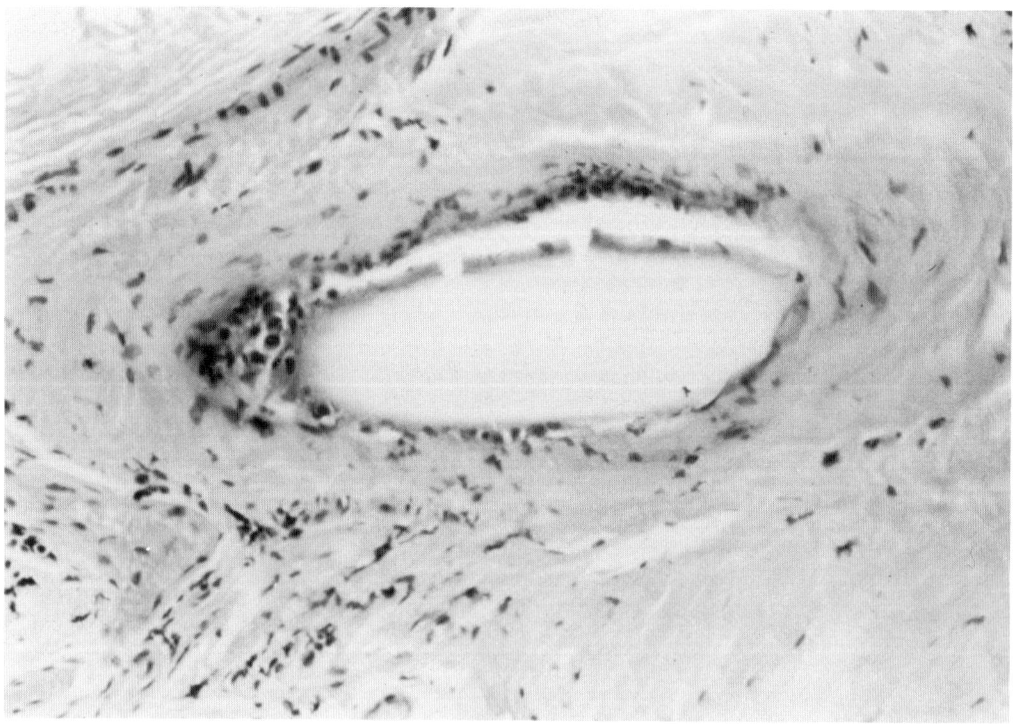

Figure 17.2: Foreign body reaction to multifilamented suture material (low power).

formed collagen bundles should be as strong as normal connective tissue. However, it is doubtful that the resulting fibrous tissue can resist the inevitable collagen metabolic disorder with the passage

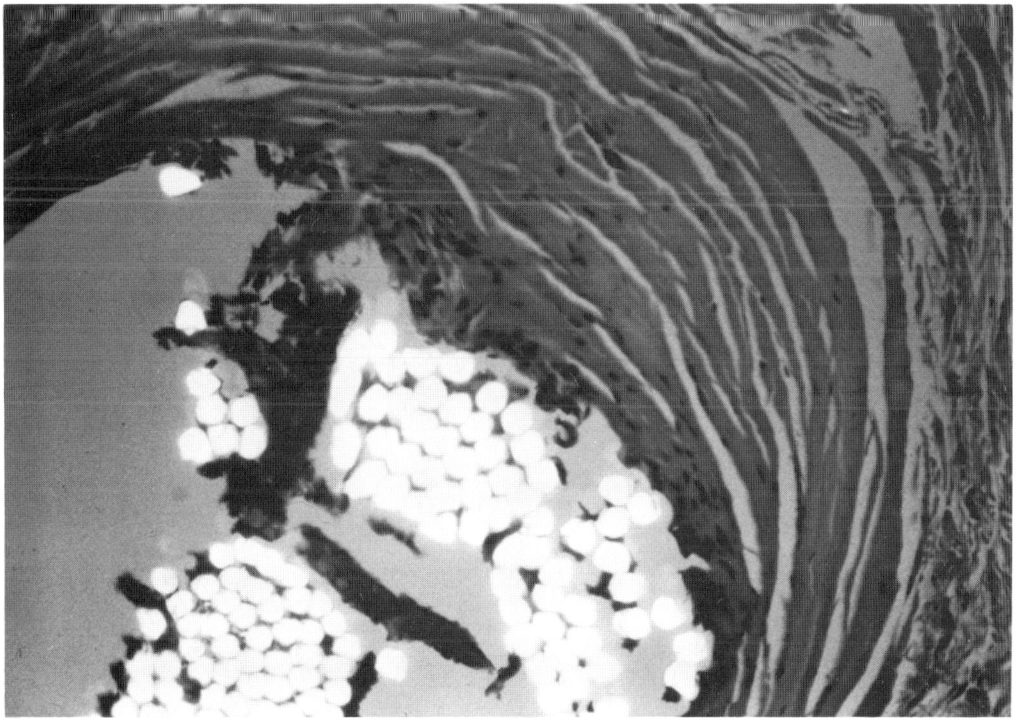

Figure 17.3: Foreign body reaction to multifilamented suture material (high power and polarized light).

of time. Furthermore, our animal experimentation as well as the experiments of other investigators[12,14] have shown that such fibrous tissue, in the case of ventral hernia, cannot resist intra-abdominal pressure and cannot prevent hernia formation.

Resistance to infection

Decades ago, surgeons learned that use of multifilamented braided suture materials, by excluding macrophages but not bacteria, frequently resulted in infection, foreign body granuloma and sinus tract formation[15]. Figure 17.2 is a micrograph of tissue with embedded mesh removed from a patient who had developed a chronic draining sinus tract after an inguinal hernia repair with Marlex mesh. At first glance, the presence of foreign body reaction and granuloma can easily be blamed on the use of biomaterial. However, when examined at higher magnification and under polarized light (Figure 17.3), it becomes apparent that the foreign body granuloma was caused by the multifilamented suture material used to fix the mesh.

Biomaterials that contain pores or spaces less than 10 μm in any of their three dimensions may increase the chance of infection and sinus tract formation[14,16]. Bacteria averaging 1 μm in size can hide in such small spaces and proliferate while protected from neutrophilic granulocytes averaging 10–15 μm in size.

Macroporous biomaterials with pore sizes larger than 10 μm, such as Marlex mesh, do not promote or harbour infection. Furthermore, when the surgical field becomes infected, a monofilamented biomaterial such as Marlex mesh does not have to be removed. In these situations, drainage of the wound is all that is needed for the management of the infection. Microporous biomaterials such as expanded PTFE (Gore-Tex), polyester mesh (Mersilene), multifilamented polypropylene mesh (Surgipro) and PTFE mesh (Teflon) can promote or harbour infection. Figure 17.4 is a CT scan sinograph from a patient who developed draining sinus tract three months after a bilateral inguinal

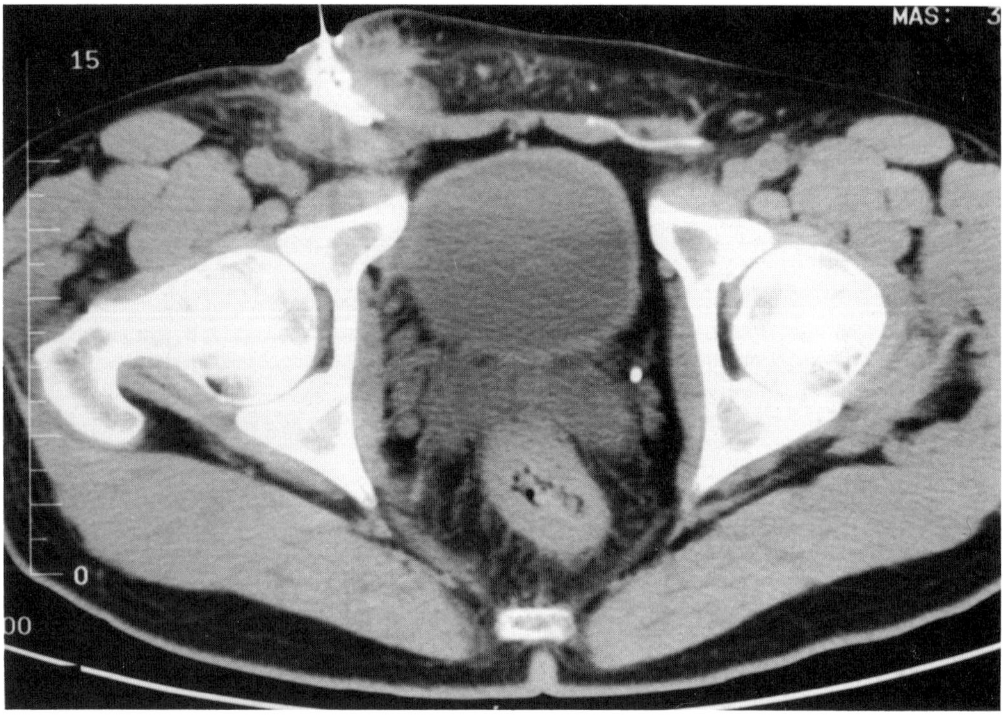

Figure 17.4: CT scan sinograph of sinus tract formation in the right groin after bilateral hernia repair with PTFE patch.

hernia repair with expanded PTFE soft tissue patch. The patch was spontaneously extruded eight months later in spite of long-term massive antibiotic therapy. In the event of infection, the microporous biomaterial needs to be removed, as in the case of infected vascular grafts.

Rapid fibrinous fixation

Rapid fibrinous fixation of biomaterials by the host's endogenous fibrin 'glue' is desired if seroma formation is to be prevented.

This fixation characteristic, which is the function of molecular permeability of macroporous biomaterials, decreases the chance of seroma collection[17] by eliminating potential dead space between the mesh and the host tissue. Furthermore, adequate molecular permeability results in the formation of proper scaffolding for future fibrocytic infiltration into the substance of the mesh[18].

Host tissue incorporation

Complete incorporation of the mesh with the host tissue is an important requirement if a solid repair is to be expected. The degree of host tissue infiltration into the biomaterial depends on pore size, surface texture and anatomical location.

Pore size

Tissue incorporation of synthetic prosthesis is proportional to the degree of its porosity[18]. Fibrocytic and collagen infiltration of the host tissue into the mesh with adequate porosity occurs in about one month[18]. Complete incorporation requires a pore size of 75–100 μm. Monofilamented polypropylene

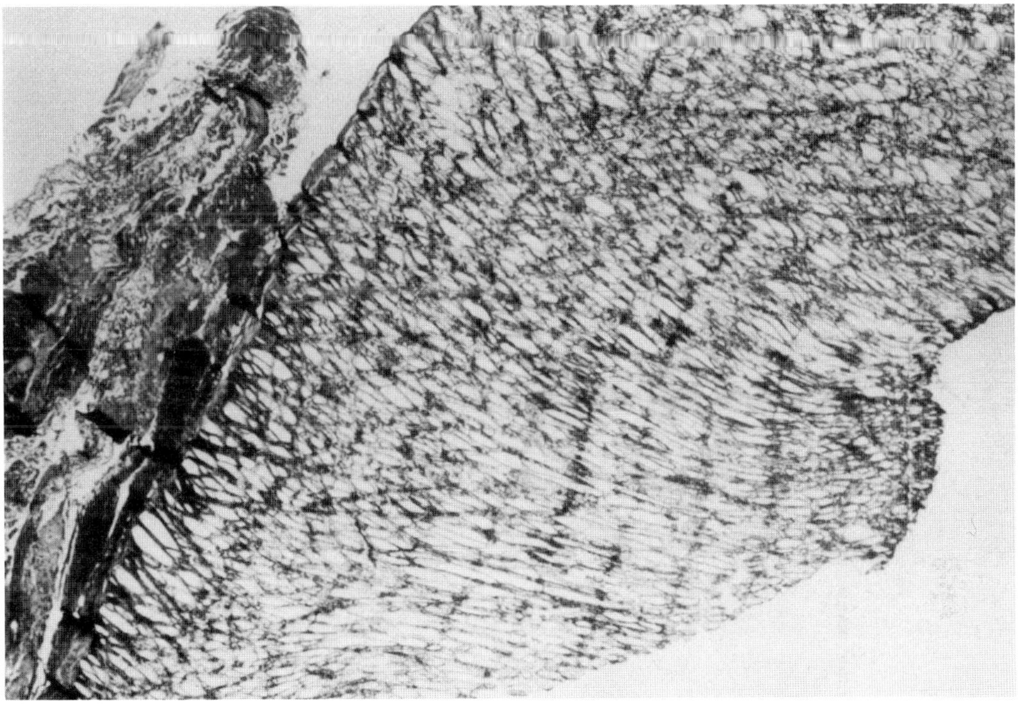

Figure 17.5: Complete host tissue incorporation of Marlex mesh.

mesh with a pore size larger than 100 μm produces complete infiltration of the host tissue into the entire thickness of the mesh (Figure 17.5). Biomaterials that contain pores or spaces of less that 75 μm attract more histiocytic than fibrocytic infiltration from the host tissue[19]. This abundance of histiocytes over fibrocytes is the reason for the formation of young and loose granulation tissue in and around such material.

Surface texture

A greater degree of fibrous tissue reaction and infiltration is associated with a textured surface prosthesis[20]. Slight roughness of the surface of the individual fibres of Marlex mesh, as well as the texture of its weave, stimulates fibroplasia and furthers the host tissue incorporation.

Anatomical location

Experimental studies have shown that the best incorporation results from placement of the mesh between two abdominal muscle layers. Less ingrowth was noted with mesh placed between peritoneum and abdominal muscles. The least infiltration was achieved by mesh between the abdominal aponeurotic tissue and the subcutaneous fat (onlay graft)[21].

Figure 17.5 is an example of host tissue infiltration into the thickness of a piece of Marlex mesh, which was removed from a patient three years after its implantation.

Figure 17.6 is an example of inadequate host tissue incorporation of a microporous expanded PTFE soft tissue patch removed four years after its implantation from the same patient as in Figure 17.5.

Based on the results obtained from animal experiments and clinical human experience it appears that monofilamented polypropylene mesh (Marlex and Prolene) is far superior to other available synthetic materials. It is completely inert, resists infection and sinus tract formation, has rapid fibrinous fixation, becomes completely incorporated into the host tissue and, in the event of infection, does not have to be removed.

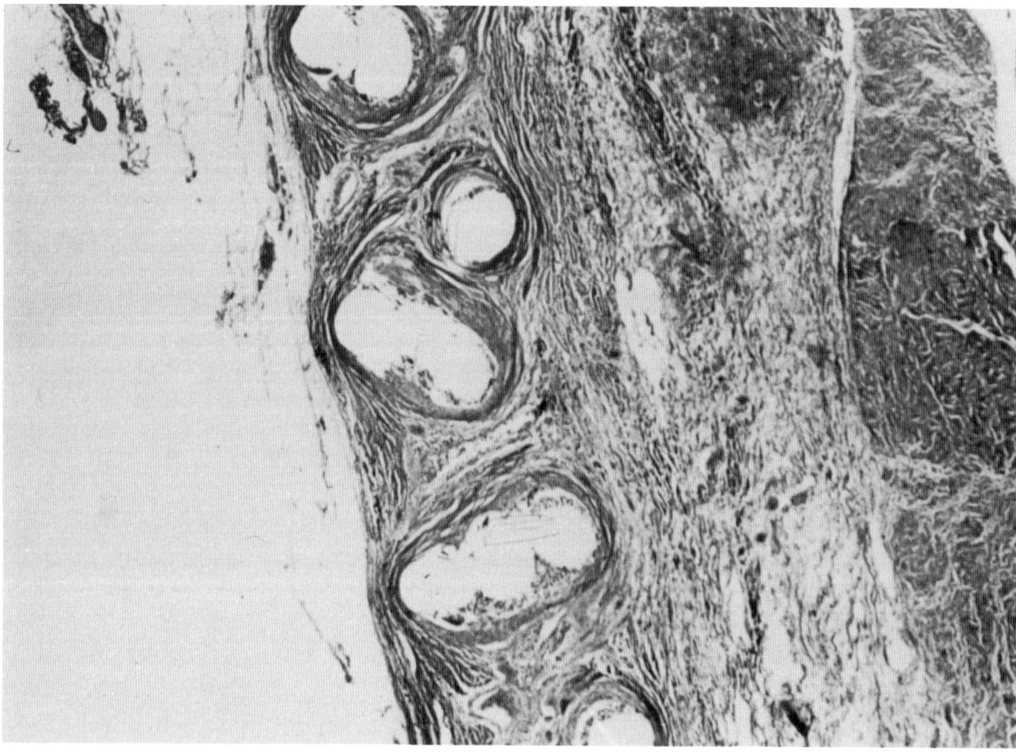

Figure 17.6: Incomplete host tissue incorporation of PTFE patch.

Biomaterials in common use today are monofilamented polypropylene mesh (Marlex) (Figure 17.1c), multifilamented polypropylene mesh (Surgipro) (Figure 17.1e), multifilamented polyester mesh (Mersilene) (Figure 17.1b), multifilamented polytetrafluoroethylene (PTFE) mesh (Teflon) (Figure 17.1a) and expanded PTFE soft tissue patch (Gore-tex) (Figure 17.1d). Except for the monofilamented polypropylene mesh, the biomaterials are either purely microporous (pore sizes less than 10–75 μm in at least one of the three dimensions), such as expanded PTFE soft tissue patch, or contain microporous components such as multifilamented biomaterials (PTFE mesh, polyester mesh and multifilamented polypropylene mesh).

Because of their microporosity, these meshes can cause a histiocytic reaction and promote or harbour infection. Mersilene, which is a multifilamented Dacron mesh, has gained popularity in Europe. However, because of the high incidence of infection with coated or uncoated Dacron sutures[22] and its multifilamented structure, it is less than ideal for the repair of abdominal wall hernias; moreover, in the event of infection, it may have to be removed[23]. Mersilene mesh is pliable and handles more easily when used for preperitoneal inguinal or incisional hernia repair, but its risk–benefit ratio should be carefully calculated when being considered for use. Furthermore, if the surgeon chooses to use the simpler stapling technique for fixation of the mesh in the preperitoneal approach, the slight stiffness of Marlex is better than the pliability of Mersilene.

The use of mesh for the repair of ventral hernias has come under special scrutiny because of the propensity to form intestinal adhesions when in direct contact with the intestines, which may lead to biomaterial-related intestinal fistula formation[24,25].

Our animal studies support the experimental results of other investigators indicating that all currently available absorbable and non-absorbable biomaterials adhere to the adjacent intestines[26,27]. It has been suggested by some authors[28,29] that covering the intestinal side of a non-absorbable mesh with a layer of absorbable mesh would prevent adhesions and the formation of biomaterial-related intestinal fistulas. It is reasoned that a mesothelial lining would occur and prevent fistula formation before absorption was complete. Because of the lack of histological evidence, the postulated effectiveness of such a combination could not be substantiated by our study.

Since adhesion of intestine to biomaterial is the first stage of biomaterial-related intestinal fistulas, its prevention is a logical step toward the elimination of this complication. Our animal studies show that a composite made of a layer of porous polypropylene (polypropylene mesh) on the parietal side and a layer of a non-porous material such as polypropylene sheeting on the intestinal side has the selective property of allowing infiltration of the host tissue to one side yet preventing adhesions of bowel to the other. Such a composite provides complete incorporation of the porous layer while preventing encapsulation and unlikely extrusion of the solid layer. These composites might also be applicable to the repair of chest wall and diaphragmatic defects and to intraperitoneal laparoscopic hernioplasties if the latter prove superior to the open 'tension-free' repair.

Conclusions

Pioneered by Francis Usher in 1958, the first generation of Marlex mesh made of polyethylene (a Phillips petroleum product) was introduced. It provided the strength and inertness lacking in other prostheses, but could not be easily sterilized and thus proved unsatisfactory. In 1962, polypropylene Marlex was developed. This material not only provided all the advantages of polyethylene but also permitted sterilization by autoclaving.

Polypropylene is produced by closely controlled polymerization of prolene, a derivative of propane gas, and has the excellent chemical resistance of hydrocarbon polymers. It has an outstanding hinge life[30], excellent stress crack resistance, burst strength of more than 172.5 kPa (25 p.s.i.) suture retention of 4.86 kg (10.7 lb) (warp) and 3.1 kg (6.9 lb) (course), and stretchability of 60% (warp) and 20% (course). Long-term studies have shown that the tensile strength of polypropylene implanted in tissue remains unchanged[30–32]. Our animal studies show that Marlex mesh coupled with a layer of non-porous material such as polypropylene sheeting can produce an adhesion-free composite.

References

1. George CD, Ellis H. The results of incisional hernia repair: a twelve-year review. *Ann R Coll Surg Engl* 1986; **68**: 185–93.
2. Amid PK, Shulman AG, Lichtenstein IL. Critical scrutiny of the open 'tension-free' hernioplasty. *Am J Surg* 1993; **165**: 369–71.
3. Shulman AG, Amid PK, Lichtenstein IL. The safety of mesh repair for primary inguinal hernias: results of 3,019 operations from five diverse surgical sources. *Am Surg* 1992; **58**: 255–7.
4. Martin RE, Max CE. Primary inguinal hernia repair with prosthetic mesh. *Hospi Medica* 1984; **1**: 1.
5. Barnes JP. Inguinal hernia repair with routine use of Marlex mesh. *Surg Gynecol Obstet* 1987; **165**: 33–7.
6. Capozzi JA, Berkenfield JA, Cheaty JK. Repair of inguinal hernia in the adult with Prolene mesh. *Surg Gynecol Obstet* 1988; **167**: 124–8.
7. Tinkler LF. Inguinal hernia repair using local anaesthesia. *Ann R Coll Surg Engl* 1985; **67**: 268.
8. Cumberland O. Ueber die Verschliessung von Bauchwunden und Brustpforten durch Versenkte Siberdrahtnetze. *Zentralbl Chir* 1900; **27**: 257.
9. Scales JT. Discussion on metals and synthetic materials in relation to soft tissues; tissue reaction to synthetic materials. *Proc R Soc Med* 1953; **46**: 647.

10. Usher FC, Allen JE, Crosthwait RW, Cogan JE. Polypropylene monofilament. A new, biologically inert suture for closing contaminated wounds. *JAMA* 1962; **179**: 780.

11. Wagner MW. Evaluation of diverse plastic and cutis prostheses in a growing host. *Surg Gynecol Obstet* 1970; **130**: 1077.

12. Lamb JP, Vitale T, Kaminski DL. Comparative evaluation of synthetic meshes used for abdominal wall replacement. *Surgery* 1983; **93**: 643–8.

13. Brenner J. Implantation of Vicryl patch for inguinal hernia. Presented at the International Frascia Congress, Hamburg, Germany, May 1991.

14. Amid PK, Shulman AG, Lichtenstein IL. Selecting synthetic mesh for the repair of groin hernia. *Postgrad Gen Surg* 1992; **4**: 150–5.

15. Elek SD, Conen PE. The virulence of *Staphylococcus pyogenes* for man. Study of the problems of wound infection. *Br J Exp Pathol* 1957; **38**: 573.

16. Neel III HB. Implants of Gore-Tex. *Arch Otolaryngol* 1983; **109**: 427–33.

17. Arnaud JP, Eloy R, Adloff M, Grenier JF. Critical evaluation of prosthetic materials in repair of abdominal wall hernias. New criteria of tolerance and resistance. *Am J Surg* 1977; **133**: 338–45.

18. White RA. The effect of porosity and biomaterial on the healing and long-term mechanical properties of vascular prostheses. *ASAIO Trans* 1988; **11**: 95–100.

19. White RA, Hirose FM, Sproat RW, Lawrence RS, Nelson RJ. Histopathologic observations after short-term implantation of two porous elastomers in dogs. *Biomaterials* 1981; **2**: 171–6.

20. Taylor SR, Gibbons DF. Effect of surface texture on soft tissue response to polymer implants. *J Biomed Mater Res* 1983; **17**: 205–27.

21. Dabrowiecki S, Svanes K, Levken J, Grong K. Tissue reaction to polypropylene mesh: a study of oedema, blood flow, and inflammation in the abdominal wall. *Eur Surg Res* 1991; **23**: 240–9.

22. Edlich RF, Panek PH, Rodeheaver GT, Turnbull VG, Kurtz LD, Edgerton MT. Physical and chemical configuration of sutures in the development of surgical infection. *Ann Surg* 1973; **177**: 679–88.

23. Stoppa RE, Rives JL, Warlaumont CR, *et al.* The use of Dacron in the repair of hernias of the groin. *Surg Clin North Am* 1984; **64**: 269–85.

24. Kaufman Z, Engelberg M, Zager M. Fecal fistula a late complication of Marlex mesh repair. *Dis Colon Rectum* 1981; **24**: 543.

25. Schneider R, Herrington Jr JL, Granada AM. The mesh repair of a diaphragmatic defect later on into the distal esophagus and stomach. *Am Surg* 1970; **45**: 339.

26. Law NW, Ellis H. Adhesion formation and peritoneal healing on prosthetic materials. *Clin Materials* 1988; 3: 95–101.

27. Reisfeld D, Schechner R, Wetsel W. Traumatic lumbar hernia. *Surg Rounds* 1989; **12**: 69–72.

28. Wantz GE. Incisional hernioplasty with Mersilene. *Surg Gynecol Obstet* 1991; **172**: 129–371.

29. Loury JN, Chevrel JP. Traitement des eventrations. Utilization simultanee du treillis de polyglactine 910 et de dacron. *Presse Med* 1983; **34**: 2116.

30. Smith DS. The use of prosthetic materials in the repair of hernias. *Surg Clin North Am* 1971; **51**: 1387.

31. Postlethwait, RW. Long-term comparative study of non-absorbable sutures. *Ann Surg* 1970; **171**: 892.

32. Usher CF. Hernia repair with Marlex mesh. In: Nyhus LM, Harkins HN, eds. *Hernia*. Philadelphia: JB Lippincott, 1964: 752.

18

Prosthetic Materials and Adhesion Formation

RICCARDO ANNIBALI AND ROBERT J FITZGIBBONS Jr

Theodor Billroth, famous European surgeon of the last century, once said: 'If we could artificially produce tissues of the density and toughness of fascia and tendon, the secret of the radical cure of hernia would be discovered'[1]. Today, prosthetic meshes are widely used for hernia repairs. The relative importance of the type of mesh on the safety and effectiveness of the repair, and consequently which material is to be preferred, is still debated. An important aspect of this discussion is the relationship between placement of a prosthetic patch and the development of intraperitoneal adhesions, together with their possible prevention.

Foreign bodies and adhesion formation

Mechanical trauma, thermal injury, infections, tissue ischaemia and foreign materials are the most important factors responsible for adhesion formation[2]. In 50–68% of cases the foreign material was talc; others were sutures, cotton lint, filaments of dressings, starch, extruded gut contents and, obviously, prosthetic grafts. A combination of different materials has also been noted (usually talc and thread)[3,4].

The common pathway leading to adhesion formation is inflammation that produces exudates containing high quantities of fibrinogen[5–7]. Fibrin clots develop, which cause adherence, at least temporary, between surfaces otherwise unattached. Granulation tissue results after colonization of the fibrin network by fibroblasts, macrophages and new blood vessels. A healthy and well-vascularized peritoneum (even with a defect) has an effective fibrinolytic system, due to a form of plasminogen activator, which is able to absorb completely the newly developed fibrinous attachments[2,8]. Prosthetic materials can considerably impair the fibrinolytic activity with two different mechanisms (Figure 18.1):

- Tight suturing and grafting induce peritoneal ischaemia. Ischaemic tissues are potent stimuli to adhesion formation and actively inhibit fibrinolysis in adjacent peritoneal tissue[5,7–10]. Thus, retention of vascularization is essential for proper, adhesion-free peritoneal healing[5,11,12].
- Mesothelial cell proliferation seems to be another important factor for adhesion prevention[13,14]; its reduction, observed in infected wounds and in those where a prosthetic mesh is applied, corresponds to decreased fibrinolytic activity[14].

Prosthetic materials

A variety of different non-absorbable and absorbable prosthetic materials has been used for repairing abdominal wall defects (Table 18.1).

Non-absorbable *silver prostheses* were first employed at the beginning of the century in Germany[15] and came into use in the USA in 1903[16]. This metal, however, had limited tensile power and was

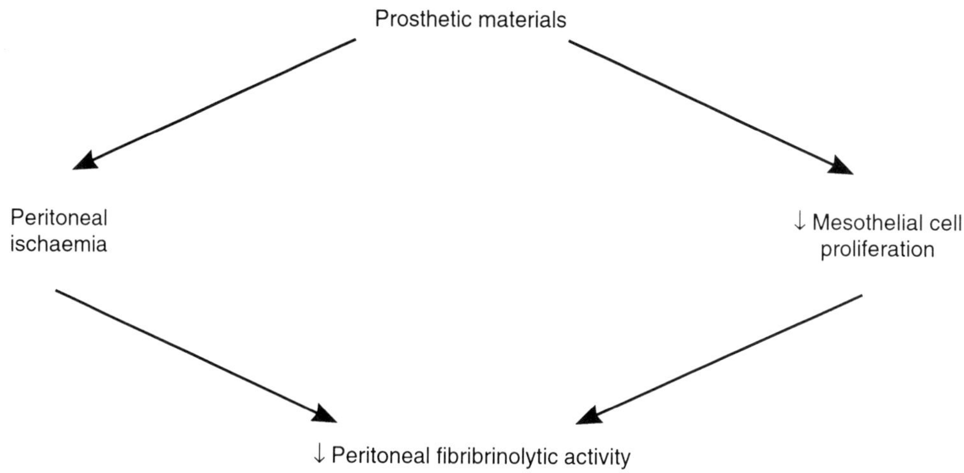

Figure 18.1: Impairment of fibrinolytic activity by prosthetic materials.

Table 18.1: Prosthetic materials for hernia repair

Non-absorbable
• Silver
• Stainless steel
• Tantalum
• Nylon net
• Polypropylene (Marlex, Prolene)
• Expanded polytetrafluoroethylene (ePTFE, Teflon, Gore-Tex)
• Polyester fibre cloth (Dacron, Mersilene)
• Polyester fibre sheeting (Mylar)
• Polyvinyl cloth (Vinyon-n)
• Acrilic cloth (Orlon)
• Carbon fibres
Absorbable
• Polyglactin mesh (Vycril)
• Polyglycolic acid (Dexon)

found to corrode and oxidize when in contact with tissue fluids, losing its strength and hardening over time[17]. Moreover, it tended to fracture, with fragments migrating to cause fistulas[1].

Tantalum mesh, first reported by Burke in 1940 and Koontz in 1948[18,19], solved the problem of corrosion and oxidation, but still tended to fragment with repeated flexion within the tissues. Serious complications related to the fragments have been reported, such as erosion of the skin and peritoneum, ulceration and bowel fistulas[1,20].

Stainless steel mesh also does not oxidize and was used mainly in the middle of this century to repair defects in the abdominal wall. It has been recently reintroduced in Europe for the same purpose, as an improved, pliable and solid mesh, named Toilinox[21]. Stainless steel, as tantalum, provides resistance to infection and a good fibrous ingrowth within the mesh. Should the mesh be removed because of infection or recurrence, however, the whole body wall would have to be removed with it and replaced, because of the strong adherence[1].

Subsequently, synthetic meshes derived by carbon polymers became available. The initial experience with nylon nets was not satisfactory, as this material tended to dissipate when reacting with the tissues, failing to resist intra-abdominal pressure and herniation. The employment of other materials, such as polyethylene, acrylic cloth (Orlon), polyester sheeting (Mylar), polyvinyl cloth (Vinyon-N) and sponge (Ivalon), for abdominal wall defects did not gain wide popularity because of the poor resistance to infection, with frequent abscess formation and need for subsequent removal[1].

Perhaps the most important development in the history of prosthetic mesh was obtained in 1958 by Usher, who reported good results with the use of a woven polypropylene mesh in incisional hernias[22]. The original product was modified in 1962, with the construction of a knitted mesh which was more malleable and could be stretched along both its axes to fit better the defect to cover. In addition, the problem of unravelling after cutting, observed with the first prototype, was eliminated[1]. Usher used this mesh widely for repairing extensive abdominal defects[23]. This type of mesh subsequently gained wide popularity also in Europe, especially in France[24]. Today, polypropylene mesh (Marlex, Prolene) is the most widely used prosthetic patch in the repair of hernias[1,17,25–27]. It is composed of a monofilament, arranged in a network fashion with large square pores of about 620 μm per side, to allow the infiltration of fibroblasts and production of dense collagen fibres as a result of a mild foreign body reaction. It has intrinsic good strength, and additional inguinal floor reinforcement occurs when fibrous ingrowth takes place. Observation for as long as 20 years in patients with conventional preperitoneal inguinal hernia repairs suggests that this material is durable[28].

Inflammatory reaction to polypropylene mesh has proven to be responsible for dense scar formation in some cases[17,29]. Complications have also been reported, including wound sepsis, mesh extrusion, erosion into intra-abdominal organs and bowel fistulas[30–33]. These considerations have stimulated a search for other prosthetic materials. Two of them became more viable with polypropylene mesh: the expanded polytetrafluoroethylene and polyester fibres.

The initial clinical experience with meshes woven from solid *polytetrafluoroethylene (PTFE, Teflon)* was unfavourable and discouraging[34]. The discovery in the 1970s of a new process to produce this material into an expanded microporous form (*ePTFE, Gore-Tex*) open new possibilities[35]. The pore size of less than 10 μm should reduce cellular penetration and fibre ingrowth. First applications were in cardiovascular surgery, Gore-Tex being used as a pericardial membrane substitute and material for vascular grafts. Since the early 1980s ePTFE has been widely used as a replacement for abdominal wall defects.

Polyester fibre mesh (Dacron, Mersilene) is a thin and pliable wide-meshed net, which allows early fixation as a result of the quick development of connective tissue through its fibres. It is well tolerated by the body and evokes and moderate fibrotic response[1,36,37].

Carbon fibres dissolve in a relatively short time, and fragments are removed by macrophages. They stimulate a considerable ingrowth of dense collagen fibres, which tend to orientate themselves along the lines of stress. Their potential carcinogenicity, however, has limited their wide use.

Theoretically, the ideal prosthesis should be strong, pliable, durable, inert, hypoallergenic, sterilizable, non-carcinogenic, stable in body fluids and resistant to infection. It should not stimulate a foreign body reaction, but allow host tissue infiltration and ingrowth for rapid incorporation, thus preventing distortion and migration and reinforcing the repair. The prosthesis should not be associated with adhesions between its abdominal surface and intra-abdominal organs, and should preferably be permeable to body fluids to prevent seroma formation[1,38–40]. In order to evaluate which mesh could best satisfy these requirements, a number of single and comparative studies to analyse the outcome of different meshes have been reported. Most studies compare the use of *polypropylene* and *expanded PTFE* to repair abdominal wall defects[14,26,27,41–43]. Three main parameters have been commonly evaluated:

- patterns of fibrous ingrowth and development of adhesions
- resistance to infection
- incidence of seroma formation.

Table 18.2: Prosthetic materials: fibrous ingrowth

	Marlex	*ePTFE*
Foreign body reaction	++or+++	+
Fibroblasts ingrowth	Extensive	< 10%
Host tissue incorporation	Complete, with dense collagen fibres (strong scar)	Encapsulated by regular and evenly distributed collagen fibres
Mesothelial cells growth pattern	Irregular	Continuous layer
EM	Rough surface	Smooth surface

Table 18.2 summarizes the features of the two different materials on which most authors agree. It must be noted, however, that different opinions are found in the literature, regarding both the specfic features of these materials and their true significance.

Patterns of fibrous ingrowth and adhesion formation

Wagner proved Marlex mesh to be the least reactive after examining several plastic prosthetic materials, including ePTFE[41]. Usher found Marlex to be intact at four years in an experimental study[44]. Elliott and Juler, on the other hand, reported microporous PTFE to be less reactive than Marlex in a rabbit study; according to these authors, this positive finding was due to a rapid fibroblastic cellular ingrowth. On the contrary, the higher foreign body reaction of polypropylene would have been responsible for its fragmentation in some areas when studied with polarized light microscopy. This phenomenon, associated with marked inflammation and dense scarring tissue production, would have caused distortion and dislocation of the Marlex mesh implant in the groin area. Expanded PTFE sheets, however, were incorporated into host tissue with little distortion and retained a flat orientation of scar tissue; it would stimulate the host to produce a 'neofascial' structure[42].

Interestingly, Amid has come to completely different conclusions. He has shown that polypropylene mesh is very well tolerated, has rapid host tissue fixation and becomes completely incorporated into the host tissue, whereas the penetration of fibroblasts from the host issue into the depth of expanded PTFE was only about 10% four years after its implantation (if associated with a superimposed infection, this was further decreased)[43]. The finding that penetration of fibroblasts from the host tissue into the depth of ePTFE is only about 10% has been confirmed by a study of Law and Ellis[14]. These authors also observed that Marlex mesh was incorporated by dense collagen fibres with a mild foreign body reaction, whilst collagen penetration of the interstices of the ePTFE patch was regular and evenly distributed. Mesothelial cells were observed in an irregular pattern over the Marlex patch, and presented as a continuous layer after four weeks on the ePTFE mesh. This has been attributed to the different appearance of the two meshes at low power scanning micrographs: the peritoneal surface of Marlex mesh was irregular but that of ePTFE was smooth. According to Taylor and Gibbons, a rounded and smooth surface stimulates encapsulation, whereas a rough one prevents it[45]. Bauer and Lamb, in separate papers, have also reported a better fibrous tissue annexation of PTFE over polypropylene, with better imbedding in fibrous tissue and a more complete incorporation into a healing wound[17,27]. Again, what seems to be an adverse factor of polypropylene for proponents of ePTFE, namely roughness of the surface or the weave of the fabric, according to Amid is a positive aspect that increases fibroblastic reactions and host tissue incorporation[43]. Actually, a criticism raised about hernia repair with PTFE is that it is based entirely on the strength of the prosthesis, as fibrous ingrowth is reduced[28]. Moreover, both Monaghan and Van der Lei have independently noted that a poorly secured ePTFE patch prevents collagen ingrowth, with an increased incidence of buttonhole hernias between sutures at the patch–fascia interface[46,47]. According to Van der Lei, this was due to the short internodal space of ePTFE patches, insufficient to allow good ingrowth[47]. Monaghan points out that poor collagen ingrowth means poor anchorage of the graft with tissue reaction alone, and recommends a running suture at the edge of the graft to prevent herniation between interrupted sutures[46]. Other advantages claimed for expanded PTFE compared with polypropylene included a lower rate of adhesion formation and a lower infection rate[17,26,48]. In Goldberg's experimental study, however, expanded PTFE increased the formation of postoperative peritoneal adhesion, possibly because it incited some degree of inflammatory and foreign body reaction[49]. Jenkins noticed the same rate and density of adhesions to both ePTFE and Marlex when these prostheses were used to repair abdominal defects in rats[50].

Resistance to infections

Marlex has been regarded as the prosthesis of choice in contaminated wounds[30,51,52], mainly because of its wide pores which should not harbour bacteria. In fact, Amid maintained that chances of infection are increased in meshes (such as ePTFE or Dacron) with pores smaller than 10 μm, as bacteria averaging 1 μm in size can hide in such small spaces and proliferate, sheltered from granulocytes[43]. Brown's opinion was contrasting: microporous structure and reduced wetting of ePTFE offer a less hospitable nidus for bacteria and improved resistance to infection with less adhesion formation[26]. Law and Ellis, however, observed the same maximum adhesion formation stimulated by the combination of infection and either ePTFE or polypropylene mesh, two and four weeks after the implantation[14,51]. DeBord has also reported a high incidence (9.6%) of infection following repair of large ventral incisional hernias with ePTFE[38].

Seroma formation

It has been said that polypropylene, being a more porous material, allows better communication of fluid collections (such as macromolecular substances or seromas) between the preperitoneal space and the infected peritoneal cavity then ePTFE[53]. In fact, a high incidence (42%) of seroma formation after repair of inguinal and incisional hernias has been reported by Monaghan[46]. There is evidence, however, that sealing of the peritoneal cavity occurs within 12 hours with or without mesh employment, and no drainage should be possible after that time[54]. A final observation is that ePTFE is not transparent like polypropylene, and does not allow staple placement under direct vision during laparoscopic hernia repair – with the possible risk of vascular and nerve injury. There seems to be general agreement that the use of Marlex at direct contact with intra-abdominal viscera involves a higher risk of fistula formation[30–33,43].

Dacron has been used both in the USA and in Europe, especially in France by the groups of Rives and Stoppa[37,55]. Hanson, after comparing abdominal wall implants of polydimethylsiloxane–Dacron and Marlex in rats whose peritoneal cavity had been contaminated with faeces, reported a significantly lower incidence of infections in the Dacron group. He attributed this result to the different host response to the two meshes: Dacron laminate was encapsulated, whilst Marlex interface was obviously characterized by tissue ingrowth. This difference would justify the different responses to the infection. Once more, fibrous ingrowth was seen not as a sign of biocompatibility but as a factor promoting bacterial proliferation and adhesion formation.

Absorbable meshes have been proposed for temporary peritoneal coverage in contaminated cases after extensive sepsis[1,43]. Favourable results with implantation of a *polyglactin (Vicryl) mesh* for inguinal hernia have been reported by Brenner[56]. In 1983, however, Lamb had reported that a Vicryl mesh was not detectable 12 weeks after the implantation in rabbit abdominal wall. At three weeks, the mesh showed peritoneal covering but there was no demonstrable fibrous tissue growth over the abdominal wall defect. The material was considered by the author to be unsatisfactory for safe and successful hernia repair[27]. Similar results were obtained by Amid in another experimental implantation study on rabbits[43]. *Polyglicolic acid mesh (Dexon)* did not induce a strong fibrous response, and consequently an adequate support to the abdominal wall, in a previously mentioned comparative study conducted by Law[14].

In conclusion, a survey of the literature generates some confusion. If one had to draw a conclusion, it might be suggested that polypropylene is best employed within the preperitoneal space, whilst ePTFE responds better to the need of intraperitoneal placement, in direct contact with intra-abdominal viscera. An additional element, however, should be taken into consideration: the difference in adhesion formation between laparotomy and laparoscopy.

In 1990 Luciano completed an experimental randomized study comparing postoperative adhesions in rabbits subjected to laser incisions over one uterine horn and over the peritoneal surface of either lower quadrant, by laparotomy or laparoscopy[57]. He demonstrated that in the laparotomy group postoperative adhesions were present not only on the tissues involved with initial injury but also at the laparotomy incision. In addition, adhesions were often found where no apparent injury had been inflicted. No adhesions were observed in the laparoscopy group. Filmar, on the other hand, reported no significant difference between the two procedures in postoperative adhesion formation in an animal model comparable to the one used by Luciano[58] The difference may be explained in that Filmar inflicted the injury with sharp scissors with subsequent bleeding which was not immediately controlled. These results support a number of clinical observations in which the incidence of adhesion formation was over 50% following open laparotomy for infertility (discovered at a second-look operation). When the procedure was accomplished laparoscopically, the incidence was considerably lower[57]. These conclusions are supported by the results of an experimental study on the swine model conducted by our group at Creighton University[59].

Laparoscopic surgery decreases the incidence of adhesion formation by eliminating incisions, reducing the amount of blood loss, preventing talc shed in the abdominal cavity, allowing precise dissection with magnification, and eliminating traumatic micro-injuries caused by the use of sponges and lint.

Prevention of adhesion formation

Several types of adjuvants have been tried to decrease the formation of adhesions. They belong to different classes.

The *high viscosity instillates* recall fluids into the peritoneal cavity, creating a sort of 'hydroflotation bath'. The aim is to reduce apposition of the serosal and peritoneal surface, thus decreasing adhesion formation during the period of epithelial regeneration[60]. They are also thought to prevent fibrin deposition. The most popular substance in this class is 32% dextran 70 (molecular weight 70 000) or Hyskon. It proved to be effective at high dosage in animal studies[61]. Human studies, however, gave contradictory results. Both a prospective randomized multicentre trial[62] and a retrospective study[63] demonstrated beneficial effects of 32% dextran 70, but two other human studies failed to reveal an advantage[64]. Moreover, various allergic reactions have been reported as side-effects following peritoneal instillation of Hyskon, though these were not frequent[60].

Another class of adjuvants is that of *mechanical barriers*. These are materials interposed between two surfaces to prevent their adherence. Various kinds of barriers have been employed: fascia, peritoneum, omentum, tunica vaginalis, vena cava, cellophane, Teflon, Silastic, nylon, etc. Reabsorbable materials have been preferred, to reduce the potentiating effect of foreign bodies on bacterial virulence. Two of them have gained some popularity. *Oxidized cellulose* (Surgicel) was first tested in laboratory animals: in two studies it did not promote the formation of adhesions when left in the abdominal cavity after surgery[65,66], but in another one adhesion formation was increased[67]. Subsequent modifications in the degree of oxidation, porosity and density led to the development of a new reabsorbable and biocompatible barrier called *Interceed* (TC7)[68,69]. Interceed has a finer knit pattern, which allows pores in the fabric to close in a few hours, as a result of swelling of the fibres. A significant reduction in adhesion formation was achieved in two rabbit studies, and subsequently confirmed in a human study conducted on 74 infertility patients treated for bilateral pelvic side-wall adhesions with laparotomy adhesiolysis and follow-up second-look laparoscopy. The

Table 18.3 Adhesion prevention: pharmacological methods

- Calcium channel antagonist
- Heparin
- Tissue plasminogen activator (t-PA)
- Sodium tolmetin in hyaluronic acid
- Carboxymethylcellulose (CMC)
- Non-steroidal anti-inflammatory drugs (NSAIDs)
- Prostacyclin analogues (Iloprost)
- Steroids
- Antihistamines

deperitonealized area of one side was covered with Interceed and the other served as a control. The covered area had a 90% improvement over control side-walls in preventing adhesion formation. In a swine study conducted at Creighton University, the average percentage of the surface area of prosthetic patches covered by adhesions compared with a composite patch of oxidized regenerated cellulose and polypropylene (Prolene, Interceed) was not significantly different[59]. Moreover, other authors report an increase in *de novo* intraperitoneal adhesion formation caused by Interceed in a murine model[70].

Several *pharmacological substances* have also been employed to try to reduce adhesion formation in experimental studies (Table 18.3). Potential good results, however, have been hampered by the difficulty of delivering the drug with effective concentration at the potential site of adhesion formation.

Conclusions

Despite promising data, we have to admit that a definitive solution to the problem of adhesion formation after intraperitoneal placement of synthetic prostheses has not yet been found. It is for this reason that most surgeons prefer the preperitoneal approach. Presumably, by covering the prosthesis with peritoneum, adhesions formed directly to the prosthesis with possible intra-abdominal organ erosion is prevented. It is not unlikely, however, that, with the development of future technology, safer and more reliable materials for intraperitoneal placement will be provided.

References

1. Read RC. Prostheses in abdominal wall hernia surgery. In: Bendavid R, ed. *Prostheses and abdominal wall surgery*. Austin: Landes Medical Publishers, 1993: (in press).
2. Breland U, Bengmark S. Peritoneum and adhesion formation. In: Bengmark S, ed. *The peritoneum and peritoneal access*. London: Wright, 1989: 122–9.
3. Weibel M, Majno G. Peritoneal adhesions and their relation to abdominal surgery. *Am J Surg* 1973; **126**: 345 53.
4. Myllarniemi H. Foreign material and adhesion formation after abdominal surgery. *Acta Chir Scand Suppl* 1967; 377.
5. Ellis H. The aetiology of post-operative abdominal adhesions an experimental study. *Br J Surg* 1962; **50**: 10–16.
6. Ellis H. The cause and prevention of postoperative intraperitoneal adhesions. *Surg Gynecol Obstet* 1971; **133**: 497–511.
7. Raftery AT. Regeneration of peritoneum. A fibrinolytic study. *J Anat* 1979; **129**: 659–64.

8. Buckmann RF, Buckmann PD, Hufnagel HW, Gervin AS. A physiologic basis for the adhesion-free healing of deperitonealized surfaces. *J Surg Res* 1976; **21**: 67–76.

9. Buckmann RF, Woods MC, Sargent L, Gervin AS. A unifying pathogenetic mechanism in the etiology of intraperitoneal adhesions. *J Surg Res* 1976; **20**: 1–5.

10. Gervin AS, Puckett CL, Silver D. Serosal hypofibrinolysis: a cause of postoperative adhesions. *Am J Surg* 1973; **125**: 80–8.

11. Robbins GF, Brunschwig A, Fook FW. Deperitonealization: clinical and experimental observations. *Ann Surg* 1949; **130**: 266.

12. Ellis H, Harrison V, Hugh TB. The healing of peritoneum and normal and abnormal conditions. *Br J Surg* 1965; **52**: 471–6.

13. Renvall S, Lehto M, Pentinen R. Development of peritoneal fibrosis occurs under the mesothelial cell layer. *J Surg Res* 1987; **43**: 407–12.

14. Law NH, Ellis H. Adhesion formation and peritoneal healing on prosthetic materials. *Clin Mater* 1988; **3**: 95–101.

15. Geopel R. Uber die verschliessung von bruchpforten durch einheilung geflochtener fertiger silberdrahtnetze. *Verh Deutsch Ges Pathol* 1900; **29**: 4.

16. Bartlett W. An improved filigree for the repair of large defects in the abdominal wall. *Ann Surg* 1903; **38**: 47–62.

17. Bauer JL, Salky BA, Gelernt IM, Kreel I. Repair of large abdominal wall defects with expanded polytetrafluoroethylene (PTFE). *Ann Surg* 1987; **206**: 765–9.

18. Burke GL. The corrosion of metals in the tissues; and an introduction to tantalum. *Can Med Assoc J* 1940; **43**: 125–8.

19. Koontz AR. Preliminary report on the use of tantalum mesh in the repair of ventral hernias. *Ann Surg* 1948; **127**: 1079–85.

20. Lam CR, Szilagy DE, Puppendahl M. Tantalum gauze in the repair of large postoperative ventral hernias. *Arch Surg* 1948; 57: 234–44.

21. Validire J, Imbaud P, Dutet D, Duron JJ. Large abdominal incisional hernias: repair by fascial approximation reinforced with a stainless steel mesh. *Br J Surg* 1986; **73**: 8–10.

22. Usher FC, Ochsner J, Tuttle Jr LLD. Use of Marlex mesh in the repair of incisional hernias. *Ann Surg* 1958; **24**: 969–74.

23. Usher FC, Fries JG, Oschner JL, Tuttle UD. Marlex mesh – a new plastic mesh for replacing tissue defects. *Arch Surg* 1959; **78**: 138–45.

24. Stoppa RE, Warlaumont CR. The preperitoneal approach and prosthetic repair of groin hernia. In: Nyhus LM, Condon RE, eds. *Hernia* 3rd ed. Philadelphia: JB Lippincott, 1989: 199–225.

25. Smith DS. The use of prosthetic materials in the repair of hernias. *Surg Clin North Am* 1971; **51**: 1387.

26. Brown GL, Richardson JD, Malangoni MA, Tobin GR, Ackerman D, Polk HC. Comparison of prosthetic materials for abdominal wall reconstruction in the presence of contamination and infection. *Ann Surg* 1985; **201**: 705–11.

27. Lamb JP, Vitale T, Kaminski DL. Comparative evaluation of synthetic meshes used for abdominal wall replacement. *Surgery* 1983; **93**: 643–8.

28. Filipi CJ, Fitzgibbons RJ, Salerno GM, Hart RO. Laparoscopic herniorraphy. *Surg Clin North Am* 1992; **72**: 1109–24.

29. Toy FK, Smoot RT. Toy–Smoot laparoscopic hernioplasty. *Surg Laparosc Endosc* 1991; **1**: 151–5.

30. Voyles CR, Richardson JD, Bland KI, *et al.* Emergency abdominal wall reconstruction with polypropylene mesh. Short-term benefits versus long-term complications. *Ann Surg* 1981; **194**: 219–23.

31. Schneider R, Herrington Jr JL, Granada AM. Marlex mesh in repair of a diaphragmatic defect later eroding into the distal esophagus and stomach. *Am Surg* 1979; **45**: 337–9.

32. Kaufman Z, Engelberg M, Zager M. Fecal fistula: a late complication of Marlex mesh repair. *Dis Colon Rectum* 1981; **24**: 543–4.

33. Stone HH, Fabian TC, Turkelson ML, Jurkiewicz MJ. Management of acute full-thickness losses of the abdominal wall. *Ann Surg* 1981; **193**: 612–18.

34. Gibson LD, Stafford CE. Synthetic mesh repair of abdominal wall defects. *Am Surg* 1964; **30**: 481–6.

35. Soyer T, Lempinen M, Cooper P, Norton L, Eisemann B. A new venous prosthesis. *Surgery* 1972; **72**: 864–72.

36. Arnaud JP, Eloy R, Weill-Bousson M, *et al.* Resistance et tolerance biologique de 6 protheses inertes utilisees dans la reparation de la paroi abdominale. *J Chir* 1977; **113**: 85–100.

37. Stoppa RE, Rives JL, Warlamount CR, Palot JP, Verhaeghe P, Delattre JF. The use of Dacron in the repair of the hernias of the groin. *Surg Clin North Am* 1984; **64**: 296–85.

38. DeBord JR, Wyffels PL, Marshall S, Miller G, Marshall WH. Repair of large ventral incisional hernias with expanded polytetrafluoroethylene prosthetic patches. *Postgrad Gen Surg* 1992; **4**: 156–60.

39. Cumberland VH. A preliminary report on the use of prefabricated nylon weave in the repair of ventral hernia. *Med J Aust* 1952; **1**: 143.

40. LeBlanc KA, Booth WV. Repair of primary and secondary inguinal hernias using an expanded polytetrafluoroethylene patch. *Contemp Surg* 1992; **41**: 29–32.

41. Wagner MW. Evaluation of diverse plastic and cutis prostheses in a growing host. *Surg Gynecol Obstet* 1970; **130**: 1077–81.

42. Elliott MP, Juler GL. Comparison of Marlex mesh and microporous Teflon sheets when used for hernia repair in the experimental animal. *Am J Surg* 1979; **137**: 342–5.

43. Amid PK, Shulman AG, Lichtenstein IL. Selecting synthetic mesh for the repair of groin hernia. *Postgrad Gen Surg* 1992; **4**: 150–5.

44. Usher FC. Hernia repair with Marlex mesh. In: Nyhus LM, Condon RE, eds. *Hernia*. Philadelphia: JB Lippincott, 1978: 561–80.

45. Taylor SR, Gibbons DF. Effect of surface texture on soft tissue response to polymer implants. *J Biomed Mater Res* 1983; **17**: 205–27.

46. Monaghan RA, Meban S. Expanded polytetrafluoroethylene patch in hernia repair: a review of clinical experience. *Can J Surg* 1991; **34**: 502–5.

47. Van der Lei B, Bleichrodt RP, Simmermacher RK, *et al.* Expanded polytetrafluoroethylene patch for the repair of large abdominal wall defects. *Br J Surg* 1989; **76**: 803–5.

48. Murphy JL, Freeman JB, Dionne PG. Comparison of Marlex and Gore-Tex to repair abdominal wall defects in the rat. *Can J Surg* 1989; **32**: 244–7.

49. Goldberg JM, Toledo AA, Mitchell DE. An evaluation of the Gore-Tex surgical membrane for the prevention of postoperative peritoneal adhesions. *Obstet Gynecol* 1987; **70**: 846–8.

50. Jenkins SD, Klamer TW, Parteka J, Condon RE. A comparison of prosthetic materials used to repair abdominal wall defects. *Surgery* 1983; **94**: 392–8.

51. Law NW, Ellis H. A comparison of polypropylene mesh and expanded PTFE patch for the repair of contaminated abdominal wall defects – an experimental study. *Surgery* 1991; **109**: 652–5.

52. Schmitt Jr HJ, Grinnan GLB. Use of Marlex mesh in infected abdominal war wound. *Am J Surg* 1967; **113**: 825–8.

53. Goris RA. Ogilvie's method applied to infected wound disruption. *Arch Surg* 1980; **115**: 1103–7.

54. Boyd WC. Use of Marlex mesh in acute loss of the abdominal wall due to infection. *Surg Gynecol Obstet* 1977; **144**: 251–2.

55. Rives J. Surgical treatment of the inguinal hernia with Dacron patch. *Int Surg* 1967; **47**: 360–1.

56. Brenner J. Implantation of Vicryl patch for inguinal hernia. Presented at the International Fascia Congress, Hamburg, Germany, May 1991.

57. Luciano AA. Laparotomy versus laparoscopy. In: di Zerega GS, Malinak LR, Diamond MP, Linsky CB, eds. *Treatment of post surgical adhesions.* New York: Wiley–Liss, 1990: 35–44.

58. Filmar S, Gomel V, McComb PF. Operative laparoscopy versus open abdominal surgery: a comparative study on postoperative adhesion formation in the rat model. *Fetil Steril* 1987; **48**: 486–9.

59. Salerno GM, Fitzgibbons Jr RJ, Corbitt RJ, Hart RO, Filipi CJ. Laparoscopic inguinal hernia repair. In: Zucker KA, ed. *Surgical laparoscopy update.* St Louis, Mo: Quality Medical Publishing, 1993: 373–94.

60. Diamond MP, Hershlag A. Adhesion formation/reformation. In: di Zerega GS, Malinak LR, Diamond MP, Linsky CB, eds. *Treatment of post surgical adhesions.* New York: Wiley–Liss, 1990: 23–33.

61. Mazuji MK, Fadhi HA. Peritoneal adhesions. *Arch Surg* 1965; **91**: 872.

62. Adhesion Study Group. Reduction of post-operative pelvic adhesions with intraperitoneal 32% Dextran 70: a prospective, randomized clinical trial. *Fertil Steril* 1983; **40**: 612–19.

63. Rosenberg SM, Board JA. High-molecular-weight dextran in human infertility surgery. *Am J Obstet Gynecol* 1984; **148**: 380–5.

64. Diamond MP, De Cherney AH, Linsky CB, Cunningham T, Constantine B. Assessment of carboxymethylcellulose and 32% Dextran 70 for prevention of adhesions in a rabbit uterine horn model. *Int J Fertil* 1988; **33**: 278–82.

65. Larsson B, Nisell H, Granberg I. Surgicel – an absorbable hemostatic material – in prevention of peritoneal adhesions in rats. *Acta Chir Scand* 1978; **144**: 375–8.

66. Raftery A. Absorbable haemostatic materials and intraperitoneal adhesion formation. *Br J Surg* 1980; **67**: 57.

67. Hixson C, Swanson LA, Friedman CI. Oxidized cellulose for preventing adnexal adhesions. *J Reprod Med* 1986; **28**: 662.

68. Diamond MP, Linsky CB, Cunningham T, Constantine B, di Zerega G, DeCherney AH. A model for sidewall adhesions in the rabbit: reduction by an absorbable barrier. *Microsurgery* 1987; **8**: 197–200.

69. Interceed (TC7) Adhesion Barrier Study Group. Prevention of postsurgical adhesions by Interceed (TC7), an absorbable adhesion barrier: a prospective, randomized multicenter clinical study. *Fertil Steril* 1989; **51**: 933–8.

70. Hanney AF, Doty E. Murine peritoneal injury and de novo adhesion formation caused by oxidized-regenerated cellulose (Interceed*[TC7]) but not expanded polytetrafluoroethylene (Gore-Tex* Surgical Membrane). *Fertil Steril* 1992; **57**: 202–8.

19

Rationale for the Use of e-PTFE in the Intraperitoneal Position

FREDERICK K TOY

The Gortex peritoneal onlay laparoscopic hernioplasty has been performed on 170 patients with a total of 212 hernioplasties over the past 32 months, from February 1991 to August 1993. In this

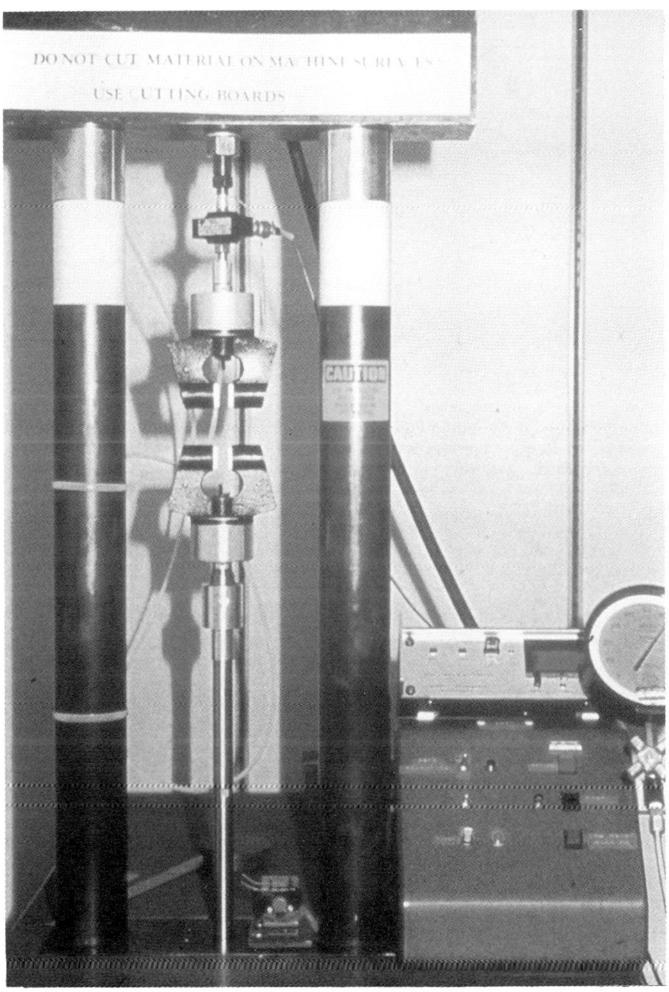

Figure 19.1: Standard testing machine used by industry to measure materials' tensile strength.

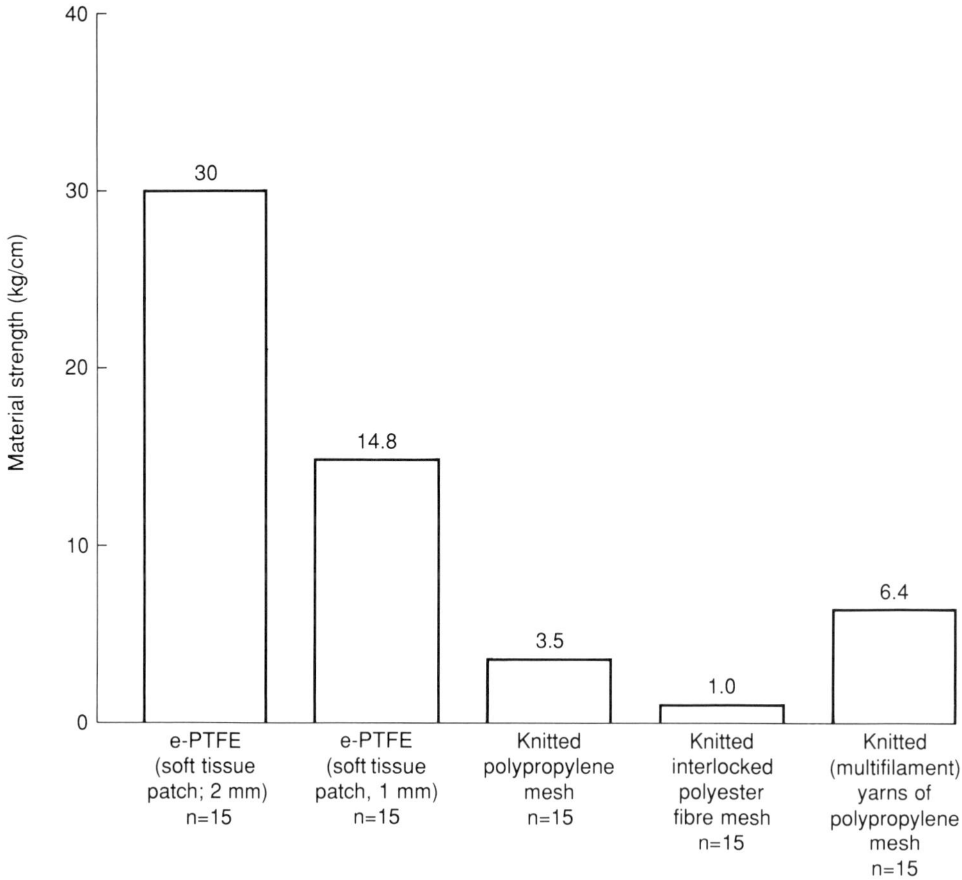

Figure 19.2: Material strength comparison.

chapter I discuss my rationale for choosing e-PTFE rather than the other prosthetic biomaterials available for this procedure.

Choosing one prosthetic biomaterial over another should be made after a sound and thorough review of the experimental and clinical data available. This comparison of biomaterials is divided into mechanical and biological characteristics. The mechanical characteristics are strength, fixation retention and durability. The biological characteristics are infectability, adhesion formation and erosion/fistulization.

In setting the criteria of an ideal biomaterial, strength and fixation/retention are of obvious concern and importance, not only during the initial postoperative phase but also in the long term. A biomaterial must be able to serve its intended use over the life span of the patient, with no major complications. Therefore, durability is of importance as well.

To evaluate the strength, the various biomaterials were analysed on a standard testing machine (Figure 19.1). Ultimate tensile-strength testing illustrates the ability of a material to withstand application of forces at high rates. The 1 mm e-PTFE is two to 14 times stronger than the polypropylene or polyester mesh materials (Figure 19.2). It should be noted that all of these biomaterials have adequate tensile strength and have been super-engineered for their intended application. It is a commonly stated misbelief among many surgeons that the dense fibrous incorporation of the macromesh materials is necessary to increase the strength of the repair. There

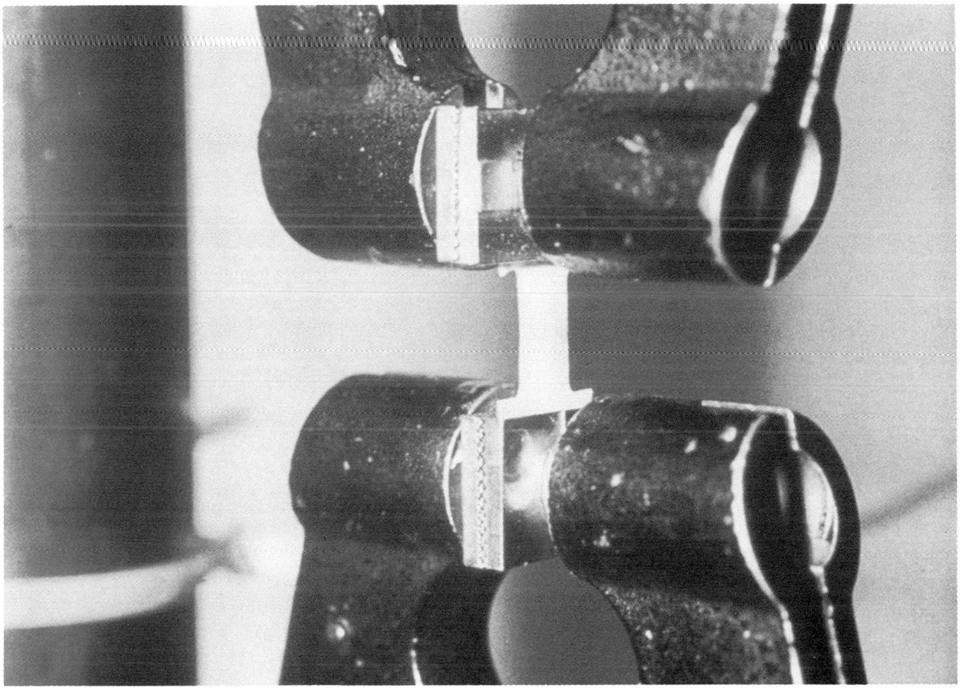

Figure 19.3: Biomaterial placed in the testing machine.

is a large volume of study on wound repair[1–8] that has revealed that this dense fibrous reaction forms in concentric whorls of fibrous tissue instead of the normal longitudinal fibres of fascia. This scar tissue never regains the strength of normal tissue, and it is converted from elastic, pliable tissue to a contracted, unelastic, brittle mass.

The materials were also tested to determine fixation retention values. Fixation retention is important because of the high impact forces the material may experience *in vivo* (ie coughing, sneezing, muscle contraction, etc.) Fixation retention testing defines the resistance of a biomaterial to the pull-out of sutures or staples at very high rates. Rectangular samples of prosthetic material were placed in the testing machine (Figure 19.3) in which a pin passes through the material and is then pulled apart at a high rate. The force at which the material failed was recorded. Fixation retention for the 1 mm e-PTFE (0.9 kg/PIN) is equivalent to or several times stronger than the meshes (0.32 kg/PIN) (Figure 19.4).

To evaluate durability, a test was designed to mimic the different forces that would be placed on a material *in vivo* over time. Muscle contraction, flexing, sneezing and coughing can all produce significant strain on a material. Therefore, a material must not only be strong and have adequate fixation retention, but be durable as well. The material was placed in a device similar to the fixation pull-out test. A static load of 8 lb (3.6 kg) was applied, with an intermittent load of 16 lb (7.2 kg) applied every second. Each cycle was recorded until the material failed. The durability of 1 mm e-PTFE (1320.9 cycles) is considerably greater than the meshes (50–0.1 cycles) (Figure 19.5).

In conclusion, considering the mechanical characteristics, the 1 mm e-PTFE is stronger, has better fixation retention values and is more durable than any other biomaterial available. These features, as well as good handling characteristics, can better meet the demands of a wide variety of repairs and applications than the mesh materials.

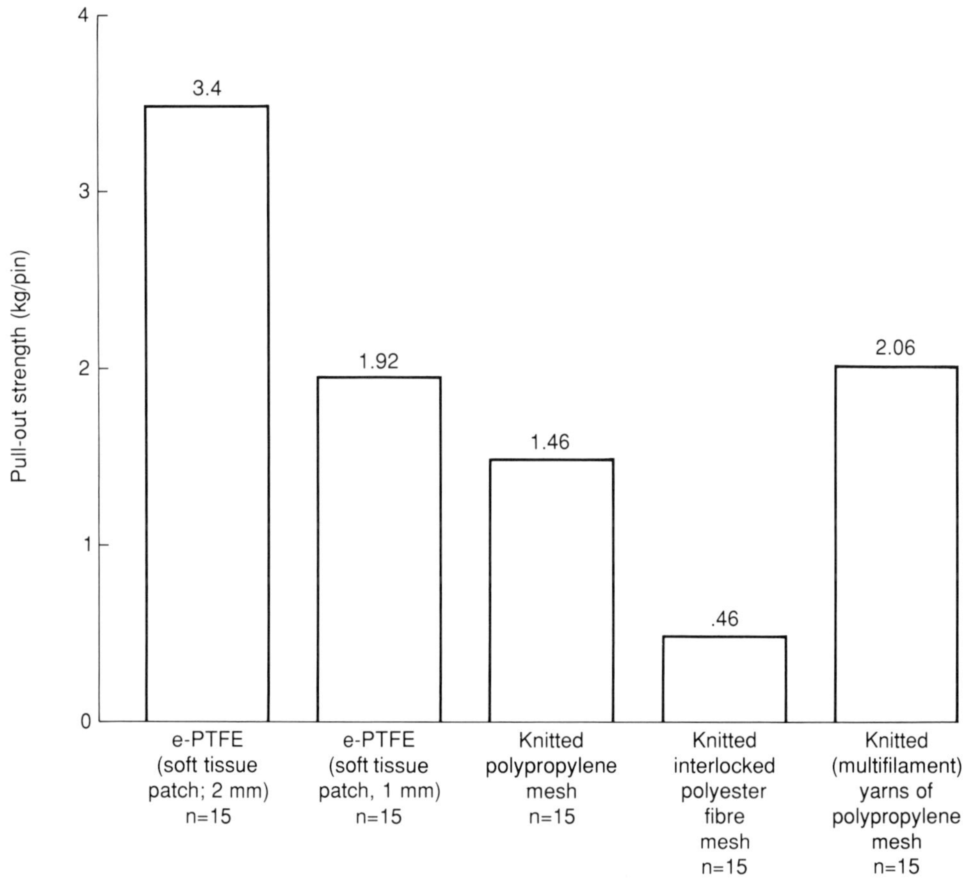

Figure 19.4: Fixation retention strength comparison.

Biological response

Biocompatibility of an implanted material encompasses not only the nature of the response from the surrounding tissue but also the inherent characteristic of the material itself. The e-PTFE is inert, preventing significant inflammatory responses, with a microstructure that provides latticework for tissue ingrowth. Monofilament, as well as multifilament, mesh materials elicit a mild to severe inflammatory response with encapsulation of the material. It must be understood that *ingrowth* and *encapsulation* are microscopic terms. Ingrowth is characterized by infiltration of blood elements, fibrin and proteinaceous material throughout the microstructure. This is followed by histiocytes and fibroblasts, with deposition of collagen in the interstices, providing firm anchorage (Figure 19.6). At the interface, there is fibrous tissue attachment to the material surface (ie e-PTFE). Encapsulation is characterized by infiltration of acellular blood elements only (fibrin, proteinaceous material). There is minimal localized attachment of tissue to material surface and no collagen deposition into the interstices. The fibrous tissue encircles the material and prevents cellular migration in the interstices. The material is isolated, and there is no incorporation by host tissue (ie polypropylene meshes).

During the normal healing of any wound, there are three phases: inflammation, granulation tissue formation and rebuilding process. Natural host tissue healing events take place when e-PTFE soft tissue patch (pore size/internodal space average 22 μm (17–41 μm)) (Figure 19.7) is placed in a wound for the repair of a wall defect or hernia. Serous fluid and blood cells infiltrate the e-PTFE structure. White blood cells (WBCs)/leucocytes (average diameter 14–20 μm) surrounded and

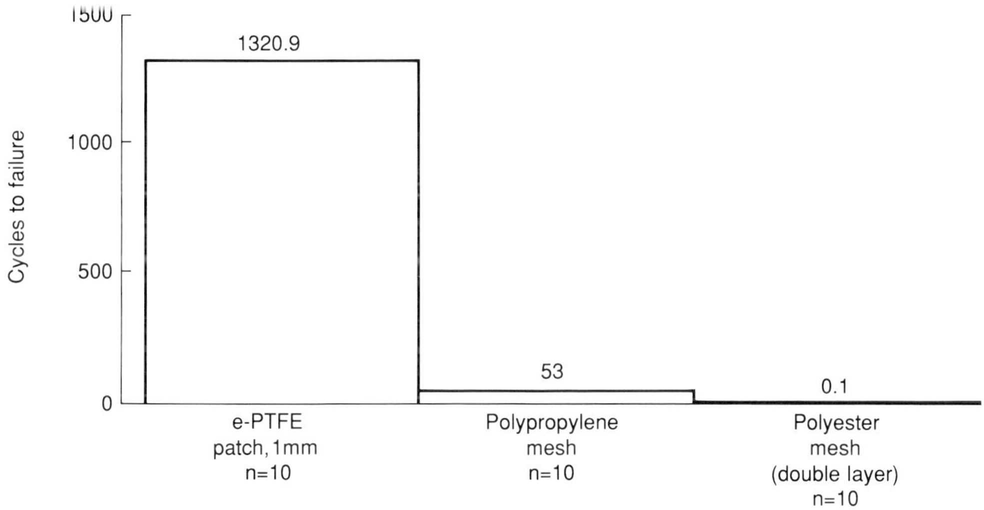

Figure 19.5: Cyclic flex analysis.

infiltrate the e-PTFE within the wound. Fibroblasts (average 15 μm wide × 50 μm long) appear within the material, usually between 14 and 28 days (as early as seven days) postoperatively and produce collagen along the e-PTFE structure and deposit collagen into the interstices of the e-PTFE. The tissue around the e-PTFE exhibits minimal contracture because of the specific orientation of the collagen fibres. The collagen fibres align in parallel with the e-PTFE surface and perpendicular to the surface within the material (Figure 19.8). Such biaxial alignment may be associated with minimal contracture of the tissues surrounding the e-PTFE. The resulting scar tissue is smooth and pliable. Other foreign implant materials (eg sutures and meshes, with pore sizes ranging from approximately 2 to 10 mm between filaments and 0–10 μm between filaments at points of contact) are also surrounded by collagen fibres and fibre bundles. These collagen fibres are parallel and concentrically aligned, encapsulating the individual mesh fibres (Figure 19.9). In contrast to the biaxial alignment of the collagen fibres with e-PTFE, the concentric alignment around the mesh filaments and the parallel alignment of the collagen fibres between the mesh filaments through the thickness of a mesh may be related to the reported distortion and scar contracture of mesh materials.

In experimental studies as well as in clinical observations, e-PTFE was found to have complete fibroblastic cellular ingrowth through the interstices of the material at eight weeks, with only minimal inflammatory reaction. With the parallel orientation of the scar tissue, the e-PTFE retained a flat orientation of graft to the fibrous tissue, forming a 'neofasica'. In contrast, polypropylene meshes has rapid formation of dense scar tissue with marked inflammatory tissue reaction. The fibrous tissue is concentrically aligned around the mesh fibres, causing the graft to become encased in a whorled mass of dense scar. Contracture of the scar tissue caused graft distortion and loss of anatomical position. This is felt to be a contributing factor to recurrences when prosthetic meshes are used.

Infectibility

The incidence of wound infection with a standard anterior groin repair has been approximately 1% for primary repairs and 3% for recurrent repairs[9]. The incidence has been even lower with

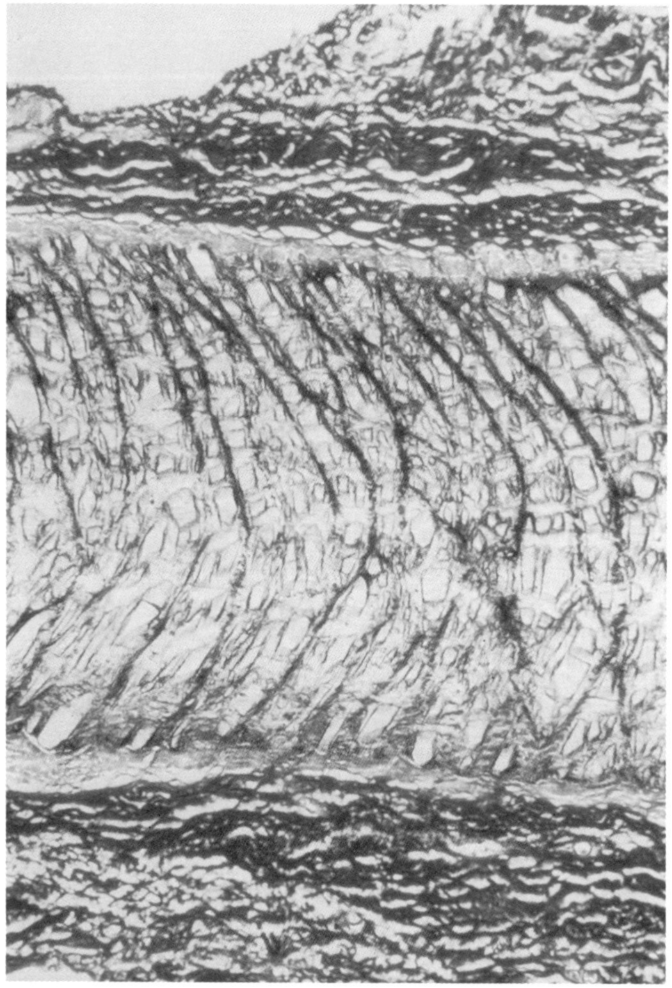

Figure 19.6: Onlay inguinal hernia repair: 25 months' implant duration. Good collagen penetration of 45% of thickness of the soft tissue patch wall is observed from both surfaces in localized regions throughout the material thickness. ×25

laparoscopic hernioplasties, as one would expect, as no incisions are required in areas carrying a high burden of skin bacteria. The prosthetic material in a laparoscopic hernioplasty is passed into the peritoneal cavity or preperitoneal space via trocars and should never touch the skin. This makes the debate of infectibility somewhat irrelevant in choosing a prosthetic for laparoscopic hernioplasty. However, for wound contamination to progress to wound infection, the concentration of organisms has to be 10^6 per gram of tissue for most pathogens. The host's defence system will immobilize and phagocytose and, with delay in the subsequent wound healing phases, try to rid the wound of bacteria with and without the help of antibiotics.

When a prosthetic material is introduced into the wound, the concentration of micro-organisms necessary to turn the wound contamination into infection significantly decreases (ie 10^3 per gram tissue decrease)[10]. Bacteria and tissue cells are competing to reach the prosthetic material. Whichever (bacteria or tissue cell) arrives at the foreign material first will penetrate, adhere to and populate the prosthesis to the greater degree. The host tissue defence mechanism works similarly to normal wound healing, using neutrophils and macrophages to immobilize and phagocytose foreign material and

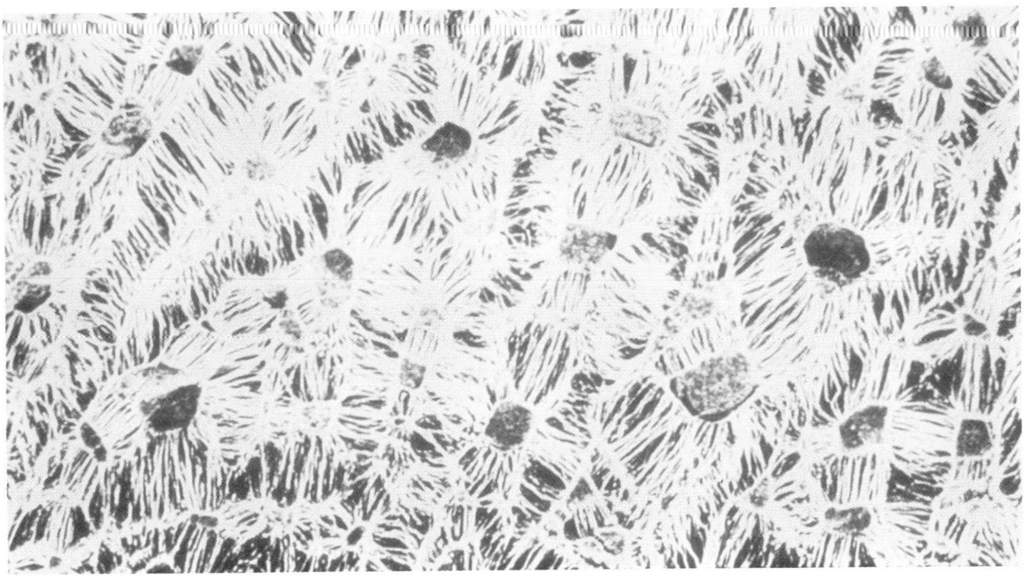

Figure 19.7: Surface view of a Gore-Tex soft tissue patch.

bacteria. Depending on the physical structure of the prosthesis and localized infection, the host may be able to resolve the infection.

Tissue ingrowth within the e-PTFE is important because it fills the internodal void spaces, thus limiting access to bacteria. The hydrophobic nature of the e-PTFE appears to slow initial bacterial advance into the material and inhibit 'wicking' of the micro-organisms. Wicking is the fluid-phase transport of bacteria. The e-PTFE structure (average pore size 22 μm) seems to prohibit harbouring of bacteria and limits them (the bacteria) to the periphery of the e-PTFE. This reaction seems to prevent the rapid spread of infection. As a result, WBCs (neutrophil average size 14 μm) gain ready access to the bacteria and appear to play an active role in ridding the wound of bacteria, while fibrous tissue keeps contamination localized.

In comparison, mesh materials are considered to be macroporous. Some regions between the weave filaments at points of contact are too small for WBC and fibroblastic penetration. However, these spaces remain large enough to harbour bacteria and permit bacterial access ('wicking') along material filaments. This wicking effect can complicate and potentially inhibit the success resolution of infection.

Elek *et al.*[10] demonstrated that, when foreign bodies are present, fewer organisms are required to produce a clinical infection. The foreign body acts synergistically by decreasing the concentration of bacteria necessary to produce an infection. The adherence of bacteria to a foreign body is a very complex process, involving stereospecific interaction between bacterial ligands and receptor sites on the foreign body surface[11]. Sugarman[12] showed that the magnitude of the adherence is related to the type of bacteria and foreign body involved in the interaction. Brown *et al.* demonstrated that the e-PTFE patches consistently had 100-fold fewer organisms per square centimetre than did the polypropylene meshes in the absence of antibiotics or with antibiotics administered after contamination with *Staphylococcus aureus*. They concluded that e-PTFE is more resistant to the production of clinical infection if contamination occurs intraoperatively. This conclusion is supported by a great deal of clinical experience, particularly in the vascular literature, where PTFE has been used since 1976[13–21]. This was felt to be secondary to the porous structure (22 μm) and the hydrophobic properties of e-PTFE, which result in a less hospitable nidus for bacterial adherence.

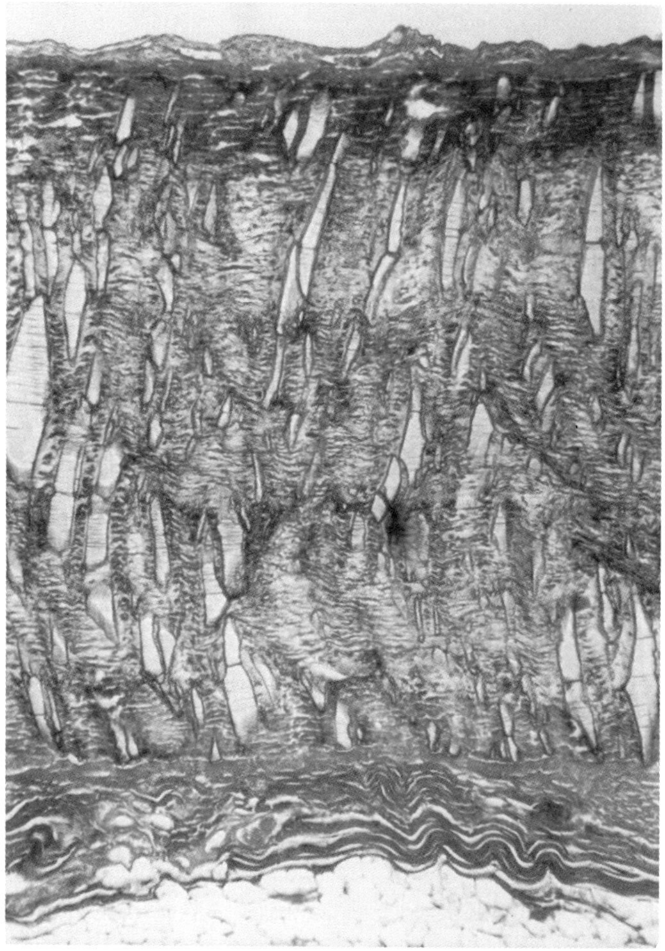

Figure 19.8: (a) Collagen fibrils laid down along the soft tissue patch surface and perpendicular to the surface within the internodal spaces (incorporation). Full-thickness abdominal wall repair, rabbit model, three-month implant. × 25.

Adhesions

Adhesions may be categorized in three ways:

- *fibrinous*, which resolve spontaneously within a few weeks
- *omental*, which cause no persistent problem for the patient
- *fibrous*, which may form into tendinous bands capable of constricting visceral organs.

The chief concerns regarding peritoneal adhesions is eventual bowel obstruction. An estimated 30% of all intestinal obstructions are caused by adhesions. Experimental studies and clinical experience with repairs of full-thickness abdominal wall defects have shown a lower incidence and grade of visceral adhesions formation and/or adhesion-related complications with e-PTFE when compared to mesh material[10,21–27]. Peritoneal injury and all types of foreign materials will stimulate adhesion formation. In experimental studies, laparotomy incisions closed with monofilament suture had a 30% incidence of adhesions. The incidence of adhesions to e-PTFE, polypropylene mesh and polyester mesh was 36%, 82.4% and 100%, respectively (Figure 19.10). Lennox and Ellis[22] showed

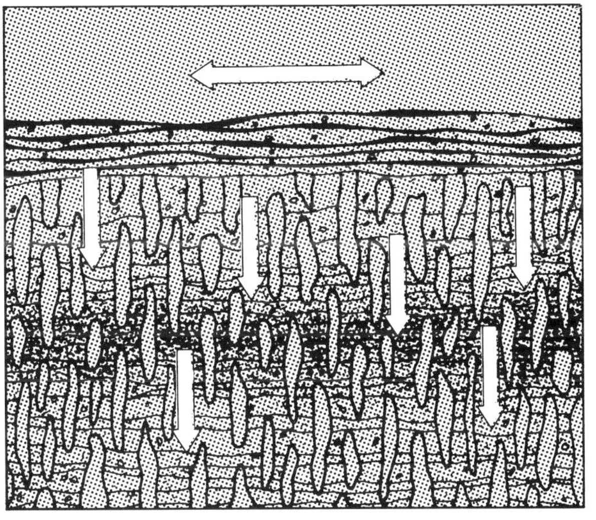

Figure 19.8: *continued* (b) Schematic depicting biaxial alignment of collagen fibrils around and within the soft tissue patch.

that fibrinous adhesions are replaced by fibrous tissue at about ten days, which then remain permanent. This conversion is prevented by the fibrinolytic activity of the peritoneum, which is divided equally between the mesothelial and submesothelial layers.

Studies by Law and Ellis[22] demonstrated that e-PTFE would support a continuous layer of mesothelial cells on the peritoneal surface. The collagen penetration of the interstices of e-PTFE was regular and evenly distributed. The mesothelial cells would first appear at approximately two weeks after implantation and became a continuous layer at approximately four weeks. With Marlex mesh, the mesothelial cells were observed in an irregular pattern and were found only in association with fatty or omental adhesions. Law and Ellis demonstrated that adhesion formation to e-PTFE and the mesh materials is inversely related to the number of mesothelial cells on the peritoneal surface. In the presence of infection, mesothelial cells are found infrequently with a reduction in fibrinolytic activity, such that the fibrinous adhesions are not removed and develop into dense fibrous adhesions that are permanent. This was confirmed in infected wound studies by Brown *et al.* and Law and Ellis[23], in which there was increase in adhesions with both e-PTFE and polypropylene mesh in the presence of infection.

If adhesions form to the e-PTFE, they usually include and originate at the line of fixation, which is a point of mechanical rigidity, tissue compression and/or tissue ischaemia. The adhesions to the e-PTFE have been reported to be of a filmy nature and easily dissectable. The smooth surface of the e-PTFE and associated mild foreign-body response appear to provide minimal interference with peritoneal healing and neomesothelialization. The chemical nature and physical structure of mesh materials are likely factors in the formation of adhesions. Because of their rigidity and rough surface structure, meshes can irritate and injure the underlying tissue structures, causing inflammatory fibroplasia and a moderate foreign-body response. The re-formation of the mesothelial layer is somewhat retarded and incomplete, as a result of the irregular surface and dense scar formation around the mesh filaments. The incidence of adhesions in experimental trials of mesh materials ranges from 80% to 90%.

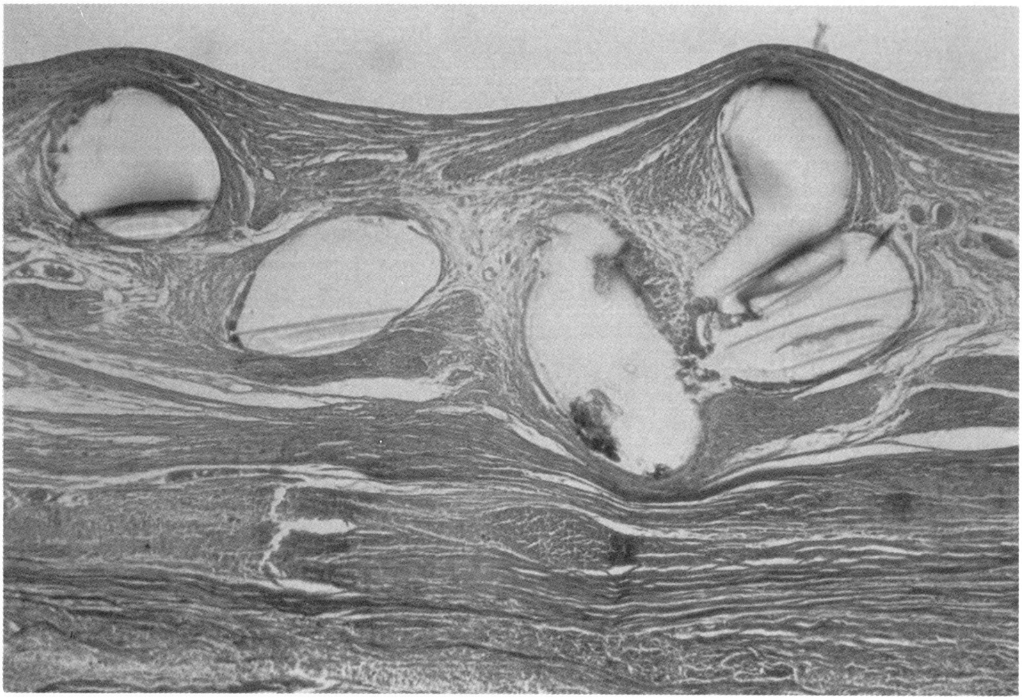

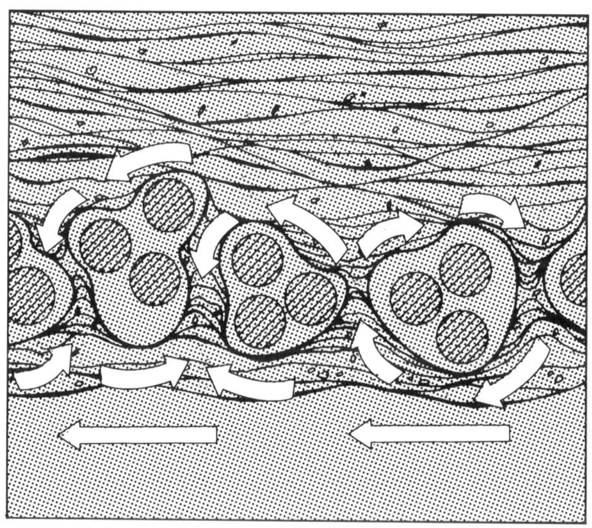

Figure 19.9: (a) Parallel and concentric alignment of collagen fibril bundles around polypropylene mesh. Collagen fibril bundles are laid down around and between each of the polypropylene filaments (encapsulation). Full-thickness abdominal wall repair, rabbit model, three-month implant. × 25. (b) Schematic depicting parallel and concentric alignment of collagen fibril bundles around polypropylene mesh.

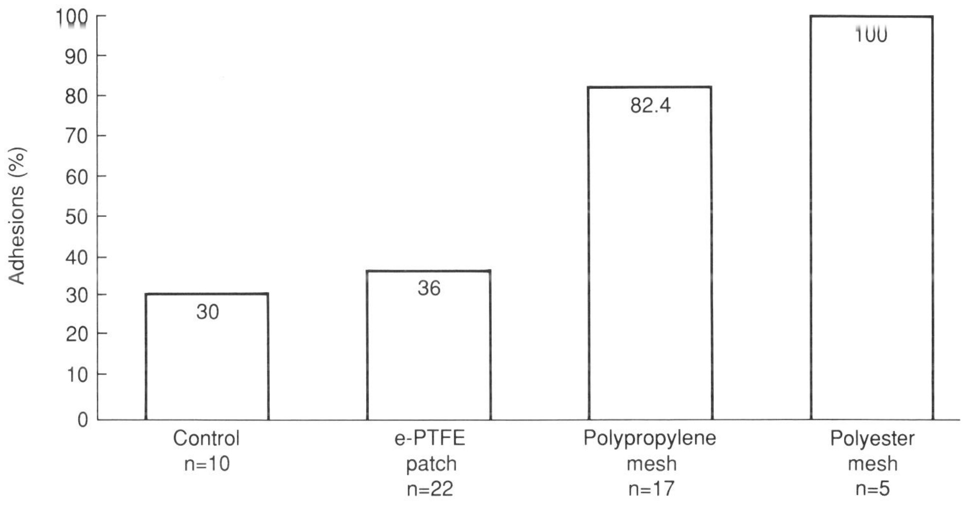

Figure 19.10: Visceral adhesions at 12 weeks postoperatively.

Erosion-fistulization

Erosion of abdominal viscera resulting in obstruction, abscess and fistula formation is the cardinal determining factor for choice of prosthetic material in the peritoneal position. Experimental studies and clinical experience with polypropylene mesh are replete with complications of erosion and fistulization[23,27–35].

e-PTFE has been used in the peritoneal cavity for vascular bypass since 1976 and for hernia repair since 1983, with no clinical cases of bowel strangulation or fistula formation reported. In addition, e-PTFE has been used for the repair of diaphragmatic defects, slings for repair of rectal prolapse, bladder and urethral suspension, and bands for vertically banded gastroplasties. In all of these procedures, the e-PTFE is placed adjacent to hollow viscus organs, with no reports of erosion or fistulization. On the contrary, erosions and fistulization have been seen in all of these procedures with the use of polypropylene meshes. The mechanism for erosion and fistula formation is similar to that for adhesion formation, with the addition of time.

Mesh materials have a moderate to severe inflammatory and foreign-body response. They do not promote neomesothelialization and, therefore, cause dense fibrous adhesions. The mesh materials also have a rigid and abrasive surface. If bowel, with its continuous wall motion (peristalsis), is densely adherent to this rigid, abrasive surface, in time it will erode through the wall and fistulize.

On the contrary, e-PTFE is inert, has a mild inflammatory and foreign-body response, and promotes rapid proliferation of mesothelial cells on the peritoneal surface. It also has a smooth, pliable, non-abrasive surface which does not promote erosion and fistula formation.

Economics

Economics is certainly an important consideration when choosing any medical supplies, especially in today's environment of competitive marketing. It is often said that the e-PTFE is more expensive than the polypropylene meshes. When compared, indeed it was. When comparing products by their

Table 19.1: Comparison of costs of patches

Product	*Size*	*Price [per cm²]*
Gore-Tex soft tissue patch	7.5 cm × 10 cm × 1 mm (3 × 4 in)	$115 [$1.53]
Marlex mesh	7.5 × 15 cm (3 × 6 in)	$90 [$0.80]
Surgi-Pro	7.5 × 12.5 cm (3 × 5 in)	$46 [$0.49]
Prolene	(6 × 11 cm)	$36 [$0.55]

Gore-Tex is a registered trademark of W.L. Gore & Associates Inc. Marlex is a registered trademark licensed to C.R. Bard Inc. Surgi-Pro is a registered trademark of United States Surgical Inc. Prolene is a registered trademark of Ethicon Inc.

Table 19.2: Comparison of time costs*

Difference between 40 and 60 minutes' operating room time	$318
Anaesthesia time	15
Additional expense	$333
Difference between 30 and 60 minutes' operating room time	$678
Anaesthesia time	52
Additional expense	$730

* Nanticoke Memorial Hospital, Seaford, Delaware

closest available sizes, e-PTFE was found to be $25 more expensive than Marlex (the most commonly used polypropylene mesh today) and $79 more than the cheapest mesh. When comparing by square centimetre, e-PTFE is 48% more expensive than Marlex and 68% more expensive than the cheapest mesh (Table 19.1).

Several points need to be made when looking at the economic impact of prosthetic choice. The use of e-PTFE does not require as much peritoneal dissection, no peritoneal flaps have to be elevated, and no peritoneal closure is required, as is with the transabdominal preperitoneal repair (TAPP). It is also a much easier dissection than with the extraperitoneal repair. The stapled peritoneal onlay with e-PTFE takes easily 20–30 minutes less operative time. I found at my hospital (Nanticoke Memorial Hospital, Seaford, Delaware) that the savings for 20 and 30 minutes of operating time were $333 and $730, respectively (Table 19.2).

It is quite obvious that the increased cost of e-PTFE is made up for several times by the savings in operating time.

In addition, a considerable number of bowel obstructions and fistulas have been reported at the major endoscopic and hernia meetings recently. They were all associated with the use of the polypropylene meshes, either as peritoneal onlay or transabdominal preperitoneal laparoscopic repair. Just one of these complications per year would grossly negate any cost saving with the polypropylene meshes.

Conclusions

In summary, e-PTFE is the strongest, has the best fixation retention strength, has the best durability, is the most inert, has the least inflammatory response, has the least foreign-body response, has minimal adhesions, has no reported bowel erosions or fistulizations, and is economically competitive when compared to all other biomaterials available for laparoscopic hernioplasty.

References

1. Elliott MP, Juler GL. Comparison of Marlex mesh and microporous Teflon sheets when used for hernia repair in the experimental animal. *Am J Surg* 1979; **137**: 342–4.
2. Madden JW, Peacock EE Jr. Studies on the Biology of Collagen During Wound Healing. III. Dynamic Metabolism of Scar Collagen and Remodeling of Dermal Wounds. *Ann Surg* 1971; **174**: 511.
3. Peacock Jr EE, Van Winkle Jr W. *Surgery and Biology of Wound Repair*, 2nd ed. Philadelphia: WB Saunders, 1976.
4. Douglas DM. The healing of aponeurotic incisions. *Br J Surg* 1962; **104**: 273.
5. Howes EL, Soroy JW, Harvey SC. The healing of wounds as determined by their tensile strength. *JAMA* 1929; **92**: 242.
6. Levenson SM, Geeve EF, Crowley W, Oates JF, Beard CW, Rosen H. The healing of rat skin wounds. *Ann Surg* 1965; **161**: 293.
7. Mason ML, Allen HS. The rate of healing of tendons. An experimental study of tensile strength. *Ann Surg* 1941; **113**: 424.
8. Rovee DT, Miller CA. Experimental role of breaking strength of wounds. *Arch Surg* 1968; **96**: 43
9. Nyhus LM, Condon RE, eds. *Hernia*, 3rd ed. Philadelphia: JB Lippincott, 1989.
10. Elek SD, Conin PE. The virulence of Staphylococcus pyogenes for man: a study of the problem of wound infection. *Br J Exp Pathol* 1957; **38**: 573–9.
11. Franson TR, Sheth NK, Rose HD, Sohule PG. Scanning electron microscopy of bacterial adherent to intravascular catheters. *J Clin Microbiol* 1984; **20**: 500–5.
12. Sugarman B. *In vitro* adherence of bacteria to prosthetic vascular grafts. *Infection* 1982; **10**: 2–11.
13. Schmitt DD, Bandyk DF, Pequet AJ, Towne JB. Bacterial adherence to vascular prostheses. A determinant of graft infectability. *J Vasc Surg* 1986; **3**: 732–40.
14. Rosenman JE, Pearce WH, Kempczinski RF. Bacterial adherence to vascular grafts after *in vitro* bacteremia. *J Surg Pres* 1985; **38**: 648–55.
15. Voyles CR, Richardson JD, Bland KI, *et al.* Emergency abdominal wall reconstruction with polypropylene mesh. *Ann Surg* 1981; **194**: 219–23.
16. Bhat DJ, Tellis VA, Kohlberg WI, Driscoll B, Veith FJ. Management of sepsis involving expanded polytetrafluoroethylene grafts for hemodialysis access. *Surgery* 1980; **87**: 445–50.
17. Connolly JE, Brownell DA, Levine EF, McCart M. Complications of renal dialysis access procedures. *Arch Surg* 1984; **119**: 1325–8.
18. Gifford RRM. Management of tunnel infections of dialysis polytetrafluoroethylene grafts. *J Vasc Surg* 1985; **2**: 854–8.
19. Raju S. PTFE grafts for hemodialysis access. *Ann Surg* 1987; **206**: 666–73.
20. Tellis V, Weiss P, Matas A, Veith F. Skin flap coverage of polytetrafluoroethylene vascular access graft exposed by previous infection. *Surgery* 1988; **103**: 118–21.
21. Tellis VA, Kohlberg WI, Bhat DJ, Driscoll B, Veith FJ. Expanded polytetrafluoroethylene graft fistula for chronic hemodialysis. *Ann Surg* 1979; **189**: 101–5.
22. Lennox MS, Ellis H. Fibrinolysis and adhesions formation in the peritoneum. *2nd International Symposium on the Surgery and Biology of the Greater Omentum*.
23. Law NH, Ellis H. Adhesion formation and peritoneal healing on prosthetic materials. *Clin Mater* 1988; **3**: 95–101.

24. Usher FC, Gannon JP. Marlex mesh. A new plastic mesh for replacing tissue defects. *Arch Surg* 1959; **78**: 131–7.

25. Boyd WC. Use of Marlex mesh in acute loss of the abdominal wall due to infection. *Surg Gynecol Obstet* 1977; **44**: 251–2.

26. Saxen L, Myllarniemi H. Foreign materials and postoperative adhesions. *N Engl J Med* 1968; **279**: 200–2.

27. Stone HH, Fabian TC, Turkleson ML, Jurkiewicz MJ. Management of full thickness losses of the abdominal wall. *Ann Surg* 1981; **193**: 612–18.

28. Schneider R, Herrington Jr JL, Granada A. Marlex mesh in repair of a diaphragmatic defect later eroding into the distal esophagus and stomach. *Ann Surg* 1979; **45**: 337–9.

29. Kaufman Z, Engelberg M, Zager M. Fecal fistula: a late complication of Marlex mesh repair. *Dis Colon Rectum* 1981; **24**: 543–4.

30. Voyles CR, Richardson JD, Bland KI, *et al.* Emergency abdominal wall reconstruction with polypropylene mesh. Short-term benefits versus long-term complications. *Ann Surg* 1981; **194**: 219–23.

31. Mathes SJ, Stone HH. Acute traumatic losses of abdominal wall substances. *J Trauma* 1975; **15**: 386–90.

32. Cerise EJ, Busuttil RW, Craighead CC, Ogden WW. The use of mersilene mesh in repair of abdominal wall hernias: a clinical and experimental study. *Ann Surg* 1975; **181**: 728–34.

33. Dayton Mt, Buchele BA, Shirazi SS, Hunt LB. Use of an absorbable mesh to repair contaminated abdominal wall defects. *Arch Surg* 1986; **121**: 954–60.

34. Murphy JL, Freeman JB, Dionne PG. Comparison of Marlex and Gore-Tex to repair abdominal wall defects in rats. *Cn J Surg* 1989; **32**: 244–7.

35. Van da Lei B, Bleichrodt RP, Simmmermocher RKJ, Van Schilfgaarde R. Expanded polytetrafluoroethylene patch for the repair of large abdominal wall defects. *Br J Surg* 1989; **76**: 803–5.

20

Biological Implant Materials: a Chemical, Physical and Bacteriological Study

DALILA GRECO, E CHIESARA, F CASA, L MARABINI, G ORTISI AND C TOSI

The human body can be thought of as a complex ecosystem in which cells and inert biological materials develop a strict union and after these combinations live a single future that sometimes lasts a long time.

Many questions need to be answered, particularly how biologically inert materials modify and deteriorate after being used as implants. This is a very important problem and requires the attention of an interdisciplinary group[1,2], but is very hard to accomplish when studying complex molecules such as polymers and copolymers.

When studying complex molecules and copolymers, the authors prefer to carry out physical studies such as monitoring of physical properties[3–5]. The physical parameters of *tensile strength, elongation at failure, elastic rebound* and *crushing strength* that we have studied for many years are a good index to describe deterioration of implant materials, especially of silicon rubber[6]. In 1991 we began a study, using electron microscopy, of the morphological deterioration of implant materials after undergoing stress tests.

The most interesting and noteworthy results were obtained from the bacteriological test, and they are presented in this chapter.

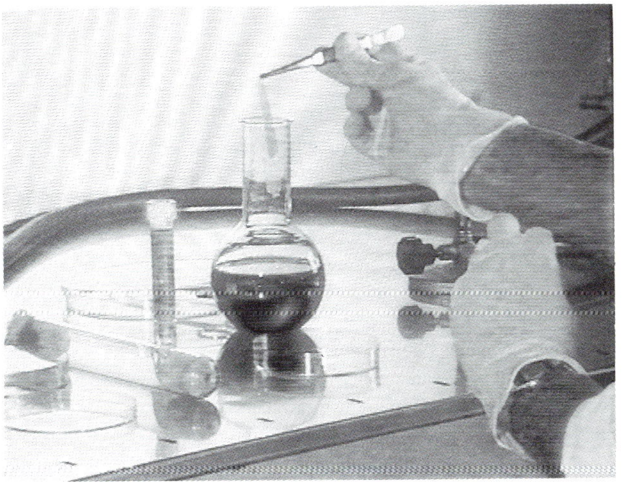

Figure 20.1: Incubation of materials in medium with strains of high adhesivity.

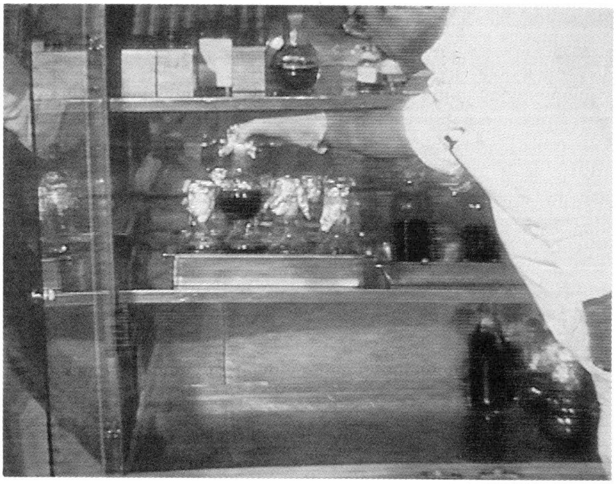

Figure 20.2: Materials stored in thermostatum.

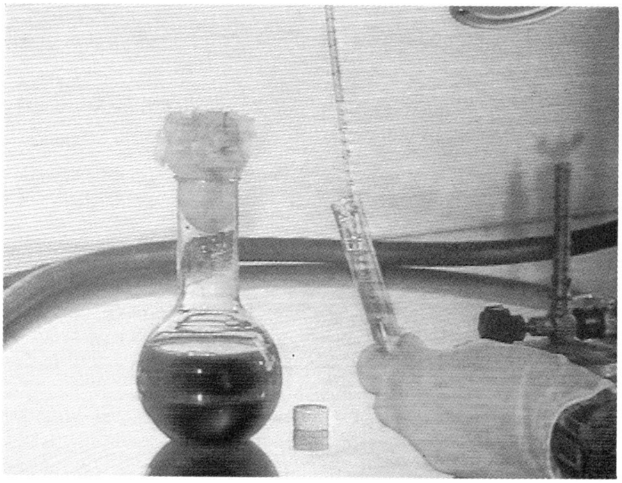

Figure 20.3: Reinoculation.

The tests

The experiments were conducted to study the effect of bacteria on waste biological implant materials. The materials tested included silicon sheeting, micro-structured mammary prostheses, meshes for parietal reconstruction (Mersilene, polypropelene [Marlex], Dacron, Gore-Tex). They were incubated in sterile medium and high adhesivity strain (Figure 20.1) and then stored in a thermostatum at 37 °C (Figure 20.2). After two weeks the media were reinoculated (Figure 20.3).

After 90 days, samples were removed and brought into contact with TSA plates (Figure 20.4) in order to assess the number of colonies per square centimetre after a first washing and again after 24 hours of washing (Table 20.1). Mesh materials were studied after 60 days of incubation.

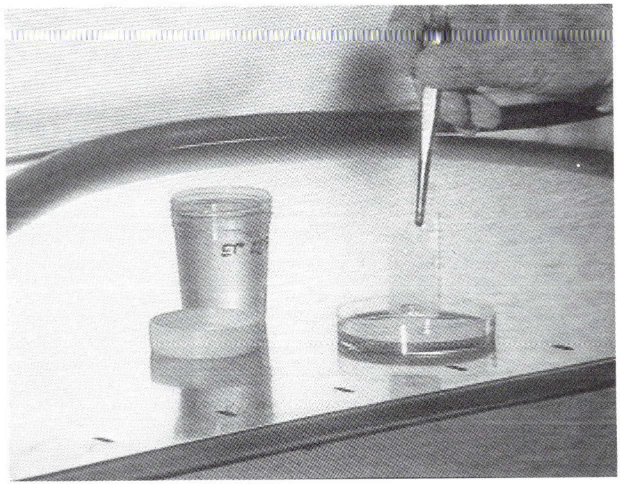

Figure 20.4: Silicon rubber adhesivity test.

Table 20.1: Number of colonies per square centimetre on silicon sheeting after contact with TSA plates

Bacteria	*Time 0*	*1st washing*	*After 24 hours' washing*
Escherichia coli	> 100	38	11
Pseudomonas aeruginosa	> 100	0	0
Streptococcus faecalis	> 100	50	2
Staphylococcus epidermidis	> 100	4	1
Staph. aureus	> 100	35	11
Broth	0	0	0

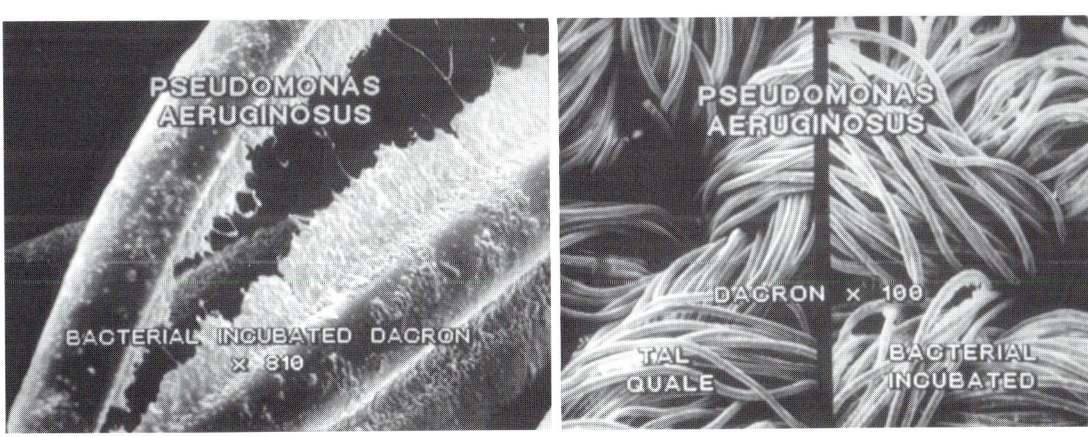

Figure 20.5: Electron micrographs showing the high adhesivity of *Pseudomonas aeruginosus* to Dacron. × 100; × 810

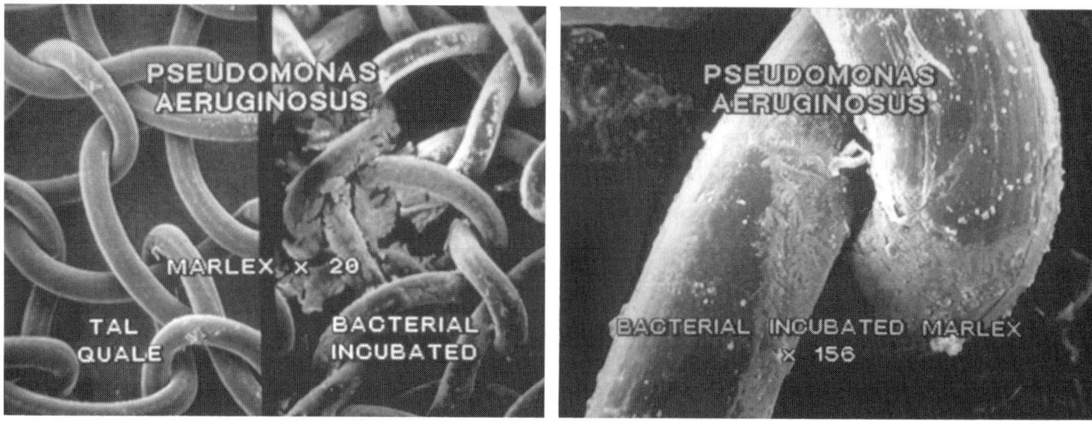

Figure 20.6: Electron micrographs showing the high adhesivity of *Ps. aeruginosus* to polypropelene [Marlex]. (a) × 20; (b) × 150

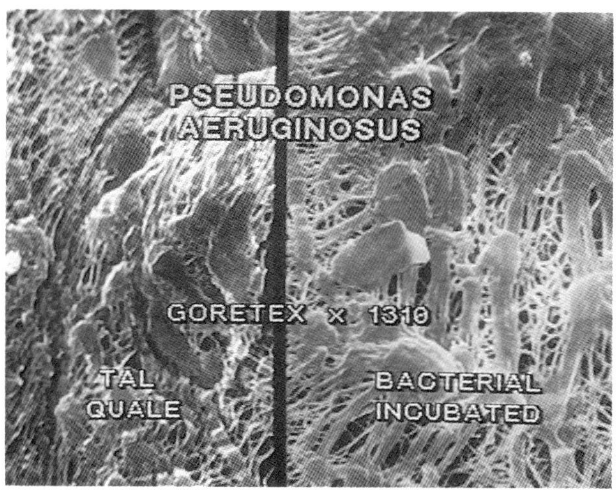

Figure 20.7: Electron micrograph showing no adhesivity of *Ps. aeruginosa* to ePTFE. × 1310

Initially we studied a large number of strains coming from pathogens high adhesivity strains:

- *Escherichia coli*
- *Staphylococcus epidermidis*
- *Staphylococcus aureus*
- *Pseudomonas aeruginosa*
- *Streptococcus faecalis*

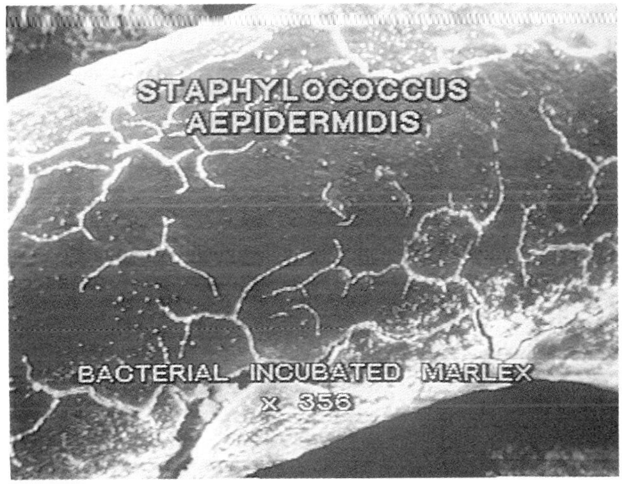

Figure 20.8: Electron micrograph showing high adhesivity of *Staph. epidermidis* to ePTFE. × 10 400

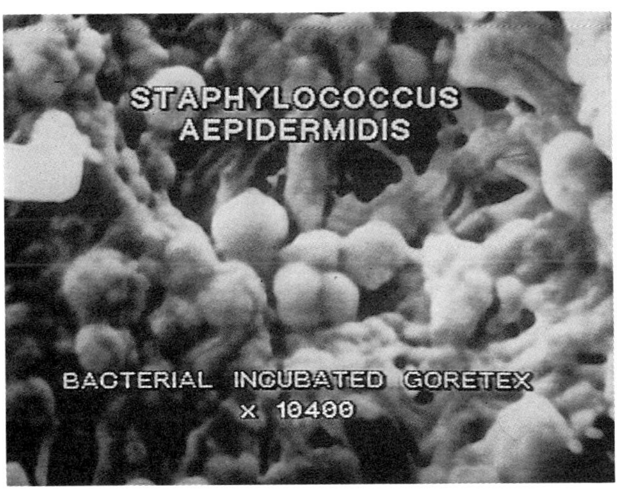

Figure 20.9: Electron micrograph showing the corrosive action of *Staph. epidermidis* on Marlex. × 356

We next studied in detail *Ps. aeruginosa* and *Staph. epidermidis.*

Results

The data we obtained demonstrate:

- high adhesivity of *Ps. aeruginosa* to Dacron (Figure 20.5)
- low adhesivity of *Ps. aeruginosa* to polypropylene (Marlex) (Figure 20.6)

- no adhesivity of *Ps. aeruginosa* to e-polytetrafluoroethylene (ePTFE) (Figure 20.7)
- high adhesivity of *Staph. epidermidis* to ePTFE (Figure 20.8)
- corrosive action of *Staph. epidermidis* for polypropylene (Marlex) (Figure 20.9).

This microbiological test is the best that we can use to study the deterioration of mesh materials.

The main important factors arising from our experiments are that there is

- triangle material, bacterium, biology, in which a saprophytic bacterium such as *Staph. epidermidis* becomes a very dangerous killer for prosthetic materials.

Conclusions

From our studies we conclude that mesh materials can be employed but only when using strictly aseptic surgical techniques to prevent contamination with *Staph. epidermidis.*

References

1. Greco D, Casa F, Marabini L, Brattina L. Modificazioni indotte nello stato di reticulozione del d-metilpolisilossano dall'uso della colla di fibrina umana nel corso di impianto biologico. In: *VI Congresso Nazionale SIATEC Societa' Italiana Applicazioni Tecnologiche in Chirurgia*. Milan: Editor Monduzzi, 1990: 585–90.
2. Greco D, Casa F, Tosi G, Ortisi G, Sala C, Marabini L. Silicon modification after radiation and biological implant. In: *Second World Week of Professional Updating in Surgery and in Surgical and Oncological Disciplines of the University of Milan*. Milan; Editor Monduzzi, 1990: VII, 157–61.
3. Crawford DT, Bains JW, Kethchman. A standard model for tensiometric studies. *J Surg Res* 1965; 5: 265–8.
4. Greco D, Chiesara E, Brattina L, Marabini L, Sala C. Morphological study of capsule maturation with the use of tissue glue. *Plastic Surgery* 1992; 2: 689–90.
5. Hench LL, Ethridge EC. *Biomaterials and Interfascial Approach*. New York: Academic Press, 1982.
6. Hench LL. Biocompatibility of silicates for medical use. In: Corey ER eds. *Silicon Chemistry*. Chichester: J Wiley, 1988.

21

Open Versus Laparoscopic Groin Herniorrhaphy: Economic Realities

IRA M RUTKOW

Review of current opinion

To appreciate the socioeconomic impact of groin hernia repair on American health care (est. $1 trillion in 1993), it is essential to have an understanding of the numbers of surgical operations performed annually in the USA[1]. According to data from the National Center for Health Statistics (Hyattsville, Maryland) the five most common major surgical operations performed by general surgeons in 1991 were:

1 groin hernia, 680 000

2 cholecystectomy, 571 000

3 lysis of peritoneal adhesions, 339 000

4 appendectomy, 255 000

5 partial excision of large intestine, 220 000.

To provide a basis for comparison, other general surgical operations include:

- mastectomies, 118 000
- umbilical hernias, 80 000
- incisional hernias, 70 000
- carotid endarterectomy, 67 000
- colostomy, 63 000
- thyroidectomy, 47 000
- abdominal aortic aneursymectomy, 35 000
- aortoiliofemoral bypass, 29 000.

In a study published in 1987, the Metropolitan Life Insurance Company found that the local hospital and physician charges for a groin hernia operation averaged $4400[2]. More than likely, this figure has increased over the last six years, but, using the $4400 amount, it can be noted that the actual performance of groin herniorrhaphies accounts for almost $3 billion in yearly health care revenue. Therefore, it is self-evident that the present debate regarding the technical merits of varying hernia repairs (ie open versus laparoscopic) is one with enormous economic implications.

Traditional sutured methods of inguinal and femoral herniorrhaphy (Bassini, McVay or Cooper ligament, Shouldice or Canadian, Nyhus or preperitoneal iliopubic tract, etc.) have long been criticized for their well-known postoperative complications. Foremost among these difficulties have been a notoriously slow and painful recovery process. Due to tension-creating approximations of musculoaponeurotic tissues, patients are frequently restricted from significant lifting for as long as six to eight weeks, until sufficient tensile strength has developed in the wound to diminish the chance of recurrence. Consequently, there is a general inability of patients to resume normal day-to-day activities within a reasonable amount of time. This failure to return to work in less than one week's time remains a tremendous detriment to the continued use of the 'old-fashioned' sutured anterior herniorrhaphy. Because of these and other concerns, it was obvious that new and more innovative surgical approaches would have to be formulated for groin hernia repair.

Among the most novel of the new hernioplasty techniques has been the use of synthetic materials in order to strengthen the intrinsically weak groin area. In the late 1950s and early 1960s Usher began to report on the use of a monofilament knitted polypropylene mesh (Bard Marlex) in the repair of inguinal and incisional hernias[3]. He used the mesh prosthesis to buttress and reinforce a standard sutured anterior hernia repair. Usher demonstrated that this synthetic material had considerable tensile strength, was rapidly incorporated into fibrous tissue and was not associated with an increase in infection.

In 1974, Lichtenstein proposed eliminating a tissue weakness or defect with a cylindrical rolled plug made out of Bard Marlex mesh[4]. He treated femoral and recurrent inguinal hernias with this simple technique. Eleven years later, Shockett reaffirmed the principles proposed by Lichtenstein when he described the concept of implanting a rolled piece of Bard Marlex mesh beneath the floor of the inguinal canal by slipping it through the internal ring or a defect in the direct space[5]. Shockett hypothesized that fibroblastic activity through the mesh's interstices would cause it to become a permanent barrier against future herniation, irrespective of the natural progressive degeneration that any surrounding tissue would undergo.

In 1986, Lichtenstein introduced the term 'tensionless' hernioplasty, and since then the management of groin hernias has undergone an amazing evolution[6]. He showed that the single most important factor in both recurrences and complications of herniorrhaphy is ill-conceived attempts at approximating normally unapposed tissues under tension. The presence of tissue tension in a hernia repair is now known to account for virtually all of the short- and long-term pain associated with such an operation. Lichtenstein and his associates described an operative technique that consisted of a sutured onlay patch of Bard Marlex as the primary hernia repair. The importance of their concept is that the mesh prosthesis is not used to buttress or support an anterior sutured herniorrhaphy but *is* the actual repair. No attempt is made to approximate weakened tissue with sutures. Therefore, any distortion of normal anatomy via tension on a suture line is totally avoided. This technique was found applicable to all types of primary indirect and direct inguinal hernias.

The next logical step in the evolution of the prosthetic-based groin hernia repair was initiated by Gilbert in the late 1980s[7]. He utilized a 'sutureless' plug procedure for the treatment of small to moderate sized indirect inguinal hernias, both primary and recurrent. Gilbert took a flat piece of polypropylene mesh, which he slit and folded into a cone-like configuration. This prosthetic plug was positioned into the internal ring where it would hold the hernia in place.

Gilbert's mesh plug repair is most notable for its simplicity and ease of performance. There is virtually no disturbance of normal anatomy. The sphincter-like action of the internal ring and the sling and shutter mechanism of the inguinal canal are preserved. Needle and suture holes, which may gradually enlarge or tear through and lead to a recurrence, are completely eliminated. Dissection is kept to a minimum and any chance of nerve injury is decreased. Gilbert's concept provides for a tension-free repair and closely resembles the act of placing a cork in a bottle.

Rutkow and Robbins expanded on Lichtenstein's 'tensionless' concept and Gilbert's plug technique by standardizing the mesh plug method for *all* primary and recurrent groin hernias[8,9]. In almost 1700 patients with over four-year follow-up they were able dramatically to decrease not only recurrence rates but also, and most importantly, operative morbidity and short- and long-term complications. As a consequence, individuals are able to resume their normal day-to-day activities more quickly and return to work sooner.

Utilizing the Rutkow–Robbins anterior approach mesh plug method, an average herniorrhaphy takes less than 20 minutes to perform. Completed under epidural or local anaesthesia, the patient has minimal discomfort and is allowed to return to most work-related activities within 48–72 hours. Recurrence rates remain under 1%, and complications – especially the problem of postoperative discomfort – have been virtually eliminated.

In addition to the advent of prosthetic-based herniorrhaphies, the other 'innovative' method of performing groin hernia repairs is through a laparoscope[10]. Following the remarkable success of laparoscopic cholecystectomy – especially reduced recovery time, decreased pain, improved cosmesis and overall cost-effectiveness – it was felt that these advantages could possibly be incorporated into a laparoscopic hernia repair. Accordingly, over the last two years the laparoscope companies and the surgeons who represent them have been conducting large-scale public relations efforts and massive advertising campaigns to convince other surgeons and the lay public of the necessity to perform hernia repairs via laparoscopy.

Certainly, for laparoscopic hernias, there has been a relatively small follow-up period as well as a limited number of procedures available for evaluation. In addition, the laparoscopic techniques themselves are constantly changing, which makes it difficult to focus on one particular method and attempt to complete a valid, prospective, randomized clinical trial.

Throughout all these controversies laparoscopic hernia repair has been touted as having the following benefits over a *sutured* anterior hernia repair:

- minimal invasion with small incisions
- decreased postoperative pain
- quick recovery and return to work
- ability to lessen overall health care costs.

In reality, minimal invasion means the extreme disadvantage of having to use the more dangerous general, as opposed to epidural or local anaesthesia. When the length of the multiple small incisions for a laparoscopic hernia repair is compared with the length of one incision for an anterior repair, the total lengths of incisions closely approximate one another (with the Rutkow–Robbins mesh hernia plug method, their one incision measures less than 6 cm). The standard groin incision for an anterior repair is always located within the 'bikini' line. This is in contrast with those for the laparoscopic repair which are located higher up and, consequently, more clearly visible on an exposed abdominal wall. Neither is it evident that a patient is able to engage in normal day-to-day activities more rapidly after a laparoscopic repair than following several currently existing open techniques. In the Lichtenstein, Gilbert or Rutkow–Robbins mesh-based repairs, patients are permitted to begin such activities using their own discretion, which is usually within 24–48 hours after surgery.

Despite the now-constant barrage of advertising pamphlets and brochures, there is little in the surgical literature to indicate that laparoscopic herniorrhaphy should be considered to be the current standard in groin hernia repairs[11]. Most cogently, it is not likely that a laparoscopic hernia repair can lessen health costs. Since most of the 680 000 hernia operations performed every year in the USA are already completed on an outpatient (ambulatory) or same-day basis, the concept of a laparoscopic approach decreasing facility or hospital costs by shortening the stay would appear to be nonsensical. This is in direct contradistinction to other types of laparoscopic surgery (ie cholecystectomy, bowel resection, etc.) where a lengthy in-patient stay, necessitated by traditional surgical techniques, has been truly shortened. In fact, the laparoscopic approach for hernia repair ultimately costs more because a considerable amount of expensive equipment must be purchased in order to perform the laparoscopic operation.

The preceding paragraph presents a very important point which cannot be stressed too strongly in view of what is occurring in present-day American politics and the drive toward reform of the health care system. Laparoscopic instrument makers and surgeons who use their equipment are attempting to incorporate as many surgical operations under the umbrella of laparoscopic surgery as possible. For many types of operations this is a reasonable approach which truly decreased in-patient days and postoperative discomfort. However, in hernia surgery there already exist several operative techniques that unarguably decrease a patient's time in a hospital or surgical facility and decidedly lessen their postoperative discomfort. This makes it possible for an individual to return to normal activities in as short a period as one to two days.

Some surgeons who perform laparoscopic surgery and manufacturers of laparoscopy equipment disregard the availability of these efficient and less painful mesh-based hernia repairs and, instead, concentrate all of their arguments using the 'old-fashioned' open *sutured* hernia repair for their comparison.

Quantitative comparison outlining procedural cost

There are several economic factors which need to be defined relative to the cost of a hernia procedure:

- surgeon's fee
- anaesthesiologist's fee
- facility fee

For any groin hernia repair, a patient and his insurance carrier must contend with these three separate items. For the health care system, the most perplexing question is which of these items can be reduced in cost. Facility fees, because of the 'high technology' involved in a laparoscopic hernia repair, must be carefully scrutinized. Two major components make up what a facility charges: fixed overheads (ie rent or mortgage, personnel salaries including nurses, and equipment common to each operation, including clamps, scissors, mesh, etc. Within this equipment is a rather hefty one-time expense for such laparoscopic items as camera, television screen, insufflation devices, etc.); and soft overheads (what I define as 'throw-aways' for each procedure, including caps, gowns, gloves, medication, sutures, etc.)

At The Hernia Center the soft-overhead costs for performing a mesh-plug repair (including the mesh) is $175 per case. If we were to do laparoscopic hernia repairs, these soft costs would have to be increased by another $400–$500 per operation. According to a survey of various laparoscopic equipment companies, our expenses for the disposable items needed to complete a laparoscopic hernia repair would be:

- one Verres needle ($22–$28 cost range)
- one 5 mm trocar ($58–$73)
- two 12 mm trocars ($147–$206)
- one hernia stapler ($136–$170)
- one reload for the stapler ($27–$49).

Items for which I have not included individual prices within the economic equation of open *vs* laparoscopic hernia repair are the fixed expenses. They are obviously quite high but are more a function of how many cases are performed over the lifetime of the equipment. The more cases, the lower the per-case price. However, the initial set-up for laparoscopic hernia equipment (ie camera, video monitor, insufflation apparatus, etc.) costs between $25 000 and $50 000. This is in stark contrast to the $0 start-up cost of performing a mesh-based repair.

It is well recognized that an average laparoscopic repair takes approximately 45–90 minutes to complete, as against 20 minutes for a mesh plug hernia repair. This extra operating room time must also be factored into the cost equation of open *vs* laparoscopic hernia repair. In addition, the added operating time will be reflected in an increased anaesthesiologist fee because their professional charge is calculated on the basis of 15-minute units. Surgeons, too, have been known to increase their professional fees because of the longer time necessary to complete laparoscopic surgery.

Having outlined these cost, some 'real-life' figures need to be explained so that the true economic realities of performing laparoscopic hernia repairs can be fully appreciated. At The Hernia Center, recently completed negotiations with various health care establishments managed care networks, compensation carriers, Blue Cross and Blue Shield, etc. have yielded an average facility reimbursement for a hernia repair of from \$750 to \$900 per case. This is the total fee the facility collects regardless of whether the repair is open, laparoscopic, mesh-based, sutured or non-sutured. There has been no company willing to pay an 'extra' fee because of the use of laparoscopic technology.

It is inherently obvious, then, that if our soft costs alone for a laparoscopic hernia are in the vicinity of \$650 per case (\$175 for caps, gowns, gloves, medications, sutures, mesh, etc. plus \$475 for laparoscopic disposables), and this is prior to factoring in the enormous fixed costs (mortgage, salaries, laparoscopic non-disposable equipment, etc.), it becomes financially untenable to complete a laparoscopic hernia repair. Conversely, a mesh-plug repair with soft costs of only \$175 per case allows for much greater flexibility in the ability to negotiate a satisfactory facility fee arrangement. As an aside, it should be noted that the most recent outpatient (ambulatory) surgical facility fee schedule issued by Medicare provides for a reimbursement of approximately \$500 per hernia case. Since individuals over the age of 65 represent such a high percentage of hernias completed in the USA (26%), it would be economically impossible to perform laparoscopic hernia repairs on this large segment of our society.

In order for a laparoscopic hernia repair to be financially attractive to the USA's 'overall' health care system, it would have to be able to return patients to work faster than after open hernia repairs (ie reduce time out of work and decrease loss of wages and disability payouts). This would be the only way in which it could reduce costs because a laparoscopic hernia repair incurs facility charges that are so high. Since with modern mesh-based repairs patients are returning to normal activities within 48–72 hours, and a laparoscopic repair cannot claim a faster recovery time, there is no possibility of a laparoscopic repair decreasing overall health care costs when contrasted with an open repair. It can only *increase* costs!

Some recent writings on laparoscopic hernia repair are beginning to state that, perhaps for primary unilateral hernias, a laparoscopic technique is not justified on cost. Instead, what is currently being touted is the advantage of laparoscopic hernia repair for bilateral, recurrent and doubtful hernias. However, the same economic equations that pertain to unilateral repairs are essentially applicable to bilateral herniorrhaphies. Besides which, less than 15% of hernia repairs in the USA are completed on a bilateral basis. There are no economic justifications for performing bilateral hernia repairs via a laparoscope. With regard to recurrent hernias, published data on the Lichtenstein[12], Gilbert[13] and Rutkow–Robbins [14] mesh-based repairs show them to be performed just as easily on recurrent hernias as on primary defects. This being so, there would again be no economic justification in performing laparoscopic repair of recurrent hernias.

Personal observations

What the manufacturers of laparoscopic equipment have failed to acknowledge is that, by prematurely encouraging the mass use of the unproven and costly laparoscopic hernia repair, they are able to increase their company's profits, but at the possible expense of overall patient safety and welfare, and with increasing costs to our health care system.

Clearly, laparoscopic surgery will have an important place in the overall armamentarium of any surgeon. What is not evident is that every known surgical operation should be or can be converted to reside under the umbrella of laparoscopy. This is certainly the case for hernia repair. The modern mesh-based methods of open repair (Lichtenstein, Gilbert, Rutkow–Robbins) have a much wider economic and practical appeal than a laparoscopic approach.

Simply because an operation can be done laparoscopically does not mean that it is necessarily the most expedient method. The obvious case in point is laparoscopic hernia repair. Laparoscopic surgery is here to stay, but that does not mean that hernia repair need be accomplished in a laparoscopic manner. In the changing socioeconomic environment that grips Washington and federal policy-makers, it is unlikely that the added costs of laparoscopic hernia surgery will ever pass muster.

References

1. Rutkow IM, Robbins, AW. Demographic, classificatory, and socioeconomic aspects of hernia repair in the United States. *Surg Clin North Am* 1993; **73**: 413–26.
2. Anonymous. Costs of three common surgical procedures: 1987 update. *Stat Bull* July–September 1989: 20.
3. Usher FC, Cogan JE, Lowry TI. A new technique for the repair of inguinal and incisional hernias. *Arch Surg* 1960; **81**: 847–52.
4. Lichtenstein IL, Shore JM. Simplified repair of femoral and recurrent inguinal hernias by a 'plug' technique. *Am J Surg* 1974; **128**: 439–44.
5. Shockett E. Routine rapid preperitoneal Marlex mesh buttressing in the repair of all inguinal hernias. *Contemp Surg* 1985; **26**: 22–7.
6. Lichtenstein IL, Shulman AG. Ambulatory outpatient hernia surgery, including a new concept, introducing tension-free repair. *Int Surg* 1986; **71**: 1–7.
7. Gilbert AI. Inguinal hernia repair: biomaterials and sutureless repair. *Perspect Gen Surg* 1991; **2**: 113–19.
8. Robbins AW, Rutkow IM. The mesh-plug hernioplasty. *Surg Clin North Am* 1993; **73**: 501–11.
9. Rutkow IM, Robbins AW. 'Tension-free' inguinal herniorrhaphy: a preliminary report on the 'mesh plug' technique. *Surgery* 1993; **114**: 3–8.
10. Arregui M, Navarrete J, Davis CJ, Castro D, Nagan RF. Laparoscopic inguinal herniorrhaphy: techniques and controversies. *Surg Clin North Am* 1993; **73**: 513–27.
11. Rutkow IM. Laparoscopic hernia repair: the socioeconomic tyranny of surgical technology. *Arch Surg* 1992; **127**: 1271.
12. Lichtenstein IL, Shulman AG, Amid PK. The cause, prevention, and treatment of recurrent groin hernia. *Surg Clin North Am* 1993; **73**: 529–44.
13. Gilbert AI. Sutureless repair of inguinal hernia. *Am J Surg* 1992; **163**: 331–5.
14. Rutkow IM, Robbins AW. 1669 mesh plug hernioplasties. *Contemp Surg* 1993; **43**: 141–7.

22

Economics of Hernia: the Hospital's Perspective

RONALD N RINER

Laparoscopic surgical procedures have become very common. More than 500 000 cholecystectomies are performed annually in the USA. In fact, laparoscopic cholecystectomies are currently replacing open cholecystectomy in the management of gall bladder disease. Whilst initial results of laparoscopic cholecystectomy suggest that this type of surgical procedure is performed safely, there are many questions that remain concerning the economics of these procedures. My comments in this chapter are related to the economics of hernia repair and my perspective is from a national vantage point. As Vice President of Medical Affairs, I am the Chief Medical Officer for the Daughters of Charity National Health System, the largest not-for-profit Catholic health care system in the USA. We have 43 acute care hospitals with over 60 facilities and close to 14 000 acute care beds. Approximately 10 000 physicians practise at Daughters of Charity facilities. Our physicians are, by and large, a private practice fee-for-service group of clinicians, covering a wide geographic area from the west coast to the east coast of the USA.

Laparoscopic surgery (minimally invasive surgery) has been one the most impressive developments affecting the practice of surgery over the past several years. Duodenal ulcer repair, appendectomy, hysterectomy, prostatectomy, laminectomy and lung tumour removal are now capable of being performed by minimally invasive surgery. Inguinal hernia repair is currently in the forefront of discussion, and my comments here relate to the various aspects of laparoscopic inguinal hernia repair.

Market size

Approximately 5% of the population experiences inguinal hernias. Men are more likely than women to have a hernia, and the problem increases with ageing. Many of these individuals eventually come to surgery, and over 500 000 hernia repairs are performed annually in the USA. Because of the many operations that are done among the actively employed, the economic impact (10–15 million work-days lost each year) has far reaching implications. In 1991, in the USA, about 5% of inguinal hernias were repaired laparoscopically. There are some individuals who predict that, by 1996, about 75% of inguinal hernias will be repaired laparoscopically.

Operational impact

What are the effects of this new technology on the operation of a multi-hospital national health system? The first implication has been that most of this type of activity has been done on an outpatient basis. Many of our hospitals have dedicated surgical centres, day care surgical centres and recovery centres, but the vast majority of hernia repairs are done outside the confines of the acute care facility. Patients go home within several hours of the procedure. This fact alone has led to major restructuring of the facilities to accommodate the types of surgical procedures that are being performed by this new type of technology. Inpatient beds go empty as there is increasing demand for outpatient procedures.

Laparoscopic procedures may also be completed more quickly than the open procedure, although other surgeons debate this issue. Indeed, some laparoscopic procedures take more time to perform than traditional open surgery.

Environmental issues

Obviously, in 1993 environmental issues are of major concern. Waste disposal is an ever-increasing problem for our facilities. This type of technology uses numerous materials and instruments that previously had been reusable. Now they are viewed as 'disposable'.

Effect of limited number of suppliers

As a national health system, we are accustomed to negotiating national contracts with our suppliers to achieve economies of scale. Whilst there are a number of companies focused on endosurgery, the market is dominated by a few suppliers. Domination by small numbers of suppliers can result in reduced competition, which makes it much more difficult to negotiate favourable contracts on a national level.

Consumer push marketing

Consumers have become increasingly aware of the benefits of minimally invasive surgery and are asking physicians to perform this technique instead of 'open surgery'. The benefits identified by consumers include a minimal hospital stay or an outpatient procedure, shortened recovery time and speedier return to work, less pain and a few small incisions as opposed to a larger scar. This consumer push has in no small way been compounded by active marketing on the part of individuals and hospitals using this type of technology.

Accreditation and risk management issues

The development and growth of laparoscopic procedures has made it necessary to focus on risk management. The critical risk management issues being addressed by hospitals and medical staff include the following:

- determining the safety of new equipment
- controlling approval of experimental procedures
- ensuring adequate training of personnel to perform new procedures and use new equipment
- tracking adverse outcomes
- extending risk management activities from the usual inpatient situation to the outpatient setting.

Additionally, few hospitals have adequately addressed the accreditation implications of this new technology. As more and more procedures, such as herniorrhaphy repair, adopt this technique, the issue of who is qualified to perform the various endosurgical procedures must be clarified. This issue has sparked major debate between and among various disciplines.

Financial implication

The significant reduction in the length of stay for many of the procedures performed by laparoscopic technology has led to a shift from inpatient to outpatient setting, and has caused a significant drop in inpatient days. Depending on the patient mix involved, this could adversely affect the financial state of a hospital. Secondly, operating times can be longer with laparoscopic procedures, thereby decreasing the frequency with which an operating room can be used. The need for general anaesthesia for laparoscopic hernia repair is a theoretical disadvantage over conventional repair. Capital costs for this new equipment are relatively minor compared with capital expenditure for instrumentation such as a cardiac catheterization laboratory or an operating room. We are talking in terms of \$50 000–\$70 000 rather than \$1 000 000–\$2 000 000. In general, supply costs for laparoscopic procedures appear to be higher, especially in view of the non-reusable nature of the equipment employed.

Recent hospital survey

Several months ago, in anticipation of preparing this chapter, I did a very informal survey of our 43 hospitals. I received responses from 23. In 1991, the 23 respondent hospitals performed 4319 open-surgery hernia repairs, and in 1992 they performed 4329 such procedures. In 1991, they performed 94 laparoscopic hernia repairs. This was done at only five of the 23 hospitals responding. However, by 1992, 379 procedures had been performed in 12 hospitals. Even now, despite the large number of our hospitals, the proportion of laparoscopic hernia repairs is not large.

I also asked our hospitals to provide me with *cost* as well as *charge* data. Of the 23 hospitals responding, only a few could provide me with information about 'true cost' as opposed to charge. Based strictly on a few hospitals reporting, it would appear that inpatient *costs* for open herniorrhaphy in 1992 were approximately \$4341. The *charge* for that procedure was approximately \$8765. If the procedure was performed in an outpatient setting, the *cost* was \$1231 and the *charge* was \$2550. Again, based on a few hospitals reporting, inpatient laparoscopic hernia repair *cost* \$4085–\$4400, with *charges* of \$9493. If the hernia repair was done laparoscopically on an outpatient basis, the *cost* was \$1938 with a *charge of* \$4464.

It would appear that the cost of these procedures, if done by open-surgery repair or by laparoscopic technique, is approximately 50% of the charges. In our system, laparoscopic hernia repair accounted for only 10% of total hernia repairs, one hospital in our system performing the vast majority of those laparoscopic repairs.

What, therefore, are the lessons that we have learned thus far? Hospital stays may certainly be shorter. Unquestionably there is a move from the inpatient to the outpatient setting for these procedures. It would appear that the costs and charges for laparoscopic hernia repair may actually exceed the cost and charges for an open hernia repair. Whilst it is generally accepted that most patients undergoing open-surgery inguinal herniorrhaphy remain off work and avoid heavy labour for six to eight weeks compared with the one week with laparoscopic repair, there are those who challenge that concept. This latter issue needs to be clarified by additional investigation. It would also appear, from existing data, that recurrent hernias have developed in fewer than 2% of individuals undergoing laparoscopic hernia repair. The incidence of perioperative complications with the laparoscopic technology seems to be comparable to that of the open procedure.

Conclusions

I believe that there are some hard economic questions to answer. The challenge for a clinician is to consider all new technologies in the light of clinical efficacy and cost benefits. There is a need to balance carefully the requests of patients with the needs of society. Herein is the challenge for our profession today. We need to look at clinical guidelines for the use of new technology. We must emphasize the final results to support the development of new technologies and we must be honest in our assessment of the economics of these new technologies. Whilst we have used laparoscopic cholecystectomy as a starting point for discussion of laparoscopic inguinal hernia repairs, and whilst it is true that 75% of cholecystectomies are done laparoscopically, does that necessarily mean that all laparoscopic procedures are preferable to open procedures? The challenge, therefore, as one tries and endorses these new technologies is to prove not only to ourselves as professionals but to society as well that the new technology has its place, both financially as well as clinically.

23

Disability Income and Loss of Productivity

FRANK T CROSSLAND AND JOSEPH A PERKINS

M-J Insurance is an independent insurance agency located in Indianapolis. Its sister company, Benefit Design and Administrators, is a third party administrator that adjudicates medical, dental and disability claims. The focus of this chapter is the cost implications – to employer and employee – of disability.

Insurance claims for disability

In the last five years the insurance industry has seen a significant increase in the number of claims filed for disability. Several factors are attributable to this increase, two major one being medical technology and previously unrecognized causes of disability, such as stress-related disorders. There is a philosophy in our industry that the keys to effective disability management are prevention, early intervention and a strong return-to-work ethic. One of the insurance carriers with whom M-J Insurance does business is UNUM Life Insurance Company of America, a leader in the disability market. Life Insurance Company of America, Cincinnati, OH UNUM recently conducted a study of a company with about 800 employees, which had experienced a large increase in the number of long-term disability claims filed by women aged 40–45, who had been employed by the company for fewer than two years. UNUM discovered that the claims were mainly attributed to long work shifts and extended periods of standing and lifting. As a result of this study the employer has created a task force to adhere to a formal strategy for disability management. This is an example of an employer taking a proactive role in managing disability claims[1].

Worker's compensation

Worker's Compensation costs are no different from employer-sponsored disability costs: they continue to rise. According to the US Department of Health and Human Services, Worker's Compensation cost as a percentage of payroll has increased from 1% in 1970 to a conservative estimate of 2.3% in 1990. In 1982 employers paid approximately $23 billion in Worker's Compensation and by 1990 that figure had doubled to $50 billion. From 1980 to 1988 Worker's Compensation had increased by 191%[1]

Work time lost

Work days lost is another issue. The Bureau of Labor statistics indicates that the number of work days lost per 100 employees has increased from 47.9 days in 1972 to 78.7 days in 1989[1]. A variety of factors have contributed to this increase: the establishment of OSHA in 1972 and confrontation among trial lawyers, unions, employers, insurance companies, and, as mentioned, medical technology.

The following assumptions were made when preparing the data in this chapter:

- the short-term disability benefit is 60% of earnings to a maximum of $500 per week; Plan is assumed to be day 1 for an accident and day 8 for sickness, with benefit paid to a maximum of 26 weeks
- replacement costs were calculated using $105 per day for clerical workers and $145 per day for skilled blue collar workers
- in calculating Worker's Compensation state laws vary; for this analysis Indiana state law was assumed.

Table 23.1 gives weekly disability income benefit provided by the employer, Table 23.2 lists replacement costs to the employer and Table 23.3 gives worker's compensation payable to the employee. Table 23.4 compares weekly wage and Worker's Compensation benefit in the state of Indiana, from 1991 to 1994.

Table 23.1: Weekly disability income benefit provided by employer

	Days of disability			
	5	*10*	*20*	*30*
Professional (Earnings $80 000) Weekly income costs	$500	$1000	$2000	$3000
Clerical (Earnings $22 500) Weekly income costs	$260	$520	$1040	$1560
Skilled blue collar (Earning $31 000) Weekly income costs	$358	$716	$1432	$2148

Table 23.2: Replacement costs to employer

	Days of disability			
	5	*10*	*20*	*30*
Professional (Earnings $80 000) Replacement costs	$0	$1600	$4800	$8000
Clerical (Earnings $22 500) Replacement costs	$0*	$450	$1350	$2250
Skilled blue collar (Earnings $31 000) Replacement costs	$0	$725	$2175	$3625

* May vary from employer to employer, depending upon extent of support staff available.

Conclusions

This study demonstrates that there is a significant difference in cost to an employer when an employee is disabled and unable to work. Many large employers fund their own weekly income benefits, which an employee can receive for generally up to 26 weeks. If the employee has a 'key' position, the employer may also see the need to replace the disabled worker, which will increase the cost further. Therefore, it becomes very important to an employer to get the disabled worker back to work as quickly as possible.

Table 23.3: Worker's Compensation payable to employee

	Days of disability			
	5	*10*	*20*	*30*
Professional (Earnings \$80 000) Worker's Compensation	\$281	\$562	\$1125	\$1688
Clerical (Earnings \$22 500) Worker's Compensation	\$206	\$412	\$822	\$1234
Skilled blue collar (Earnings \$31 000) Worker's Compensation	\$281	\$562	\$1125	\$1688

Table 23.4: State of Indiana Worker's Compensation temporary total disability benefits

	Maximum wage/week	*Maximum benefit/week*
July 91	\$492	\$328
July 92	\$540	\$360
July 93	\$591	\$394
July 94	\$642	\$428

Reference

1. Disability Management. March, 1992. Employee benefit plan review. p. 32.

Part II: Open hernia repairs

24

Ring(s) Closure of Indirect Inguinal Herniation

RAYMOND C READ

Whereas the external ring in the external oblique aponeurosis was palpated and used as a venue for directors and other instruments applied by the ancients to assist in taxis for replacement of hernial contents into the abdomen, the internal ring was not identified until the beginning of the nineteenth century when Astley Cooper wrote his first text on hernia[1]. This remarkable surgical anatomist was given the ultimate accolade by Halsted in his second report on hernia[2], 'From a clinical, anatomical and pathological standpoint, the work of Sir Astley Cooper on hernia is undoubtedly the greatest of all, and very little has been added to our knowledge of hernia of all kinds since his book appeared'.

Astley Cooper, in describing for the first time the transversalis fascia, pointed out that there was a ring within it which allowed transmission of the cord into the inguinal canal. He called that ring the 'internal abdominal ring' in his second book[3], and stated regarding it in his second edition[4], 'thus then it appears that the internal ring is not a circumscribed aperture but the external abdominal ring is formed by the separation of two portions of fasciae which have different attachments and distributions at the crural arch'.

The clearest demonstration of these two layers in forming the internal ring perhaps was given by Lytle of Sheffield in 1945[5]. He described the classic ring in the transversalis fascia and then reported a deeper ring in what he called the preperitoneal fascia but, as we know today, is actually the posterior lamina of Cooper's transversalis fascia. Lytle felt that, in the repair of the internal ring, both of these rings should be identified with the inferior epigastric vessels passing between them. The processus vaginalis in indirect herniation should be ligated above them and then separate suturing of both rings should be employed to reconstruct the defect. Fowler, in Australia in 1975[6], confirmed and extended Lytle's observations, stating, 'the preperitoneal fascia of the groin is distinct from the transversalis fascia although often mistaken for it; special features include the fascial ring or secondary internal ring which appears to have been confused in the past with the transversalis fascial opening or internal ring proper'. (In Chapter 5, I have pointed out that reanalysis would suggest that Fowler's preperitoneal fascia ring is simply the extra ring in the posterior layer of transversalis fascia.) Fowler went on to point out that the 'preperitoneal fascial ring or secondary internal ring occupies the position fairly constantly superolateral to the transversalis fascial ring or internal ring proper. In many children it is found to be fully 0.5 to 1 cm or more from the transversalis opening, a surprising distance.'

We now know that the internal spermatic fascia comes, not from the anterior layer of transversalis fascia surrounding the internal ring, but from the posterior lamina at the deeper ring. Therefore, one needs to have the concept of an inner inguinal canal extending between these two rings and lined by fascial connections. If these are not disrupted, ligation of the peritoneal protrusion is not high enough; furthermore, extraperitoneal fat, a so-called lipoma, can be retained within this inner inguinal canal and form a starting point for a recurrence that is actually a retention of the original indirect herniation.

It is remarkable how many cases of recurrent indirect inguinal herniation occur, again in the indirect position. This was pointed out by Postlethwait in 1971[7] when he stated that, in 300 cases of recurrent groin herniation, an indirect residual sac was found in more than half of them. It has always been interesting to me that recurrent indirect inguinal herniation tends to be found in the same position in the cord anatomically as the original processus vaginalis. This indicates again that the recurrence through the defect is being funnelled by a persistent inner inguinal canal that has not been disrupted and is formed by the transversalis fascial layers coming together. This retention of the inner inguinal canal can occur even with preperitoneal repair from the posterior approach if the surgery is conducted superficial to the inferior epigastric vasculature, which lies between the two layers of transversalis fascia. It is easy to mistake the depth of the operation because fat may accompany these vessels and this may be considered to be the preperitoneal fat. The posterior lamina of Cooper is translucent although a definite tough membrane, as I described earlier in the proceedings.

The importance of really high ligation above the two rings was emphasized by Henry[8] when he described his experience with the preperitoneal approach. He illustrated the true and the false neck of the peritoneal protrusion, pointing out that, if the ligation occurs at the more distal false neck, recurrence is frequent. It is interesting that, when Bassini first described the modern operation[9], he explanted the cord laterally, dividing the internal oblique and transverse layers up to within 2.5 cm (1 inch) of the anterior superior iliac spine, in order to get a high ligation. He reported ligating the processus vaginalis in indirect herniation within the iliac fossa, flush with the general peritoneal cavity. He can be considered to be the first surgeon working within the preperitoneal space, but of course he approached it from the classic anterior exposure.

Henry said, 'the true neck of the sac and the correct site for high ligation is some distance from the false neck of the internal ring proper'. Ligation of the sac at the anatomical level of the classic transversalis internal ring can result in a residual funnel of sac being missed by the operator. This is a likely cause of recurrent hernia in a substantial number of cases. Much of the success of the Shouldice operation can, I believe, be attributed to their 'destruction' of the internal ring(s) and complete freeing of the peritoneal protrusion. Astley Cooper has to bear some of the responsibility for failing to emphasize this inner inguinal canal, even though he did report on two layers of transversalis fascia[3]. In his days, the word 'peritoneum' was held to include everything between the peritoneal layer we now define and the musculoaponeurotic layers of the abdominal wall. This convention has persisted in anatomical work since. Astley Cooper also started the idea of reporting fascial layers and rings, without adding the vasculature in those drawings of the two layers of transversalis fascia. This stylistic convention has held sway until the last 50 years when photography and better artwork have depicted what is actually seen rather than what is expected to be there.

Bassini's earth-shaking work so dominated the field for the following half century that the emphasis was placed to an extreme on simple removal of the processus vaginalis without much concern about the defect in the internal ring. This was especially true in children and young adults, because it was considered that the muscles were so strong, what with the shutter mechanism, the normal overlap of the internal ring by the internal oblique muscles and the tightening of the crura of the ring with contraction of the transversus abdominus, that no separate closure of the transversalis ring was necessary. Furthermore Bassini's repair became corrupted into a more superficial fixation of the internal oblique muscle either anterior or posterior to the cord down to the inguinal ligament without repair of the transversalis fascia and the internal ring itself. The results, especially in young recruits entering military service during the two World Wars, were unsatisfactory. The Bassini operation fell into disrepute, largely because it was misapplied (or, better stated, it was not performed properly). Recurrence after direct hernia was so great that it was suggested by some that operation should not be performed in these cases, which were becoming more prevalent anyway as the population aged and smoking increased. Trusses were again recommended.

Harrison clearly pointed out the problem in 1922[10] when he stated, 'When we consider the dozens of hundreds of men who first show a hernia [indirect] at 50 and 60 after their active life is over, the hypothesis [ie the primacy of the peritoneal sac] becomes improbable to say the least'. The emphasis then returned in inguinal hernia repair to repair of the transversalis fascial internal ring itself along with the processus vaginalis. The has gone so far now with the modern Bassini (the

Shouldice operation) that surgeons have pointed out that removal of the sac itself is of no significance if the defect in the transversalis fascia is properly repaired. Many surgeons anyway, once releasing the peritoneum completely, would invert the sac without opening it. I have generally felt that the sac should be opened because, otherwise, one cannot determine that there is no remaining sliding component, etc. Another advantage of opening the sac is that the finger can be inserted into the peritoneal cavity, as originally recommended by Bassini, and all other potential defects (certainly femoral) palpated. Because we are seeing an increasing number of patients who have multiple groin herniation, we now accept Fruchaud's concept that there is a common muscular fascial bony defect in the groin, including the passage of the cord and of the femoral vessels into the leg, which needs to be taken care of when any type of groin herniation is being dealt with[11].

The first isolated closure of the internal ring, as performed by Marcy in 1892[12], followed Bassini's contribution. Some authorities have said that he performed this operation as early as 1872, after he returned from working with Lister in England and introduced antisepsis to the USA[13]. However, careful analysis of his writings indicates that the ring he was talking about at that time was actually the external ring, and his operation was conducted without division of the external oblique aponeurosis and without exposure of the inguinal canal. He used the dilated external ring as his entry point. His 1892 contribution is described in his book on hernia[12]. This is an excellent approach today in selected cases, especially in the young with incomplete herniation (bubonocele). This operation is conducted routinely in children. I believe that, when isolated ring closure is performed at the internal ring, we should do as Marcy did: make the closure medial so that the obliquity of the inguinal canal is, if anything, increased. The idea of putting sutures lateral to the cord, popularized by Harkins in the early 1950s[14], is not to be recommended; I believe Bassini's principle of medial suturing to be better (as also adopted by Halsted), if necessary explanting the ring laterally. It is important, however, that the lateral portion of the internal ring be exposed well. Failure of the transversalis fascia in this area may extend to the femoral sheath, and prevascular herniation can be present along with inguinal defects themselves. If these other hernias are not taken care of, the patients may return to the surgeon soon after his procedure. Again, the Shouldice surgeons have stressed lateral explantation of the cord if necessary. Closure of these internal rings can be performed using an umbrella plug prosthesis, as recommended by Gilbert and Rutkow.

Even though, as I mentioned above, Postlethwait and Henry had been concerned about indirect recurrences, my own data suggest that today the commonest recurrence following isolated closure of the internal ring is direct. This, I believe, occurs because the decision to do an isolated closure of the ring is unwise if there is good evidence of more generalized weakness of the floor of the inguinal canal. McVay stressed this point[15] – he used isolated closure of the ring in a surprising number of his operations, perhaps a third, whereas he did his Lotheissen–Cooper's ligament repair in the other two-thirds (the so-called complete operation). The strength of the inguinal floor should be tested both externally and internally when other potential groin orifices are being 'fingered'.

Closure of patent processus vaginales poses a problem in laparoscopic herniorrhaphy because the surgeon runs into the problem of asymptomatic patent indirect sacs, which are known to be present in 20% of men at autopsy. Should these be closed? In general, yes. However, herniation at this orifice demands repair of the fascial ring as well. This is why plugging of the peritoneal protrusion alone has proved unsatisfactory. In some instances, repair of the peritoneal defect 'alone' may succeed because the surrounding fascial layers are inadvertently included.

References

1. Cooper AP. *The Anatomy and Surgical Treatment of Inguinal and Congenital Hernia*. London: Longman, 1804.
2. Halsted WS. The radical cure of inguinal hernia in the male. *Johns Hopkins Hosp Bull* 1893; **4**: 17.

3. Cooper AP. *The Anatomy and Surgical Treatment of Crural and Umbilical Hernia*. London: Longman, 1807: 3–4.

4. Cooper AP. *The Anatomy and Surgical Treatment of Abdominal Hernia*, 2nd Am ed. Rev. by CA Key. Philadelphia; Lea & Blanchard, 1844: 17–58.

5. Lytle WJ. The internal inguinal ring. *Br J Surg* 1945; **32**: 441.

6. Fowler R. The applied surgical anatomy of the peritoneal fascia of the groin and the 'secondary' internal inguinal ring. *Aust NZ J Surg* 1975; **45**: 8.

7. Postlethwait RW. Causes of recurrence after inguinal herniorrhaphy. *Surgery* 1971; **69**: 772–5.

8. Henry AK. Operation for femoral hernia by a midline extraperitoneal approach: with a preliminary note on the use of this route for reducible inguinal hernia. *Lancet* 1936; **1**: 531.

9. Bassini E. Nuovo metodo per la cura radicale dell'ernia inguinal. *Atti Congr Assoc Med Ital* 1887; **2**: 179.

10. Harrison PW. Inguinal hernia: a study of the principles involved in surgical treatment. *Arch Surg* 1922; **4**: 680.

11. Fruchaud H. *Anatomie chirurgicale des hernies de l'aine*. Paris, G. Doin, 1956.

12. Marcy HO. *Hernia*. New York: Appleton, 1892.

13. Ellis H. Lord Lister and the compound fracture. *Contemp Surg* 1979; **15**: 67.

14. Bruce J. Discussion of Nyhus IM, Stevenson JK, Listerud MB, Harkins HN. Preperitoneal herniorrhaphy: a preliminary report in fifty patients. *West J Surg Obstet Gynecol* 1959; **67**: 48.

15. McVay CB. Preperitoneal hernioplasty. *Surg Gynecol Obstet* 1966; **123**: 349.

25

Bassini Repair

GEORGE E WANTZ

American and European Bassini inguinal hernioplasties differ. In the American operation the cremaster muscle and the posterior wall of the inguinal canal are not divided, and the repair consists of suturing the conjoint tendon to the shelving portion of the inguinal ligament. In the European operation the cremaster muscle in the inguinal canal is excised and the posterior wall of the inguinal canal completely divided, thereby permitting a thorough survey and assessment of the anatomical parts to be sutured. The repair then approximates with interrupted sutures Bassini's 'triple layer' consisting of internal oblique abdominal muscle, the transverse abdominal muscle and the transverse fascia to the inguinal ligament and iliopubic tract. The European Bassini hernioplasty, therefore, resembles the Shouldice hernioplasty because the dissections are identical and the repairs approximate identical structures, albeit and Shouldice repair is more refined.

Pondering on this subject led to me the discovery of a remarkable atlas by A Catterina, which he claims describes and depicts the authentic Bassini operation[1]. The atlas was widely published throughout Europe but not in North America – which explains the discrepancy.

The Operation of Bassini by Catterina

Attilio Catterina was Professor of Surgery at Genoa. He had been a protégé and then a colleague of Bassini for many years. Indeed, he had actually translated into German Bassini's Italian description of the procedure for publication in the *Langenbäck Archives* in 1890. This was the publication that ignited the worldwide enthusiasm for the Bassini hernioplasty. Catterina was very fond of Bassini and considered him as his 'great master'. He understood the Bassini hernioplasty very well and was eminently qualified to describe it.

Catterina became disturbed because everywhere the Bassini operation was incorrectly performed, modified and criticized. He ascribed most of the blame for this to Bassini because Bassini's descriptions and illustrations were incomplete and imprecise. Also, Catterina failed to mention what he surely must have known – that Bassini never specifically described dividing the cremaster muscle and posterior wall of the inguinal canal. Nevertheless, Catterina was bent on setting the record straight. Consequently, he travelled widely, explaining and performing the correct way to do the operation. In his travels he encountered in Innsbruck a talented surgeon–artist by the name of O Gaigher whom he persuaded to illustrate an atlas he proposed on the Bassini hernioplasty.

The atlas, with beautiful life-sized coloured plates depicting the precise technical details of the operation, was published in Bologna in 1932, Berlin in 1933, Paris in 1934, London in 1934, Madrid in 1935, but curiously never in North America. Noteworthy is the fact that in the atlas Catterina states that two important steps in the operation which were omitted by surgeons everywhere were division of the cremaster muscle and division of the posterior wall of the inguinal canal.

The atlas was not completely unnoticed in North America because it was reviewed: the German edition in the *New England Journal of Medicine*, the *Journal of the American Medical Association* and the *American Journal of Surgery*, and the French edition in the *Journal of the American Medical Association*. The reviewers, whose names were not given, failed to grasp the significance of the book and none of the reviews was enthusiastic. Until recently, the surgeons of North America have been unaware of the atlas and of Bassini's intent. Furthermore, the atlas is rare in the USA. The Berlin and Bologna editions are in the library of the New York Academy of Medicine. The London edition is in the National Archives, in the antique book collection of the University of Kansas and in the library of the Mayo Clinic in Rochester, Minnesota. This last is not surprising because the Mayo brothers wrote a foreword for the London edition, at Catterina's request. Recently, I acquired two copies of the London editions.

The house that Bassini built fell down and was rebuilt.

Surgeons employing a corrupted form of the Bassini operation consistently obtained poor results. 'The house that Bassini built fell down', Brandon's well known comment in *The Lancet*, is appropriate[2]. Although the incorrect Bassini operation continued to be done in America and Great Britain, and by some in Europe, most European surgeons were performing Catterina's Bassini operation, were obtaining good results and were little interested in other procedures. In North America, however, the corrupt Bassini operation was abandoned by surgeons, who recognized the poor results, in favour of McVay's Cooper ligament repair, Marcy's simple ring closure and Nyhus's preperitoneal approach.

Meanwhile, and without fanfare, surgeons at the Shouldice Hospital in Toronto evolved a technique of inguinal hernioplasty that was ultimately to sweep the world because of its exceptionally good results and very fast recovery time. The Shouldice surgeons were unaware of Catterina's atlas and that their operation bore a very close resemblance to the authentic Bassini procedure. The Shouldice inguinal hernioplasty should be called the Shouldice–Bassini inguinal hernioplasty. The Shouldice surgeons had unwittingly returned the Bassini operation to prominence and grace.

Advantages and disadvantages of the Shouldice–Bassini operation

The Shouldice–Bassini inguinal hernioplasty has many advantages. Many, I included, consider the procedure to be the quintessential operation in surgery. It is a joy to perform and eminently suitable for unassisted local anaesthesia in day surgery centres. Its reputations for being unintrusive and for producing good results with minimal discomfort are legendary. For example, in my personal experience, 6.0% of the patients (mainly physicians and lawyers) return to work the same day as the operation, and 72.0% miss three or fewer days of work. Recovery rates such as these are hard to beat. Patients claim that the entire event was a 'piece of cake'.

The Shouldice–Bassini hernioplasty has been justly criticized because it does not address the femoral region, and very likely actually causes some femoral hernias through excess suture tension on the femoral sheath. Fortunately, femoral recurrences are infrequent. The procedure is also inadequate for recurrent hernias (my recurrence rate was 6.0% for a single recurrence) and probably inadequate for combined indirect and direct hernias (3.5% recurrence rate).

Another disadvantage is that much experience is required to obtain recurrence rates for primary hernioplasties in the range of 1.0%. For surgeons not specialized in the procedure, recurrence rates in the range of 4.0–8.0% are to be expected. Most of these recurrences will be in the first year or at the pubic tubercle, both of which I view as the result of inadequate surgical technique.

The Shouldice–Bassini hernioplasty may also be criticized because it is an anterior repair. During an anterior repair the sensory nerves are handled and the inguinal canal and the spermatic cord are necessarily dissected. Therefore, the chances of residual neuralgias and testicular atrophy are increased. In posterior repairs these complications are greatly decreased.

Another just criticism is the fact that the repair is not anatomical because it uses the inguinal ligament to reconstruct the posterior wall of the inguinal canal. The inguinal ligament is movable in its central portions and an unsteady structure. Moreover, it is not part of the posterior wall of the abdomen but is, instead, the lowermost edge of the most superficial myoaponeurotic layer of the abdomen. To use it to repair the innermost layer of the abdomen is illogical. This criticism, although true, is pedantic since the repair unquestionably works.

Finally, the Shouldice–Bassini hernioplasty, along with all the classic hernioplasties, does not address the issue of continued deterioration of the tissues, which occurs in everybody with age. Recurrence will always continue to occur years after the original operation. True recurrence rates can never be known. Recurrence curves are asymptotic.

Recurrence rates

The Bassini hernioplasty is rarely performed anymore except perhaps in Italy. Reported experience is old and the authors do not specify the Bassini technique used, the experience of the surgeons or the number of surgeons involved. The recurrence rates reported are, therefore, unreliable. However, for the record, the reported average recurrence rate was 10.3% (Table 25.1)[4]. Bassini himself reported a recurrence rate of 3.8% in 1890.

Glassow reported the recurrence rate of individual surgeons known to have exceptionally large personal experience with the Shouldice–Bassini hernioplasty[3]. The average of the collected results was 1.5% (Table 25.2). These recurrence rates are exceptional and, of course, can not be compared to the results reported in the paragraph above.

M Kux is the only known surgeon who has specifically compared the results of the authentic Bassini operation with those of the Shouldice–Bassini. His data have not been published yet, although

Table 25.1: Bassini hernioplasty: recurrence rate (average 10.3%)

Author	*Year*	*No.*	*Recurrence rate* (%)
Bassini	1890	206	3.8
Bellenger	1967	1102	25.0
Callum	1974	186	7.5
Scheibe	1974	309	2.6
Hoare	1975	281	3.6
Carlin	1980	269	11.1
Magnusson	1983	125	9.6
Vayre	1983	305	7.2
Stoppa	1984	91	22.5

Table 25.2: Shouldice hernioplasty: recurrence rates (average 1.5%)

		Recurrences	
Author	*No. of operations*	*No.*	%
Barwell	1566	28	1.8
Berliner	1084	12	1.1
Burson	2000	70	3.5
Devlin	787	7	0.9
Dunn	2949	34	1.2
Shearburn	953	7	0.7
Wantz	2470	23	0.9

the paper has been accepted for publication in the *American Journal of Surgery*. However, Kux told me that the recurrence rate for the Bassini operation was 8.7%, whilst that for two groups of Shouldice operation was 3.6% and 2.3%. The results are significant and indicate that the Shouldice–Bassini operation is better than the pristine Bassini operation.

Finally and most importantly, it must be remembered that, in any discussion of classic hernioplasties, success can*not* be measured by recurrence rates. *There are too many variables.* The quality of the surgery, the quality of the tissues and the degree of tension are more important than the chosen technique.

References

1. Wantz GE. The operation of Bassini as described by Attilo Catterina. *Surg Gynecol Obstet* 1989; **168**: 67–80.
2. Brandon WJM. Inguinal hernia: the house that Bassini built. *Lancet* 1945; **Feb. 10**: 167–71.
3. Glassow F. Inguinal hernia repair using local anaesthesia. *Ann Coll Surg Engl* 1984; **66**: 382–7.
4. Pietri P, Gabrielli F. Recurrent inguinal hernia. *Int Surg* 1986; **71**: 164–8.

26

The Shouldice Operation

ROBERT BENDAVID

The Shouldice Hospital was established in 1945 and, since then, more than 215 000 operations have been carried out on all forms of external abdominal wall hernias. To date, 2118 recurrences have been identified, accounting for a recurrence rate of 0.98%. In 1991, for example, 7364 operations were performed, of which 957 had been for recurrences. Of all patients seen, 12% revealed a secondary hernia which, by itself, could have required surgery. This fact underlines the necessity of carrying out a search for additional, simultaneous hernias.

The Shouldice repair for inguinal hernia is an operation that draws from many of the steps introduced in the last 100 years by many of the eminent contributors to surgery, among them:

- Championniere, Marcy, Bassini – ligation of the sac
- Bassini, Marcy, McVay – division of the inguinal floor
- Condon – inclusion of the iliopubic tract in closure
- Marcy, Bassini, Halsted, McVay – closure of the inguinal floor.

The Shouldice operation is generally carried out under local anaesthesia using 1% procaine (Novocain) to a volume of 200 ml. Preoperative medication consists of diazepam (10–20 mg orally) and meperidine (Demerol) (25–100 mg i.m.)

Surgical aspects

The most important aspect of the Shouldice operation lies in the dissection, which will demonstrate the presence of all possible hernias – inguinal (direct and indirect), femoral, prevesical and interstitial. The careful dissection, besides revealing hernias, will also bring about exposure of the structures necessary for an adequate herniorrhaphy (Figure 26.1). This skin is infiltrated, along a line joining the anterior superior iliac spine to the pubis, with 1% procaine (Novocain). The incision is made, superficial bleeders are controlled and the external oblique aponeurosis exposed.

At this stage 20–30 ml procaine (Novocain) is injected deep to the aponeurosis, allowing infiltration of the ilioinguinal and iliohypogastric nerves. The aponeurosis is incised along the direction of the fibres from the superficial inguinal ring to a level just lateral to the deep inguinal ring. At this stage, the ilioinguinal, iliohypogastric nerves, as well as the genital branch of the genitofemoral nerve are clearly identified and in turn, infiltrated with 1 ml procaine (Novocain) each.

The cremaster muscle is now picked up with forceps and incised longitudinally from the level of the pubic crest to the deep inguinal ring, yielding a medial and lateral flap. This medial flap is resected. The lateral flap is divided and each stump (lateral – near the internal ring and medial near the pubis) is doubly ligated with a resorbable suture.

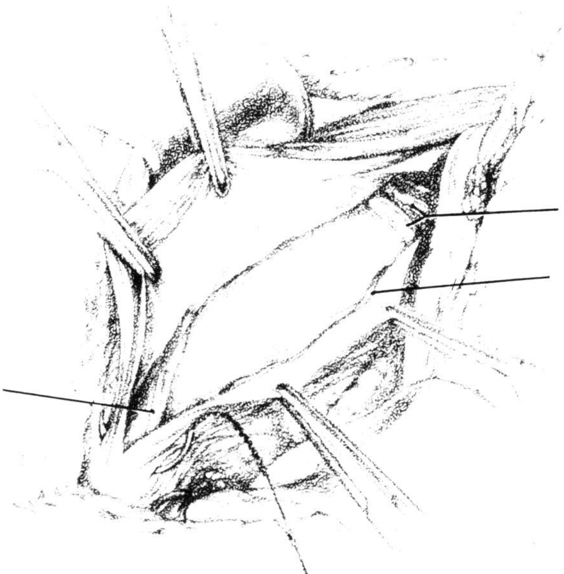

Figure 26.1: Dissection completed. The first suture picks up the transversalis fascia laterally (iliopubic tract), then crosses to include the lateral edge of the rectus abdominis, transversalis fascia, transversus abdominis and internal oblique. (By permission of Encyclopedie Medico-Chirurgicale)

Dissection on the medial aspect of the spermatic cord will reveal, without difficulty, an indirect sac which will be freed circumferentially beyond the deep inguinal ring. The sac is then opened, ligated near the base, the excess peritoneal sac resected so that the stump springs back into the preperitoneal space of Bogros to disappear. If an indirect sac is absent, identification of a peritoneal protrusion, which is peeled off the spermatic cord and allowed to retract, will confirm the absence of an indirect hernial sac.

Resection of an indirect sac, a well established practice by all, may in fact not be necessary[4]. This belief was confirmed by Welsh and Ryan who presented a series of more than 3000 sliding inguinal hernias and proved that simply freeing a sac and returning it to the preperitoneal space was adequate[1,2,3]. The important step was the reconstruction of the inguinal floor, which acts as a barrier to reprotrusion. In that series, 11 recurrences were recorded, only one being a true recurrence, the others being femoral or direct inguinal hernias forming subsequently.

Examination of the inguinal floor is now possible. If any doubt exists, the patient may be asked to strain or cough to reveal a direct hernia if one is present. The next step consists in incising the inguinal floor from the level of the deep inguinal ring to the pubic crest. (In female patients, the incidence of direct inguinal hernias is 0.2%, so the floor need not be incised as frequently[4,5].) This is done by incising the transversalis fascia on the medial aspect of the deep ring to avoid injuring the inferior epigastric vessels. To enter the preperitoneal space of Bogros, the posterior lamina must also be incised to reveal the glistening preperitoneal fat, which is dissected away deep to the posterior aspect of the inguinal wall. In so doing, one notices medially the transversus aponeurotic arch and, deep and medial, the lateral portion of the rectus muscle. Laterally, the transversalis fascia is clearly identified, carefully avoiding injury to the iliopubic vein, on the deep aspect of the fascia. The fascia cribriformis, an extension of the fascia lata, is now incised below the inguinal ligament from the

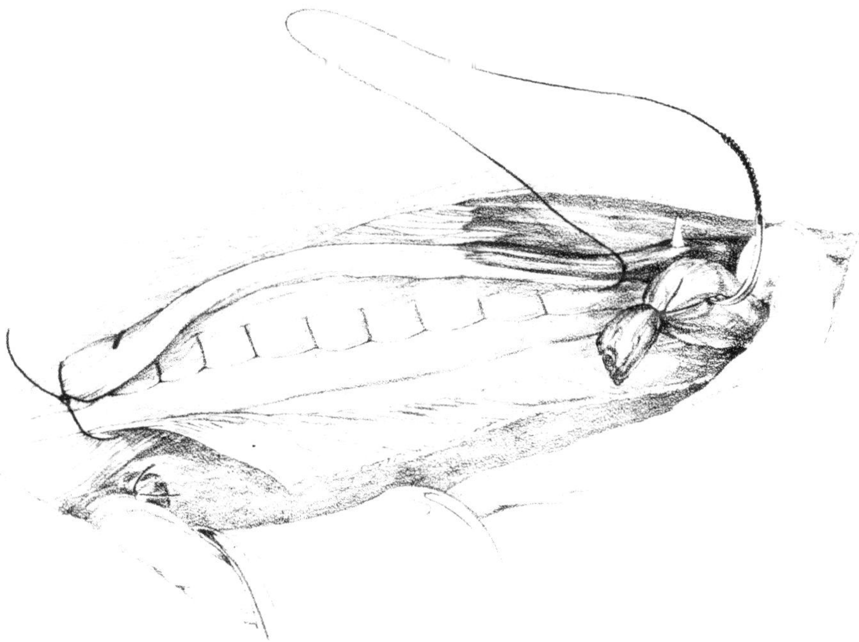

Figure 26.2: First line of suture picks up the cremasteric stump laterally, before reversing as line two, towards the pubic crest. (By permission of Encyclopedie Medico-Chirurgicale)

level of the femoral vein to the pubic crest. This manoeuvre will allow examination of the femoral ring from above and below the inguinal ligament. Dissection is now complete and repair may begin.

Traditionally, wire suture (gauge 32 and 34) is used for the inguinal repair. The aim is to lay down four lines of sutures. The first suture will provide lines one and two. A second suture will provide lines three and four. The first suture is inserted into the transversalis fascia, near the pubis, crosses over to the other side to incorporate the lateral portion of the rectus muscle, transversalis fascia, transversus abdominis muscle and internal oblique, and a knot tied (Figure 26.2). The long end of this first suture will be a continuous suture, advancing toward the deep inguinal ring. Halfway, the rectus muscle becomes too distant and is no longer incorporated. Laterally, the cremasteric stump is included to provide a new sling about the spermatic cord. The suture now reverses its course toward the pubic crest and in so doing will include the shelving edge of Poupart's ligament (Figure 26.3). Near the pubis, a knot is tied. The first and second lines are completed.

The second suture is now readied and will provide the third and fourth lines. The third line begins near the deep inguinal ring, goes through the internal oblique and transversus abdominis, then across to the inner aspect of the external oblique aponeurosis, which it picks up along a line parallel to the inguinal ligament and, in fact, creating a new artificial inguinal ligament (Figure 26.4). This third line proceeds to the level of the pubic crest and then reverses its course toward the deep inguinal ring. The medial 2 cm of the external oblique aponeurosis will be laid down on the medial aspect of the floor of the canal to reinforce a site known to be subject to breakdown and recurrence. This fourth line continues still toward the deep inguinal ring where a knot will be tied, completing the fourth line. The spermatic cord is allowed to be placed on the new inguinal floor and the external oblique aponeurosis closed over it (Figure 26.5). The medial cremasteric stump is anchored near the pubic crest to prevent a low-lying testicle. A sedulous follow up, as long as 35 years, reveals a recurrence rate of 1.46% (Table 26.1). Table 26.2 reveals results as obtained by various authors.

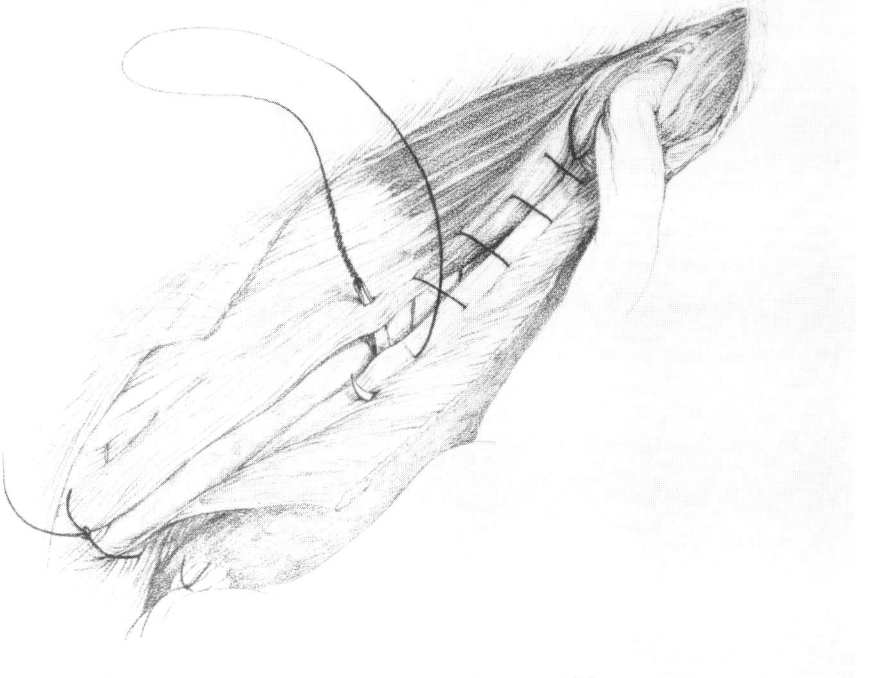

Figure 26.3: Line two picking up the ligament of Poupart. (By permission of Encyclopedie Medico-Chirurgicale)

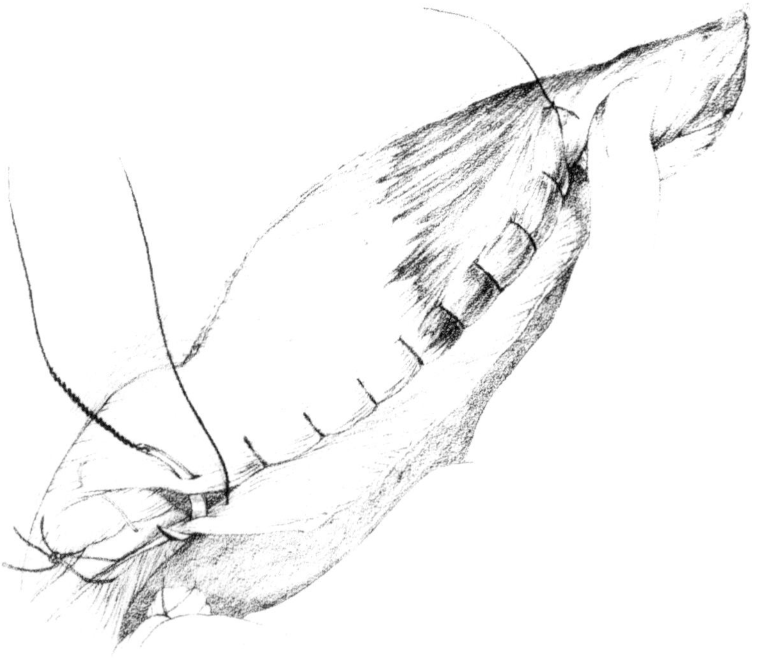

Figure 26.4: Line three which begins near the deep inguinal ring and proceeds towards the pubic crest. (By permission of Encyclopedie Medico-Chirurgicale)

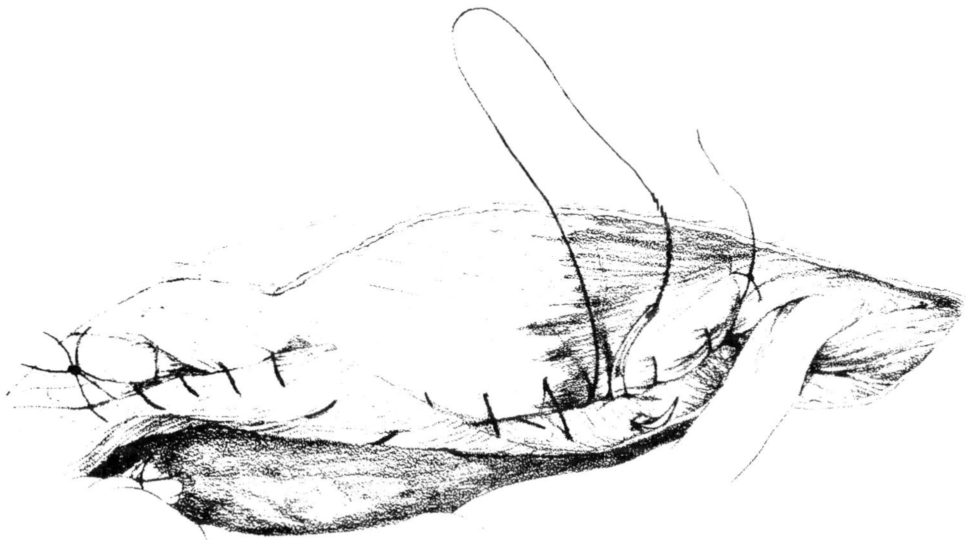

Figure 26.5: Line four. Note the medial portion of the external oblique aponeurosis covering the medial aspect of the inguinal floor. (By permission of Encyclopedie Medico-Chirurgicale)

Table 26.1: Follow up: 35 years of follow up of 2748 repairs on 2270 patients at Shouldice Hospital

1955	3	
1956	4	
1957	1	= 8 in 2 years
1958	3	
1959	3	
1960	2	= 16 in 5 years
1961–1965	8	= 24 in 10 years
1966–1975	7	= 31 in 20 years
1976–1980	9	= 40 in 35 years
Recurrence rate after 35 years: 1.46%		

Complications

Complications are invariably of a minor nature except for testicular atrophy. Infections are rarely over 1%; this is due to the fact that most operations are elective, on healthy individuals. Patients with a known infective source are first treated with antibiotics and their surgery delayed. Haematomas represent 0.3%; these haematomas are unusual, and when indicated they are evacuated and a search for bleeders is carried out. Rarely are the haematomas deep to the inguinal floor. Testicular atrophy is seen in 0.1% of primary herniorrhaphies and in 0.9% of recurrent herniorrhaphies. Hydrocele formation was well identified (0.7%) and published by Obney[6]. Dysejaculation, a painful, burning, searing sensation, is probably of the order of 0.25%[7]. Phlebitis, atelectasis, pneumonitis and

Table 26.2: Recurrence rate following the Shouldice operation

Author	*Number of cases*	*Percentage followed up*	*Years of follow up*	*Recurrence*
Shearburn	550	100	13	0.2%
Volpe	415	50	3	0.2%
Wantz	2087	–	5	0.3%
Myers	953	–	18	0.7%
Devlin	350	–	6	0.8%
Flament	134	–	6	0.9%
Wantz	2454	–	1–20	1.0%
Shouldice Hospital	2748	–	35	1.5%
Moran	121	–	6	2.0%
Berliner	591	–	2–5	2.7%

pulmonary embolism are practically non-existent, thanks to early ambulation and the regimen of light exercises after surgery.

Mortality is of the order of 0.009% and has never been a direct result of surgery. Twenty deaths have been recorded through the years, due to myocardial infarction (15 cases, average age 70), cerebrovascular accident (one case, 66 years) and four undetermined causes (ages 56, 66, 70, 78).

Conclusions

The Shouldice repair is based on a sound anatomical dissection and reconstruction. The operation is safe, can easily be carried out under local anaesthesia and is marred by few complications.

References

1. Welsh DRJ. Bilateral sliding inguinal hernias. *Postgrad Gen Surg* 1992; **4**: 114–16.
2. Ryan EA. An analysis of 313 consecutive cases of indirect sliding inguinal hernias. *Surg Gynecol Obstet* 1956; **102**: 45–58.
3. Ryan EA. Recurrent hernias; an analysis of 369 consecutive cases of recurrent inguinal and femoral hernias. *Surg Gynecol Obstet* 1953; **96**: 343–54.
4. Glassow F. High ligation of the sac in indirect inguinal hernia. *Am J Surg* 1965; **109**: 460–3.
5. Glassow F. Inguinal hernia is the female. *Surg Gynecol Obstet* 1963; **116**: 701
6. Obney N. Hydroceles of the testicle complicating inguinal hernias. *Can Med Assoc J* 1956; **75**: 733–6.
7. Bendavid R. Dysejaculation: an unusual complication of inguinal herniorrhaphy. *Postgrad Gen Surg* 1992; **4**: 139–41.
8. Bendavid R. The Shouldice method of inguinal herniorrhaphy. In: Nyhus LM, Baker RJ, eds *Mastery of surgery*, 2nd ed. Boston Toronto London: Little, Brown, 1992; pp 1584–94.

27

Cooper Ligament (McVay) Repair

ROBB H RUTLEDGE

The indirect, direct and femoral hernia sacs are within inches of each other. Rather than using a different repair for different types of hernias, why not use a hernia repair that works for all adult groin hernias? Your recurrence rates will be lower if you repair all possible defects at the original operation. There are several ways this can be done. My preference has been a Cooper ligament repair.

Why a Cooper ligament repair?

Advantages

The Cooper ligament repair restores normal anatomical planes and provides the best anchor for a strong reconstruction of the posterior wall. It closes the femoral canal and displays the femoral vessels to protect them from injury. It is the only anterior repair that closes the complete myopectineal orifice and repairs all the hernias that can occur in the groin[1,2].

Disadvantages

The Cooper ligament repair is more extensive than most hernia operations, and patients have a slower convalescence. There are also concerns about tension, vascular injuries and thromboembolic complications.

I agree with the first two disadvantages but I strongly disagree about the last three. They can be avoided by a generous relaxing incision and careful technique around the femoral vessels.

Historical background

The story of the Cooper ligament repair really should begin with Sir Astley himself[3]. In 1784, at the age of 16 years, he was apprenticed to Mr Henry Cline, the leading surgeon at St Thomas' Hospital in London. One night when Astley was attending one of Mr Cline's lectures on hernias he realized that he, himself, was the subject of that complaint. He ran home, dashed upstairs to his room, threw himself on the bed, elevated his legs on the bedpost and waited for Mr Cline to come home. When Mr Cline arrived, he confirmed the diagnosis and fitted young Astley with a truss that he wore faithfully for five years. He apparently had no further trouble.

This episode stimulated Cooper's interest in hernias. In 1804 he published his classic hernia work and dedicated it to Mr Cline[4]. In this book, Cooper demonstrated the anatomical defects of groin hernias. He described the transversalis fascia and the superior pubic ligament which later bore his name. Anaesthesia and asepsis were unknown then, and Cooper recommended surgery only for incarceration. He did not use his own ligament in his repairs.

A relaxing incision is an essential part of a Cooper ligament repair[5]. Although Anton Wolfler did not use the Cooper ligament in his hernia surgery, he is given credit for doing the first relaxing incision. He reported his method in the Festschrift for Theodor Billroth in 1892. Wolfler made a relaxing incision in the anterior rectus sheath whenever he noted tension approximating the rectus sheath to the inguinal ligament[6].

In 1897, Georg Lotheissen, another of Billroth's pupils, was the first to suture the conjoined tendon to the Cooper ligament. He was operating in Innsbruck on a 45-year-old woman with twice recurrent inguinal hernia following previous Bassini repairs. Her inguinal ligament was destroyed, so he anchored the conjoined tendon to the Cooper ligament instead. He then used this method without a relaxing incision for both inguinal and femoral hernias[7].

In 1938, while he was a medical student at Northwestern, Chester McVay, unaware of Lotheissen's work, became involved in an anatomical study with Barry Anson. They pointed out that the normal insertion of the transversus abdominis and the transversalis fascia was on the Cooper ligament, not the inguinal ligament. From these dissections McVay developed his technique of a Cooper ligament repair, and reported this from Ann Arbor in 1942 when he was a surgical resident[8]. He used a relaxing incision and recommended this repair for direct, large indirect, and femoral hernias. He did not use it for small or medium-sized indirect hernias, believing that reconstruction of the posterior wall was unnecessary in those cases[9,10].

In 1958, McVay reported 580 hernia repairs done without using the inguinal ligament[11]. This was the report that got me started. His overall recurrence rate was 2.4%, with 91% follow-up ranging from one to eleven years. He did only an abdominal ring repair for small or medium indirect hernias, believing that that was all they needed. His recurrence rate in this group was 3.2%. He did a Cooper ligament repair for direct, large indirect, and femoral hernias. His recurrence rate with these more difficult hernias was only 0.85%. This is the only report that I have seen that had a higher recurrence rate for the easier, indirect repairs.

McVay felt that the causes of recurrences after his abdominal ring repairs were direct recurrences due to misjudgment or later deterioration of the posterior wall, missed femoral hernias, and technical problems around the internal ring. It seemed to me that his abdominal ring repair was not enough. A more complete repair on the small and medium indirect hernias should give better results.

Surgical management

Since 1959, I have done a Cooper ligament repair for all groin hernias in adults, primary or recurrent, regardless of the presenting defect. Throughout this time there have been only two significant changes in operative technique. First, because of some indirect recurrences along the cord, I stopped transplanting the spermatic cord subcutaneously in 1972 and since then have left it in its natural position. Second, since 1989 I have routinely used a Marlex mesh patch to close the relaxing incision defect[12–15].

General anaesthesia has been preferred, and perioperative antibiotics are given. A Foley catheter is inserted immediately before the operation and removed in the recovery room.

Surgical technique

A low, almost transverse incision is made. The external oblique is opened through the external ring. The cord is dissected free in the canal but no dissection is done medial to the pubic tubercle. The posterior wall of the canal is taken down and the Cooper ligament dissected free. The spermatic cord is retracted superiorly with a Deaver retractor and the deeper portion of the Cooper ligament is cleared.

Then starting lateral to the femoral artery, the anterior femoral fascia is developed. Working medially, the anterior surface of the femoral artery and vein are cleaned off. Then the fat and lymph nodes are cleared from the femoral canal and any collaterals to the obturator circulation are divided and ligated so that they will not be torn during the repair.

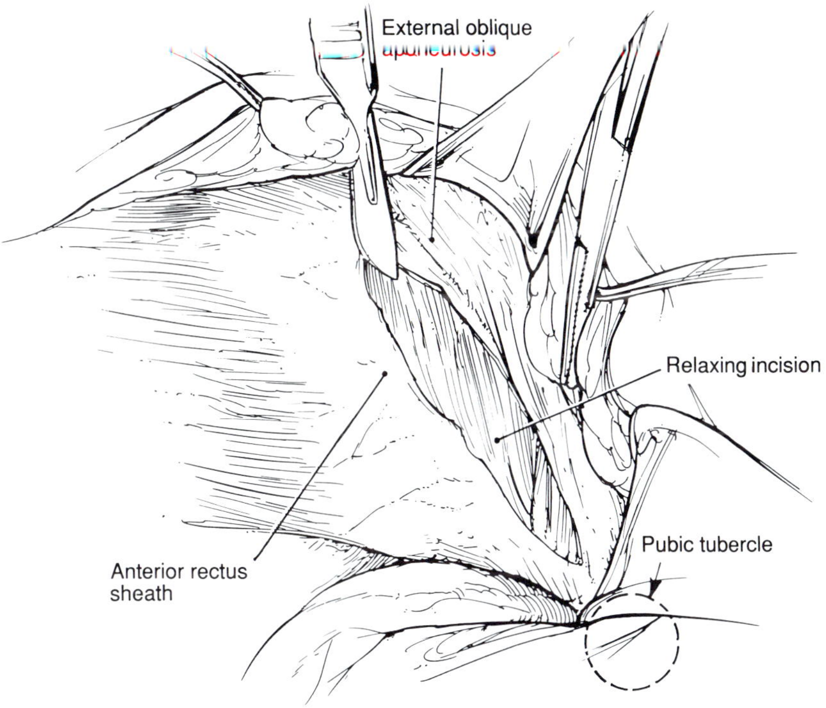

Figure 27.1: See text.

After the inferior dissection is completed, the transversus abdominis arch is freed from the underlying preperitoneal tissues. Then a relaxing incision is made at the point of fusion of the external oblique aponeurosis and the anterior rectus sheath. This begins at the pubis and goes at least 10 cm (4 inches) superiorly (Figure 27.1).

The patient is placed in the Trendelenburg position to decrease the chance of intestinal injury. The spermatic cord is opened and the cremaster fibres are divided at the internal ring. Indirect sacs are opened and explored to evaluate any intra-abdominal pathology. Small indirect sacs are removed, and the peritoneum is closed. Large indirect sacs are transected at the internal ring and the distal portion is left in place to avoid ischaemic orchitis. If no indirect sac is apparent, the anteromedial portion of the cord is dissected superiorly to identify and ligate the small peritoneal tab that is always present. The external spermatic artery is divided as it comes off the inferior epigastric so that the cord can be moved laterally during the repair. The preperitoneal tissue and any direct sac are imbricated with a continuous 0 chromic catgut suture. This must be done carefully to prevent any intestinal injury.

The repair is begun by bringing the transversus abdominis arch down to the Cooper ligament. I use an Allis clamp on the transversus abdominis arch to be sure I get a good bite of it, not merely the overlying internal oblique. This layer of interrupted sutures starts at the pubic tubercle and continues laterally to the medial edge of the femoral vein. About ten sutures are used (Figure 27.2).

The femoral canal is closed by two or three transition sutures between Cooper's ligament and the anterior femoral fascia. The lateral suture is placed just lateral to the last suture in the Cooper ligament. The medial two or three are medial to this and go between the Cooper ligament sutures (Figure 27.3).

The repair is continued laterally between the transversus abdominis arch and the anterior femoral fascia going beyond any indirect sac so the cord comes out obliquely laterally at the new internal ring. No sutures are placed lateral to the cord. This layer is 0 silk. The sutures are tied medial to

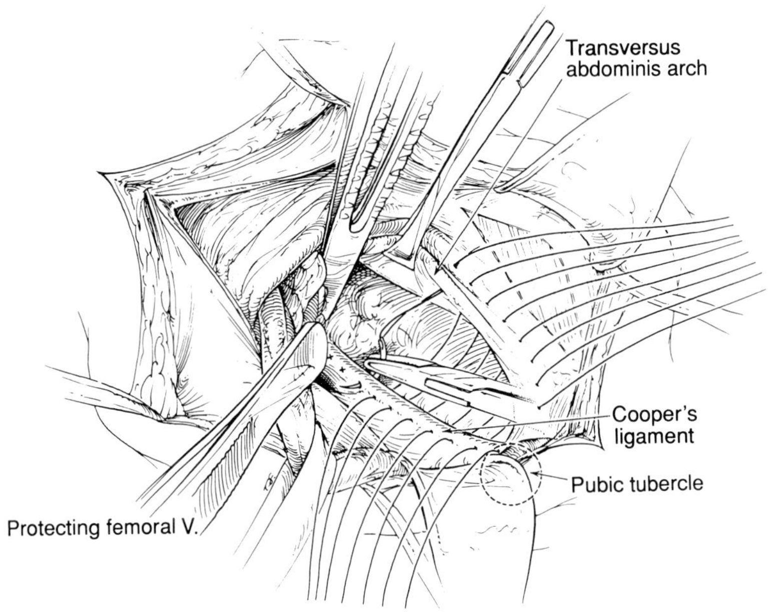

Figure 27.2: See text.

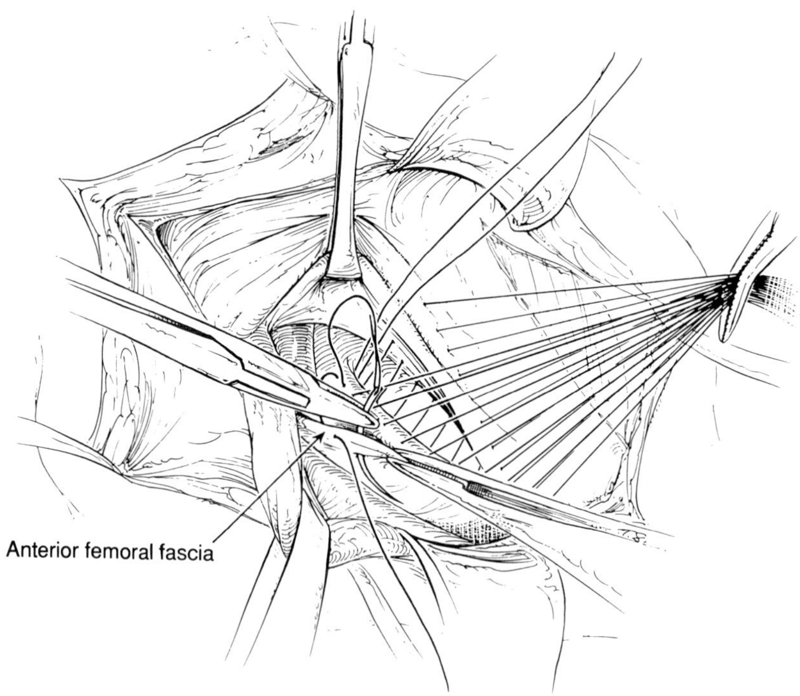

Figure 27.3: See text.

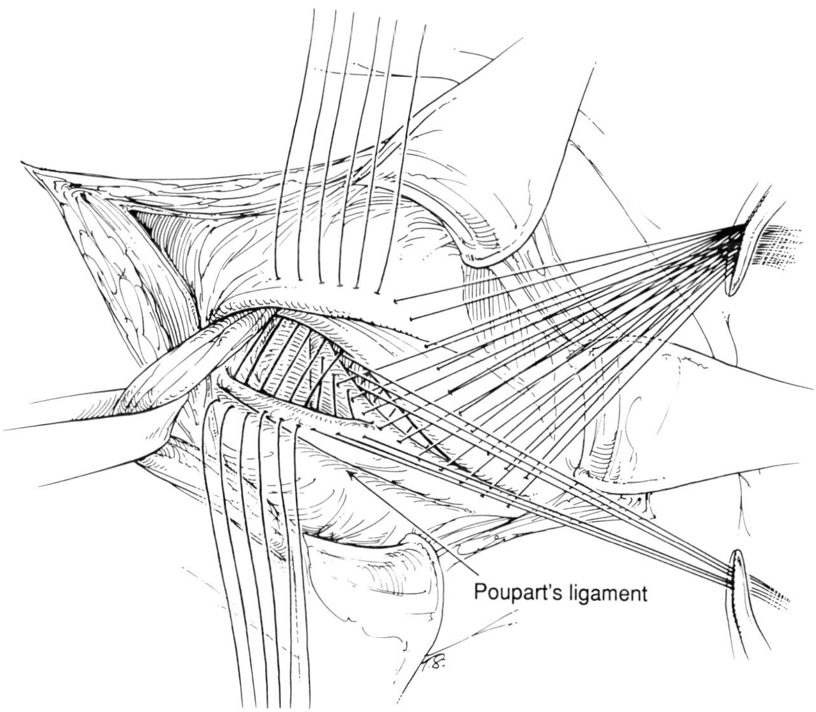

Figure 27.4: See text.

lateral and the patient is brought up out of the Trendelenburg position (Figure 27.4). The new internal ring is snug. It admits only a Kelly clamp.

The relaxing incision defect can be secured in place with some interrupted sutures, but I have preferred to fill the defect with a Marlex mesh patch that has been soaking in a double antibiotic solution and suture this in place with a continuous 0 Prolene (Figure 27.5). About 10% of the time I reinforce this basic repair with an onlay graft of Marlex mesh (Figure 27.6).

The cord is returned to its natural position, and the external oblique is closed over the cord with continuous 2–0 Vicryl. The new external ring is quite loose. The skin is closed with 4–0 subcuticular Dexon suture and sterile adhesive strips.

Special considerations

Recurrent hernia

Recurrent hernias are repaired as just described from an anterior approach. Beginning laterally in clean tissues the previous repair is dismantled completely, regardless of the type of recurrence. A long relaxing incision is made, the spermatic cord is carefully preserved and a Cooper ligament repair is done. If indicated, either in inlay or an onlay prosthetic graft can be added for reinforcement.

Bilateral hernias

Bilateral hernias are usually repaired at the same operation through two separate incisions, leaving a broad area between them to minimize scrotal swelling.

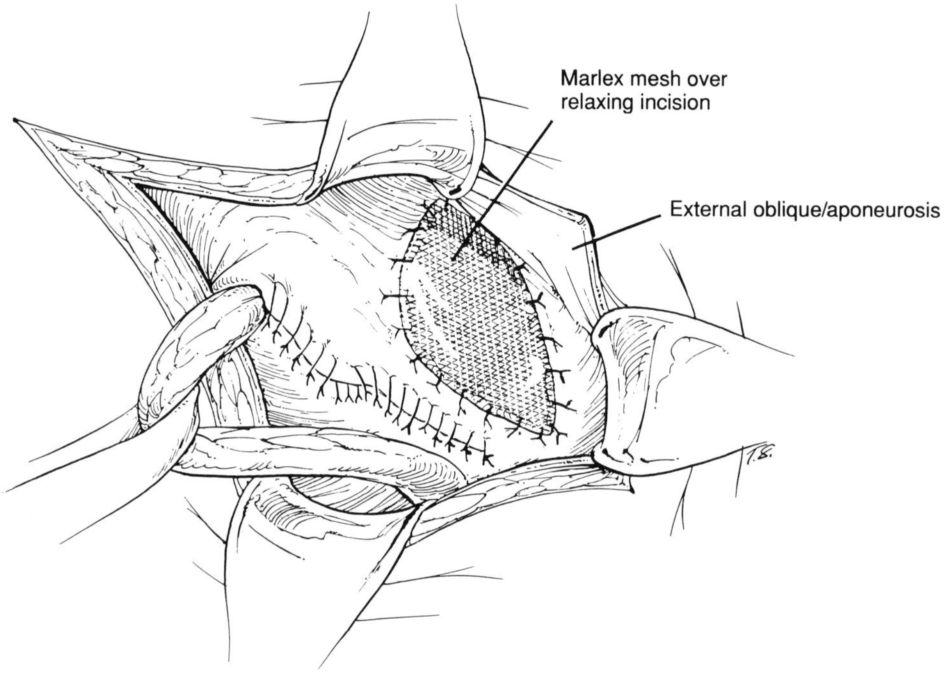

Figure 27.5: See text. Mesh is currently sutured in place with continuous 0 Prolene.

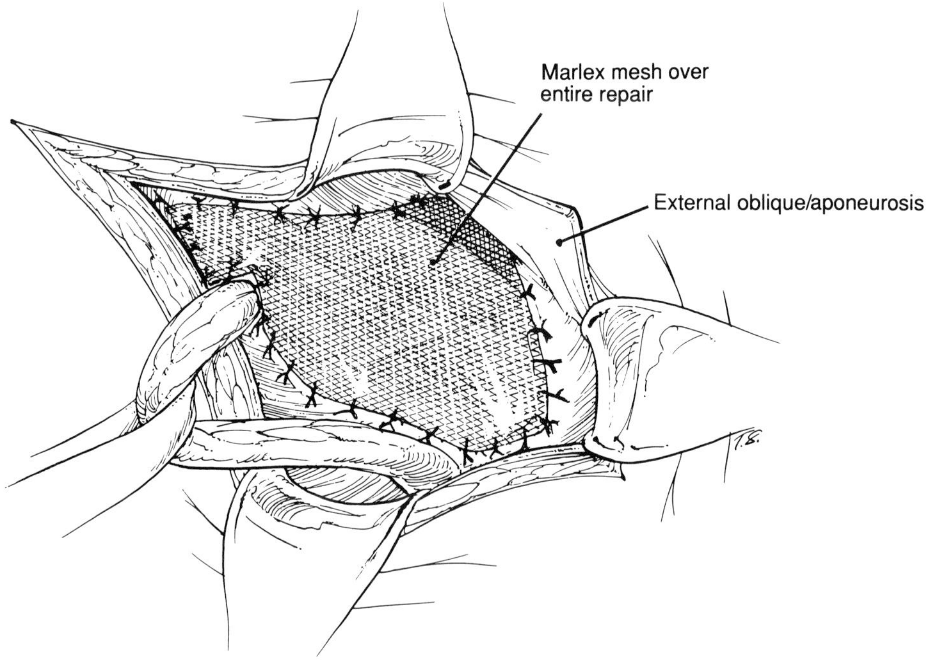

Figure 27.6: See text. Mesh is currently sutured in place with continuous 0 Prolene.

Tension

Tension need not be a problem if an adequate relaxing incision is made. This starts right at the pubis and extends at least 10 cm (4 inches) superiorly. If there is tension, I make the incision longer. If there is still a problem, McVay pointed out that you can divide some aberrant aponeurotic fibres lateral to the pyramidalis[16]. Occasionally, this is quite helpful.

Personal series

At my last complete study, I reported on 1142 hernia repairs done between 1959 and 1984[13]. Twenty-eight patients with 34 repairs were lost, giving a follow up of 97%. The only operative death was in a 65-year-old man with a proven myocardial infarction on the fourth postoperative day. There were 167 late deaths, leaving 747 patients with 906 hernia repairs to be examined. I personally examined 80% of these patients and talked to the remaining 20% on the telephone.

There were 18 recurrences, giving a 2% overall recurrence rate. Seventeen of these were indirect along the cord in a subgroup of 147 repairs done with a transplanted cord. I stopped using that technique in 1972. Excluding the group with the transplanted cord, the recurrence rate was 0.13% for 759 repairs followed up for an average of 7.4 years.

The only three recurrences in the 127 recurrent repairs were indirect along the cord in the subcutaneously transplanted group. There has been no recurrence in a recurrent repair otherwise.

My total experience through 1992 includes 1582 Cooper ligament repairs (Table 27.1). Although another complete follow up has not been done, I continue to follow my patients closely and am aware of the results. I believe that the recurrence rates are essentially unchanged.

Table 27.1: Cooper ligament repair 1959–1992 (1582 repairs)

	1351 Primary No. (%)	*231 Recurrent No.* (%)
Direct	482 (35)	133 (58)
Indirect	818 (61)	90 (39)
Femoral	51 (4)	8 (3)
Total	1351 (100) (85% of total)	231 (100) (15% of total)

Discussion

More extensive operation

The biggest disadvantage of a Cooper ligament repair is that it is a more extensive operation. The patients have a slower convalescence and generally have more discomfort for the first postoperative week. Although some go home the afternoon of surgery, most patients spend one night in the hospital. They are advised to stay home for one week and to walk daily for exercise. More vigorous activities are encouraged in several weeks.

In March 1993, I examined all of my hernia patients from 1992. This included 52 patients with 60 hernia repairs. There were no recurrences, no draining sinus tracts and no testicular problems. Four patients complained of some incisional discomfort but none was taking any medication or having any evaluation for a pain problem.

Fifteen of the patients were retired. Of those patients doing desk or standing work, 89% were back at work within two weeks; 50% of those doing heavy work were off for nearly six weeks.

Over all, 33% of patients had resumed all of their usual activities by two weeks and 88% had by four weeks. Retired patients resumed usual activities sooner than employed patients. Patients with recurrent or bilateral repairs tended to have a slower recovery. The personal interview showed that there was a great variation in individual motivation.

Although the recovery is slower than with laparoscopic repairs, the difference is not as great as advertised.

Vascular and embolic problems

Vascular injuries and thromboembolic problems are cited as dangers of a Cooper ligament repair[17–19]. Careful technique around the femoral vessels should prevent both of these concerns. The chances of vascular injury are minimal because the vessels are seen and protected. The deep layer of the repair is stopped at the medial edge of the femoral vein to prevent venous constriction and decrease the risk of thrombophlebitis.

In my series of 1582 Cooper ligament repairs there has been no vascular injury. Only two patients have had pulmonary emboli that required heparin therapy. Phlebograms on each of these patients did not show the operative side to be the source. One patient had a flare-up of a recurrent superficial phlebitis. A fourth patient had a transient venous constriction with swelling of his leg. This subsided with elevation and elastic support. No anticoagulants were used. His leg was then asymptomatic for the remaining six years of his life. The femoral vessels need not be a problem if careful technique is used.

Summary

Although a Cooper ligament repair is a more extensive operation than most hernia repairs, it can be done safely with minimal morbidity and a very low recurrence rate. It restores anatomical planes and provides the best anchor for a strong reconstruction of the posterior wall. It displays the femoral vessels to protect them from injury. It closes the complete myopectineal orifice, thereby repairing all of the hernias that can occur in the groin. A generous relaxing incision and careful technique around the femoral vessels are required. Many surgeons would choose a Cooper ligament repair for direct, large indirect, and femoral hernias only. I have used it for all groin hernias in adults, primary or recurrent, regardless of the presenting defect. I believe it is the strongest hernia repair done today.

References

1. Fruchaud H. *Anatomie chirurgicale des hernies de l'aine*. Paris: G Doin, 1956.
2. Wantz GE. *Atlas of Hernia Surgery*. New York: Raven Press, 1991: 4.
3. Cooper A. *Lectures on the Principles and Practice of Surgery*. London: E Portwine and JT Cox, 1835.
4. Cooper A. *The Anatomy and Surgical Treatment of Inguinal and Congenital Hernia*. London: JT Cox, 1804.
5. Ponka JL. The relaxing incision in hernia repair. *Am J Surg* 1968; **115**: 552.
6. Wolfler A. Zur radikaloperation des freien leistenbruches. In: Festschrift Theodor Billroth, ed. *Beitrage zur Chirurgie*. Stuttgart: Verlag von Ferdinand Enke, 1892: 552.
7. Lotheissen G. Zur radikaloperation der schenkelhernien. *Zentralbl Chir* 1898; **25**: 548.
8. McVay CB, Anson BJ. A fundamental error in current methods of inguinal herniorrhaphy. *Surg Gynecol Obstet* 1942; **74**: 746.
9. Halverson K, McVay CB. Inguinal and femoral hernioplasty, a 22 year study of the authors' methods. *Arch Surg* 1970; **101**: 127.
10. McVay CB. The anatomic basis for inguinal and femoral hernioplasty. *Surg Gynecol Obstet* 1974; **139**: 931.

11. McVay CB, Chapp JD. Inguinal and femoral hernioplasty. *Ann Surg* 1958; **148**: 499.

12. Rutledge RH. Cooper's ligament repair for adult groin hernias. *Surgery* 1980; **87**: 601.

13. Rutledge RH. Cooper's ligament repair: a 25 year experience with a single technique for all groin hernias in adults. *Surgery* 1988; **103**: 1.

14. Rutledge RH. Cooper's ligament repair. *Surg Rounds* 1989; **12**: 17.

15. Rutledge RH. The Cooper ligament repair. *Surg Clin North Am* 1993; **73**: 451.

16. McVay CB. *Anson and McVay Surgical Anatomy* 6th ed. Philadelphia: WB Saunders, 1984: 556.

17. Nissen HM. Constriction of the femoral vein following hernia repair. *Acta Chir Scand* 1975; **141**: 279.

18. Normington EY, Franklin DP, Brotman SL. Constriction of the femoral vein after McVay inguinal hernia repair. *Surgery* 1992; **111**: 343.

19. Schamberger RC, Ottinger LW, Malt RA. Arterial injuries during inguinal herniorrhaphy. *Ann Surg* 1984; **200**: 83.

28

The Lichtenstein Open Tension-free Hernioplasty

PARVIZ K AMID, ALEX G SHULMAN AND IRVING L LICHTENSTEIN

Weakening of the transversalis fascia, the sole support of the inguinal floor, due to collagen deficiency resulting from impairment of prolene hydroxilation is considered to be an important aetiological factor in adult groin hernias[1–5]. Using this already defective tissue, and especially under tension, is counter-productive, while its total reinforcement with a sheet of biomaterial and employment of a 'tension-free' technique is a more effective approach[6].

All standard methods of hernia repair involve suturing together tissues that are not normally in apposition. This violates the basic surgical principle that tissue must never be approximated under tension and accounts for an unacceptable number of failures. From June 1984 to June 1992 3250 primary inguinal hernias have been repaired at the Lichtenstein Hernia Institute by the open 'tension-free' technique using Marlex mesh. All patients were male, from 20 to 88 years of age (median age 52). The patients were followed for from one to eight years by physician examination. The follow-up rate was 87%. There were four recurrences. 44.4% of patients had indirect, 43.1% had direct, and 12.5% had a combination of indirect and direct inguinal hernias; 11.41% of patients had sliding hernias. 78.5% were of normal weight to 9 kg (20 lb) overweight, 19.7% were 9–23 kg (20–50 lb) overweight, and 2% were more than 23 kg (50 lb) overweight.

Operative technique

The procedure is carried out under local anaesthesia. After skin incision, the external oblique aponeurosis is opened in the direction of its fibres and the lower leaf is freed from the spermatic cord. The spermatic cord with its cremaster covering is freed from the floor of the inguinal canal and the pubic bone for a distance of approximately 2 cm beyond the pubic tubercle. The anatomical plane between the cremasteric sheath and the aponeurotic tissue attached to the pubic bone is avascular, so there is no risk of damaging the testicular blood flow by this manoeuvre. When elevating the cord, care is taken to include the external spermatic vessels and the genital nerve together with the cord (Figure 28.1). This ensures that the genital nerve, which is always in juxtaposition with the external spermatic vessels, is preserved. Cutting or ligation of the genital nerve can cause inordinate and incapacitating neuralgia for years[7]. The ilioinguinal and iliohypogastric nerves are also preserved. To thin the spermatic cord, the spermatic fat pad (lipoma of the cord), if present, is excised. The cremasteric fibres, if needed, are transversely incised at the level of the internal ring over clamp avoiding the nerve. Complete stripping and excision of the cremasteric fibres from the spermatic cord is unnecessary. This may result in injury to the nerves and small blood vessels and kinking of the vas deferens and increase the likelihood of postoperative neuralgia[8], ischaemic orchitis, infertility and dysejaculation[9].

Indirect hernial sacs are freed from the cord to a point beyond the neck of the sac. Opening the sac allows for digital examination of the femoral ring, and the sac is then inverted into the abdomen without ligation which may cause more postoperative pain[10,11]. To minimize the risk of postoperative

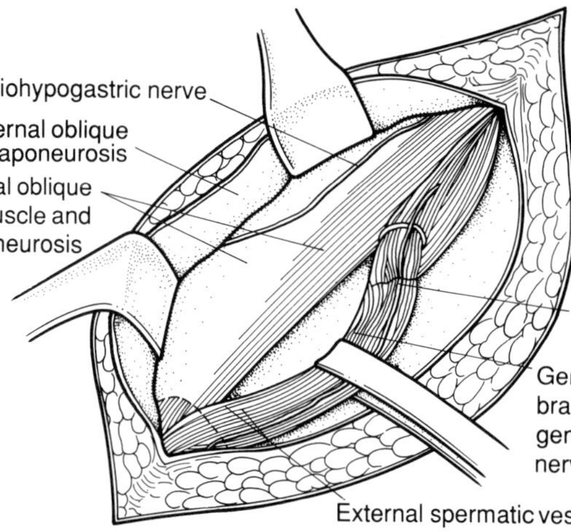

Figure 28.1: Spermatic cord is placed in between the two tails of the mesh.

ischaemic orchitis because of extensive dissection, complete scrotal hernia sacs are transected at the mid-point of the canal, leaving the distal section in place. The anterior wall of the sac is incised in order to prevent postoperative hydrocele formation[12]. In the event of direct hernias, the femoral ring is evaluated through a small opening in the floor of the inguinal canal. When large, the direct sac is inverted using an absorbable suture. The external oblique aponeurosis is separated from the underlying internal oblique muscle high enough to accommodate a 6–8 cm wide patch that can overlap the internal oblique muscle and aponeurosis by at least 2–3 cm above the upper border of Hesselbach's triangle. A manufacturer's pre-cut sheet of Marlex mesh 8 × 16 cm is used. Marlex is the preferred choice of biomaterial because its slight roughness stimulates fibroplasia[13] and its widely spaced monofilamented fibres do not promote or harbour infections[14,15]. If necessary, it is trimmed narrower for 1–2 cm to match the varying sizes of the inguinal floor. The medial end of the mesh is rounded to the shape of the medial corner of the inguinal canal.

With the cord retracted upward, using a running suture of non-absorbable monofilamented material, the rounded corner is sutured to the aponeurotic tissue over the pubic bone overlapping the bone by 1.5–2 cm (Figure 28.2). This is a crucial step in the repair because failure to overlap this bone may result in recurrences. The periosteum of the bone is avoided. This suture continues to attach the lower edge of the patch to the shelving margin of Poupart's ligament up to a point just lateral to the internal ring.

If a concomitant femoral hernia is present, the medial portion of the lower edge is sutured to Cooper's ligament. Because of the very low incidence of femoral hernia, routine attachment of the mesh to Cooper's ligament is not necessary. However, if deemed necessary, the entire myopectineal orifice can be covered by this modification[16]. A slit is made at the lateral end of the mesh, creating two tails – a wider one (two-thirds) above and a narrower (one-third) below. The upper wide tail is grasped with a haemostat and passed cephalad from underneath the spermatic cord. This manoeuvre positions the cord between the two tails of the mesh (Figure 28.2). The wider upper tail is crossed and placed over the narrower one and held with a haemostat. The crossing of the two tails produces a configuration similar to that of the normal transversalis fascia sling, which is assumed to be largely responsible for the normal integrity of the internal ring (Figure 28.3).

The upper leaf of the external oblique aponeurosis is retracted upward; the upper edge of the patch is sutured to the internal oblique aponeurosis or muscle, whichever is available, using a few interrupted absorbable sutures while avoiding injury to or entrapment of the iliohypogastric nerve. Sharp retraction of the upper leaf of the external oblique during this phase of the repair is important

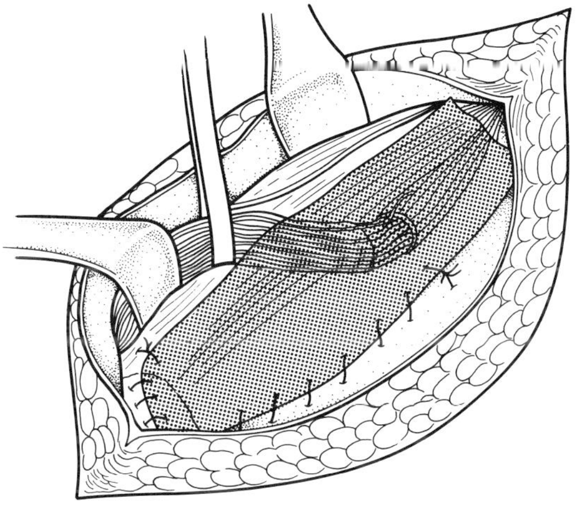

Figure 28.2: Medial end of the patch overlaps the pubic bone 1.5–2 cm.

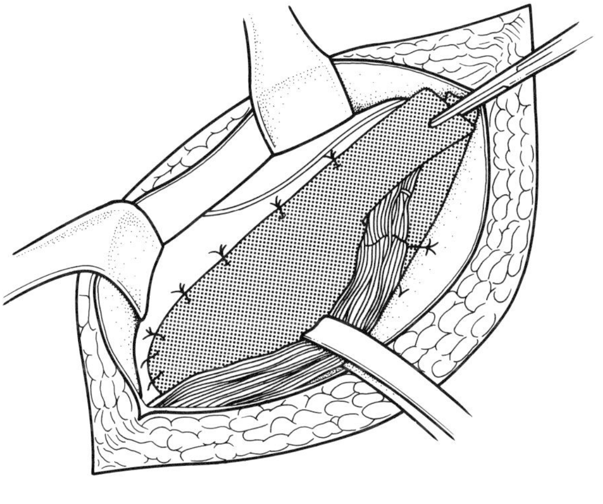

Figure 28.3: Crossing of the two tails.

because it achieves the appropriate amount of laxity for the patch. When the retraction is released, the mesh buckles slightly. This desirable laxity ensures a true tension-free repair and is taken up when the patient strains on command during the operation or resumes an upright position.

Using a single non-absorbable monofilamented suture, the lower edges of each of the two tails are fixed to the shelving margin of Poupart's ligament just lateral to the completion knot of the lower running suture (Figure 28.4). This creates a new internal ring made of mesh. The excess patch on the lateral side is trimmed, leaving approximately 3–4 cm of mesh beyond the internal ring. This is tucked underneath the external oblique aponeurosis, which is then closed over the cord using absorbable suture material.

Patients are discharged within a few hours of their operation with minimal postoperative pain, for which mild analgesics are prescribed. Unrestricted activity is encouraged. They return to their normal unrestricted activities after two to ten days (Table 28.1).

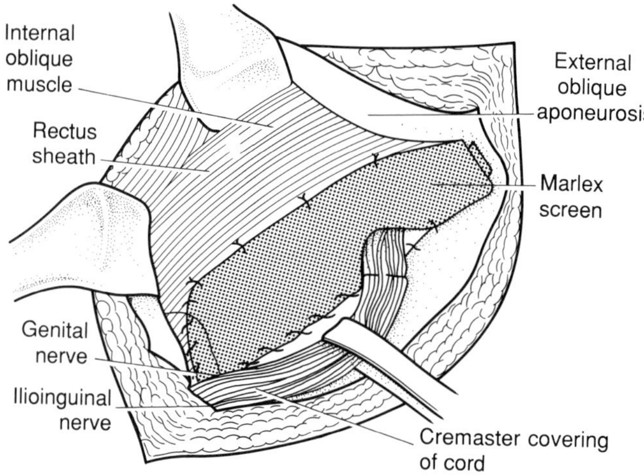

Figure 28.4: The lower edges of the two tails are sutured to the shelving margin to create a new internal ring made of mesh.

Table 28.1: Return to work after surgery

Time after surgery	*Manual workers*	*Office workers*
Less than 1 week	10.8%	45.2%
1 week	40.9%	30.7%
10 days	20.8%	16.9%
2 weeks	17.6%	4.7%
More than 2 weeks	9.9%	2.5%

Results

A computerized follow-up system is used. Recorded in the data sheets are preoperative, operative and postoperative information including classification, complications, and return to work for manual workers and office workers. Our personal series include 3250 consecutive patients with primary inguinal hernias. The patients have been followed up from one to eight years (mean of four years) with a physician examination follow-up rate of 87%. Unreliable[17,18] mail or telephone follow-up was not used and patients lost to follow-up were excluded from our series. There has only been one major complication, a case of orchitis. There has been no chronic postoperative neuralgia or seroma formation requiring aspiration.

Four recurrences due to technical errors were encountered in patients who were operated on early in the evolution of this technique. Three recurrences occurred at the pubic tubercle area because of failure to overlap the bone with the mesh. One recurrence resulted from total disruption of the mesh from the inguinal ligament because the mesh was too narrow. There have been no recurrences in those patients who were operated on within the last three years. A multicentre study[19] involving five groups[20–24] of published surgeons with a special interest in hernia surgery showed recurrence rates of zero to 0.7%, a rejection rate of zero, and an infection rate of less than 0.5%.

A survey of 70 different surgeons without a special interest in hernia surgery, who performed 22 300 'tension-free' hernioplasties, showed similar results with regard to postoperative recurrence, rejection and infection rates, as well as postoperative pain and recovery period.

Conclusions

Open 'tension free' hernioplasty is a safe, simple and effective procedure. Patients are discharged from the hospital within hours of their operation and return to unrestricted work or daily activities within two to ten days depending on their motivation and jobs. Table 28.1 shows the disability period after the open 'tension-free' operation in manual workers and office workers. The fact that the results of surgeons without a special interest in hernia repair were identical to those with a special interest in this subject is a testament to the simplicity, safety and effectiveness of open 'tension-free' hernioplasty. However, the use of mesh does not always in itself guarantee success. For the procedure to be successful, the mesh must be wide enough and correctly secured without tension on either the tissues or the mesh itself.

References

1. Wagh PV, Leverich AP, Sun CN, White HJ, Read RC. Direct inguinal herniation in men: a disease of collagen. *J Surg Res* 1974; **17**: 425.
2. Peacock Jr EE. *Wound repair*. 3rd ed. Philadephia: WB Saunders, 1984.
3. Berliner SD. An approach to groin hernia. *Surg Clin North Am* 1984; **64**: 197–213.
4. Read RC. A review: the role of protease–antiprotease imbalance in the pathogenesis of herniation and abdominal aortic aneurysm in certain smokers. *Postgrad Gen Surg* 1992; **4**: 161–5.
5. Ajabnoor MA, Mokhtar AM, Rafee AA, Taha AM. Defective collagen metabolism in Saudi patients with hernia. *Ann Clin Biochem* 1992; **29**: 430–6.
6. Peacock EE. Here we are again: behind again! *Am J Surg* 1989; **157**: 187.
7. Lichtenstein IL, Shulman AG, Amid PK, Montllor M. Cause and prevention of post-herniorrhaphy neuralgia: a proposed protocol for treatment. *Am J Surg* 1988; **155**: 786–90.
8. Gatt MT, Chevrel JP. The treatment of neuralgia following inguinal herniorrhaphy: a report of 47 cases. *Postgrad Gen Surg* 1992; **4**: 142–7.
9. Bendavid R. 'Dysejaculation': an unusual complication of inguinal herniorrhaphy. *Postgrad Gen Surg* 1992; **4**: 139–41.
10. Smedgerg SGG, Broome AEA, Gullmo A. Ligation of the hernia sac? *Surg Clin North Am* 1984; **64**: 299.
11. Shulman AG, Amid PK, Lichtenstein IL. Ligation of hernial sac a needless step in adult hernioplasty. *Int Surg*. In press.
12. Wantz GE. Complications of inguinal hernial repair. *Surg Clin North Am* 1984; **64**: 287–97.
13. Taylor SR, Gibbons DF. Effect of surface texture on soft tissue response to polymer implants. *J Biomed Mater Res* 1983; **17**: 205–27.
14. Amid PK, Shulman AG, Lichtenstein IL. Selecting synthetic mesh for the repair of groin hernia. *Post Grad Gen Surg* 1992; **4**: 150–5.
15. Neel III HB. Implants of Gore-Tex. *Arch Otolaryngol* 1983; **109**: 427–33.
16. Celdran A, Vorwald P, Merono E, G-Ureña MA. A single technique for polypropylene mesh hernioplasty of inguinal and femoral hernias. *Surg Gynecol Obstet* 1992; **175**: 359–61.
17. Panos RG, Beck DE, Maresh JE, Harford FJ. Preliminary results of a prospective randomized study of Cooper's ligament versus Shouldice herniorrhaphy technique. *Surg Gynecol Obstet*. 1992, **175**. 315–18.
18. Abramson JH, Gafin J, Hopp C, *et al.* The epidemiology of inguinal hernia: a survey in western Jerusalem. *J Epidemiol Community Health* 1978; **32**: 59.

19. Shulman AG, Amid PK, Lichtenstein IL. The safety of mesh repair for primary inguinal hernias: results of 3,019 operations from five diverse surgical sources. *Am Surg* 1992; **58**: 255–7.

20. Lichtenstein IL, Shulman AG, Amid PK, Montllor MM. Cause and prevention of post-herniorrhaphy neuralgia: a proposed protocol for treatment. *Am J Surg* 1988; **155**, 786–90.

21. Martin RE, Max CE. Primary inguinal hernia repair with prosthetic mesh. *Hospi Medica* 1984; **1**: 1.

22. Barnes JP. Inguinal hernia repair with routine use of Marlex mesh. *Surg Gynecol Obstet* 1987; **165**: 33–7.

23. Capozzi JA, Berkenfield JA, Cheaty JK. Repair of inguinal hernia in the adult with prolene mesh. *Surg Gynecol Obstet* 1988; **167**: 124–8.

24. Tinkler LF. Inguinal hernia repair using local anaesthesia. *Ann R Coll Surg Engl* 1985; **67**: 268.

29

Sutureless Hernia Repair

ARTHUR I GILBERT

An operation that damages or destroys normal tissues to repair others should be rethought and replanned

The sutureless repair of inguinal hernia in concept embodies three factors:

- the internal ring is a convenient passageway to the retromuscular preperitoneal space
- prosthetic mesh provides an effective and safe barrier
- the body's inherent forces are sufficient to secure the mesh repair.

This technique requires two swatches of prosthetic mesh, each placed in its appropriate tissue plane. One swatch is positioned immediately posterior to the internal ring between the peritoneum and the transversalis fascia. There it prevents protrusion of the peritoneal sac, instantly curing the indirect hernia. To prevent the formation of an incipient direct hernia the second swatch is positioned immediately anterior to the canal's intact posterior wall. Sutures are unnecessary: both pieces of mesh are secured in place by the body's own hydrostatic and intra-abdominal pressures (Pascal's principle). The same dynamic forces that created the hernia are harnessed to repair it. The technique is simple and is used for most indirect and certain direct inguinal hernias[1].

Materials

The only satisfactory material to use for the sutureless repair is polypropylene mesh. It is a knitted monofilament configuration available in sheets (30 × 30 cm, 12 × 12 in) which can be cut to the desired size, or in individually packaged sterile pieces (6.25 × 20 cm, 2½ × 4½ in) (Prolene, Ethicon; Marlex, Bard). Polypropylene's most desirable feature is its memory. Regardless of how its conformation is changed, it inherently attempts to retain its flat contour. Foreign body giant cell response and inflammatory tissue reaction are identical for polypropylene mesh and suture material. By eliminating the need for sutures, both the destructive needle holes in tissue and tension on tissues are avoided.

Two valuable anatomical features are preserved – the sling mechanism of the internal ring and the shutter feature of the transversus aponeurotic arch. Avoided are the recurrent direct hernias most frequently encountered at the pubic tubercle (type 5), which incidentally are iatrogenic. Clearly this type of recurrence is due to failure to reinforce successfully the inferior portion of the posterior wall or follows the breakdown of tissues sutured together under tension. The other common iatrogenic error avoided is excessive tightening of the internal ring, frequently creating full-floor recurrent direct hernia (type 4). To avoid these errors, the intact posterior wall is reinforced by placing the mesh flat against it. It will be held flat beneath the sutured external oblique aponeurosis. Fibroblastic and collagen ingrowth through the mesh ensures that the posterior wall is fortified and protected.

Technique

It is recommended that the procedure be done with a local or regional anaesthetic. A combination of 30 ml of 3% chloroprocaine (Nesacaine), 50 ml of 0.5% bupivacaine (Marcaine) and 8 ml of 8.4% sodium bicarbonate makes the local anaesthetic formula. It is invaluable for the patient to be awake, initially to assist by demonstrating the full extent of tissue damage and later to confirm the immediate success of the repair.

A low inguinal incision is made. Thorough dissection of the elements of the canal is performed. The presence or absence of a peritoneal sac, the size of the internal ring and the integrity of the posterior wall are the three elements to be reconciled in any inguinal hernia before deciding which repair is most appropriate. For the peritoneal sac of an indirect hernia, either the entire sac is dissected free and is invaginated or, for a sac firmly attached to the distal cord, its proximal portion is divided and ligated after its neck is dissected from adhesions to the cord and the investing fibres of the transversalis fascia. Although high ligation of the sac is not essential, high dissection of the sac is critical and essential to the success of this procedure. By performing the high dissection, the peritoneal layer is freed from the endopelvic fascia and posterior surface of the abdominal wall musculature. Where a potential space existed, an actual space is created. To position it in the preperitoneal space, a swatch of Prolene mesh 6.3 × 6.3 cm (2½ × 2½ in) is shaped into the form of an umbrella (Figure 29.1). After the peritoneal sac is invaginated within the abdominal cavity, the umbrella plug graft is passed through the internal ring to be situated between the peritoneum and the transversalis fascia. In the preperitoneal space the umbrella plug opens and completely blocks the peritoneum from escaping through the internal ring. Once positioned, the graft becomes firmly secured in place when the patient performs the Valsalva manoeuvre. The greater the patient strains, the flatter and better the graft becomes seated.

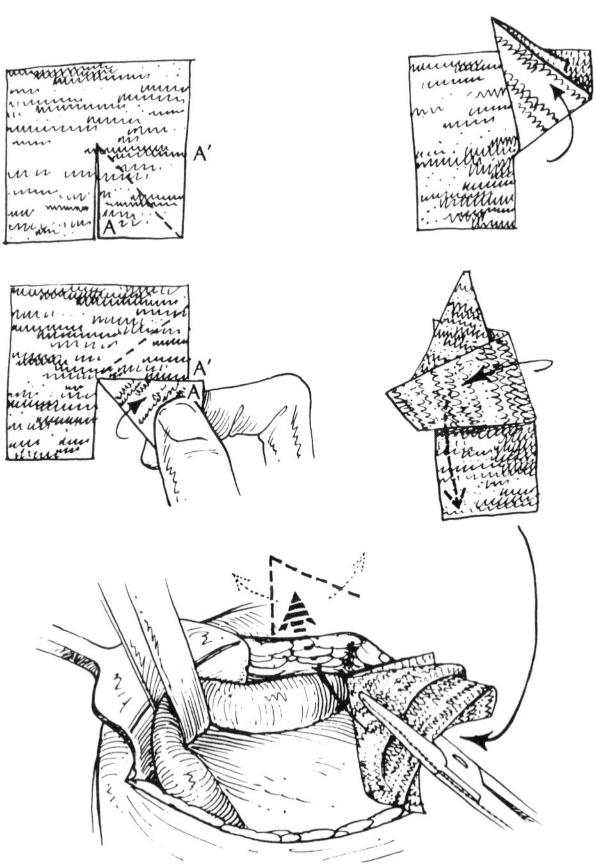

Figure 29.1 Creating the umbrella plug.

The second swatch of Prolene mesh is placed as an overlay graft against the posterior canal wall and brought comfortably round the spermatic cord by dividing its lateral portion into two tails. With the second swatch of mesh flat against the posterior wall, the cord and the ilioinguinal nerve are replaced in their bed and the external oblique aponeurosis is closed over them with an absorbable suture. The overlay graft is held flat between the posterior wall and the external oblique aponeurosis. The external oblique layer has no bearing on the repair; it simply covers the cord and the graft and holds them flat in place. Both grafts are held flat in their functional position when the patient strains, coughs, or performs the Valsalva manoeuvre.

Results

From September 1987 through December 1992, 1003 primary and 99 recurrent hernias were repaired by the sutureless technique: 742 were repaired under local anaesthesia, 320 with epidural, 12 with spinal, and 28 with general. Of the 1102 total repairs there have been three recurrences. All three were lateral and superior to the repair, and presented as interstitial defects led by fatty degeneration or lipomas in those areas. All three followed the repair of recurrent hernia. In the total series there were six infections, 15 seromas, 15 haematomas, and one case of testicular swelling which has subsided. In no case was there testicular atrophy or significant neuralgia.

Conclusions

The sutureless technique is used for primary and recurrent inguinal hernias. It is simple and safe, and its effectiveness can be immediately verified. Postoperative discomfort has been minimal. About one-third of patients take nothing for pain, one-third use only paracetomol (acetaminophen), and one-third use propoxyphene napsylate and paracetomol (acetaminophen) tablets. All patients are encouraged to resume their normal unrestricted activities immediately, and for the most part do so by the second postoperative day.

Reference

1. Gilbert AI. An anatomic and functional classification for the diagnosis and treatment of inguinal hernia. *Am J Surg* 1989; **157**: 331–3.

30

Groin Hernia Repair by Extraperitoneal Bilateral Mesh Prosthesis and Midline Subumbilical Approach

RENÉ E STOPPA AND O BOUDOURIS

Some surgeons called this method 'giant prosthetic reinforcement of the visceral sac' (GPRVS). We have used it since 1967 as the most extensive prosthetic repair of groin hernias.

A prosthesis . . . Why?

There are *historical reasons*. Before the introduction of laparoscopic procedures hernia surgery aimed to prevent hernias recurring for professional and economic reasons and prosthetic repair was yet an almost absolute weapon against recurrences when using GPRVS.

There are *anatomical reasons* for using prosthetic material. We followed Henri Fruchaud[1], who, after others, united all types of groin hernia, whatever their superficial emergences, as being the consequence of the weakness of the myofascial layer in the area of the myopectineal hole, the weak zone of the groin. The transversalis fascia, the deep pressure proof layer of the groin, can be properly reinforced or replaced by an unabsorbable mesh – a sort of artificial endoabdominal fascia – placed (underlaying) between the wall and the peritoneum (*see* Figure 30.1)

Appropriate materials are now available with proper features, such that the size of the prosthesis can be as large as needed for GPRVS. One must use a mesh, easily penetrated by the connective tissue, not an impervious sheet, not incorporated; EPFE is rather a sheet than a mesh. Following experimental French studies[4], polyester (Dacron) mesh is our preference: it meets the biological criteria, is cheap, and is available in very large sizes (up to 50 × 30 cm). Polypropylene meshes, equally well tolerated but less pliable, are less convenient. Absorbable meshes are not recommended where unabsorbable material is much more logical.

On good use of the mesh

Aiming the ultimate radical efficiency among repair techniques, I do not use patches: even though they are tensionless repairs, they cannot regularly resist the intra-abdominal pressure which has a component tearing force at the level of stitches. I prefer giant bilateral underlay, widely wrapping the visceral sac – thus rendering it unextensible – and, at the same time reinforcing, posteriorly, the weak area of the adjacent wall. When using very large mesh prosthesis, no direct repair of hernial orifices, and no direct fixation of the prosthesis are necessary, owing to Pascal's hydrostatic principle (Figure 30.3). If you intend to use intra-abdominal pressure – the force that created the hernia – to act in favour of repair, the wider the prosthesis the safer the repair. Lastly, I must underline that the extraperitoneal position of the mesh prevents the formation adhesions of the abdominal viscera and maintains the characteristics and benignity of an extra-abdominal procedure to GPRVS.

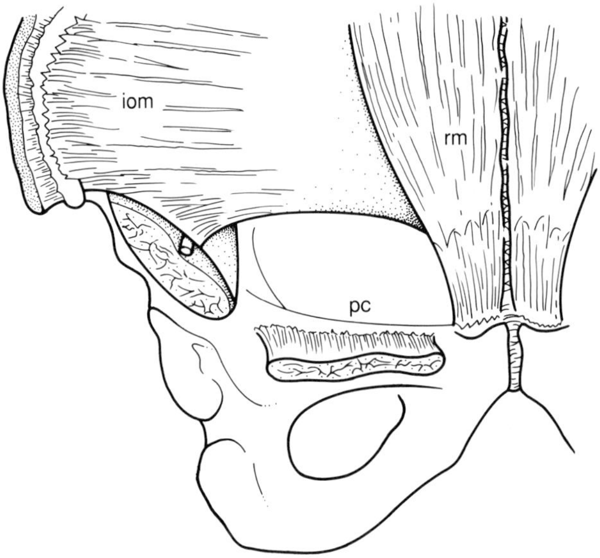

Figure 30.1: Schematic representation of Fruchaud's myopectineal orifice, the weak area of the inguinal wall tightened to the intra-abdominal pressure only by the transversalis fascia. iom, internal oblique muscle, pm, psoas muscle; pc, pectineal crest; rm, rectus muscle.

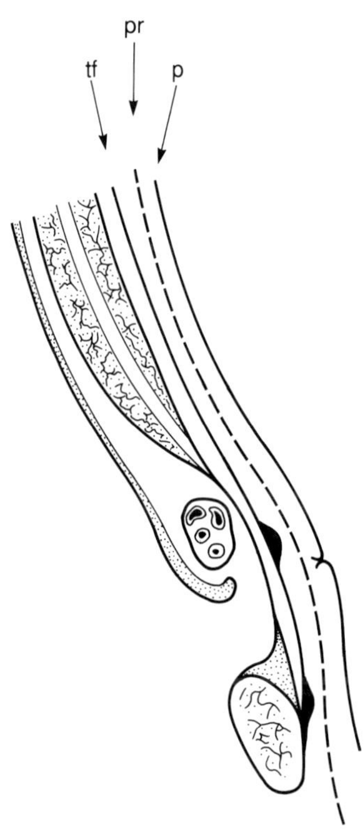

Figure 30.2: Schematic sagittal cross-section of the groin region, after GPRVS repair, showing the position of the mesh prosthesis (pr) between peritoneum (p) and transversalis fascia (tf).

Midline subumbilical preperitoneal route (proposed by Cheatle[5], defended by Henry[6], and spread by Nyhus' *Hernia* book[7,8]) is a well known easy one, most pleasingly dealing with normal anatomy and avoiding any risk of injuring the distal testicular vascularization in recurrent hernias. Through

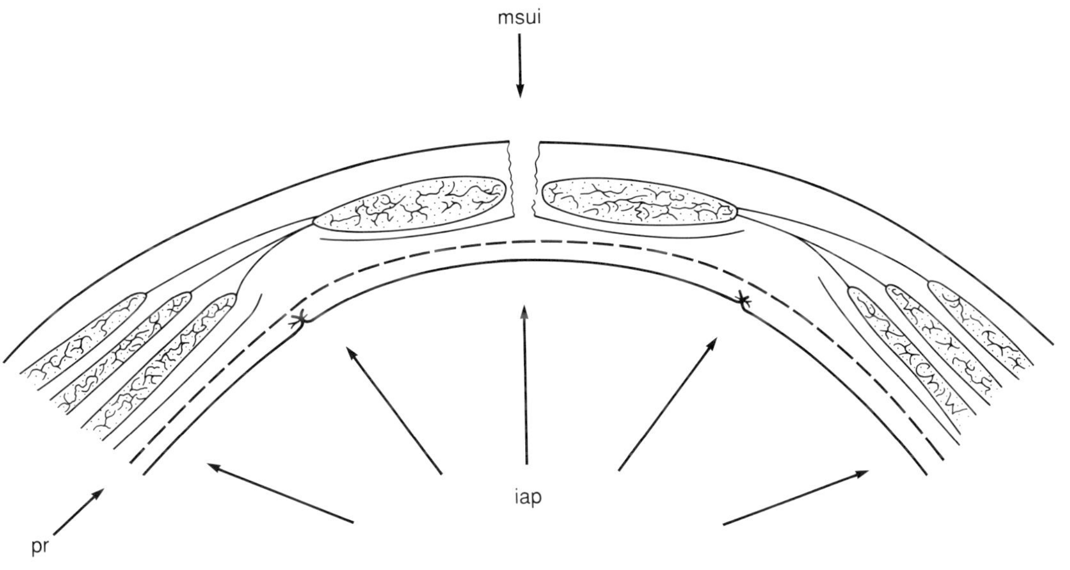

Figure 30.3: Schematic horizontal cross-section of the lower part of the abdominal wall, showing how the intra-abdominal pressure (iap) presses the prosthesis (pr) against the wall (following Pascal's hydrostatic principle), after GPRVS through a midline subumbilical uncision (msui).

this approach, cleavable retroparietal preperitoneal spaces are a perfect site – in size and depth – for the placement of large mesh underlays.

GPRVS personal technique

This is a well-established method. It is usually performed using general anaesthesia, although spinal or peridural anaesthesia are also convenient. G. Wantz uses sometimes only local and frequently a stand-by anaesthesia for unilateral GPRVS. The duration of the procedure is 20–45 minutes, a short one for a bilateral repair.

I have already published details of the GPRVS technique[9,12] and shall only recall, here, the main steps:

- Midline subumbilical extraperitoneal incision.
- Quick easy retrofascial cleavage, and at first reaching hernial sacs – none of which is easily missed – and adequately treating them.
- Parietalization of the spermatic cord components, to avoid slitting the mesh.
- Having performed the retroparietal cleavage and parietalization of the cord on one side of the patient, repeat it on the opposite side.
- Cut the mesh to suit the patient, grasp it with a 8 curve long Rochester clamps for handling, unfolding, and placing it.
- Wrap the visceral sac in the mesh, using the clamps to push it into place.
- Lastly, close the wall and the skin.

The operation is over. Remember: no direct repair of hernial orifices, no direct fixation of the mesh prosthesis. That makes this operation very simple.

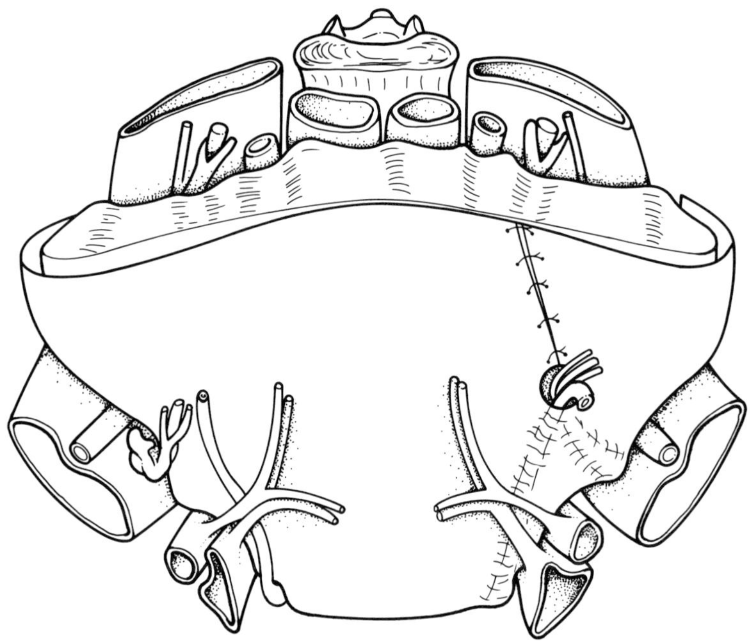

Figure 30.4: Schematic representation, from a horseman view, of the mesh prosthesis wrapping the inferior part of the visceral sac after GPRVS. At left the cord components have been parietalized; this is far better than slitting the mesh, to let the cord pass through, as represented at right.

Postoperative course

GPRVS is a safe, simple and comfortable operation, followed by a fast recovery and a short hospital stay (two to four days). In my 1981 series (C. Warlaumont thesis), complication rates were:

- seromas and haematomas 1.3%
- hydroceles 1.5%
- sepsis 1.1%.

The incidence of postoperative sepsis is the same for both prosthetic and non-prosthetic repairs. Though being no longer a scarecrow, septic accidents must remain an object of careful prevention and treatment.

Prevention

All members of the team must contribute to carrying out a precise plan, which consists of applying the normal rules of all high quality surgery. Before the operation: selection of sepsis-free patients and disinfection. During the operation: staff discipline, antibiotic monotherapy flash in every case with potential risk. After the operation: precise survey of clinical sepsis indicators, echographic control of the wound if necessary.

Treatment

Patent sepsis treatment must preferably be early and this is the surgeon's responsibility. When the sepsis is superficial, the wound must be opened immediately. When the abcess is in contact with the prosthesis, widely incise the wall, without removing the mesh; treat the local infection, in the most classic manner, so that the mesh will be secondarily incorporated in the scar connective tissue. When, exceptionally, a late sinus presents, make a fistulography, then thoroughly excise the sinus, without removing the mesh.

Technical variations

One can use a horizontal skin incision for cosmetic purposes. When the content of a scrotal hernia is irreducible, a separate high scrotal incision is helpful to free the sliding sac or the adherent viscera. Suction drainage should be placed in distal abandoned sacs, or in front of the mesh, if necessary. The unilateral Wantz operation is a half-cut bilateral GPRVS, developed as a one-day surgery repair[13–14].

Late satisfactory results

In my 1981 series of 2108 patients, with a follow up of one to 12 years, the recurrence rate was 1.1%. In my 1986 series of 522 patients, with one to five years of follow up, the recurrence rate was 0.56%. Interestingly, for the purpose of patient controls, all recurrences appeared within the first six months after the operation.

Indications for GPRVS

This method has been imagined, and is still now mostly used, for *recurrent hernias*. For *primary repair*, I use it for hernias that will be difficult to treat or are at high risk of recurrence: prevascular, multiple, voluminous, sliding; in obese or cirrhotic patients or those making efforts. Over all, these indications comprise 30% of all repairs in my practice. In *unilateral hernias*, I propose to use GPRVS when the diagnosed hernia is a scrotal one, or a large direct one, or the patient is obese or hard working. I consider as incentives the following datas: a contralateral hernia appears within ten years following a unilateral repair, in 10–30% of the operated patients . . . on another hand my personal experience showed a 12% rate of undiagnosed contralateral hernia when performing a GPRVS for a clinically unilateral hernia . . . and one can add to these an unreported number of undiagnosed associated hernias . . . Lastly a scrupulous surgeon may use Wantz' excellent operation as an alternative to GPRVS[13,14] in unilateral difficult hernias.

Contraindications

The risk of sepsis is an absolute one, related to dermatosis or recent regional septic accident. Others are not absolute, such as a midline subumbilical scar, or a history of iliocaval venous thrombosis which can be overcome with some more difficulty, or contraindicated general or spinal anaesthesia, which obliges the surgeon to use local anaesthesia.

Conclusions

GPRVS, widely wrapping the visceral sac, through a midline subumbilical route, into a giant bilateral piece of unabsorbable mesh is usually a simple and regularly efficient gesture. I think this method is of greatest value in complex and difficult hernias. Now we must continue to personalize hernia repairs, so that I should be surprised if all hernias will be proposed for a laparoscopic repair in the future.

Summary

This is the ultimate and most radical remedy against difficult hernias of the groin, and has been used for more than 25 years. The principles of the method are:

- reinforcing the transversalis fascia and, at the same time, widely wrapping the visceral sac into a mesh prosthesis, thus rendering it unextensible.
- using a very large bilateral piece of mesh, which makes it unnecessary to repair hernial orifices or to fix the prosthetic mesh.
- using the preperitoneal subumbilical midline approach for the preperitoneal cleavage, parietalization of the cord components, and placement of the mesh.

Some comments include sepsis risk, late satisfactory results, personal indication and contraindications of GPRVS. Even if some similarity can be found in the principles, this method differs from laparoscopic prosthetic repairs, when its main step is wrapping the visceral sac – a very simple gesture – and not repairing the wall. Thus open GPRVS does not need any fixation of the mesh, different from laparoscopic careful stitching or stapling of the prosthesis.

References

1. Fruchaud H. *Anatomie chirurgicale des hernies de l'aine*, Paris: Doin Ed, 1956.
2. Petit J, Stoppa R *et al.* Evaluation expérimentale des réactions tissulaires autour des prothèses de la paroi abdominale en tulle de Dacron. *J Chir* 1974; **197**: 667.
3. Arnaud JP, Eloy R, Weil-Bousson M, *et al.* Resistance et tolérance biologique de 6 prothèses 'inertes' utilisées dans la réparation de la paroi abdominale. *J Chir* 1977; **113**: 85.
4. Soler M, Verhaeghe P, Essomba A, *et al.* Le traitement des éventrations post-opératoires par prothèse composée (Polyester-Polyglactine 91). Etude clinique et expérimentale. *Ann Chir* 1993;
5. Cheatle GL. An operation for inguinal hernia. *BMJ* 1920; **2**: 68.
6. Henry AK. Operation for femoral hernia by a midline extraperitoneal approach. *Lancet.* 1936; **19**: 531.
7. Nyhus LM, Condon RE, Harkins HN. Clinical experiences with preperitoneal hernia repair for all type of hernia of the groin. *Am Surg* 1960; **100**: 234.
8. Nyhus LM. The preperitoneal approach and iliopubic tract repair of inguinal hernia. In: Nyhus LM, Condon RE, eds. *Hernia*, 3rd ed. Philadelphia and Toronto: JB Lippincott, 1989
9. Stoppa R, Petit J, Abourachid H. Procédé original de plastie des hernies de l'aine. L'interposition sans fixation d'une prothèse en tulle de Dacron par voie médiane pré-péeritonéale. *Chirurgie* 1973; **99**: 119.
10. Stoppa RE, Rives JL, Warlaumont CR, *et al.* The use of Dacron in the repair of hernias of the groin. *Surg Clin North Am* 1984; **64**: 269.
11. Stoppa RE, Warlaumont CR. The preperitoneal approach and prosthetic repair of groin hernia. In: Nyhus LM, Condon RE, eds. *Hernia*, 3rd ed. Philadelphia and Toronto: JB Lippincott, 1989.
12. Stoppa RE, Warlaumont CR. The midline preperitoneal approach and the prosthetic repair of groin hernia. In: Nyhus LM, Baker RJ, eds. *Mastery of Surgery*, 2nd ed. Boston: Little, Brown, 1992.
13. Wantz GE. Giant reinforcement of the visceral sac. *Surg Gynecol Obstet* 1989; **169**: 408.
14. Wantz GE. *Atlas of hernia surgery*. New York: Raven Press, 1991.

31

Groin Hernia: When is Surgery Necessary?

STANLEY D BERLINER

Change is inevitable, and hernia surgery is no exception. However, some things do not change over the years. During our training days we are programmed to think certain ways, good and bad. If you ask third-year medical students what is most important in taking a history from the patient with a hernia, they properly reply 'everything'. If you ask third-year surgical residents when is surgery necessary for a groin hernia, many respond: 'as soon as you have made the diagnosis'. Is this indeed a fact?

Confirming the diagnosis of groin hernia

Once the diagnosis of a groin hernia is confirmed, two questions need to be addressed.

- Are the patients symptoms consistent with the clinical findings?
- If the patient is asymptomatic, is surgery necessary?

A groin ligament strain often prompts a consultation for a hernia. It can be difficult to examine these people in the acute phase. If in doubt, the wise plan of action is to delay a final diagnosis for four to six weeks. Having told a patient he has a groin strain, it is embarrassing to have him return several months later with an obvious hernia. A chronic or subacute adductor tendinitis can be a disabling problem, and it is not uncommon in progestional athletes. I have operated on some of these people for concomitant indirect inguinal hernias. Surgery does not relieve the pain.

It is not unusual for the family physician or gynaecologist to refer a patient to the surgeon with a multitude of abdominal complaints, *hoping* that a hernia will be found. I have learned not to say to the patient 'you do not have a hernia'; I will say, 'I do not find a hernia at this time. Come back if you become aware of a swelling'.

There are instances where the symptoms do not correlate with the clinical findings. It is explained to the patient and the family that the hernia needs correction to prevent incarceration or strangulation, but the operation will not alter the complaints of back pain, sciatica, impotence, flatulence, constipation, etc.

The happy patient is the one whose lump and whose symptoms have disappeared. It might save much heartache to delay elective surgery for a pertinent work-up. I feel most comfortable when the patient with a hernia presents with a history of increasing symptoms as the day progresses and is symptom-free while resting. Searing pain is an early symptom caused by the hernia protruding through the external ring with nerve impingement. Once the size of the hernia stabilizes, the burning usually abates.

Use of the truss

If I am in doubt about the patient with a moderate sized direct hernia and much pain, I instruct him wear a truss for about a week. If the symptoms are relieved, it is reasonable to expect that surgery will be successful. Small direct hernias seldom give trouble. If asymptomatic and not enlarging, they can be managed with judicious neglect.

Hernia surgery may have to be postponed because of a more pressing medical situation.

A chronic or subacute adductor tendinitis can be a disabling problem, and is not uncommon in professional athletes. Surgery does not relieve the pain.

The truss is not an obsolete device. It was championed by Ambroise Paré in the mid sixteenth century. Paré was court physician and surgeon to four French kings. The truss did two things. It decreased mortality. And since the barber surgeons in the provinces were accustomed to performing orchiectomy with herniotomy, it protected virility. This maintained population stability and perhaps encouraged growth so that head tax payments to the king would not suffer. If the hernia is symptomatic and reducible, most patients do well with a truss as a temporizing procedure.

Femoral hernias

All femoral hernias require surgery. It is an acquired disease. The femoral cone is a normal anatomical variant dependent on the configuration of the pelvis and on the mode of insertion of transversus fibres on the superior pubic ramus. An increase in intra-abdominal pressure can trap preperitoneal and intraperitoneal contents in the narrow and unyielding distal femoral ring. Of 159 femoral hernias, 16% were irreducible and required urgent correction, 18% required emergency surgery for acute incarceration and 5% required a bowel resection[1].

Inguinal hernias

Inguinal hernias in women are almost always indirect and require operation. Patients may be referred by the gynaecologist for persistent abdominal pain. There is no detectable pelvic pathology, and they are told that they may have a hidden hernia. This is seldom the case, with two exceptions. In one, there is a thickening in the region of the external ring. If this is coupled with a history of pain related to the menstrual cycle, surgery is worthwhile. The usual findings are small chocolate cysts in the hernia sac and adjacent tissues. If this endometrioma is localized, the complaints are relieved. The other situation is typified by a young, healthy airline stewardess who presented with a two-year history of intermittent episodes of severe lower abdominal pain lasting several minutes. A mass was never seen, and work-up was negative. She localized the pain to the site of the internal inguinal ring. Surgery revealed an indirect sac. I have had five such cases. Following surgery the attacks, presumably from momentary incarceration, have not recurred.

The attitudes of the surgeon and primary care physician play a major role in the decision for or against surgery. It is unfortunate that some family physicians wait until an emergency arises before they refer the patient to the surgeon. On the other hand, primary care physicians have the advantage of knowing the total patient, not just the groin pathology. They can best evaluate the hernia and its symptoms. For example, they must weigh the risks of elective surgery in a patient with unstable angina against the risks of an emergency operation in that individual.

Assessing the results

Having undertaken surgery, how are we going to evaluate our results? There are essentials we must record if we want to progress from clinical impression to some degree of scientific evaluation.

Follow-up period

We need to know the mean follow-up time, not the median or average follow-up time. A series followed from one to five years has an average follow-up of three years. The mean follow-up time, which is the sum total of months the entire group was followed divided by the total number of

Table 31.1: Results of 530 Posterior wall hernioplasties, 1972 through 1974

Mean follow-up time (months)	*Failures in primary repairs* (%)	*Failures in recurrent repairs* (%)	*Percentage followed by personal examination*
12	2/454 (0.44)	1/76 (1.3)	100
24	5/444 (1.1)	2/76 (2.6)	98
60	6/412 (1.5)	4/70 (5.7)	91

patients in the series, may be only two years. The numbers of patients followed by personal examination is important. More than one-third of my pubic tubercle failures were asymptomatic and unaware of the recurrence at the time of their annual follow-up visit. The type of repair performed relative to the pathology encountered is significant. Any repair we undertake for a small indirect hernia will yield brilliant results.

It is comforting to know that other centres have done the same operation with good long-term results. It took 25 years for much of the surgical world to recognize that McVay's low recurrence rates with a Cooper's ligament repair did not hold up in certain circumstances. My failure rate with this technique for direct and recurrent hernias was 11%. On the other hand, the excellent results of the posterior wall hernioplasty of the Shouldice variety have been replicated world wide.

Storing data on computer

Personal record keeping and follow up can be facilitated by the use of a computer stored database system. New software makes it simple to create your own personalized data bank. Follow-up is a tedious task for the busy general surgeon. It requires office personnel with the instincts of a Sherlock Holmes, the charm of a head waiter and the tenacity of an insurance salesman. After five years, my follow-up of groin hernias by personal examination drops to the low 90% level (Table 31.1). After ten years, follow-up by personal examination approaches 80%. One exception was a series of 44 Henry operations for incarcerated and strangulated femoral hernias[2]. With a mean follow-up time of six years, follow-up by personal examination was 100% because most of the patients were permanent residents in a state mental institution.

Patients lost to follow-up

Patients lost to follow-up must be suspect for recurrence. In a retrospective review of 720 Bassini and McVay repairs done prior to 1972, 68 cases were located with great difficulty and refused to come in for examination. We learned that 21 had had a recurrence of their hernia and had either seen another surgeon or were living with a truss. Most of these patients had McVay repairs for recurrent or multiply recurrent hernias. Therefore the failure rate in this 'almost lost to follow-up group' was 31%.

In my various series, from one-half to three-quarters of 1% of patients die annually of unrelated causes and are removed from the follow-up files. These patients are comfortably placed in the 'cured' category.

References

1. Berliner SD. The femoral cone and its clinical implications. *Surg Gynecol Obstet* 1990; **171**: 11–14.
2. Berliner SD. Burson LC, Wise L. The Henry operation for incarcerated and strangulated femoral hernias. *Arch Surg* 1992; **127**: 314–16.

32

Pitfalls and Complications of Inguinal Hernia Repair

ARTHUR I GILBERT

The road to successful hernia surgery is filled with traps and pitfalls. Some are obvious, others are subtle. Classically these include seroma or haematoma formation, infection, recurrence of the hernia, testicular atrophy and postoperative neuralgia. No complication is completely avoidable, but each can be minimized by the surgeon's awareness.

Seroma or haematoma formation

The incidence of clinically significant seroma, considering all types of hernia repair, is about 1%. It is higher when prosthetic grafts are used. Increased incidence of seroma formation, however, is a small price to pay for the value gained from implanted prosthetic grafts. Older patients, particularly those who have compromised cardiac output, have a higher incidence of seroma formation. To minimize this complication in prosthetic hernioplasties in all age groups the mesh should be implanted at the deepest layer of the dissection. Seromas and haematomas occur more frequently following recurrent hernia repairs, presumably related to the loss of contractility of scarred lymphatics and capillaries. Wound drainage to prevent seroma formation is rarely helpful. A seroma typically presents between the fourth and sixth postoperative days, long after a suction drain would have been removed. Treatment for a seroma is aspiration once or twice; after that the remainder of the effusion usually is reabsorbed. The formation of a permanent hydrocele following a seroma is infrequent.

The incidence of haematoma also is about 1%. It can be minimized by observing certain matters of preoperative evaluation. A personal or family history of abnormal bleeding deserves investigation. Aspirin should be stopped ten days before the procedure. A preoperative coagulogram should include a prothrombin time, partial thromboplastin time and a platelet count. Anticoagulants are withdrawn four or five days before the procedure, and a prothrombin time checked before the operation. The partial thromboplastin time will help discover other coagulopathies, especially those with deficiencies of higher clotting factors. The critical level for platelets is 50,000.

Intraoperative and postoperative bleeding problems are related to the lack of complete surgical haemostasis. When entering the groin the superficial epigastric vessels are encountered. They lie between Camper's and Scarpa's fascia. If divided, lasting haemostasis is best obtained by ligation not coagulation. The external spermatic vessels lie in the lateral flap of the cremasteric fascia. The pubic branch of the obturator artery lies low in the canal; when it is divided and left unattended it forms the classic corona mortis. Deep to the posterior wall and inferomedial to the true neck of an indirect sac are the deep epigastric vessels. These frequently are punctured when sutures are used to invaginate the posterior wall in a type 4 hernia[1]. (Figure 32.1). The deepest vessels of concern are the deep circumflex iliac and external iliac vessels. If the above vessels are injured, bleeding can usually be controlled by gentle pressure after removing the needle and suture. If the deep circumflex iliac or external iliac is injured, it may be necessary to open the posterior wall and gain control with vascular clamps.

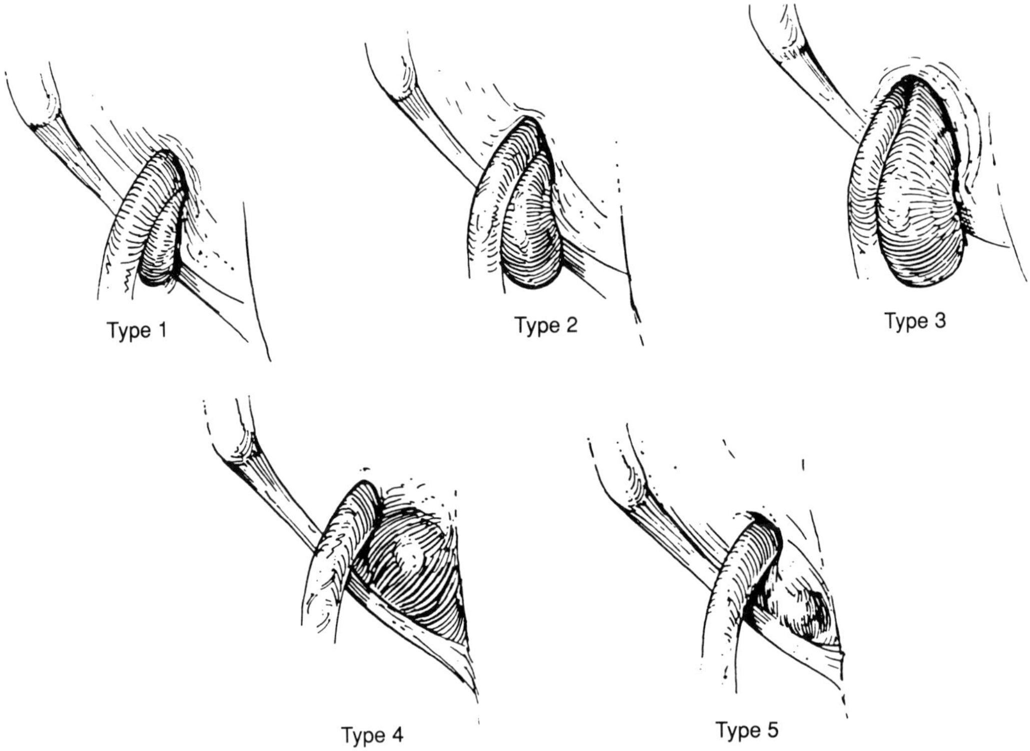

Figure 32.1: Type 1,2 and 3 are indirect hernias. Types 4 and 5 are direct hernias.

Haematoma of the wound is treated by draining it. Ecchymosis of the scrotum occurs often and alarms the uninformed patient. Small haematomas in the spermatic cord rarely require drainage. Much acrimony can be spared by alerting the patient to this predictable eventuality. A scrotal haematoma large enough to create skin tension is probably best drained. This decision is made, balancing the risk of opening a new path for infection against pressure breakdown of scrotal skin with its sequelae.

Infection

The recurrence rate related to infection is much lower following mesh repairs than after pure tissue repairs. In a report from the Shouldice Clinic dealing with recurrent hernias, primary repairs that became infected had an incidence of recurrence four times greater than non-infected cases[2]. Persistent infection and sinus formation are related to the use of multifilament suture material such as silk or cotton. When monofilament suture is used in a mesh repair, it is unnecessary to remove the mesh in most infected cases. Drainage and specific antibiotic treatment usually will solve the problem. If the mesh has been placed flat, it becomes protected by tissue ingrowth on both surfaces. Plugs and other graft materials placed in apposition (double layer of mesh) make protective tissue ingrowth more difficult and often retain the persistent nidus of infection. These must be removed if permanent healing is to occur. Perioperative prophylactic antibiotics do not significantly reduce the incidence of infection; they do not have a significant impact on the cost of care. One dose of a first generation cephalosporin and its access route cost more than $70. In a prospective study of almost 2500 hernia repairs, the incidence of infection was close to 1% in all groups whether the hernia was primary or recurrent, repaired with or without prosthetic mesh, or whether perioperative antibiotics were given.

Recurrence associated with indirect hernia

Errors that explain recurrence associated with the repair of an indirect hernia include:

- inadequate dissection of the peritoneal sac
- improper closure of the internal ring
- failure to recognize an associated hernia
- failure to evaluate the posterior wall correctly
- iatrogenic damage to the posterior wall.

Inadequate dissection of the peritoneal sac

The neck of the sac must be freed from the cord and from investing fibres of the transversalis fascia. It is important to dissect the neck and 'shoulders' of the sac to be certain no part of the peritoneum remains attached to the endopelvic fascia surrounding the true internal ring (Figure 32.2). Management of the sac is a matter of personal preference. Some surgeons ligate and resect it; others simply invaginate it. Resection requires cutting and ligating the peritoneum; both cause significant postoperative pain.

Improper closure of the internal ring

When the internal ring is left too loose, it allows protrusion of the peritoneum or a properitoneal lipoma (lipoma theory of Cloquet). When the internal ring is closed too tightly, it causes protrusion of the posterior wall medial to it. This encourages the development of a type 4 hernia. Closure of the external oblique beneath the spermatic cord in a Halsted I repair places the superficial ring directly over the deep ring, and so the obliquity of the canal responsible for its protective sling mechanism is lost.

Failure to recognize associated hernias

These occur in 7–15% of cases. When repairing an indirect hernia, a direct inguinal and a femoral component must be searched for and treated. The normal cone of the femoral canal should not be overevaluated. The usual content of a normal femoral canal is a fat pad and lymph nodes, the so-called node of Rosenmueller or Cloquet.

Failure to evaluate the posterior wall correctly

A defect or deficiency in the wall may not always be evident. One must weigh not reinforcing every posterior wall against repairing too many. If 20% of patients who have indirect hernia repairs later develop direct hernias, reinforcing the posterior wall in every patient means that unnecessary extensive surgery is done in 80% of cases, many of which iatrogenically create posterior wall defects.

Damage to the posterior wall

This is caused by needle holes and necrosis on tissue due to excess tension. No text can teach how much tension is too much. This is learned by personal experience and by following one's own results for many years. Most iatrogenically created hernias are type 5. According to Postelthwait's series, 60% occur at the pubic tubercle. Breakdown due to tension on sutured tissue is blamed; however,

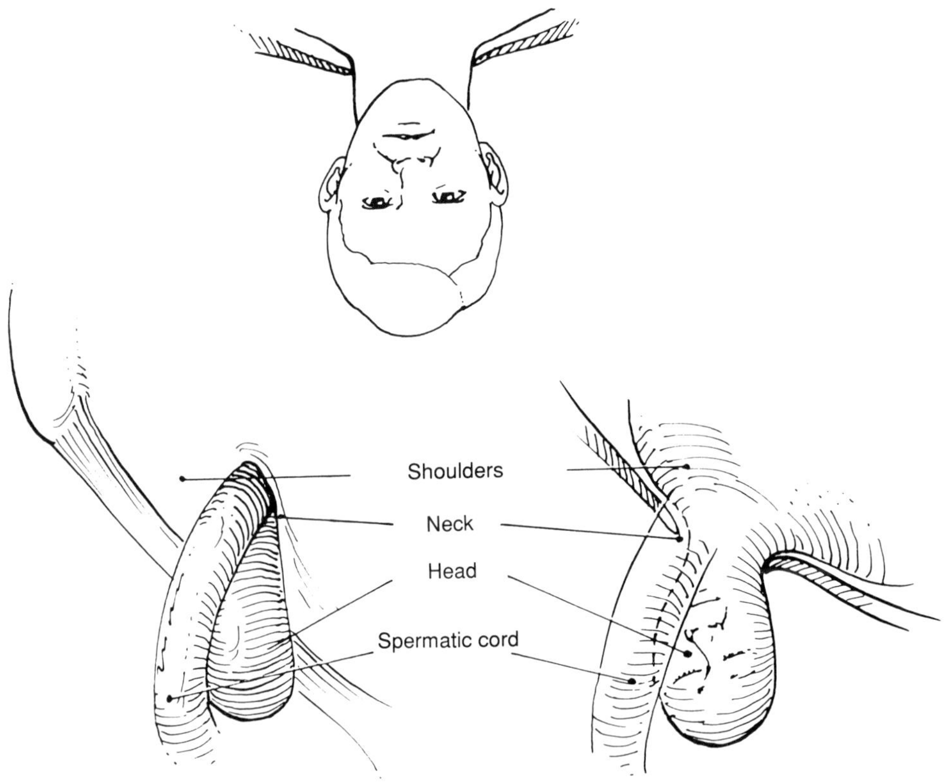

Figure 32.2: An indirect peritoneal sac can be personified as a human head seen upside down. By dissecting the true neck and shoulders of the peritoneum beneath the posterior wall, the properitoneal space is developed.

the majority are created in a Bassini-type operation by failure to close the defect at the inferior angle of the canal. Common causes of this error are related to using an incision that is too high (cephalad) and too transverse in the interest of being cosmetically more acceptable.

Recurrence associated with direct hernia

- The use of the inguinal ligament as an anchor structure subjects it to unnatural tension. This causes tearing and results in breakdown of the repair.
- Cooper's ligament is a fixed structure that lacks the resilience to withstand the functional pressures developed between it and the transversus arch after a McVay repair.
- Repair by invagination of the posterior wall alone carries a 20% failure rate. If reinforcement is done with a prosthetic mesh, the failure rate is reduced significantly[1,3]. The posterior wall can be envisaged as a trampoline that is equally resilient throughout (Figure 32.3). A single suture in it will cause an abnormal fixed point. If it is necessary to suture the posterior wall at all, an entire line should be used or the entire wall reinforced by a prosthesis. Read showed that relaxing incisions are more beneficial for direct repairs than for indirect repairs, this being due to the slide effect of the stretched posterior wall[4].
- Failure to use a relaxing incision or using too short a relaxing incision in a pure tissue technique can cause recurrence associated with direct hernia repair.

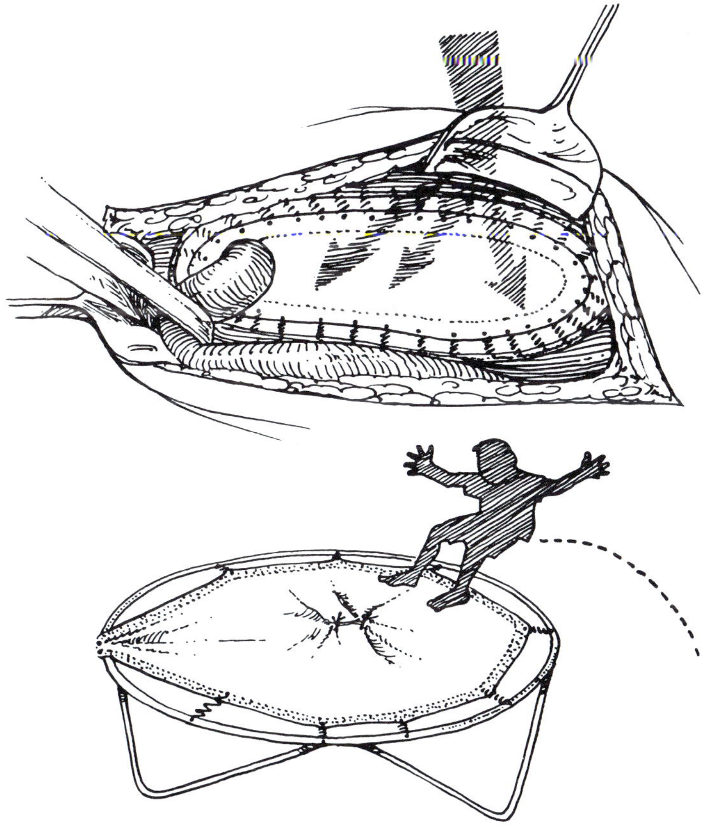

Figure 32.3: The resilient posterior inguinal wall is analogous to a trampoline.

- Failure to recognize a coexistent indirect, interstitial or femoral hernia results in a failed repair.
- If a prosthetic mesh that is not large enough is used, a failed repair can be anticipated.

The essence of prevention of recurrence lies in a working knowledge of the anatomy of the area; clear evaluation of the internal ring, the peritoneal sac and the posterior wall; avoidance of general anaesthesia whenever possible; use of relaxing incisions to minimize or reduce any degree of tension noted in sutured repairs; appreciating the trampoline effect of the posterior wall; being liberal in the use of prosthetic materials; and recognizing that simultaneous repair of bilateral hernias carries a higher complication rate and a higher failure rate than when done separately[5].

Testicular atrophy

The matter of testicular swelling and atrophy is very disappointing to patients and physicians alike. It is one of the main causes of lawsuits following hernia surgery. Venous occlusion proximal in the cord is done therapeutically by ligation of the internal spermatic vein to resolve a varicocele. Wantz has argued that closure of the internal ring is not the cause of testicular swelling; rather he blames trauma and venous thrombosis in the distal cord for undesirable sequela of the testicle[6]. Division of the neck of the sac, leaving the distal sac undisturbed, minimizes testicular swelling. When doing a hernia repair, making the external ring too tight is more injurious than a tight internal ring. The venous return more distal in the cord is affected. If damage to the cord is suspected or traumatic handling of tissues is unavoidable, intravenous steroids given intraoperatively seem helpful in reducing the frequency and intensity of reactions in the testicle. As a rule, it is unwise to remove the testicle from the scrotum. It is preferable not to do hydrocelectomy and hernia repair simultaneously. Larger hernias have more adhesions, consequently they have a higher degree of postoperative testicular swelling. Patients advised to delay their operation allow enlargement of their hernias. Extensive fibrous scarring occurs between the neck of the sac and the cord. This increases the chance of testicular swelling when the hernia is eventually repaired.

Postoperative neuralgia

Postoperative neuralgia is the most difficult postoperative problem to solve. It is reported most frequently in compensation and liability cases. Patients typically are depressed and many express job dissatisfaction. All operations tried for relief usually fail. Laparoscopic hernia repair is not immune to postoperative neuralgias, especially the lateral femoral cutaneous nerve that is involved with stapling techniques. A local anaesthetic and steroid injection can be tried once or twice. If it is ineffective, it is pointless to continue. It has been my observation that these matters are best treated by outwaiting them. The patient eventually finds a different job or is stimulated to a better attitude. A final plea is to exclude the term 'entrapment' from medical parlance. Actually it is a misnomer unless it describes a syndrome of burning pain associated with trophic changes in the distribution of the inguinal nerve. Postoperative neuralgia of some degree is a matter that follows most herniorrhaphies. The term 'entrapment' is extremely inflammatory to any patient and can do nothing but lead to unnecessary lawsuits.

Conclusions

Laparoscopic hernia repair (LHR) can be currently described as a procedure being investigated. Considering that the majority of general surgeons have learned and use laparoscopic cholecystectomy (LC), one needs to examine the pitfalls that have kept LHR from becoming equally popular and accepted comfortably by the same surgeons. Its various techniques have been sufficiently exposed, courses have been taught, and results have appeared in the peer review literature as well as monthly surgical periodicals.

In Florida, which the US medical industry considers a progressive state, a personal survey of LHR was done by polling the membership of the Florida Surgical Society. It showed that LHR is currently used in about 10% of repairs. Comments from surgeons who responded included the following concerns: general vs local anaesthesia, technically more difficult than LC and open hernia repair, serious complications, high immediate failure rate, unknown long-term success rate, and too expensive.

References

1. Gilbert AI. Prosthetic adjuncts to groin hernia repair: a classification of inguinal hernias. *Contemp Surg* 1988; **32**: 128–35.
2. Glassow F. The surgical repair of inguinal and femoral hernias. *Can Med Assoc J* 1973; **108**: 308–13.
3. Shulman AG, Amid PK, Lichtenstein IL. The safety of mesh repair for primary inguinal hernias: results of 3,019 operations from five diverse surgical sources. *Am Surg* 1992; **58**: 255–7.

4. Read RC. Influence of a relaxing incision on suture tension in Bassini's and McVay's repairs. *Arch Surg* 1981; **116**: 440–5.

5. Palumbo LT, Shape WS. Primary inguinal hernioplasty in the adult. *Surg Clin North Am* 1971; **51**: 1293–307.

6. Wantz GE. Complications of inguinal hernial repair. *Surg Clin North Am* 1984; **64**: 287–98.

33

Genitofemoral Neuralgia

JAMES R STARLING

Most cases of primary inguinal herniorrhaphy are executed successfully, with excellent patient satisfaction and return to normal activity. Esoteric complications can occur, but, fortunately, these are rare. Persistent pain (neuralgia) and pricking, burning sensations (paraesthesias) in the inguinal region caused by ilioinguinal, iliohypogastric or genitofemoral nerve entrapment after herniorrhaphy are exceedingly rare but, when persistent, may result in severe patient morbidity.

That peripheral nerve trauma can occur despite great care being taken is demonstrated by the observation that 10–15% of patients will develop neurapraxia and report hypoaesthesia after herniorrhaphy, which may last up to six months postoperatively. Additionally, pain in the distribution of the peripheral nerves can continue weeks after the incisional pain abates. This unwelcome pain pattern in the inguinal region fortunately subsides in most cases.

It has been emphasized routinely that the ilioinguinal nerve must be identified as the primary peripheral sensory nerve when performing an inguinal herniorrhaphy through a conventional anterior inguinal incision. The iliohypogastric nerve is mentioned sparingly. Few references prior to 1984 have emphasized the importance of the branches of the genitofemoral nerve or the fact that this nerve can be involved by entrapment neuropathy. Only recently have some surgeons mentioned attention to the genital branch of the genitofemoral nerve in their description of operative technique[1,2].

Genitofemoral neuralgia is an unusual clinical entity, resulting in severe pain and paraesthesia in the distribution of the genitofemoral nerve. The syndrome of genitofemoral neuralgia (causalgia) was first reported by Magee in 1942[3] and by Lyon in 1945[4]. Of the ten instances of genitofemoral neuropathy reported by these authors, eight occurred after an appendectomy, one after a psoas abscess and one after blunt groin trauma. Genitofemoral neurectomy effectively alleviated symptoms in eight of these ten patients.

Entrapment of the ilioinguinal or iliohypogastric nerve by suture placement, adhesions or actual formation of a cicatricial neuroma after transection of a nerve can occur and result in severe, debilitating postoperative pain. Occasionally, it may be necessary to re-explore a postoperative hernia incision to perform a neurectomy of the ilioinguinal (iliohypogastric) nerve or to excise the neuroma. The common differential diagnosis of ilioinguinal (iliohypogastric) neuralgia includes entrapment of neighbouring nerves.

The surgical literature infrequently mentions genitofemoral neuralgia. Patients who suffer from this syndrome may previously have had repeated groin explorations for ilioinguinal or iliohypogastric entrapment, or may have had chronic pain treated by repeated local injections, nerve stimulators or pain and antidepressant medication. Symptoms usually occur immediately after the primary operation.

Since 1981, 29 patients have had a retroperitoneal genitofemoral neurectomy at the University of Wisconsin Clinical Science Center and the Veterans Administration Hospital. Twenty of these patients were diagnosed after primary inguinal herniorrhaphy. Nine patients developed signs of genitofemoral entrapment after a perforated appendix, blunt trauma or nephrectomy.

Anatomy

The inguinal region, which includes the inguinal canal, spermatic cord, and surrounding skin and subcutaneous tissue (including the femoral triangle of Scarpa), receives sensory innervation from the T11 and 12 nerves and the ventral divisions of the L1 and 2 spinal nerves. The cutaneous branches of the lumbar plexus include the iliohypogastric, ilioinguinal, genitofemoral, lateral femoral cutaneous and obturator nerves (Figure 33.1). The spermatic sympathetic plexus contains the sensory fibres for the testes.

The genitofemoral nerve arises from the L1 and 2 vertebral plexus and consists mainly of sensory fibres with a motor component to the cremaster muscle (cremasteric reflex). It lies within the fascial lining of the abdomen by piercing the psoas muscles and the psoas fascia near its medial border opposite the L3 or L4 vertebra (Figure 33.2). It descends under the peritoneum on the surface of the psoas major muscle, crossing obliquely behind the ureter. At a variable distance above the inguinal ligament, the nerve divides into the genital (external spermatic) and femoral (lumboinguinal) branches. Great variation of nerves is not uncommon, with free communication between branches of the genitofemoral nerve or the ilioinguinal and iliohypogastric nerves. The femoral branch (lumboinguinal) is the cutaneous nerve to the femoral triangle. Branches of the femoral nerve descend laterally to the external iliac artery, behind the inguinal ligament, through the fascia lata into the femoral sheath. The femoral nerve supplies the skin over the upper part of the femoral triangle and communicates with the intermediate cutaneous nerve of the thigh. The genital branch (external spermatic) crosses the lower end of the external iliac artery and enters the inguinal canal through the internal inguinal ring. It supplies the cremaster muscle and traverses the inguinal canal to the end of the skin of the scrotum. In women, the genital branch accompanies the round ligament of the uterus and ends in the skin of the mons pubis and labium majus.

The ilioinguinal and iliohypogastric nerves are formed by branches of T12 and L1 nerves. The ilioinguinal nerve runs subperitoneally at first and then pierces the transversus abdominis muscle. The iliohypogastric nerve passes between the internal oblique and transversus abdominis muscles. The ilioinguinal and iliohypogastric nerves gradually pierce the internal oblique muscle, and lie between it and the external oblique muscle as they near the internal inguinal ring. Within the inguinal

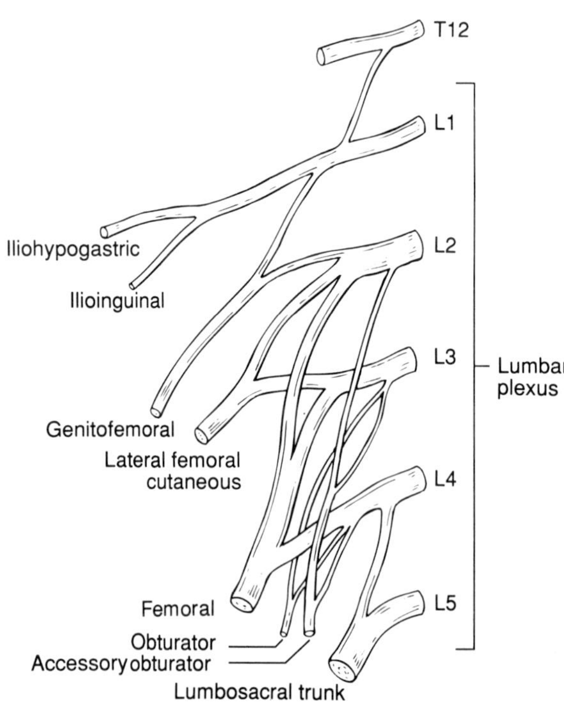

Figure 33.1: Origins of the ilioinguinal, iliohypogastric and genitofemoral peripheral nerves.

canal they usually lie on the anterior surface of the spermatic cord. A frequent anatomical variation is an aberrant inguinal sensory trunk of the ilioinguinal nerve, which descends with the genital branch of the genitofemoral nerve.

Diagnosis

The clinical features of genitofemoral neuralgia consist of intermittent or constant pain in the inguinal region, with radiation of pain to the genitalia and upper thigh. Pain can be aggravated by walking, stooping or hyperextension of the hip, and may be helped by recumbency and flexion of the thigh. Tenderness along the inguinal canal or the inguinal ring may be detected, and hyperaesthesia in the distribution of the nerve may be present. The major differential diagnosis of genitofemoral neuralgia includes entrapment of or damage to the ilioinguinal or iliohypogastric nerves. The latter condition is usually characterized by burning pain over the lower abdomen that radiates down into the inner portion of the upper thigh and into the scrotum or labia majora. The pain can occasionally be reproduced by gently tapping over an area of point tenderness (Tinel sign) or by extending the thigh or hip.

Because communication between the genitofemoral and ilioinguinal (iliohypogastric) nerves causes overlap of sensory innervation, local or specific blocks should be done to attempt to determine whether the ilioinguinal or genitofemoral nerve is specifically entrapped. If a local entrapment or neuroma is responsible for the pain, a local block of the ilioinguinal (iliohypogastric) nerve should alleviate the symptoms. If the pain is not relieved, the 1st and 2nd lumbar nerve plexus can be blocked through a paravertebral route with 0.5% bupivacaine and 0.75% lignocaine (lidocaine) with adrenaline (epinephrine) 1 : 200 000. By performing separate blocks and observing for pain relief, the distinction between genitofemoral and inguinal neuropathy can be made in most instances.

We are especially cautious in recommending remedial surgery on patients who have severe coexistent ipsilateral testicular pain.

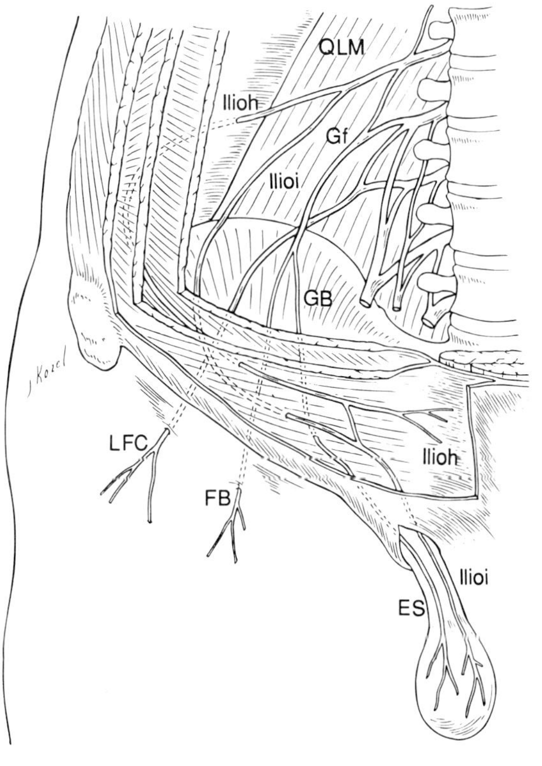

Figure 33.2: Course of the ilioinguinal, iliohypogastric and genitofemoral nerves. ES, external spermatic; FB, femoral branch; GB, qenital branch; GF, genitofemoral; Ilioh, iliohypogastric; Ilioi, ilioinguinal; LFC, lateral femoral cutaneous; QLM, quadratus lumborum muscle.

Surgical treatment

If an ilioinguinal nerve block provides complete or substantial relief of pain, surgical exploration of the inguinal incision and identification of the ilioinguinal (iliohypogastric) nerve is indicated. If the ilioinguinal nerve block does not relieve pain, a 1st and 2nd lumbar nerve block should be performed. If this results in pain relief, surgical exploration of the genitofemoral nerve should be considered. If pain is partially relieved with both blocks, staged surgical exploration of both nerves should be considered.

The genitofemoral nerve is classically approached through a transverse flank incision similar to that for lumbar sympathectomy[5]. The incision is made several centimetres lateral to and above the umbilicus, extending to the anterior axillary line. The external and internal oblique and transversus abdominis muscles are divided, if necessary. The retroperitoneum is exposed and the psoas muscle and ureter are identified. The ilioinguinal and iliohypogastric nerves course laterally to the psoas muscle on the quadratus lumborum muscle. The genitofemoral nerve can be identified as it penetrates the psoas muscle, usually as a single trunk along the medial edge. A 4 to 5 cm section of the genitofemoral nerve is excised to include the bifurcation. Because of frequent abnormal variation in the site of nerve bifurcation, both branches of the genitofemoral nerve must be identified to ensure transection of the proximal genitofemoral nerve trunk. Respective distal branches are too small to be identified precisely.

Hypoaesthesia of the scrotum (or labium majus), skin over the femoral triangle and loss of the cremasteric reflex are the only side-effects of genitofemoral neurectomy and have not caused significant morbidity. There have been a few anecdotal reports of laparoscopic genitofemoral neurectomy, and this technique may become a practical alternative to the conventional approach.

Comment

Severe pain and paraesthesia in the inguinal region, scrotum or proximal medial thigh after inguinal herniorrhaphy are rare, considering the numbers of herniorrhaphies performed each year. Severe post-herniorrhaphy pain, however, can lead to severe debility and occupational incapacity. With the exception of postoperative ilioinguinal entrapment or neuromas, little has been written about entrapment of other peripheral sensory nerves that supply the inguinal region[6]. A singular exception is trauma-induced entrapment of the lateral femoral cutaneous nerve, which may result in meralgia paraesthetica. Although initially there was considerable enthusiasm for neurolysis or neurectomy of the lateral femoral cutaneous nerve, the operation is seldom performed today because of dysaesthesia.

Before my associates' and my 1984 article[7], only 12 instances of genitofemoral neuralgia treated by neurectomy had been reported[3–5,8]. Our present series consists of 29 patients who had retroperitoneal resection of the genitofemoral nerve. Our results are unchanged since our previous publications, 70% of patients having total or significant improvement[9,10]. All patients had sensory loss in the nerve distribution without dysaesthesia. One failure, a patient who had had two previous lumbar disc operations in addition to an inguinal herniorrhaphy, suffered from pain probably of radicular origin. Continued pain in another patient may have been secondary to the rectus abdominis syndrome[6]. Most patients who are not afforded pain relief by remedial surgery will be classified as having chronic pain or myofascial pain syndromes.

References

1. Lichtenstein IL, Shulman AG, Amid PK, Montllor MM. Cause and prevention of postherniorrhaphy neuralgia: a proposed protocol for treatment. *Am J Surg* 1988; **155**: 786.
2. Tons HWCh, Kupczyk-Joeris D, Rotzscher VM, Schumpelick V. Chronic inguinal pain following Shouldice repair of primary inguinal hernias. *Contemp Surg* 1990; **37**: 24.

3. Magee RK. Genitofemoral causalgia (a new syndrome). *Can Med Assoc J* 1942; **46**: 326.
4. Lyon EK. Genitofemoral causalgia. *Can Med Assoc J* 1945; **53**: 213.
5. Laha RK, Rao S, Pidgeon CN, Dujovny M. Genito-femoral neuralgia. *Surg Neurol* 1977; **8**: 280.
6. Dawson DM, Hallett M, Millender LH. *Entrapment Neuropathies.* Boston, Mass: Little, Brown, 1983.
7. Harms BA, DeHaas DR, Starling JR. Diagnosis and management of genitofemoral neuralgia. *Arch Surg* 1984; **119**: 339.
8. O'Brien MD. Genito-femoral neuropathy. *BMJ* 1979; **1**: 1052.
9. Starling JR, Harms BA. Diagnosis and treatment of genitofemoral and ilioinguinal neuralgia. *World J Surg* 1989; **13**: 586.
10. Starling JR, Harms BA, Schroeder ME, Eichman PL. Diagnosis and treatment of genitofemoral and ilioinguinal entrapment neuralgia. *Surgery* 1987; **102**: 581.

34

Testicular Atrophy as a Risk of Open Hernia Repair

GEORGE E WANTZ

Testicular atrophy, a sequela of ischaemic orchitis, is the most important and dreaded complication of inguinal hernioplasty. It angers men of all ages and is very apt to give rise to litigation. The complication deserves more attention.

Clinical manifestations

Ischaemic orchitis always precedes testicular atrophy. Ischaemic orchitis begins insidiously and the clinical manifestations do not become apparent for two to five days. The syndrome consists of a tender, painful, swollen testicle, epididymis and spermatic cord. Usually the testicle is retracted and sometimes a mild fever is present.

The inflammatory response may resolve without sequelae or it may resolve in testicular atrophy. Usually the atrophy is evident in three to four months but sometimes a year may pass before it becomes apparent. Ischaemic orchitis is more common after recurrent hernioplasty than after primary hernioplasty, and so is the likelihood of testicular atrophy. The atrophic testicle is painless, and not prone to malignancy.

Aetiology

It is generally agreed that the pathology is thrombosis of the testicular veins with intense venous congestion of the testicle. However, the aetiology is usually an enigma, and surgeons are invariably mystified by its occurrence. The surgical literature is not helpful and suggests as possible causes too tight reconstruction of the inguinal rings, testicular anomalous blood supply and subacute infection of the urogenital tract. No wonder there are only generalizations for its prevention!

I was unclear about the complication until my experience unveiled the mystery and revealed the cause in 1981. Of the first 1682 primary Shouldice hernioplasties I performed, 11 developed ischaemic orchitis, of which two went on to atrophy. Curiously, all the patients with the complication after primary hernioplasties had had complete removal of the scrotal indirect hernias sacs. Of the first 311 recurrent Shouldice hernioplasties I performed, seven developed ischaemic orchitis, of which five went on to atrophy. This confirms the fact that ischaemic orchitis is more common and more likely to resolve in atrophy following recurrent hernioplasty than following primary hernioplasty.

The conspicuous common feature in this experience was surgical trauma to testicular veins in the cord; in the primary hernias, the trauma was to the pampiniform plexus from the dissection necessary to free a complete indirect hernia from the cord, and in the recurrent hernias it was the trauma necessary to mobilize the previously dissected and traumatized scar-encased cord from which a complete indirect hernia might have been removed.

To test these observations I proposed to limit dissection trauma to the spermatic cord by:

- never excising, if possible, the distal portion of indirect sacs
- never, if possible, dissecting beyond the pubic tubercle
- using the properitoneal approach to avoid the spermatic cord altogether whenever the spermatic cord had been previously dissected, as in recurrent inguinal hernias.

A dramatic and decisive reduction in the incidence of ischaemic orchitis resulted. Among more than 4000 primary hernioplasties in men performed since then, there was only one instance of ischaemic orchitis. Among more than 600 properitoneal recurrent hernioplasties in men performed since then, there were only two examples of ischaemic orchitis, both of which could have been anticipated. In one, the patient had a large sliding indirect hernia sac and in the other a technical mishap occurred.

The obvious conclusion is that the aetiology of the thrombosis in ischaemic orchitis is dissection trauma to the cord, and that limiting dissection of the cord greatly reduces its incidence. Had any other cause been present, surely it would have been apparent in this considerable surgical experience of a single surgeon.

At one time I believed, as some of my colleagues still do, that too tight reconstruction of the deep ring was the paramount cause of the complication. Plaintiff lawyers attach particular significance to this possibility because making inguinal rings too tight creates the image of strangulation and negligence, whereas dissection of the cord is an integral part of any anterior inguinal hernioplasty. An examination of other possible causes of ischaemic orchitis is in order.

The deep inguinal ring is not like a wedding band. Only the medial edge is fibrous. The lateral border is soft, muscular, elastic and so indistinct that it cannot be seen or palpated. It is a surgical technical impossibility to make it too tight by reconstructing the medial border. What the surgeon palpates as the deep inguinal ring is, in fact, the inguinal canal, which will necessarily be slightly diminished in diameter in all patients in whom the inguinal ligament was used for the repair of the posterior wall of the inguinal canal.

The superficial ring has fibrous and bony margins. However, the superficial ring is not reconstructed but merely reassembled. Its rigid and often eroded borders prevent otherwise.

Furthermore, ligating the testicular veins at the level of the deep ring does not cause venous stagnation. In fact, ligating the testicular veins at the level of the deep ring can be done without endangering the testicle, and is the treatment of choice for varicocele. Not surprisingly, ligating and excising a varicocele in the scrotum frequently does.

Anomalies of the testicular blood supply cannot be incriminated. None has been described; besides, the infarct of the testicle is not anaemic and arterial in origin, but, instead, congestive and venous.

Neither can subacute urogenital tract infection be accused. Were an infection a cause, suppuration would occur occasionally, but it does not.

Recommendations

It is probably impossible to eliminate this complication completely. Dissection of the inguinal canal and the spermatic cord are an essential part of every anterior inguinal hernioplasty. Also, difficult dissections and the necessity to excise an indirect hernia sac will always occur. However, dissection trauma to the spermatic cord can be reduced. This is easily accomplished by leaving the distal portion of all but the smallest of indirect hernia sacs *in situ*, if possible, and never dissecting beyond the pubic tubercle, if possible.

There will be exceptions, as, for example, in the case of an indirect sliding hernia sac. If an indirect hernia sac must be removed, the dissection should be sharp and not blunt. Bluntly stripping the sac from the cord may be the very unseen trauma that stretches, contuses and damages the delicate vein of the pampiniform plexus. Hydroceles and other pathology beyond the inguinal canal should not be dealt with at the same time as the hernia repair.

The transabdominal properitoneal approach avoid the dissection of the inguinal canal completely. It is preferred to the anterior groin approach for all patients in whom the spermatic cord has been previously dissected. This includes patients with recurrent hernias, and probably all those who have undergone previous scrotal surgery, including vasectomy. It may also be the best approach for all those worried about testicular atrophy.

Finally bilateral simultaneous inguinal hernioplasty is not recommended if an indirect hernia sac must be excised, for fear of bilateral testicular atrophy. Likewise, men in their reproductive years who develop ischaemic orchitis on one side should have the other side delayed a year until the final outcome of the ischaemic orchitis is known.

Further reading

Fong Y, Wantz GE. Prevention of ischemic orchitis during inguinal hernioplasty. *Surg Gynecol Obstet* 1992; **174**: 399–402.

Wantz GE. Testicular atrophy as a risk of inguinal hernioplasty. *Surg Gynecol Obstet* 1982; **154**: 570–1.

Wantz GE. Testicular atrophy and chronic residual neuralgia as risks of inguinal hernioplasty. *Surg Clin North Am* 1993; **73**: 571–81.

35

Risks to Fertility with Laparoscopic Mesh Repair

DEMETRIUS LITWIN

Infertility as a risk of hernia surgery has been poorly studied and possibly underestimated. During residency training we are taught that there is little risk to fertility from conventional groin hernia surgery unless there is transection of the vas deferens or testicular devascularization. Even then, the risks are considered to be minimal because it is unlikely that a patient will sustain injury to both sides.

Infertility, however, is a common problem and is said to affect 15% of North American couples of childbearing age. Physical causes are found in 80–90% of cases and, in approximately half of these cases, abnormal semen analysis indicates the male as the partner responsible for the infertility[1]

Operative risks

The risks to fertility with either conventional or laparoscopic groin hernia surgery are related to the dissection of the groin region. With laparoscopic approaches the testicular artery is vulnerable at the internal ring. The vas deferens is vulnerable as is crosses the pelvic floor from medial to lateral until it enters the internal ring. The vas deferens receives its blood supply from the deferential artery which arises from the inferior vesicle artery, and forms a microvascular network of vessels within the adventitial layer of the vas deferens[2].

Anatomical considerations

There are both sympathetic and parasympathetic nerves to the vas deferens, of which the sympathetic adrenergic nerves are most important. These are derived from the hypogastric nerves via the presacral nerve. These nerves are found in all three layers of the tunica muscularis of the vas deferens and are responsible for function[2]. Peristalsis of the vas deferens is probably dependent upon innervation and is solely responsible for spermatozoa transport[2,3].

There are only a few clinical reviews that entertain the possibility that fertility may be affected by groin hernia repair. A study of 8500 infertile male patients attending a fertility clinic associated with Tel Aviv University demonstrated that 565 (6.65%) had previous inguinal hernioplasty with or without associated atrophy of the testes[4]. Semen quality of these patients was markedly reduced. Similarly, in a three-year study from Kyoto University, 55 of 724 subfertile patients who presented to their infertility clinic had undergone childhood inguinal herniorrhaphy. Complete vas deferens obstruction caused by inguinal herniorrhaphy was diagnosed in 16 of these patients[5]. Both of these studies suggest there may be an association between infertility and groin hernia repair.

Investigation and studies

Just how sensitive is the vas deferens to manipulation? In a study on rats, Shandling and Janik[6] demonstrated that grasping the vas deferens with an atraumatic vascular clamp or even digital compression of the vas deferens led to an inflammatory reaction in all layers of that structure. Grasping the vas deferens with a non-toothed Adson clamp or mosquito haemostat had a more profound effect, and had led to complete muscular disruption in 30% and 100% of cases respectively when examined six weeks after the injury. Negligible healing following complete muscular disruption was found at six months. The authors concluded that clamping with a non-toothed forceps or mosquito haemostat was equivalent to transection[7]! However, even when the vas was grasped with an atraumatic vascular clamp or manipulated by digital compression, 10% showed partial obstruction when examined six months following the injury. Therefore, it was concluded that manipulation of the vas deferens should always be minimized.

In a similar study, Sandhu and Osborn conducted a fertility trial in rats, comparing different surgical techniques. They demonstrated that cord mobilization had little effect on fertility, but if the vas deferens was crushed or stripped, or a tight repair carried out at the internal ring, there was a profound effect on fertility[8]. They concluded that overzealous handling of the vas was injurious and that excessive vas mobilization led to devascularization and fibrosis.

Because the vas deferens appears to be more sensitive to injury than previously suspected, how significant is unilateral injury? Parkhouse and Hendry studied 30 subfertile males who had testicular obstruction following inguinal or pelvic surgery in childhood[9]. As expected, all patients with bilateral obstruction were azospermic. Of the 17 patients with unilateral obstruction, 11 had low sperm counts but six had normal sperm counts. However, all had high titres of antibodies to spermatozoa and were infertile, indicating that male infertility can result from either obstruction or its immunological consequences. An experimental study of infertility in mice after unilateral vasoligation also demonstrated that fertility was profoundly affected. High antisperm antibody titres occurred in the vasoligation group that did not occur in mice that underwent orchiectomy or sham surgery. Furthermore, *in vitro* fertilization of ova was inhibited by the presence of serum from the mice that underwent vasoligation[10]. Both of these studies indicate that infertility after unilateral vasectomy or vasoligation may be immunologically mediated by antisperm antibodies. It has been postulated that surgery and subsequent obstruction may affect the 'blood/testes' barrier, which may lead to sensitization.

It is apparent that unilateral testicular obstruction can significantly affect fertility. We must now ask ourselves if less severe, non-obstructing structural lesions can also contribute to male infertility? This is a difficult question to answer because of the lack of data. However, in a study of seminal vesiculography in the evaluation of male infertility, Ford found that three of 27 infertile patients had a non-obstructing structural lesion as the possible cause of infertility[11].

Conclusions

It is evident that groin surgery has the potential to affect fertility profoundly. The laparoscopic approach to groin hernia repair is not immune to these risks. Vascular injury to the testicle may occur as a result of either direct injury to the testicular artery or tight-ring closure with venous congestion. This latter risk may be increased if mesh if used and is cut to encircle the cord. Direct injury to the vas deferens may also occur, particularly since most laparoscopic repairs uncover the vas deferens with the creation of a large peritoneal flap. Care must be taken when creating the peritoneal flap to ensure that the vas deferens is dissected free from the peritoneum with its adventitial framework intact. This is especially important during reduction of an indirect hernia sac, when both the testicular vessels and the vas deferens must be peeled away from the sac.

The effect of preperitoneal mesh and resultant fibrosis is as yet completely unevaluated as a risk to fertility. Mesh placed in a preperitoneal position for laparoscopic groin hernia repair rests on the vas deferens and could possibly lead to partial or complete occlusion of the vas, or could cause functional obstruction on the basis of contractility dysfunction.

Summary

The effects of hernia repair on fertility have been poorly studied in conventional surgery, and not yet studied in laparoscopic surgery. Further evaluation is required in both minimal and conventional access approaches. It is entirely likely that the risks to fertility in both minimal access and conventional access surgery are greater than previously suspected.

References

1. Betz G. Evaluation of infertility in the female. *Urol Clin North Am* 1978; **5**: 489.
2. Ewing LL, Chang TSK. The testis, epididymis, and ductus deferens. In: Walsh DC, Gittis RF, Perlmutter AD, Stamey TA, eds. *Campbell's urology*. Philadelphia: WB Saunders, 1986: 200–33.
3. Bruschini H, Schmidt RA, Janagho EA. Studies on the neurophysiology of the vas deferens. *Invest Urol* 1977; **15**: 112.
4. Yavetz H, Harash B, Yoger L, *et al.* Fertility of men following inguinal hernia repair. *Andrologia* 1991; **23**: 443–6.
5. Matsuda T, Horii Y, Yoshida O. Unilateral obstruction of the vas deferens caused by childhood inguinal herniorrhaphy in male infertility patients. *Fert Steril* 1992; **58**: 609–13.
6. Shandling B, Janik JS. The vulnerability of the vas deferens. *J Pediatr Surg* 1981; **16**: 461–4.
7. Janik JS, Shandling B. The vulnerability of the vas deferens (II). The case against routine bilateral inguinal exploration. *J Pediatr Surg* 1982; **17**: 585–8.
8. Sandhu PS, Osborn DE. Surgical Techniques for Inguinal Surgery and its effect on Fertility in the Wistar Rat Model. *Br J Urol* 1991; **68**: 513–17.
9. Parkhouse H, Hendry WF. Vasal Injuries during Childhood and their Effect on Subsequent Fertility. *Br J Urol* 1991; **67**: 91–5.
10. Kessler D, *et al.* Infertility in mice after unilateral vasectomy. *Fertil Steril* 1985; **43**: 308–12.
11. Ford K, Carson CC, Dunnick NR, *et al.* The role of seminal vesiculography in the evaluation of male infertility. *Fertil Steril* 1982; **37**: 552–6.

Part III: Laparoscopic hernia repairs

36

A Rational Approach to Laparoscopic Hernia Repair, with Particular Emphasis on Herniotomy and/or Ring Closure

R DAVID ROSIN

It is over a century since Lawson Tait[1] stated 'Not only must the operation be in no way complicated, but it must be simplified to the utmost'. There is no doubt in my mind that laparoscopic indirect inguinal hernia repair is an uncomplicated simple method and that it will stand the test of time.

Historical perspective

Henry Marcy realized that failure to close the internal ring or low ligation of an indirect inguinal hernia sac predisposed the patient to recurrence. He stated that, even with the most accurate reconstruction, the repair was doomed to failure if this reconstruction did not include closure of the internal ring or if high ligation of the hernia sac was not accomplished[2,3]. He was the first surgeon to describe a procedure that achieved high ligation of the indirect sac and inguinal ring closure through a transabdominal approach[4,5].

Many surgeons carrying out a laparotomy for other intra-abdominal conditions will repair an indirect inguinal hernia from within when it is discovered by chance. The usefulness of incidental indirect inguinal hernia repair from within the abdominal cavity was recognized by Andrews in 1924. He closed the inguinal hernia defect by placing sutures in the peritoneum and fascia from within the peritoneal cavity. He felt that this was a far more effectual method for repair of an indirect inguinal hernia than other methods of that time[6].

High inguinal skin crease incision with opening of the peritoneum and dissection of the hernial sac from within the abdominal cavity followed by closure of the defect was in fact carried out by La Roque[7], who reported this method in 1932. He carried out 1700 procedures in this manner but, unfortunately, there is no accurate follow-up data.

Fifty years later, Ger[8] carried out transabdominal repair in certain patients undergoing laparotomy primarily for other intra-abdominal conditions. The difference with his procedure was that the hernia sac was not dissected, ligated or reduced. He placed stainless steel Michel staples into the peritoneal opening of the sac and the underlying tissue to close the sac. His longest follow up was 44 months and there had been only one recurrence. Interestingly, the last patient in Ger's report had the inguinal hernia defect repaired with the clips applied under laparoscopic guidance. The staples were applied with a special stapling device inserted through a second cannula. The patient had been followed up for three years without evidence of recurrence

Ger subsequently published a study in dogs with congenital indirect hernia[9]. In three dogs he performed a standard laparotomy and stapling of the peritoneal opening under direct vision, whilst in the next 12 the same opening was closed laparoscopically. On the 12 dogs undergoing laparoscopic repair of the congenital indirect inguinal hernia, all were apparently cured. Examination of the specimens showed that, if the staples were properly applied, they disappeared below the peritoneum.

Superficial application of staples resulted in migration with loss of effective closure. Examination of the processus vaginalis with probes showed that in five cases the sac was obliterated, and in eight dogs the size was considerably reduced. Ger noted the following advantages for laparoscopic repair:

- small incisions
- minimal dissection
- less chance of injury to spermatic cord
- decreased incidence of orchitis
- decreased incidence of bladder injury
- no ilioinguinal postoperative neuralgia
- the ability to achieve a very high ligation of the sac
- minimal postoperative discomfort
- fast recovery time
- simultaneous peritoneoscopy
- the ability to diagnose and treat bilateral hernias without extensive dissection.

In 1989, Bogojavalensky showed a video at an American meeting on laparoscopic hernia repair in which the peritoneum of the hernia sac was opened, the musculofascial defect bluntly dissected and subsequently filled with rolled-up Vicryl. Since that time, a number of surgeons have been carrying out laparoscopic hernia repairs for both indirect and direct inguinal hernias.

Rationale for herniotomy alone

In children and young adults, conventional herniotomy only is preformed for indirect inguinal hernias. In young adults many surgeons will perform a herniotomy and simple narrowing of the internal ring. It is only when the patient is older or much dissection has been performed around the internal ring that a prophylactic posterior wall repair is added. By not dissecting the internal ring, no damage is caused to the ilioinguinal nerve or the internal ring shutter mechanism.

Method

The patient is not shaved and is asked to void urine one hour prior to surgery when the premedication is to be administered. If a bladder is palpable prior to operation, the patient is catheterized to empty the bladder and then the catheter is removed.

Following antiseptic preparation of the skin and towelling, a pneumoperitoneum is induced via a Verres needle inserted subumbilically. A 10 mm port is inserted through the subumbilical incision and a peritoneoscopy performed using a 30° telescope. The diagnosis is confirmed and the other hernial orifice carefully examined. 5 mm ports are then inserted, level with the umbilicus on the right and left sides, under direct vision. If the patient is older and there is the possibility of a concurrent direct hernia, 10/11 mm ports are used.

For an indirect inguinal hernia, the sac is inverted; if this proves difficult, the inversion is aided by aquadissection performed under direct vision. We have never failed to invert an indirect sac even if very large. Once inverted, a PDS endoloop is placed around the neck of the sac and tightened. Care is taken to avoid the spermatic cord structures which are clearly seen at the base of the internal ring. The sac, once doubly ligated at this very high point, is not excised because it serves to obstruct the internal ring. If a type II hernia is present, sutures are placed lateral to the inverted sac to narrow the deep ring. After the first year, type II hernias were treated by preperitoneal mesh repair as were type III and IV hernias throughout the study.

Study period

From October 1990 until March 1993 inclusive, 75 type I inguinal hernias in young men were repaired by high ligation of the sac alone using the laparoscopic transperitoneal route. In the first year of the study, 20 type II inguinal hernias were repaired by herniotomy plus lateral ring closure, again using the laparoscopic approach (Table 36.1). From October 1991, all types II, III and IV inguinal hernias treated laparoscopically were repaired using a preperitoneal Prolene mesh (Table 36.1).

The age range for type I and II patients was 17–47 years, with a mean of 29. In the other hernia patients treated laparoscopically, the range was 31–89 with a mean of 48 years (Table 36.2). During this 30-month period, 75 type I, 20 type II (until September 1991), 12 type II (after October 1991), 65 type III and 20 type IV inguinal hernias were repaired laparoscopically, giving a total of 202 patients.

Results

The mean hospital stay was 36 hours following surgery, and return to work/normal activities was nine days. The longest follow up to date has been 30 months with a range of 3–30 months and a mean of 16 months. There have been no recurrences (0%) in type I hernias treated by herniotomy alone whereas there have been three recurrences (15%) in those type II hernias treated by herniotomy and ring closure (Table 36.3). Two of these recurred within 24 hours of surgery, indicating technical failure, whilst the third recurred two months following lifting. Because of the recurrences in the type II hernias, from October 1991 this procedure was abandoned and all type II hernias have since been treated with a preperitoneal mesh repair.

There were no operative problems from the laparoscopy, herniotomy or ring closure. One patient developed a transient hydrocele, one a mild epididymitis which resolved spontaneously and one patient postoperatively had unilateral scrotal emphysema which settled very quickly without treatment.

In patients treated with a preperitoneal mesh, there has been one inferior epigastric artery bleed controlled with clips and one port bleed controlled using a Foley catheter balloon; one other patient developed retention following bilateral hernia repairs.

Table 36.1: Laparoscopic transperitoneal inguinal hernia repairs (October 1990 to March 1993)

Type I	75
Type II (to September 1991)	20
(after September 1991)	12
Type III	65
Type IV	30
Total	202

Table 36.2: Ages of patients undergoing laparoscopic hernia repairs

Type I & II	*Age* (years)	*Type III & IV*	*Age* (years)
Range	17–47	Range	31–89
Mean	29	Mean	48

Table 36.3: Laparoscopic hernia repairs recurrences

Type	*Recurrence*
I	0%
II: before September 1991	15%
after September 1991	0%
III	0%
IV	0%

Discussion

It has been reported that, with conventional operation, the recurrence rate following indirect inguinal hernia repair is 0–7%, following direct inguinal hernia repair 1–10% and following recurrent inguinal hernia repair 5–35%[10]. The authors (Condon and Nyhus) state that these recurrences are related to failure to understand the anatomy, missing an indirect sac and poor surgical technique.

Laparoscopic hernia repair using mesh and a preperitoneal pocket is now accepted as a safe, good method for inguinal hernia repair. However, we feel that insertion of foreign material over a wide area for a simple type I congenital hernia where there is no muscle weakness is 'overkill'. We agree that type III and IV inguinal hernias should be repaired laparoscopically using the preperitoneal mesh operation. Although we abandoned herniotomy and closure for type II inguinal hernias, we feel that, with more accurate suturing taking the aponeurosis and muscles under direct vision having dissected them out rather than through the peritoneum, may provide a satisfactory repair and should be restudied. Longer follow up is needed but our results to date are very encouraging.

References

1. Lawson Tait. *BMJ* 1891.
2. Marcy HO. A new use of carbolized catgut ligatures. *Boston Med Surg J* 1871; **85**: 315–16.
3. Griffith CA. The Marcy repair of indirect inguinal hernias: 1870 to present. In: Nyhus LM, Condon RE, eds. *Hernia* 3rd ed. Philadelphia: JB Lippincott, 1989: 106–18.
4. Marcy HO. The cure of hernia. *JAMA* 1887; **8**: 589–92.
5. Marcy HO. *Hernia*. New York: Appleton Press, 1892.
6. Andrews E. A method of herniotomy utilising only white fascia. *Ann Surg* 1924; **80**: 225–38.
7. LaRoque GP. The intra-abdominal method of removing inguinal and femoral hernia. *Arch Surg* 1932; **24**: 189–203.
8. Ger R. The management of certain abdominal hernias by intra-abdominal closure of the neck. *Ann R Coll Surg Engl* 1982; **64**: 342–4.
9. Ger R, Monroe K, Duvivier R, Mishrick A. Management of indirect inguinal hernias by laparoscopic closure of the neck of the sac. *Am J Surg* 1990; **159**: 371–3.
10. Condon RE, Nyhus LM. Complications of groin hernias. In: Nyhus LM, Condon RE, eds. *Hernia*, 3rd ed. Philadelphia: JB Lippincott, 1989: 253–69.

37

Laparoscopic Inguinal Herniorrhaphy: an Individualized Approach

YVES-MARIE DION

Over the past three years, several reports have described laparoscopic treatment of groin hernias; four pioneers in this field have described their own technique[1–4]. Since this initial work, a variety of laparoscopic transabdominal preperitoneal approaches have been described, with gratifying results[5–8]. Follow-up is limited, however. We established a protocol for laparoscopic treatment of groin hernias[9] based on the Nyhus classification and preperitoneal approach[10–12].

Materials and methods

From March 1991 to December 1992, 63 patients (4 females and 59 males) of ages ranging from 18 to 71 years (median, 42) with symptomatic inguinal hernias received laparoscopic treatment. A research consent form stressed the important points about the technique, including an unknown recurrence rate, the necessity to insert a Foley catheter into the bladder, the possibility of a mesh repair and the laparoscopic entry into the abdominal cavity. Following surgery, patients are followed up every three months for two years and every six months thereafter.

The technique is individualized according to the type of hernia. We adopted Nyhus' classification of groin hernias[10].

- Type I is an indirect hernia with the sac located in a normal internal ring as encountered in the pediatric population.
- Type II is an indirect hernia with a dilated internal ring but an intact posterior inguinal wall. The inferior epigastric vessels are not displaced.
- Type III hernia represents a weakness of the posterior wall of the inguinal canal and is divided in three categories:
  IIIA, direct hernia
  IIIB, indirect hernia (internal ring dilated, medially encroaching on or destroying the transversalis fascia of the Hesselbach triangle – eg massive scrotal, sliding or pantaloon hernia)
  IIIC, femoral hernia.
- Type IV is a recurrent hernia.

Treatment is offered to adults. The paediatric population is excluded.

Laparoscopic technique

Under general anaesthesia, a Foley catheter is inserted in the bladder. After creation of a pneumoperitoneum, three trocars are inserted, one (10 mm) at the umbilicus and the other two (one 10 mm and one 5 mm) slightly inferior to the umbilicus and lateral to the rectus muscles. The

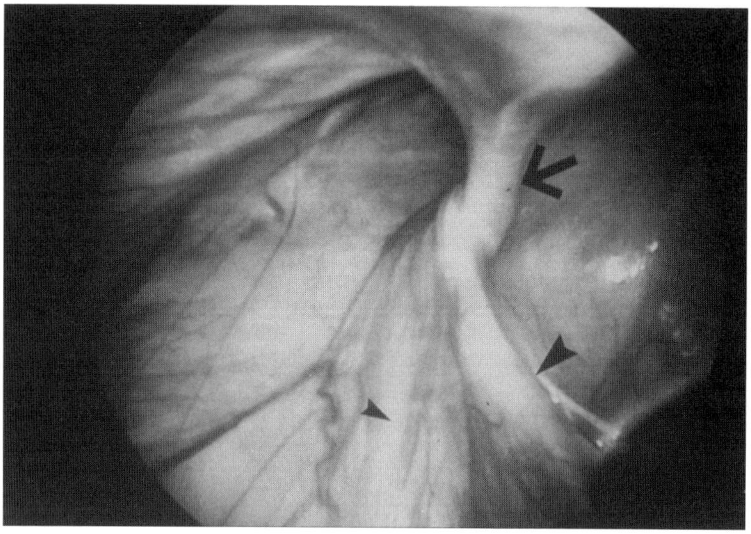

Figure 37.1: Left indirect (type II) hernia; vas deferens (large arrowhead), testicular vessels (small arrowhead) and inferior epigastric vessels (large arrow).

patient is then placed in the Trendelenburg position. The hernia is visualized (Figure 37.1) and the peritoneum incised, starting at the lateral umbilical ligament medially, arching over the inguinal defect and continuing lateral to the internal inguinal ring. The preperitoneal fat is peeled away from the transversalis fascia and conjoined tendon above and from Cooper's ligament and the iliopubic tract below. The cord is individualized from the surrounding structures, and the hernia sac is either cut at its neck in type II hernias (Figure 37.2) or reflected downward with the peritoneum in type III and IV hernias. In type II hernias we do not dissect the sac any more because it is less traumatic to cut it at its neck and leave it in the inguinal canal before closing the muscular defect. Although seromas have been described in the remaining sac, the procedure of leaving large sacs *in situ* is regularly performed by surgeons; in our series, we have not yet encountered this problem.

Once dissection is completed, repair is undertaken. In type II hernias, the upper edge of the internal inguinal ring (transversus abdominis arch) is approximated using two to four interrupted sutures of 0-Prolene (Ethicon Inc., Cincinnati, OH, USA) to its lower edge (iliopubic tract) (Figures 37.3 and 37.4), and the peritoneum is closed with haemoclips (Ethicon). Type II hernia in the female is treated by incising the round ligament before closing completely the internal ring.

The size of the newly created internal ring in the male is evaluated using forceps. The strength of the posterior wall is examined using manual palpation from outside combined with instrument palpation from inside the inguinal canal and from the posterior aspect of the canal (posterior wall). Visualization of the posterior wall is necessary at this point.

When mesh is used (Type IIIA and B, and type IV), the same dissection is performed and a piece of Prolene mesh (Ethicon Inc.) measuring approximately 12 × 7 cm, appropriately tailored, is selected. An incision is made in the lateral portion of the mesh to allow inclusion of the cord. The mesh is first fixed lateral to the cord, thereby reinforcing the internal ring. Other staples and interrupted sutures are then applied between the mesh and the conjoined tendon (and arch of the transversus abdominis muscle) above and Cooper's ligament below in a tension-free manner. Medially, the mesh is stapled and sutured to the pubic tubercle. Five or six 0-Prolene sutures and 12–15 staples are used. The peritoneum is then closed with haemoclips (Ethicon Inc.). A type IIIC hernia is closed with interrupted 0-Prolene sutures (one to three), placed between the iliopubic tract and Cooper's ligament.

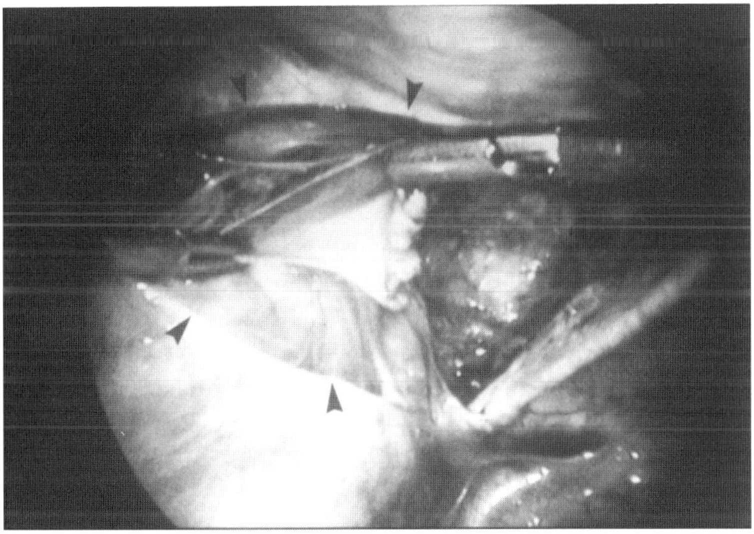

Figure 37.2: The peritoneum has been incised (arrowheads) and the indirect sac left *in situ*; two grasping forceps are opening the sac, which retracts into the inguinal canal when traction is ceased.

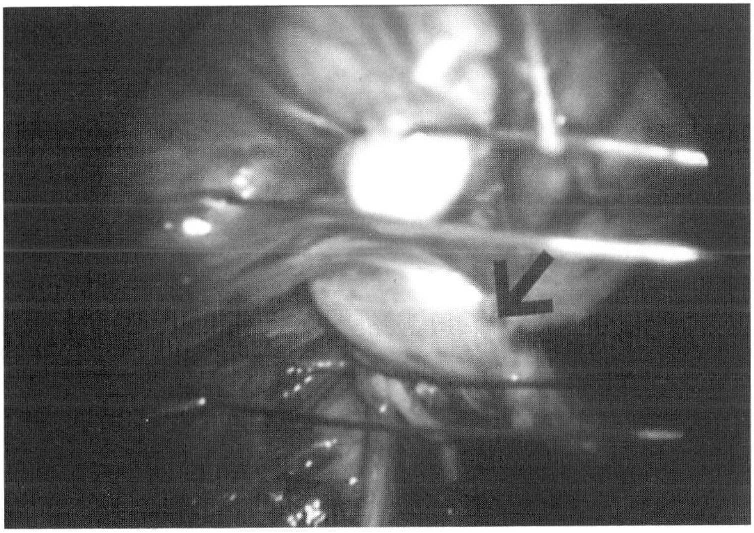

Figure 37.3: Two 0-Prolene sutures applied lateral to the cord (arrow) to approximate the upper portion of the internal ring to its lower aspect (iliopubic tract); left external iliac artery (arrow).

Results

Thirty-two patients had type II indirect hernias. Eighteen had type IIIA direct hernias. Three patients were found to have a large indirect hernia (type IIIB) with weak fascia around the internal ring orifice. Ten patients were treated for recurrent hernias (type IV). No preoperative complications were noted.

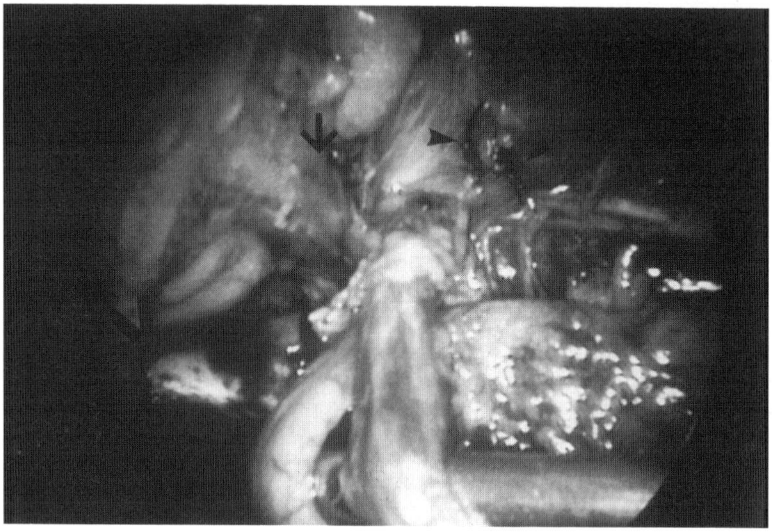

Figure 37.4: Right indirect (type II) hernia cured by application of two 0-Prolene sutures (arrowheads); similar dissection is performed in all cases to evaluate the status fo the posterior wall. The vas deferens and vessels are being elevated on a grasping forceps. Note the shiny Cooper's fascia (large arrow) and posterior wall with epigastric vessels (small arrow). For type IIIA and B and type IV hernias, a mesh is fixed with 0-Prolene sutures and staples.

Fifty-three patients (84%) took parenteral analgesia (one to five times; median, once) followed by enteral analgesics (one to six times; median, twice). Eight patients (13%) took enteral analgesia only and two (3%) did not ask for analgesia.

The median postoperative stay was two days (one to six). One patient with type IV hernia (operated for a third recurrence) had testicular pain which lasted a week, and was kept in the hospital for six days because of a generalized allergic reaction to medication. No other complications were noted. No patient complained of neuralgia. No mortality was recorded. With a median follow up of eight months (one to 21), no recurrences were noted.

Conclusions

Recent articles by Popp[2] and Schultz[4] have shown potential advantages of the laparoscopic approach over conventional techniques: pain that is less severe and of shorter duration, no muscle incision, anatomical and tension-free repair and quick return to work. We would add to this list the potential advantage provided by exploratory laparoscopy. For instance, even though it cannot be as thorough as a formal laparotomy, laparoscopy allowed us to diagnose unsuspected endometriosis in one case. An asymptomatic right colon carcinoma was also discovered during one of our laparoscopic explorations of the common bile duct.

The following are some disadvantages of the laparoscopic preperitoneal approach that can occur. The peritoneal incision made over the hernia site may invite bowel adhesion and later obstruction. So far, however, none of our patients has developed any symptoms, although scattered personal communications mention the occurrence of bowel obstruction. Recent experimental studies in piglets[13] tend to indicate that, although adhesions form, they are limited to the area of dissection and do not involve the small bowel. In a few patients who had previous operations on the contralateral side using an anterior approach, we noted adhesions of the caecum or the sigmoid to the repair, probably as a result of ligation of the sac and insertion of the finger in the abdomen to verify the integrity of the femoral ring. A complete preperitoneal approach, as advocated by McKernan[14] and Ferzli[15], would avoid the peritoneal incision. Our experience with this open approach leads us to believe that accidental breaches will be occasionally created into the peritoneum. A large sac will also have to be transsected and the peritoneum closed at this site.

Another possible complication is the use of mesh, which could become infected. Although employing mesh for treatment of different pathologies can lead to infection rates varying from 2% to 10%[10–12,16,17], Lichtenstein[18,19], using his tension-free repair on 7133 patients operated on in nine different centres, reports an infection rate of 0.03%, demonstrating that appropriate intraoperative care is an important factor in the development of mesh infection. We had no case of mesh infection in the 31 patients in whom we inserted this material.

Potential adhesions of bowel to the mesh, causing obstruction or the formation of fistulas, is unlikely to occur if the peritoneum is carefully reapproximated at the end of the procedure. Results of recent studies with dogs favour the reperitonealization of intra-abdominal mesh or mesh placement by an extraperitoneal approach because these techniques elicit less reaction than the intra-abdominal implantation of a mesh[20].

Nerve injury has been reported at a similar or even higher rate than with conventional repair. Using a preperitoneal approach, the nerves injured are the genitofemoral and the lateral femoral cutaneous[21–23]. Stapling lateral to the cord should not be performed in a plane inferior to the iliopubic tract.

We agree with Nyhus[11] that 'the only setting in which a prosthetic mesh may be used in the primary repair of groin hernias is large indirect [in reality a combined indirect and direct, later classified by him as type IIB] or direct inguinal hernias [type IIIA]'.

We do not favour the insertion of mesh in young patients in their 20s or 30s when weakness of the posterior wall is not demonstrated. A few stitches placed without tension on the enlarged internal ring (type II) cannot lead to future unexpected complications that might be related to the presence of mesh. Furthermore, most recurrences in young patients who have recurrent hernias one or two years after their original operation for indirect hernia have been direct hernias[24], demonstrating that the injury to the posterior wall after the original anterior repair was probably caused by tension on the repair.

An unexpected benefit of our technique relates to the associated cost of a laparoscopic herniorrhaphy. In our series, slightly more than 50% of the patients were treated using only 0-Prolene sutures (type II) and a few haemoclips, which makes the procedure much less expensive than when staples and mesh are used. Other studies show the same trend in terms of indirect (type II) hernia representing approximately 50% of the cases treated[25,26]. Another study demonstrates that a laparoscopic repair in the USA is more expensive than a conventional repair[25]. For instance, charges to patients for supplies and total hospital bills are $298 and $2212 for the conventional approach but $3000 and $5200 for the laparoscopic approach.

Staples are useful to fix the mesh. We still use a few sutures because *in vivo* experiments[27] have shown that different types of staples stabilize the mesh with varying resistance to a bursting stress test. A mesh fixed with 0-Prolene sutures has the highest resistance to the bursting stress test, followed by the one fixed with the Endopath EMS stapler and then by the Endo-Hernia stapler. Type II and type IIIC hernias will still be best treated by a few stitches placed in the appropriate position. At present, our operative time varies between 45 and 70 minutes. In general, it appears that laparoscopic herniorrhaphy (average time in these studies, 63–89 minutes) takes longer than its conventional counterpart[22,28,29]. Dissection requires approximately 15 minutes; repair thus accounts for most of the operative time.

Because our technique is under evaluation, we give the patients the same guidelines they would receive if operated on by a conventional method. We advise them that wound healing takes at least six weeks and to defer any strenuous activity until then. We also warn of possible adverse effects of coughing, which increases considerably (up to 220 mmHg) intra-abdominal pressure, actually more so than lifting 20 kg or exercycling[30]. As mentioned by Rignault, hernioplasty (use of a very large mesh which covers most of the lower abdomen) benefits from the intra-abdominal pressure to stabilize the mesh[31]. Herniorrhaphy, employing a relatively small mesh that covers only the inguinal region, may suffer rather from this increase in abdominal pressure.

Summary

Our technique and other transabdominal preperitoneal techniques (stapling mesh around the hernia defect) seem to be equally effective. The totally extraperitoneal laparoscopic approach gives excellent results (it is more difficult to perform that the transabdominal preperitoneal route); however, a longer follow up is necessary to evaluate the effectiveness of these operative approaches. Techniques to be avoided are the plug techniques, placement of a relatively small piece of mesh in the preperitoneal space without fixation and the simple plication of the peritoneum at the site of an indirect hernia. The intraperitoneal fixation of mesh over the hernia defect is also controversial and cannot be suggested. Nyhus' classification is sound, and a wider application is suggested because this would allow accurate comparison of the results obtained following introduction of these numerous laparoscopic treatments of groin hernias.

References

1. Ger R. Management of direct inguinal hernias by laparoscopic closure of the neck of the sac. *Am J Surg* 1990; **159**: 370–3.
2. Popp L. Transcutaneous aquadissection of the musculofascial defect and preperitoneal endoscopic patch repair. *J Laparoendosc Surg* 1991; **1**: 83–90.
3. Salerno GM, Fitzgibbons RG, Filipi CJ. Laparoscopic inguinal hernia repair. In: Zucker KA, Bailey RW, Reddick EJ, eds. *Surgical Laparoscopy*. St Louis: Quality Medical Publishing, 1991: 281–93.
4. Schultz L. Laser laparoscopic herniorrhaphy: a clinical trial. *J Laparoendosc Surg* 1990; **1**: 41–5.
5. Hawasli A. Laparoscopic inguinal herniorrhaphy: the mushroom plug repair. *Surg Endosc Laparosc* 1992; **2**: 111–16.
6. Toy FK, Smoot RT. Laparoscopic hernioplasty update. *J Laparoendosc Surg* 1992; **2**: 197–205.
7. Arregui ME, Davis CJ, Yucel O, Nagan RF. Laparoscopic mesh repair of inguinal hernia using a preperitoneal approach: a preliminary report. *Surg Laparosc Endosc* 1992; **2**: 53–8.
8. Seid AS, Deutsch H, Jacobson A. Laparoscopic herniorrhaphy. *Surg Laparosc Endosc* 1992; **2**: 59–60.
9. Dion YM, Morin J. Laparoscopic inguinal herniorrhaphy. *Can J Surg* 1992; **35**: 209–12.
10. Nyhus LM, Klein MS, Rogers FB. Inguinal Hernia. *Curr Probl Surg* 1991; **28**: 491–50.
11. Nyhus LM. Editorial. *World J Surg* 1989; **13**: 539.
12. Nyhus LM, Pollack R, Bombeck CT, Donahue PE. The preperitoneal approach and the prosthetic buttress repair for recurrent hernia. *Ann Surg* 1989; **208**: 733–7.
13. Poulos E, Eller R, Twaddel C, Russell S. Abdominal adhesions in laparoscopic hernia repair. *Proceedings from Sages*, April 1993, Phoenix, AZ.
14. McKernan JB, Laws HL. Laparoscopic repair of inguinal hernias using a totally extraperitoneal prosthetic approach. *Surg Endosc* 1993; **7**: 26–8.
15. Ferzli GS, Massaad A, Albert P. Extraperitoneal endoscopic inguinal hernia repair. *J Laparoendosc Surg* 1992; **2**: 281–5.
16. Molloy RG, Moran KT, Waldron RP, Brady MP, Kirwan WO. Massive incisional hernia: abdominal wall replacement with Marlex mesh. *Br J Surg* 1991; **78**: 242–4.

17. Simchen E, Rozin R, Yohana W. The Israeli study of surgical infection of drains and the risk of wound infection in operations for hernias. *Surg Gynecol Obstet* 1990; **170**: 331–7.

18. Lichtenstein IL, Shulman AG, Amid PK, Montllor MM. The tension free hernioplasty. *Am J Surg* 1989; **157**: 188–93.

19. Lichtenstein IL. Response to a letter to the Editor. *Am J Surg* 1990; **160**: 139–40.

20. Schlechter B, Marks J, Shillingstad R, Ponsky J. Adhesions after laparoscopic hernia repair in an animal model. *Proceedings from Sages*, April 1993, Phoenix, AZ.

21. Seid AS. Significance of groin nerve anatomy for laparoscopic hernia repair. *Proceedings from Sages*, April 1993, Phoenix, AZ.

22. Himpens J. Laparoscopic hernioplasty using a regular versus a self expanding prosthesis. *Proceedings from Sages*, April 1993, Phoenix, AZ.

23. Rosser JC, Evans D. Anatomic review in order to avoid nerve injuries associated with laparoscopic inguinal hernia repair. *Proceedings from Sages*, April 1993, Phoenix, AZ.

24. Ijzermans JNM, De Wilt H, Hop WCJ, Jeekel HJ. Recurrent inguinal hernia treated by classical hernioplasty. *Arch Surg* 1991; **126**: 1097–100.

25. Gill BD, Traverso W. Continuous quality inventory: open versus laparoscopic groin hernia repair. *Proceedings from Sages*, April 1993, Phoenix, AZ.

26. Fitzgibbons R, Annibali R, Litke B, Filipi C, Salerno G, Cornet D. A multicentered clinical trial on laparoscopic inguinal hernia repair: preliminary results. *Proceedings from Sages*, April 1993, Phoenix, AZ.

27. Dion YM, Charara J, Guidoin R. Bursting strength evaluation of an experimental hernia repair using Prolene mesh attached to tissue with EMS stapler or with US Surgical Endo Hernia. *Proceedings from Sages*, April 1993, Phoenix, AZ.

28. Newman L, Eubanks S, Lucas G, Mason E, Duncan T. Laparoscopic herniorrhaphy via the transperitoneal approach – a review of our first 151 repairs. *Proceedings from Sages*, April 1993, Phoenix, AZ.

29. Theobald DR, Mack P, Kee SG, Wong WK, Ooi PJ. Laparoscopic inguinal herniorrhaphy with preperitoneal tension-free polypropylene mesh repair. *Proceedings from Sages*, April 1993, Phoenix, AZ.

30. Twardowski ZJ, Khanna R, Nolph KD, *et al.* Intraabdominal pressures during natural activities in patients treated with continuous ambulatory peritoneal dialysis. *Nephron* 1986; **44**: 129–35.

31. Rignault DP. Properitoneal prosthetic inguinal hernioplasty through a Pfannenstiel approach. *Surg Gynecol Obstet* 1986; **163**: 465–8.

38

Animal Studies and Rationale for Intraperitoneal Repair

MORRIS E FRANKLIN Jr

Background

The Texas Endosurgery Institute, of which I am director, is an organization devoted entirely to minimally invasive surgery. We became interested in laparoscopic hernia repair in late 1989 and performed our first laparoscopic hernia repair in January 1990, about two weeks after Schultz and Corbitt began their work. We did not know of anyone else who was working on hernia repair at that time. In collaboration and consultation with Dr Dan Rosenthal it was decided to use a posterior approach and to mimic as closely as possible the work that Stoppa had done in France in the 1970s and 1980s.

We were very disappointed when our first operation took four hours and we had difficulty getting a large piece of mesh, which we though was mandatory, placed correctly. The patient did well but we were exhausted. Our efforts with the next three patients were very similar, and it occurred to us that perhaps instead of positioning the mesh in the retroperitoneal or properitoneal space we could place it intraperitoneally.

Obviously, it is essential to adhere to the principles of hernia surgery, established by Bassini, and tension-free repair is also an important factor. Whether living tissue or a prosthesis should be used to cover the defect is open to debate, but it seems that prosthetic material is being employed increasingly. We felt very strongly that it could be placed in the intraperitoneal position but we were particularly concerned about the fate of a foreign body in this cavity. Because we were worried that it could cause problems, we sought the answer in our laboratory.

The first posterior approach was reported in 1879. Cheatle and Henry popularized the method in the 1920s and 1930s, and probably did some of the first work. This approach depends on a prosthetic device, as discussed elsewhere in this volume by Stoppa, and also reported by Rignault, Rosenthal and Rives. Rosenthal has used the open preperitoneal or properitoneal approach in more than 200 cases of recurrent hernia repair, with a recurrence rate or 1.5%, and 0% in the last 100 patients. His experience was invaluable when we considered the problems and possible methods of repair.

Laparoscopically, one can make the repair by placing a curtain over the defect, or stapling the defect closed, or plugging the defect. And, of course, one can suture the defect closed, as several other writers in this work advocate. Essentially, the defective fascia transversalis is replaced with a non-absorbable impenetrable mesh, which is used to cover the potential defect. I firmly believe that it should be used to cover all areas of potential weakness. But where do we place the mesh? To position it totally extraperitoneally is a very difficult approach. A popular alternative is to place it transperitoneally (ie extraperitoneally and produce a flap) but this seems to cause all kinds of problems, the serious ones of which do not seem to have been addressed. Another possibility is the intraperitoneal approach but this is a controversial method. Our reason for undertaking animal studies was to determine what problems were caused by placing the mesh either intraperitoneally or properitoneally.

Animal studies

Our animal studies began in February 1990, after we had repaired three hernias and were not happy with how long the procedure took as well as the postoperative problems experienced. One patient complained of a lot of testicular pain, something not reported with open procedures. (This might be due to the extent of dissection required, but the cause of the problem has not yet been identified.) All the patients said that they had a lot of pain.

We studied 30 porcine models, divided into three groups.

- *Group 1*: the mesh was placed intraperitoneally. It was either sutured into place or clipped with vascular clips that we use on blood vessels and the cystic duct in laparoscopic cholecystectomy. Most of them were sutured into place with an absorbable suture, mainly 3–0 Vicryl.
- *Group 2*: the mesh was placed properitoneally either through a window (ie we created a flap and just slipped it down inside like an envelope) or via a transverse incision like most of the transperitoneal procedures done now. We made vertical incisions and did 'double doors' where we opened it up and then put it back together.
- *Group 3*: the mesh was dropped on the floor intentionally before being placed inside the animal. This group was used for confirmation that animals really do develop adhesions.

We examined the animals laparoscopically at 7, 14, 21 and 36 days, and sacrificed all but two at 36 days. The remaining two (one in each of groups 1 and 2) were kept alive and were re-examined after nearly a year.

Results

In *group 3* (the contaminated models) all the animals were well. Despite the contaminated mesh, the animals seemed well, ate the day after the procedure and had no ill-effects; however, within a week, nine out of ten had developed adhesions to the mesh. The adhesions persisted and became progressively thicker as time passed. There was no intestinal obstruction, and no fistula developed in these animals despite the contaminated mesh.

In *group 2* (the properitoneal models) we saw no migration of the mesh, although migration has been cited as a problem with this material. Similarly, there was no infection, and no fistulas although seven of the ten animals had adhesions to the peritoneal closure site. Indeed, the animals had no ill-effects.

Group 1 (intraperitoneal placement) was impressive in its lack of adhesions. Only one of the ten had light filmy adhesions between the omentum and the mesh – not covering the whole mesh but just to where its raw edge was turned up and created an omental injury.

Other animal studies

This is the first time that our studies have been reported. Other investigators have reported their studies, and they cite almost identical results. The most well known study is that of Layman, from Chattanooga, Tennessee. He studied 30 animals, using a Gore-Tex, Marlex or Prolene mesh, placed in the intraperitoneal position, to see which ones caused the most adhesions. To describe his results he used the Murphy scale: it is a scale of the amount of adhesion, the density of the adhesions and the proportion that it covers on a particular graph within a range of 1 to 4. Placing the mesh intraperitoneally but with no covering or protection, the results on the Murphy scale were: Gore-Tex, 0.7; Marlex, 1.2; and Prolene, 0.6.

Another, unpublished, study is that of Poulos and his group in Dallas, who studied 21 animals. A sham operation was performed on the left side of the abdomen, and the mesh was placed retroperitoneally (or properitoneally) on the other side. In 12 of these 21 animals, adhesions were found at the peritoneal closure site. Adhesions were present in animals in which the mesh was not completely covered, but animals in which the mesh was free were adhesion-free. Other studies have achieved very similar results.

Human studies

After obtaining clearance from our Institutional Review Board, we proceeded with (investigational) human studies. We began by placing the mesh inside. Because there were no staplers at this time, we had to suture the mesh and had no peritoneum to hold it up, which resulted in the mesh flopping back and forth. We found it easier to suture the mesh into place with transabdominal sutures attaching it to the anterior abdominal wall. We fixed the mesh with percutaneous sutures as well as intraperitoneal staples when these became available. We now use these virtually all the time. They have two roles: to hold the mesh down and spread it very evenly, and to give a second fixation point to an aponeurosis. We position the mesh where we think it should be, and transabdominally place a suture on a Keith needle. It is difficult to use the same hole with the Keith needle leaving the same site but, using some of Ed Phillips' technology, we seem to have resolved the problem: the abdominal wall is pierced with the Keith needle and then a second, 14 gauge, needle is placed to be used as a conduit to exit from the same hole. This method saves a lot of time. We now place three sutures in this way: one in the middle of the mesh and one at each end, all on the anterior abdominal wall through three separate stab wounds of less than 2 mm (Figure 38.1). Initially we removed these sutures. Now we use this method to fix the mesh to the fascia by leaving them in place, finally dissecting down subcutaneously to the fascia, actually tying the mesh to the anterior abdominal wall. There are thus two firm fixation sites, the other being, of course, Cooper's ligament.

Figure 38.2 shows what our mesh looks like when we get through. The three sutures in the anterior abdominal wall are what we used before there were staples and we were suturing it in two other places, which we found lay very nicely on the inguinal floor. We now use staples, and this Figure has a gross error: almost all of our staples were placed vertically when they were close to the nerves that everyone is rightly concerned about. The way to prevent these nerve injuries is twofold:

- We do not try to put the staples all the way into the iliopsoas muscle or into the muscular fascia; we just grasp the peritoneum.
- We orientate the staples in the direction of the nerves.

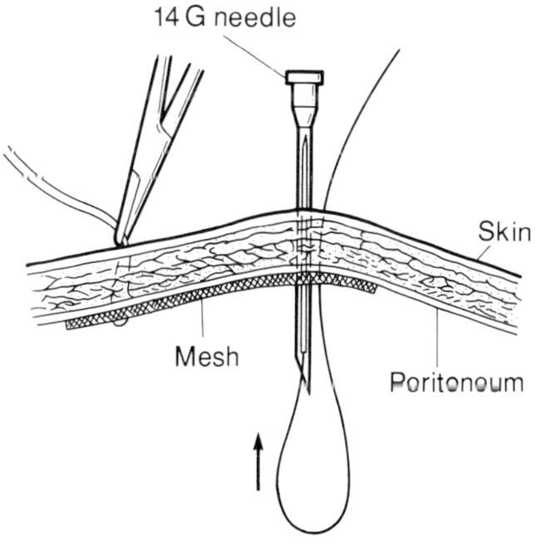

Figure 38.1: Intraperitoneal mesh in place (see text for details).

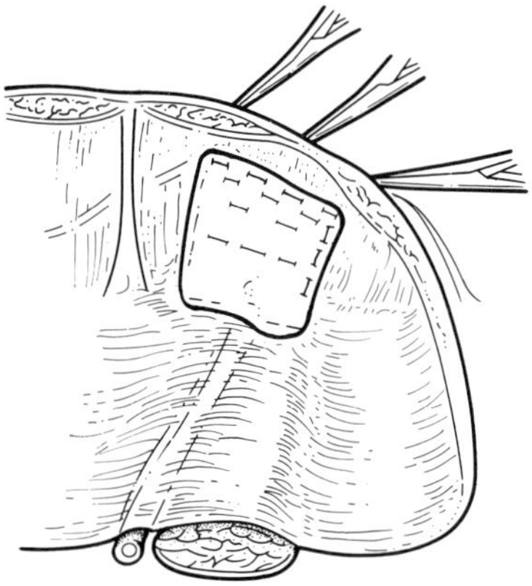

Figure 38.2: Method of insertion of transfascial sutures (see text for details).

By doing this we have had no nerve injuries (other than in the first 30 patients, two of whom suffered injury before we learned what we were doing wrong). We also do not put staples centrally around the defect; we try to staple this so that it lies flat. Visualizing the internal ring as a clock, we do not place any staples from 3 to 6 (on the right) or from 6 to 9 (on the left) around the hernia defect. In indirect hernias, we found that that is where you snag the genitofemoral nerve.

Results

We performed 201 repairs between January 1990 and April 1993. We repaired 35 recurrent hernias, 11 femoral hernias in 125 male and 17 female patients (total patients, 153).

There has been no death and no postoperative bowel obstruction, in a follow-up period of up to 40 months. Most of the patients returned home within 2–23 hours. There was one recurrence very early in the series, because we did not cover the hole. One of the reasons why we started putting in sutures was that we did not hold it in the right place and it just slipped and the patient suffered a recurrence before reaching the recovery room. There were significant haematomas in four patients and small haematomas in eight; five of our first 30 patient had transient neurapraxia. There were no nerve injuries at all in the last 90 patients. Six patients had urinary retention, so we now insert a catheter in all cases. Most of our patients are elderly and cannot empty their bladder well enough prior to the procedure.

Conclusions

The question remains: does mesh result in adhesions? It is not possible to give a definite answer but, based on our experience, mesh is unlikely to be the root cause of the problems that have been attributed to it. The mesh must be flat, the edges must be flush with the peritoneum and there must not be any raw edges. Most importantly, it is important not to cause any injury to tissue or bowel. If we could investigate all the stories about fistula formation, bowel obstruction, invasion of the bowel, and so on, we would find that there had been bowel or tissue injury of some kind that caused most of the problems – not the mesh itself. Does mesh result in adhesions? Certainly in our experience there have been no bowel adhesions, no omental adhesions, no bowel obstruction, no mesh migration, and minimal adhesions only if the edges are not flush. Obviously, there is a need for further study and investigation of this important issue.

39

Results of Laparoscopic Inguinal Herniorrhaphy, with Emphasis on the Intraperitoneal Onlay Mesh Technique

ROBERT J FITZGIBBONS Jr, RICCARDO ANNIBALI, BRADLEY LITKE, DOUGLAS CORNET AND CHARLES J FILIPI

Modern inguinal repair began with the description in 1884 by Edoardo Bassini of a procedure that combined high ligation or reduction of a hernia sac with reconstruction of the inguinal floor. Despite numerous modifications of Bassini's operation, as well as the introduction of the promising Shouldice and Lichtenstein repairs, the national recurrence rate for conventional herniorrhaphy remains at 10%[1]. The operation is considered to be relatively painful and is associated with a significant time away from work. It is for these reasons that surgeons continue to pursue alternatives to conventional inguinal herniorrhaphy.

Laparoscopic cholecystectomy has become the procedure of choice far more rapidly than any other surgical procedure[2]. Therapeutic laparoscopy was therefore destined to be expanded to other surgical fields. Laparoscopic inguinal herniorrhaphy is an example and is perhaps the most controversial of the newer therapeutic laparoscopic operations.

Laparoscopic inguinal herniorrhaphy assumes a transabdominal approach for the repair. This is not a new concept. Marcy in 1887 and Andrews in 1924 proposed intraperitoneal indirect inguinal hernia repair at the time of laparotomy performed for unrelated disease[3,4]. LaRoque in 1932 described an intra-abdominal approach as a primary method of repair. In fact, he performed this in 1700 patients[5]. The author noted that the transabdominal repair allowed closure of the internal ring and high ligation of the hernia sac with minimal dissection and a decreased postoperative recurrence rate. This was especially helpful in sliding hernias, hernias in which the viability of the sac contents was in doubt, or if concomitant intra-abdominal pathology needed to be evaluated or treated, for example ovarian cysts and appendicitis. LaRoque felt that the intra-abdominal perspective allowed him to ligate the sac as high as possible with a clear view of both sides of the internal ring. Most surgeons consider the intra-abdominal method as a primary procedure too invasive for inguinal herniorrhaphy; however, the introduction of therapeutic laparoscopy in general surgery as an alternative method to gain access to the peritoneal cavity has enabled surgeons to reconsider this approach.

Currently several different types of laparoscopic inguinal herniorrhaphies are being performed. All are based on the conventional preperitoneal inguinal herniorrhaphies popularized by Nyhus, Stoppa and Rignault[6,7]. The critical ingredient in the conventional procedure is the placement of a prosthesis after the preperitoneal space has been entered through an abdominal wall incision. The procedure is attractive because the prosthesis is placed on the abdominal side of the defect in the transversalis fascia, allowing intra-abdominal contents and pressure to actually help fix the prosthesis in place instead of being a factor in recurrence. The operation is the basis for currently accepted laparoscopic inguinal herniorrhaphies, as the preperitoneal space can be approached so easily under laparoscopic guidance.

Early laparoscopic inguinal herniorrhaphies

Schultz, Corbitt and Reich independently developed techniques for laparoscopic inguinal hernia repair that utilized polypropylene mesh 'plugs' inserted into the inguinal canal followed by closure of the peritoneal opening with staples, clips or sutures[8–10]. These procedures have become known as the 'plug and patch' techniques. Schultz and Corbitt have both abandoned these because of an excessive recurrence rate, which is not surprising because Bassini's principles of high ligation with reconstruction of the inguinal floor were not addressed.

Current laparoscopic hernia techniques

The excellent results obtained with the classic preperitoneal approach by Rignault and Stoppa encouraged laparoscopic surgeons to develop a repair that could retain the same principles and maintain the advantages of minimally invasive surgery. The laparoscopic procedures in which the preperitoneal space is opened by making an incision in the peritoneum from within the abdomen, followed by placement of a prosthesis into the preperitoneal space, are grouped under the name transabdominal preperitoneal or TAPP.

After incising the peritoneum from the medial umbilical ligament to the anterior superior iliac spine, several centimetres above the internal ring, the preperitoneal space is dissected. The inferior epigastric vessels, symphysis pubis, Cooper's ligament, iliopubic tract and the transversalis fascia are exposed. During the course of this dissection a direct sac will be reduced, defining the defect in the transversalis fascia. Indirect inguinal hernias are clearly more difficult to deal with laparoscopically. If a large sac is present, extending into the scrotum, most surgeons prefer to divide the sac just distal to the internal ring. The proximal sac is dissected off the cord structures and the distal sac is left *in situ*.

An appropriately sized prosthesis (11 × 6 cm or larger) is placed in the preperitoneal space over the hernia defect overlapping it significantly to strengthen the floor. The prosthesis can either be slit to accommodate the cord structures or simply placed over them, according to the surgeon's preference. It is stapled or sutured using the following landmarks: the symphysis pubis medially, the transversalis fascia above the internal ring superiorly, an arbitrary point approximately 1 cm medial to the anterior iliac spine laterally, the iliopubic tract inferolaterally and Cooper's ligament inferomedially. Care should be taken not to place staples or sutures inferior to the iliopubic tract when stapling lateral to the internal spermatic vessels, to prevent an inordinately high rate of postoperative neuralgias involving the lateral cutaneous nerve of the thigh or the femoral branch of the genitofemoral nerve. Finally, the peritoneum is closed over the prosthesis using staples or sutures[11].

The TAPP procedure has become the most popular technique for laparoscopic herniorrhaphy; however, it requires extensive dissection of the preperitoneal space. It is thought by many investigators to be too invasive, especially for small hernias. The TAPP operation would be greatly simplified if the prosthesis were placed intraperitoneally, avoiding the need for extensive dissection of the preperitoneal space. This assumes it would be secured using the same landmarks as the TAPP procedure, specifically the symphysis pubis medially, Cooper's ligament inferomedially, the iliopubic tract inferolaterally, the transversalis fascia superiorly and a point approximately 1 cm from the anterior iliac spine laterally. This has been termed the intraperitoneal onlay mesh technique (IPOM).

An animal study

A trial was conducted at Creighton University. Three groups of pigs with congenital indirect inguinal hernias had the IPOM procedure performed in our laboratory. The first group of 13 animals had the operation performed at the time of laparotomy, which served as a control. A second group of 13 animals had the procedure preformed laparoscopically. The animals in both groups were sacrificed at six weeks. A third group of 20 animals had the IPOM procedure performed laparoscopically and were followed for six months. All hernia repairs in all three groups were successful. In addition, it was noted that the percentage of the polypropylene patch prosthesis covered by adhesions, as well as the tenacity of these adhesions, was much less when the mesh was placed laparoscopically, compared to the control group[12].

Clinical trial

Permission was obtained from the Human Research Committee at Creighton University to begin performing this operation in patients with indirect inguinal hernias. A total of 59 IPOM procedures have now been accomplished in 56 patients. There has been one recurrence but it is small and asymptomatic and the patient has refused further therapy. The most frequent complication has been neuralgia, usually involving the lateral cutaneous nerve of the thigh but occasionally involving the distribution of the femoral branch of the genitofemoral nerve. Most of these have been transient and have resolved spontaneously. One patient did require a second laparoscopy for removal of a painful staple. As noted previously, autopsy and cadaver dissections have determined that this complication can largely be eliminated if care is taken not to place staples below the iliopubic tract when stapling lateral to the internal spermatic vessels.

The most feared complication of the intra-abdominal placement of a prosthesis is the development of adhesions, leading to bowel obstruction or other complications such as erosion of the prosthesis into intra-abdominal organs. At the time of writing, no patient has developed clinical sequelae related to adhesion. One patient developed an infection in his prosthesis and this required removal. Based on our laboratory and clinical experience, we conclude that the intraperitoneal placement of a mesh prosthesis appears to be effective for the repair of indirect inguinal hernias.

Other techniques

Many surgeons are reluctant to perform the IPOM procedure because of the fear of placing prosthetic material into the abdomen potentially in contact with intra-abdominal organs. Indeed, this must be considered an experimental operation and surgeons considering this need to so inform their patients[12].

A third technique, known as the totally extraperitoneal laparoscopic herniorrhaphy, is gaining popularity. It too is modelled after the conventional preperitoneal operation. As described by McKernan, a modified open laparoscopic approach is employed. After the skin and fascia are opened at the umbilicus, the peritoneum is left intact and dissection is begun inferiorly in the preperitoneal space of the umbilicus to one or both groins. The abdominal cavity is not entered, as the entire procedure takes place in a 'pneumoextraperitoneum'. The technique is essentially identical to the TAPP, once the critical anatomical landmarks have been identified. The procedure is more demanding than the other laparoscopic herniorrhaphies. Technical problems such as breaches in the peritoneum are not infrequent, which limits the operating space by allowing a pneumoperitoneum to develop. The small working space can be confusing to those without experience with the technique; therefore caution must be used when attempting this procedure[13].

Laparoscopic versus conventional herniorrhaphy

Scepticism exists among surgeons as to the benefits of laparoscopic herniorrhaphy. Important controversies remain and the benefits of importing laparoscopic techniques to inguinal hernia repair are not completely self-evident. The conventional operation can be performed under local anaesthesia whilst general anaesthesia is recommended for the laparoscopic approach. The significance of the local anaesthesia argument is questionable since most conventional herniorrhaphies in the USA are in fact performed under general anaesthesia. Furthermore, most conventional herniorrhaphies do not require entry into the peritoneal cavity, thus avoiding the possible risk and consequences that are inherent to laparoscopy. In addition, cost considerations are significant. At the present time, laparoscopic repair is much more expensive but this may change as the technique evolves and becomes more standardized. For these reasons, laparoscopic inguinal herniorrhaphy is still under investigation and intensive evaluation is required to prove decreased morbidity or a reduced recurrence rate before its adoption is recommended to the wider surgical community.

A multicentre trial

A multicentre trial for laparoscopic herniorrhaphy was initiated in April 1991 with Creighton University as the sponsor. Institutions in North America and Europe participated. Preliminary results of 816 herniorrhaphies in 636 patients revealed a recurrence rate of 3.2% with a minimum follow up of six months, and a median follow up over one year: 17.8% of these hernias were recurrent to begin with, and 28.3% of patients had bilateral hernias; 49% were indirect; 40% were direct; and the rest were a miscellaneous group of consisting of combined hernias, femoral hernias, etc. General and local complications are listed in Tables 39.1 and 39.2 respectively. Perhaps the most distressing complication has been neuralgia, resulting in transient or persistent leg or groin pain or numbness. This can be minimized once surgeons understand the anatomy of the nerves in the region, especially

Table 39.1: Multicentre hernia project: general complications (636 patients)

	Number (%)
Urinary	14 (2.2%)
Bleed/transfusion	1 (0.2%)
Bleed/no transfusion	6 (0.9%)
Ileus	2 (0.3%)
Adhesive small bowel obstruction	2 (0.3%)
Respiratory arrest	1 (0.2%)
Impotence	1 (0.2%)
Wound infection	1 (0.2%)
Operative mortality: postoperative myocardial infarction	1 (0.2%)

Follow up: 6 months–2 years (1 April 1993)

Table 39.2: Multicentre hernia project: local complications (n = 816)

Complications	*Number* (%)
Transient leg pain	26 (3.19%)
Persistent leg pain	8 (0.98%)
Haematoma	18 (2.20%)
Prosthesis infection	1 (0.12%)
Orchitis/epididymitis	5 (0.61%)
Transient cord or testicular pain	8 (0.98%)
Persistent cord or testicular pain	4 (0.49%)
Transient groin pain	51 (6.25%)
Persistent groin pain	15 (1.84%)
Seroma/aspiration	12 (1.47%)
Seroma/no aspiration	26 (3.19%)

Follow up: 6 months–2 years (1 April 1993)

the lateral cutaneous nerve of the thigh and the femoral branch of the genitofemoral nerve. Over all 63% of the patients were discharged the day of the surgery, and another 29% were kept overnight; 8% stayed two days or more, usually as the result of a complication or severe underlying medical illness. The recurrence rate was looked at according to the type of laparoscopic inguinal herniorrhaphy performed (ie TAPP vs IPOM vs totally extraperitoneal), and no significant difference was demonstrated. The data suggest that the learning curve for this new procedure is significant, as the recurrence rate for individual surgeons was higher in their first ten cases (Figure 39.1).

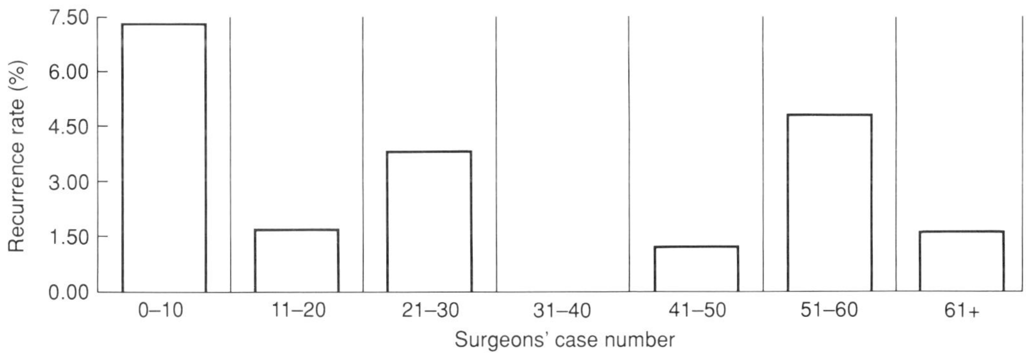

Figure 39.1: The experience of surgeons taking part in the multicentre hernia project.

Conclusions

Laparoscopic inguinal herniorrhaphy is an investigational procedure as the best technique and the exact indications are presently unclear. Laparoscopy affords an excellent exposure of the preperitoneal space which can be quite useful in repairing many inguinal hernias, especially those which are recurrent or otherwise complicated. It seems that laparoscopy will certainly have a place in the armamentarium of general surgeons caring for inguinal hernias. It is unlikely though that every inguinal hernia will best be repaired laparoscopically. However, preliminary results would suggest that further investigation is indicated.

References

1. Conceptualization and measurement of physiological health for adults. Santa Monica, California: Rand, May 1983; 3; 3–120.
2. Soper NJ, Stockman PT, Dunnegan DL, Ashley SW. Laparoscopic cholecystectomy: the new 'gold standard'? *Arch Surg* 1992; **127**: 917–23.
3. Marcy HO. The cure of hernia. *JAMA* 1887; **8**: 589–92.
4. Andrews E. A method of herniotomy utilizing only white fascia. *Ann Surg* 1924; **80**: 225–38.
5. La Roque GP. The intra-abdominal method of removing inguinal and femoral hernia. *Arch Surg* 1932; **24**: 189–203.
6. Stoppa RE, Warlaumont CR. The preperitoneal approach and prosthetic repair of groin hernia. In: Nyhus LM, Condon RE, eds. *Hernia*, 3rd ed. Philadelphia: JB Lippincott, 1989: 199–225.
7. Rignault DP. Properitoneal prosthetic inguinal hernioplasty through a Pfannenstiel approach. *Surg Gynecol Obstet* 1986; **163**: 465–8.

8. Schultz L, Graber J, Pietrafitta J, Hickok D. Laser laparoscopic herniorrhaphy: a clinical trial. Preliminary results. *J Laparoendosc Surg* 1990; **1**: 41–5.

9. Corbitt Jr JD. Laparoscopic herniorrhaphy. *Surg Laparosc Endosc* 1991; **1**: 23–5.

10. Reich H. Personal communication, 1990. Cited by Salerno GM, Fitzgibbons Jr RJ, Filipi CJ. Laparoscopic hernia repair. In: Zucker K, Reddick EJ, Bailey RW, eds. *Surgical Laparoscopy* St. Louis, MO: Quality Medical Publishing 1991: 181–93.

11. Fitzgibbons Jr RJ, Salerno GM, Filipi CJ. Open laparoscopy. In: Zucker K, Reddick EJ, Bailey BW, eds. *Surgical Laparoscopy*. St. Louis, MO: Quality Medical Publishing, 1991; 87–97.

12. Fitzgibbons Jr RJ, Salerno GM, Filipi CJ, Hunter WJ, Watson P. A laparoscopic intraperitoneal onlay mesh technique for repair of an indirect inguinal hernia (intraperitoneal onlay mesh procedure). *Ann Surg* in press.

13. McKernan JB, Laws HL. Laparoscopic repair of inguinal hernias using a totally extraperitoneal prosthetic approach. *Sugical Endoscopy*. 1993; **7**: 26–8.

Lichtenstein IL, Shulman AG, Amid PK, Montllor MM. The tension free hernioplasty. *Am J Surg* 1989; **157**: 188–93.

40

Laparoscopic Inguinal Herniorrhaphy: Transabdominal Preperitoneal Approach

MAURICE E ARREGUI, CHAD J DAVIS, DANIEL CASTRO, JORGE NAVARRETE AND ROBERT F NAGAN

Because of the remarkable success of laparoscopic cholecystectomy, the increasing popularity of minimal access surgery, the significant discomfort associated with traditional anterior hernia repairs and their relatively high recurrence rates, we and others have attempted to use the laparoscopic approach for repair of inguinal hernias[1–12]. Our own technique is based on the tensionless repair using mesh[13] and on the laparoscopic adaptation of the preperitoneal techniques of Nyhus and Stoppa[14,15] incorporating a large mesh. We feel that placing large mesh in the preperitoneal space is a much more mechanically and anatomically sound approach and may prove to be a better repair than those currently available with the open technique.

Laparoscopic inguinal herniorrhaphy is clearly in the developmental stage and numerous repairs currently exist. These include ring closure, intraperitoneal onlay mesh, plug and patch technique, iliopubic tract repair, transabdominal preperitoneal mesh repair and a totally extraperitoneal approach. With an increasing understanding of the laparoscopic approach, modifications and concepts continue to evolve, and numerous investigators have altered their technique. Because of the relative newness of laparoscopic inguinal herniorrhaphy, these techniques continue to evolve (Table 40.1). Currently, however, the most commonly used technique is the laparoscopic transabdominal preperitoneal approach using mesh. This differs from the totally extraperitoneal approach basically by requiring an incision of the peritoneum to obtain access to the preperitoneal space. Although the transabdominal preperitoneal approach is more easily performed, there exists a potential for adhesion formation secondary to the defect created in the peritoneum. Currently we perform all of our inguinal hernia repairs using an extraperitoneal approach. Most of our repairs to date, however, have been performed using the transabdominal preperitoneal approach.

Technique of transabdominal preperitoneal repair

For the technique of transabdominal preperitoneal approach using mesh, a general anaesthetic is required. Upon induction of general anaesthesia, a second generation cephalosporin is given intravenously. A Foley catheter is inserted. After preparing and draping the (unshaved) abdomen,

Table 40.1: Evolution of techniques

Schultz	Plug and patch	Properitoneal
Corbitt	Plug and patch	Properitoneal
Fitzgibbons	Intraperitoneal (all)	Properitoneal (dir)
Franklin	Properitoneal	Intraperitoneal
Arregui	Properitoneal (all)	Ring closure (type I)

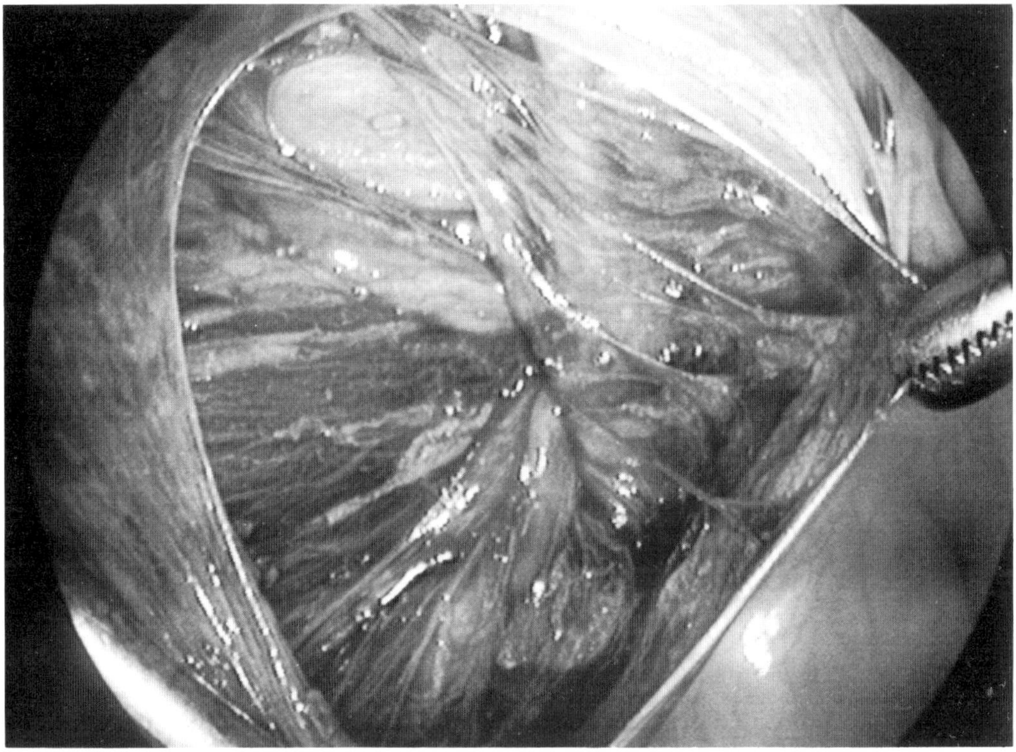

Figure 40.1: An incision made in the orifice of the left internal ring. Just deep to the preperitoneal fascia is encountered the preperitoneal fascia which forms a funnel around the hernia sac and cord structures. This forms the internal spermatic fascia.

a 1 cm incision is made in the inferior portion of the umbilicus. A Verres needle is introduced for the insufflation of carbon dioxide. An 11 mm reusable trocar is then inserted into the peritoneal cavity. Careful inspection of the peritoneal cavity will reveal contralateral hernias. If one is found, a bilateral repair is performed. One 5 mm trocar is then placed in the right lower quadrant and another in the left lower quadrant. These trocars are usually placed at or below the level of the umbilicus at the anterior axillary line. With scissors and careful use of electrosurgical cautery, the peritoneum is incised at the orifice of the internal ring.

Immediately deep to the peritoneum, the preperitoneal fascia is encountered (Figure 40.1). It is very adherent to the peritoneum as well as the vas deferens and spermatic vessels. Care must be taken to prevent injury to those structures. Medially the preperitoneal fascia separates the peritoneum from the preperitoneal space. This must be incised to get into the proper plane (Figure 40.2). Further blunt dissection is carried out to expose the epigastric vessels medially. Medially and inferiorly, Cooper's ligament is identified (Figure 40.3). Dissection is carried out to the symphysis pubis and the lower portion of the rectus abdominis muscle. Complete medial dissection requires good exposure of Hesselbach's triangle and the transversus abdominis aponeurotic arch. If a direct hernia is encountered, the attenuated transversalis fascia which forms the lining of the sac, after the peritoneum and the preperitoneal tissues have been reduced, is grasped and inverted into the preperitoneal space. With a suture or clip, it is anchored onto Cooper's ligament. The inversion of the sac eliminates the space in the inguinal area which will accumulate blood or serous fluid, which could result in a haematoma bulging outward. This could be perceived by the patient as a recurrence.

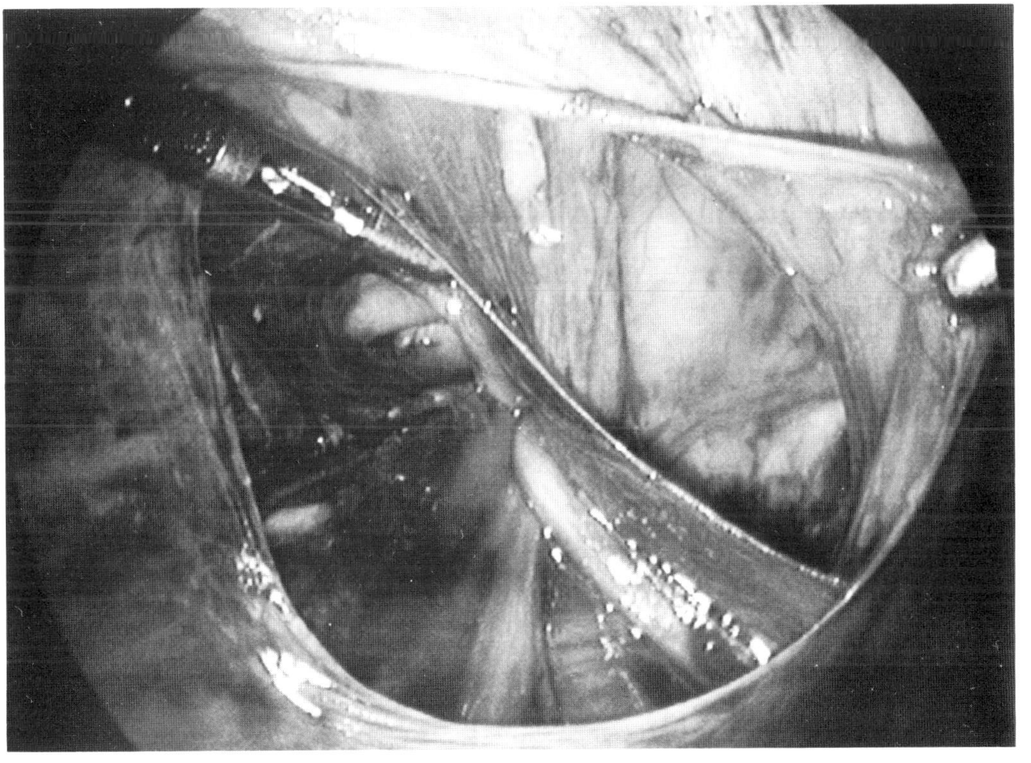

Figure 40.2: The preperitoneal fascia has been incised or bluntly dissected away to enter the proper preperitoneal plane medially. The epigastric vessels are seen. (From Arregui ME *et al.* Laparoscopic inguinal hernia repair with preperitoneal prosthetic replacement, Fig. 3. In: *Prostheses and abdominal wall surgery*, Landes Medical Publishing, 1994, in press; with permission.)

Generous lateral dissection is then carried out, separating the peritoneum off the blood supply and cord to the testicles. If separation is inadequate, it will be difficult to place a large mesh. Lateral to the epigastric vessels, the internal ring is identified. Dissection is carried lateral to the internal ring. The lateral iliopubic tract is exposed. Care must be taken not to injure the genitofemoral and lateral femoral cutaneous nerves which are located inferior to the lateral iliopubic tract (Figure 40.4). Often, a lipoma of the cord is encountered during the lateral dissection. This should be reduced or resected (Figure 40.5).

Upon complete exposure of the preperitoneal space, a large piece of mesh is placed over the myopectineal orifice of Fruchaud. This large mesh should well overlap the indirect or direct defect and should extend down below the femoral canal. The mesh measures 15 × 10 cm with the corners trimmed. The mesh can be placed on top of the cord structures and epigastric vessels or a slit can be made in the mesh to wrap round the cord structures. The mesh is then anchored using either staples or sutures (Figures 40.6 and 40.7). If sutures are used, a stitch is placed on Cooper's ligament, transversus abdominis aponeurotic arch, and lateral to the internal ring. No sutures or staples are placed between the cord structures and the lateral aspect of the iliopubic tract. This suture should be of non-absorbable material.

When the repair is completed, the peritoneum is closed using a purse-string suture of 3–0 absorbable material. The air in the preperitoneal space is allowed to escape and the mesh is checked to be certain that it is lying flat and not curling at the edges (Figures 40.8 and 40.9). The carbon dioxide is then allowed to escape. The fascial defect at the umbilical incision is closed with 2–0

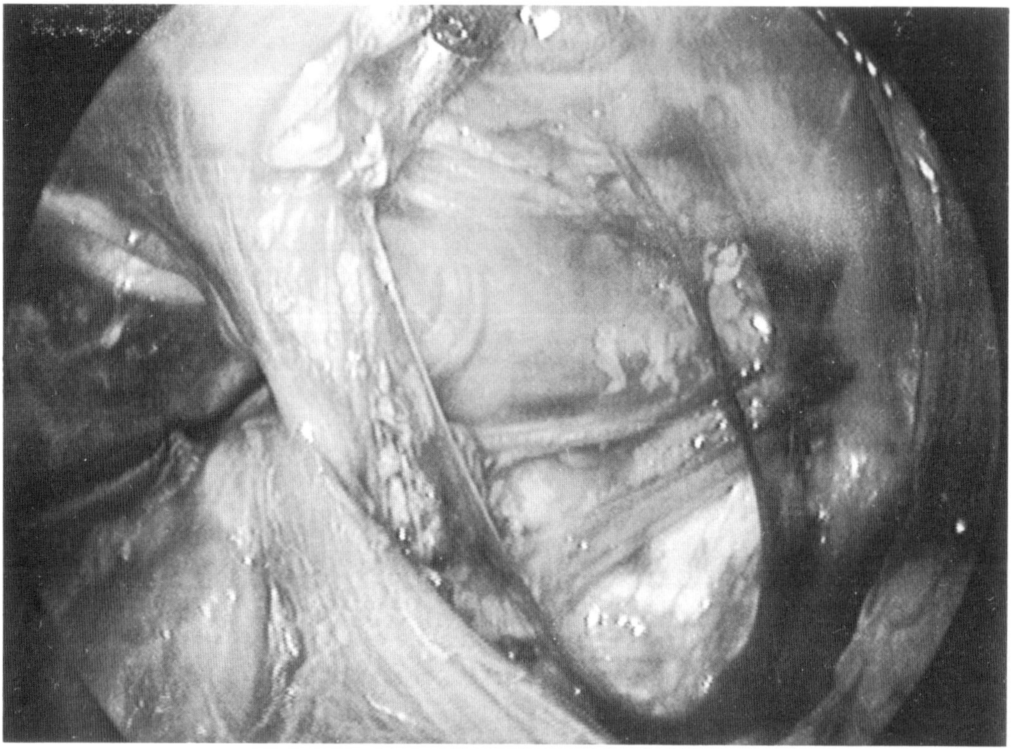

Figure 40.3: A more complete medial dissection in this patient with an indirect left inguinal hernia. The branches of the epigastric vessels and Cooper's ligament are clearly seen. (From Arregui ME, Training requirements for laparoscopic hernia repair. In: *Laparoscopy in focus*, McMahon Group, 1991, Vol 1, No 1; with permission.)

absorbable material. Any trocar incision 1 cm or greater should be closed to prevent herniation. The subcutaneous tissue is approximated with interrupted 3–0 Vicryl. Collodion is then applied to the skin as the bandage.

Results

Between October 1990 and May 1993, two of the authors (MEA, CJD) repaired 202 hernias in 156 patients: 143 males and 13 females. The age range was 12 to 83. There were 108 indirect hernias, 53 direct hernias, 34 bilateral hernias, three femoral hernias and one obturator hernia. Incidental non-clinical hernias were found during preperitoneal dissection, including nine femoral and five obturator hernias. There were 31 (15%) recurrent hernias repaired. Of these 202, 100 were repaired using the transabdominal preperitoneal technique; 90 using the laparoscopic extraperitoneal approach; and five using ring closure technique.

Recurrences

To date, there have been two recurrences. The first was in a patient who had a totally extraperitoneal repair of bilateral indirect inguinal hernias. This patient was involved in an automobile accident five weeks after surgery, and three months later manifested with a recurrent indirect left inguinal hernia. He had a single large piece of mesh placed in the preperitoneal space covering both hernias. The

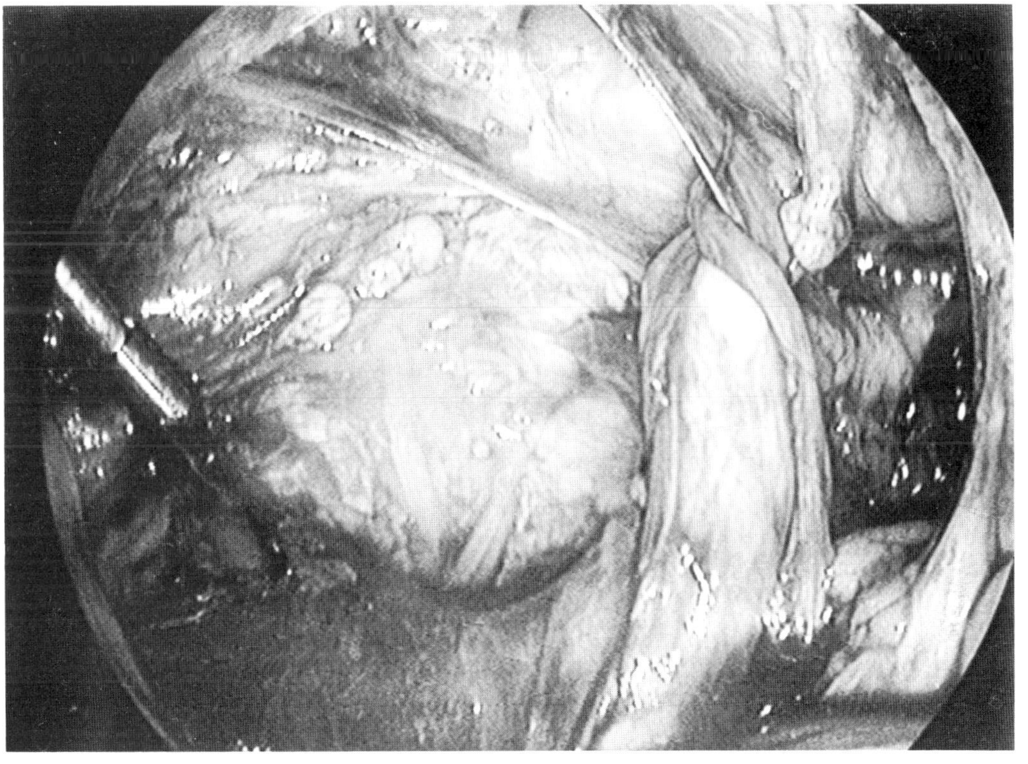

Figure 40.4: Dissection lateral to the cords and inferior to the lateral iliopubic tract exposes the femoral branches of the genitofemoral nerve in this patient with a left inguinal hernia. (From Arregui ME *et al.* Laparoscopic inguinal herniorrhaphy: techniques and controversies, Fig. 2, In: *Surgical Clinics of North America*, WB Saunders, 1993, Vol 73, No 3; with permission.)

mesh was anchored with Vicryl suture. We speculate that the impact of the auto accidents (which was severe enough to cause a cervical fracture) impelled the viscera against the mesh. This midline force probably caused the mesh to migrate and expose the orifice of the left internal ring. The mesh probably did not overlap the defect adequately and the Vicryl suture had most likely been reabsorbed by the time of his accident. This recurrence was repaired at an outside hospital using an open anterior approach.

The second recurrence, which was originally repaired with the transabdominal preperitoneal technique, was a direct hernia. This was re-explored by us laparoscopically: we found that the mesh was too small and did not adequately overlap the indirect defect. This recurrence was repaired by using a larger piece of mesh to overlap the defect properly.

Complications

We have retrospectively performed a critical review of our intraoperative and postoperative complications. We have found an intraoperative complication rate of 1.9%. The three cases comprised a patient who developed bronchospasm on induction of general anaesthesia, a patient in whom a hernia stapling device broke and a small incision was required to retrieve the tip, and a patient in whom a needle was lost in the anterior abdominal wall as it was being pulled out of the peritoneal cavity. The only conversion was in the patient who required a small incision to retrieve the broken articulating stapler tip.

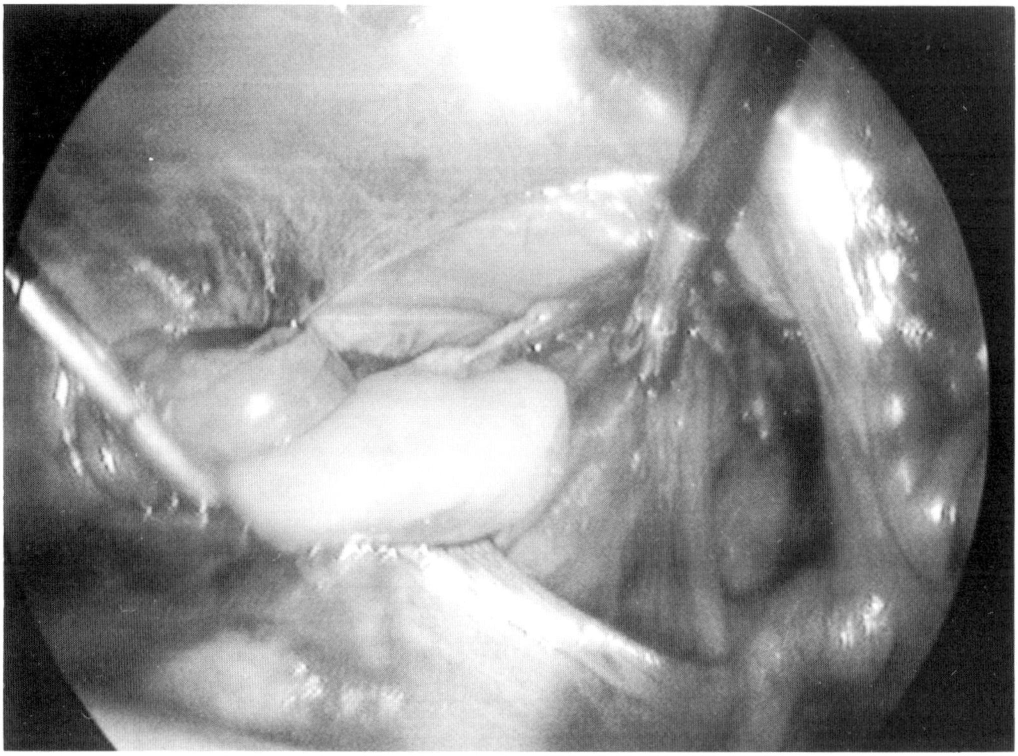

Figure 40.5: A lipoma of the cord is dissected free in this patient with a left inguinal hernia.

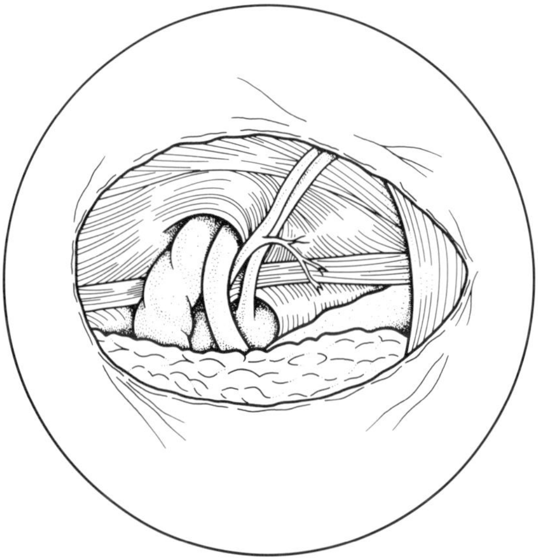

Figure 40.6: Complete dissection of the preperitoneal space. (Arregui ME *et al.* Laparoscopic mesh repair of inguinal hernia using a preperitoneal approach: A preliminary report, Fig 1, In: *Surgical laparoscopy and endoscopy,* Raven Press Ltd., Vol 2, No 1, with permission.)

There were 24 postoperative complications (15.4%). The majority of these were minor, including eight inguinal haematomas or seromas and one hydrocele. Very few of these required aspiration. Surprisingly, seven patients did complain of testicular pain which was transient in all. There were two episodes of transient lateral femoral cutaneous nerve pain; all of these resolved without intervention. There was one edididymitis, one haematuria due to the Foley catheter, one urinary retention, one urinary tract infection and one umbilical infection. In the only patient in whom a

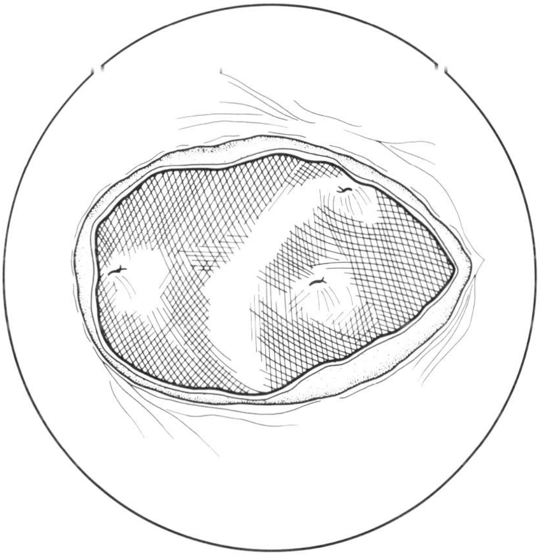

Figure 40.7: A large mesh sutured onto the anterior abdominal wall covering the myopectineal orifice of Fruchaud. (Arregui ME *et al.* Laparoscopic mesh repair of inguinal hernia using a preperitoneal approach: A preliminary report, Fig 2, In: *Surgical laparoscopy and endoscopy,* Raven Press Ltd., 1992, Vol 2, No 1; with permission.)

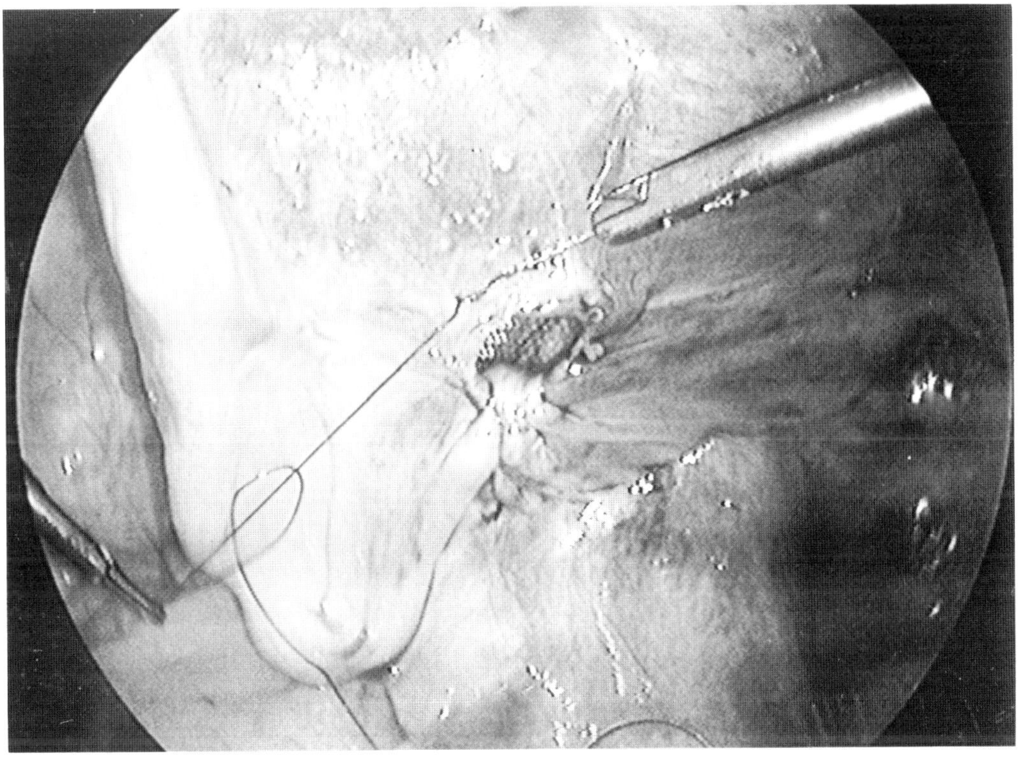

Figure 40.8: Purse-string closure of a repaired left inguinal hernia. (From Arregui ME, Laparoscopic hernia repair. In: *Laparoscopy in focus*, McMahon Group, 1991, Vol 1, No 1; with permission.)

plug was used, it was palpable in the postoperative period. However, the prominence of this plug diminished with time (Figure 40.10).

The only mortality was in an elderly patient who was hospitalized for multiple medical problems. During the hospitalization, he developed incarceration of a groin hernia during a barium enema. He

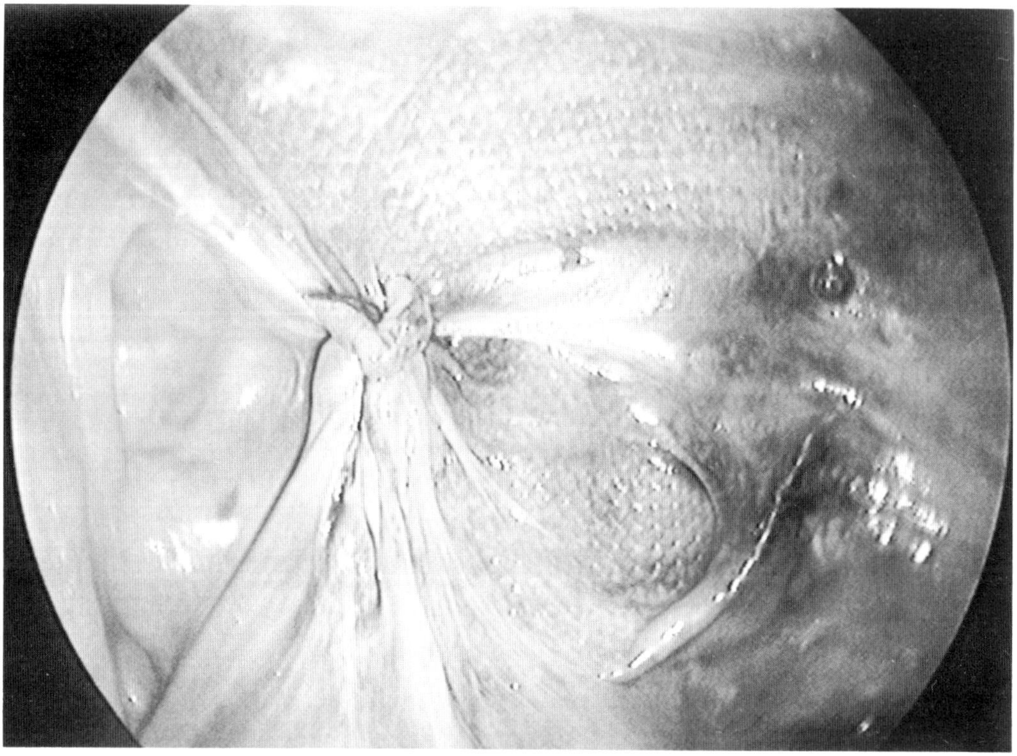

Figure 40.9: Transperitoneal inspection to be certain that the mesh is lying flat. (From Arregui ME *et al.* Laparoscopic mesh repair of inguinal hernia using a preperitoneal approach: A preliminary approach Fig 5, In: *Surgical laparoscopy* and endoscopy, Raven Press Ltd., 1992, Vol 2, No 1; with permission.)

underwent successful repair of bilateral inguinal hernias. Unfortunately, he died of disseminated histoplasmosis approximately three weeks later. This was not felt to be related to the hernia repair.

Patient satisfaction has been extremely high. They are allowed to return to work within one week of surgery without restrictions. Of those patients who underwent previous hernia repair by open technique, the vast majority felt that the laparoscopic approach was much less painful.

Multicentre review of complications

We have recently compiled information by sending questionnaires to several surgeons employing various laparoscopic techniques (Bob Fitzgibbons, Morris Franklin, Barry McKernan, Leonard Schultz and Frederick Toy, personal communication, 1993). There were 1069 hernias repaired in 866 patients. The extraperitoneal approach was used in 201 patients, transabdominal preperitoneal in 412, plug and patch in 58, intraperitoneal mesh in 300 and ring closure in five. The postoperative complication rate was 15.2%. The local complication rate was 5.3%; neurological 2.8%; urinary 2.4%; testicular 2.3%; mesh 0.8%; and miscellaneous 1%. This profile is very similar to that of our own experience. The majority of the local complications were groin haematomas, trocar haematomas, subcutaneous emphysema, hydrocele and only two cases of local wound infection. Of the 34 groin haematomas, 10 required aspiration. Blood transfusion was required for one of the nine trocar haematomas. The reported subcutaneous emphysema was asymptomatic. One of the two hydroceles did require aspiration, and one of the two wound infections was treated with antibiotics. In the miscellaneous complication, there were three incidences of small bowel obstruction; these were associated with the transabdominal preperitoneal technique. A more detailed report,

	TOTAL	24 (15.4%)

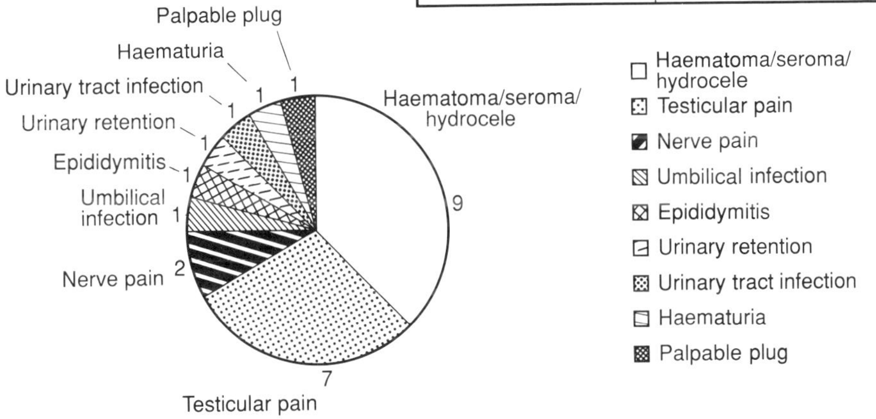

Figure 40.10: Postoperative complications of laparoscopic repair of inguinal hernias in 156 patients.

including information from additional surgeons, will be covered in another section of this book (*see* Chapter 82).

Conclusions

Although experience with laparoscopic inguinal herniorrhaphy is limited, it can be performed safely. Most of the complications reported here are minor, and are of such a nature that their occurrence is often not reported with open anterior repair. This makes it difficult to compare with the literature that discusses the complications of open hernia repair. We believe that it is important to report these minor complications or side-effects because they do affect patient comfort. In order to try to achieve the goal of reduced pain and discomfort, rapid recovery and low recurrence rates, we must pay strict attention to detail and report as accurately as possible. We feel that most of these complications, including nerve pain, haematomas and recurrences, are technical problems that will be solved with experience.

The laparoscopic extraperitoneal approach most closely mimics the open preperitoneal techniques, but is more complicated to perform and is less widely accepted than the transabdominal preperitoneal repair. The transabdominal preperitoneal repair, however, requires an incision of the preperitoneum to enter the preperitoneal space. If closure is not meticulously performed, adhesions can form – and have formed, as we have seen from our multicentre review. It has led to bowel obstruction in a very small but significant number of patients. This is the major disadvantage of laparoscopic transabdominal preperitoneal repair.

Technical considerations of the laparoscopic approach include intraperitoneal inspection, complete preperitoneal dissection, use of a large mesh, fixation of the mesh and complete closure of the peritoneum leaving a minimal defect. The place for laparoscopic herniorrhaphy is not yet certain.

However, it seems to have an advantage with recurrent hernias and bilateral hernias. Additional study and long-term evaluation is required to determine whether this approach will have any advantage over open contemporary repairs using tensionless approach with mesh.

References

1. Arregui ME, Navarrete J, Davis CJ, *et al.* Laparoscopic inguinal herniorrhaphy: techniques and controversies. *Surg Clin North Am* 1993; **73**: 513–27.
2. Arregui MR, Davis CD, Yucel O, *et al.* Laparoscopic mesh repair of inguinal hernia using a preperitoneal approach: a preliminary report. *Surg Laparosc Endosc* 1992; **2**: 53–8.
3. Arregui ME, Navarrete JL. Laparoscopic preperitoneal repair of inguinal hernias with mesh. In: Rosin D, ed. *Minimal access general surgery*. Oxford: Radcliffe Medical Press, 1993.
4. Arregui ME. Laparoscopic preperitoneal herniorrhaphy. In: Society of American Gastrointestinal Endoscopic Surgeons Annual Meeting, Monterey, CA, USA, April 18–20 1991.
5. Corbitt J. Laparoscopic herniorrhaphy. *Surg Laparosc Endosc* 1991; **1**: 23–5.
6. Franklin M. Laparoscopic hernia repair. *Laparosc Focus* 1992; **1**: 7.
7. Ger R, Monroe K, Duvivier R, *et al.* Management of indirect inguinal hernias by laparoscopic closure of the neck of the sac. *Am J Surg* 1990; **159**: 370–3.
8. Phillips EH, Carroll BJ, Fallas MJ. Laparoscopic preperitoneal inguinal hernia repair without peritoneal incision. *Surg Endosc* 1993; **7**: 159–62.
9. Salerno GM, Fitzgibbons Jr RJ, Filipi CJ. Laparoscopic inguinal hernia repair. In: Zucker KA, ed. *Surgical laparoscopy*. St Louis: Quality Medical Publishing, 1991: 281–93.
10. Schultz L, Graber J, Pietrafitta J. Laparoscopic inguinal herniorrhaphy – lessons learned after 100 cases. Video presentation to Society of Gastrointestinal Endoscopic Surgeons (SAGES). April 10–12, 1992, Washington DC
11. Schultz L, Graber J, Pietrafitta J, *et al.* Laser laparoscopic herniorrhaphy: a clinical trial – preliminary results. *J Laparoendosc Surg* 1990; **1**: 41–5.
12. Toy F. Laparoscopic hernia repair: IPOM with Gore-Tex. Presented at the Forty-third Surgical Forum, Beverly Hills, CA, USA, 18–21 March 1993.
13. Lichtenstein IL. Herniorrhaphy: a personal experience with 6,321 cases. *Am J Surg* 1987; **153**: 553–9.
14. Stoppa RE, Warlaumont CR. The preperitoneal approach and prosthetic repair of groin hernia. In: Nyhus LM, Condon RE, eds. *Hernia*, 3rd ed. Philadelphia: JB Lippincott, 1989: 199–255.
15. Nyhus LM. The preperitoneal approach and iliopubic tract repair of inguinal hernia. In: Nyhus LM, Condon RE, eds. *Hernia*, 3rd ed. Philadelphia: JB Lippincott, 1989: 154–77.

41

Transabdominal Laparoscopic Hernioplasty using Preperitoneal Mesh

SÉRGIO ROLL, AUREO L DEPAULA, PABLO MIGUEL, JOSÉ AV CARIM, FÁBIO G CAMPOS AND KIYOSHI HASHIBA

Because of the good results obtained since its introduction as a technique for cholecystectomy, laparoscopic abdominal technology has rapidly expanded its usefulness in the field of general abdominal surgery, such as hernia repair.

Inguinal herniorrhaphy according to Bassini's principles[1] is one of the most common operations performed in routine practice. Nevertheless, this approach violates a cardinal surgical principle in that the sutures of the inguinal floor are under tension, leading to various complications. Modifications of Bassini's technique over the past hundred years indicate that the ideal management for hernia repair is still elusive. The result is a painful repair leading to curtailment of the patient's routine activities for a long time, associated with significant recurrence (ranging from 0 to 21%)[2].

Three studies have demonstrated the effectiveness of using mesh in the preperitoneal space, significantly reducing recurrence. Lichtenstein[3,4] popularized the concept of 'tension-free' hernioplasty, eliminating closure with sutures under tension. This technique carries minimal discomfort, 0.25% recurrence and rapid return to normal activities. On the other hand, Nyhus[5] modified this procedure, suturing the mesh between Cooper's ligament and the transversalis fascia. In 1967, Stoppa[6] advocated the use of a larger piece of mesh (15 × 15 cm), suturing it bilaterally.

Ger[7] was the first to accomplish laparoscopic hernioplasty, in 1979. He approximated the margins of the hernial defect with clips applied by a stapler. Since then, this technique has been undergoing continual modifications and improvements.

The main technical aspects of inguinal hernia repair by laparoscopy and the results obtained in Brazil are the subject of this chapter.

Operative procedure

The patients

Between January 1991 and June 1993, 404 patient – 378 males (93.5%) and 26 females (6.5%) – with inguinal hernia underwent laparoscopic hernioplasty. Patients were included in a full-disclosure clinical study protocol and with knowledge of the actual results of the technique employed in previous cases.

Their ages ranged from 15 to 80 years (mean 46 years), and they weighed from 41 to 105 kg (90–231 lb); 65% of the patients worked in offices, 5% were athletes, 22% were manual workers and 8% were retired. In a total of 470 hernias, 384 (81.7%) were unilateral and 86 (18.3%) were bilateral. The types of defects were 148 direct (31.5%), 260 indirect (55.3%), 24 recurrent (5.1%), 35 mixed (7.4%) and three femoral (0.6%) hernias.

Anaesthesia, positioning of the team and incisions

The procedure was performed under general anaesthesia in 390 patients (96.5%) and epidural anaesthesia in 14 (3.5%). Skin preparation included the genitalia and upper thighs. The patients were placed supine and in the Trendelenburg position, with both arms next to the body to facilitate positioning of the surgical team and the equipment. Neither nasogastric intubation nor a urinary catheter was used.

The surgeon stands on the opposite side of the hernial defect; the nurse is on the opposite side, and the assistant with the camera on the same side as the surgeon, next to the patient's head.

Carbon dioxide pneumoperitoneum is induced using a Verres needle introduced through a small supraumbilical incision. The abdominal cavity pressure is maintained at about 10 mmHg. Then, a 10 mm trocar is inserted through which a viewing (0°) laparoscope is introduced. The abdominal cavity is thoroughly explored and inspected for any other diseases. Two other small incisions are made right and left just lateral to the rectus muscle at the level of the umbilicus. This stage requires extra care in order to prevent injury to the superficial epigastric vessels. A 10–12 mm trocar is placed on the side opposite the hernia and a 5 mm trocar in the other incision. If bilateral hernias are present, two 10–12 mm trocars are inserted.

Operative technique

The procedure begins by grasping the hernial sac in a cranial direction, and incising it at its base in order to separate it from the elements of the cord. This facilitates visualization of the internal ring, the iliopubic tract and the inferior epigastric vessels.

The peritoneum is dissected along the lateral margins of Hesselbach's triangle to prepare the site for perfect placement of the synthetic mesh. An open rectangular, polypropylene patch (14 × 10 cm) is placed when the region of the defect is visualized. It should cover not only the internal ring but also the region medial to the epigastric vessels and the femoral ring. The patch is then stapled on the inguinal floor. The peritoneum is sutured, covering the patch which remains in an extraperitoneal position.

Results

The operative procedure took from 30 to 190 minutes (mean 70 minutes). Two patients out of the 404 (0.5%) required conversion to standard surgery due to intraoperative perforation of the loop of the small bowel and three patient (0.7%) were reoperated for a haematoma of the inguinal region. The average hospital stay ranged from four hours to 36 days (mean 24 hours). The principal complications were: 12 cases of inguinal haematomas (2.9%), four hydroceles (0.9%), six orchitis (1.5%), 21 spermatic cord problems (5.2%), two umbilical infections (0.5%), one urinary dysfunction (0.2%), two inguinal neuralgias (0.5%) and one testicular atrophy (0.2%). These 49 complications correspond to a rate of 12.1%. Normal activity was resumed between the third to the 36th postoperative day (mean eight days). Follow-up ranged from three days to 30 months (mean 16 months) during which time five recurrences (1.2%) were noted.

Conclusions

The terminology used in the literature regarding laparoscopic herniorrhaphy is confusing when describing the various technical modifications proposed. For this reason, we have used the term 'preperitoneal transabdominal repair' for the procedure outlined in this chapter.

In this series, dissection of the hernial sac from the elements of the cord was begun by a circumferential peritoneal incision at the level of the internal ring. The sac was everted and left in the peritoneal cavity as recommended by Arregui[8]. Other options are resection with a linear stapling device[9] or suture of the sac[10]. When the sac adheres to the inguinal canal, dissection may cause varying degrees of injury to the elements of the spermatic cord; in this case, the cord and the sac should be separated, and the latter sectioned and left in the inguinal canal[11]. In the series discussed in this chapter, 32 patients (7.9%) presented with inflammation of the testicle or the cord. They were successfully managed clinically.

The patches or meshes employed most frequently are of polypropylene (Prolene or Marlex) or polyester fibres (Dacron) composed of durable, strong and non-absorbable material. The persistence of synthetic material in the abdominal cavity and inguinal region over a prolonged period may result in adhesions, erosion of adjacent structures and infection. Nevertheless, these have not been observed in the cases reported here.

The size of the mesh to be placed over the defect is a controversial subject. Most surgeons tailor the mesh according to the size of the hernial defect. Recently, however, the use of a larger sized mesh (about 14 × 10 cm) has been recommended so as to occlude the direct, indirect and femoral defects simultaneously[6,11]. This manoeuvre requires wide dissection of the preperitoneal space to accommodate the mesh properly.

The mesh can be attached in the preperitoneal space with a non-absorbable suture or with clips applied on its margins to prevent accidental migration to the scrotal pouch or the peritoneal cavity. The mesh is not stapled below the iliopubic tract, where manipulation or injury to local nerves can result in severe postoperative pain.

Closure of the peritoneum over the attached mesh should be undertaken carefully to prevent openings that would permit the constriction of intestinal loops or the formation of adhesions. For this reason we prefer to close the peritoneum using continuous non-absorbable sutures.

Early results in this series indicate that laparoscopic inguinal repair is a safe and effective procedure. Nevertheless, we have had small bowel injuries in two patients (0.5%) whose operation required conversion to standard surgery and a postoperative complication rate of 12.1%.

Local haematoma and spermatic cord problems were the main complications noted. Inguinal haematoma occurred in 12 cases (2.9%) requiring three operations (two open), all of which were successful. Twenty-one patients (5.2%) had spermatic cord problems that were managed clinically.

At 16 months' follow up, recurrence was detected in five patients (1.2%). As the major concerns of this technique are late recurrences, a longer follow up is necessary before we can draw final conclusions.

Summary

Hernioplasty by videolaparoscopy is another option for the management of inguinal hernias, depending on the results of perioperative complications and recurrence over the long term.

In our experience, this method has definite advantages over the standard technique, including the possibility of visualizing abdominal organs, a lower incidence of ilioinguinal neuralgia, greater postoperative comfort, a shorter hospital stay and early return to routine activities.

It is important to emphasize that the success of the procedure depends initially on an excellent knowledge of the inguinal region anatomy from a laparoscopic viewpoint, as well as skill in laparoscopic surgery.

The various technical aspects of laparoscopic hernioplasty with regard to the approach, the use of synthetic mesh and its attachment, are still in a developmental stage. Long-term follow-up of these patients is still needed to draw definitive conclusions, and the potential benefits of rapid postoperative recovery will have to be balanced against rates of late complications and recurrences.

References

1. Bassini E. Sulla cura radicale dell'ernia inguinale. *Arch Soc Ital Chir* 1887; **4**: 380.
2. Spaw AT, Ennis BW, Spaw LP. Laparoscopic hernia repair: the anatomic basis. *J Laparoendosc Surg* 1991; **1**: 269–77.
3. Lichtenstein IL. Herniorrhaphy. A personal experience with 6321 cases. *Am J Surg* 1987; **153**: 553–9.
4. Lichtenstein IL, Shulman AG, Amid PK, Montllor MM. The tension-free hernioplasty. *Am J Surg* 1989; **157**: 188–93.
5. Nyhus LM, Condon RE, Harkins HN. Clinical experience with pre-peritoneal hernia repair for all types of hernia of the groin, with particular emphasis to the importance of transversalis fascia analogue. *Am J Surg* 1960; **100**: 234–44.
6. Stoppa RE, Warlaumont CR. The preperitonial approach and prothetic repair of groin hernia. In: Nyhus IM, Condon RE, eds. *Hernia*, 3rd ed. Philadelphia: JB Lippincott, 1989: 199–225.
7. Ger R. The management of certain abdominal herniae by intra-abdominal closure of the neck of the sac. *Ann R Coll Surg Engl* 1982; **64**: 342–4.
8. Arregui ME, Davis CJ, Yucel O, Nagan RF. Laparoscopic mesh repair of inguinal hernia using a preperitonial approach: a preliminary report. *Surg Laparosc Endosc* 1992; **2**: 53–8.
9. Corbitt JD. Laparoscopic herniorrhaphy. *Surg Laparosc Endosc* 1991; **1**: 23–5.
10. McKernan JB, Laws HL. Laparoscopic preperitoneal prosthetic repair of inguinal hernias. *Surg Rounds* 1992; **15**: 579–610.
11. Roll S, Campos FG, Szego T. Herniorrafia inguinal por via laparoscopica. In: Creuz O, ed. *Manual de Cirurgia Video Endoscopica*. Rio de Janeiro: Ed. Revinter, 1993: 303–10.

42

Laparoscopic Extraperitoneal Prosthetic Inguinal Herniorrhaphy

J BARRY McKERNAN

Approximately 500 000 inguinal herniorrhaphy procedures are performed annually in the USA, 10–15% of these being done for hernia recurrence[1]. While the surgical literature is replete with operations for the treatment of inguinofemoral herniation, each shares the common goal of re-establishing the integrity of the inguinal floor by repairing the posterior lamina of the transversalis fascia. Most American surgeons today employ a variation of Bassini's original technique[2] and approach the inguinal floor anteriorly. A definitive preperitoneal procedure that utilizes a posterior approach to the inguinal region was first described by Cheatle in 1920[3] and was subsequently popularized by Nyhus and colleagues in the 1960s[4].

In 1975, Stoppa and associates introduced the application of a large unsutured polyester prosthesis, placed preperitoneally, for inguinal hernia repair[5]. In their extensive experience with this procedure, Stoppa and associates reported a recurrence rate of only 1.4%, with all recurrences caused by prostheses that were too small or which had split[6]. These surgeons reported that the recurrence rate with this technique was considerably lower in their experience than those for the Bassini procedure, Cooper ligament repair or inguinal patch repair.

My group has developed a laparoscopic modification of Stoppa's open procedure, and in 1991 we performed the first laparoscopic extraperitoneal prosthetic inguinal hernia repair. Since this time we have successfully employed this technique to repair over 150 indirect and direct inguinofemoral hernias, including several bilateral or recurrent defects. Before performing our extraperitoneal prosthetic repair clinically, we – along with several others, including Laws, Fitzgibbons, Arregui, Katkhouda, Litwin and Phillipi – studied and perfected the technique in the laboratory using pigs.

This chapter summarizes our herniorrhaphy procedure, patient selection criteria and postoperative management approach. A detailed description of our laparoscopic operative technique can be found in an earlier publication[7].

Preoperative management and operative technique

Preoperative preparation for our laparoscopic hernia repair procedure is straightforward. Patients arrive at the hospital the morning of surgery, after fasting from midnight. Laboratory evaluations are not included as part of our typical preoperative procedures, unless indicated by the patient's history of medical status, since routine evaluations have been shown to be of limited value for disease screening in asymptomatic, clinically normal individuals undergoing elective hernia repair[8]. All patients receive prophylactic antibiotics preoperatively and are catheterized at the outset of surgery.

For our three-port, two-handed, laparoscopic extraperitoneal repair procedure the patient is placed supine in the Trendelenburg position with arms at 90°. The surgical team consists of the surgeon, the anaesthetist, the surgical assistant (camera operator), a scrub nurse and a circulating nurse. The surgeon operates from the side opposite the hernia and the assistant is positioned opposite the surgeon.

To create the preperitoneal space, a 20 mm periumbilical or vertical skin incision is made, bluntly continuing downward through the subcutaneous tissues to expose the fascia, which is then elevated with Ochsner clamps. A 12 mm midline vertical incision is made and ½ S retractors are placed beneath the fascia. The rectus muscle is bluntly separated, retractors are placed beneath the musculature and a small tunnel in the midline is begun in the direction of the pubis between the rectus muscle and peritoneum. Stay sutures (size 0, coated Vicryl) are placed in the fascia. The Endopath 10/11 mm blunt tip trocar is inserted just beneath the rectus muscle and anterior to the peritoneum. An Olympus 10 mm OES II operating telescope with a blunt probe is placed through the 5 mm operative channel in the preperitoneal space and extended approximately 2.5 cm beyond the optics. Insufflation is started with a pressure setting of 8–10 mmHg. Insufflation pressure should be kept below 12 mmHg to prevent the development of acidosis and/or subcutaneous emphysema.

Under direct visualization to the pubis, a tunnel is dissected using the blunt probe, showing the rectus muscle anteriorly and the peritoneum posteriorly[7]. An alternative method is to use a balloon device inserted beneath the rectus muscle to the pubis that will facilitate preperitoneal dissection (Figure 42.1); approximately three-quarters of extraperitoneal dissection can be accomplished using this approach. Furthermore, with this device, there is no need for the operative telescope. After the peritoneum has been dissected free from the posterior aspect of the rectus muscle, two cannulae are placed in the midline:

- a 5 mm cannula placed approximately one fingersbreadth above the pubis
- a 10/11 mm Endopath cannula placed halfway between the pubis and the periumbilical incision.

Placement of the 10/11 mm cannula is associated with the greatest risk of invading the peritoneal cavity; therefore, to aid in its placement, we use a haemostat to bluntly dissect through the subcutaneous fat down to the fascia. The Endopath shielded trocar is placed through the fascia, the safety shield is engaged and the blunted trocar is advanced through the muscle. This manoeuvre lessens the likelihood of injuring the peritoneum.

At this point, the operative telescope is exchanged for a 0° 10 mm Olympus OES II telescope. Operating bimanually through both the 5 mm and the 10/11 mm trocars, dissection of Cooper's ligament, the iliac vein and the area of the direct defect (if evident) is accomplished. An angled (45°) 10 mm Olympus OES II telescope is then substituted and the peritoneum is further dissected from the rectus muscle cephalad using a sweeping motion to expose the internal ring and indirect sac, if present. Any lipoma is removed from the internal ring. If the indirect sac is small, it is dissected from the cord structures, but if it is large, it is entered anteriomedially, severed and ligated proximally. In this case, the distal sac, which may extend into the scrotum, is left in place.

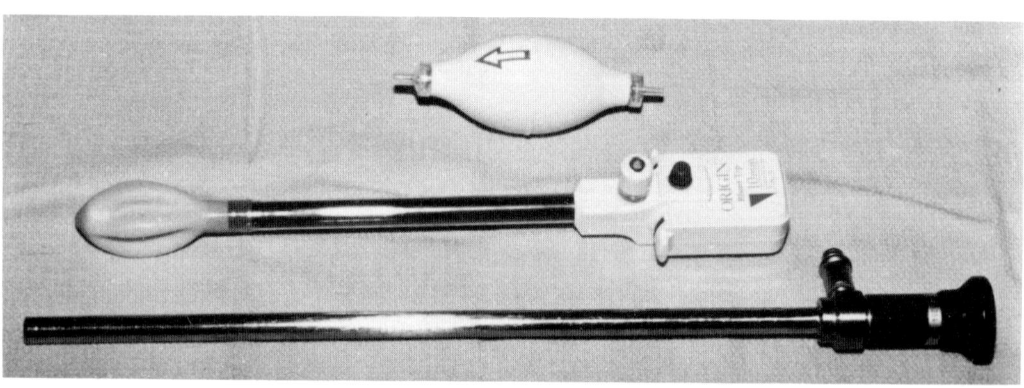

Figure 42.1: Extraperitoneal balloon device (OMS-PDB 1000; Origin MedSystems, Menlo Park, CA).

To complete repair and fortify the hernia defect, a 7.5 × 12.5 cm piece of Prolene polypropylene mesh is cut. A 1 cm cut is made vertically in the mesh 5 cm from the cephalad portion and a 1 cm hole is made for the cord structures. The vas deferens, spermatic artery and vein are carefully dissected free from the lateral pelvic wall, enabling the mesh to be placed behind the structures. The Prolene mesh cut and prepared for placement (Figure 42.2) is then inserted through the 10/11 mm cannula in proper orientation for easy positioning. The mesh is brought behind the cord structures, which are positioned to pass through the 1 cm hole (Figure 42.3). Stay sutures are cut; the mesh is then lifted into position and secured with staples (Figures 42.4 and 42.5). Great care is taken not to compromise the cord structures by deliberate placement of the first two staples. After the cut in the mesh is closed, the next staple is placed in the fascia, adjacent to Cooper's ligament in close proximity to the iliac vein, while the third is placed in the iliopubic tract cephalad or lateral to the cord structures. The mesh is then tacked along Cooper's ligament, along the iliopubic tract, cephalad or lateral anteriorly in the posterior aspects of the rectus muscle.

In the case of a bilateral hernia, two identical 7.5 × 12.5 cm pieces of Prolene mesh are placed on either side and then tacked together at the pubis. With an extremely large direct defect, an additional 5 × 15 cm piece of mesh can be placed cephalad to the pubis and connected with staples to the two pieces of mesh that had been inserted previously in the area of the direct defects. The mesh is tacked around the opening of the facial defect in addition to the previously described placement of staples. Further modification may be necessary in the presence of a large femoral hernia in which the fascia has been attenuated next to the iliac vein. A ligature (size 0, Ethibond Endoknot) is placed through Cooper's ligament and the mesh close to the iliac vein.

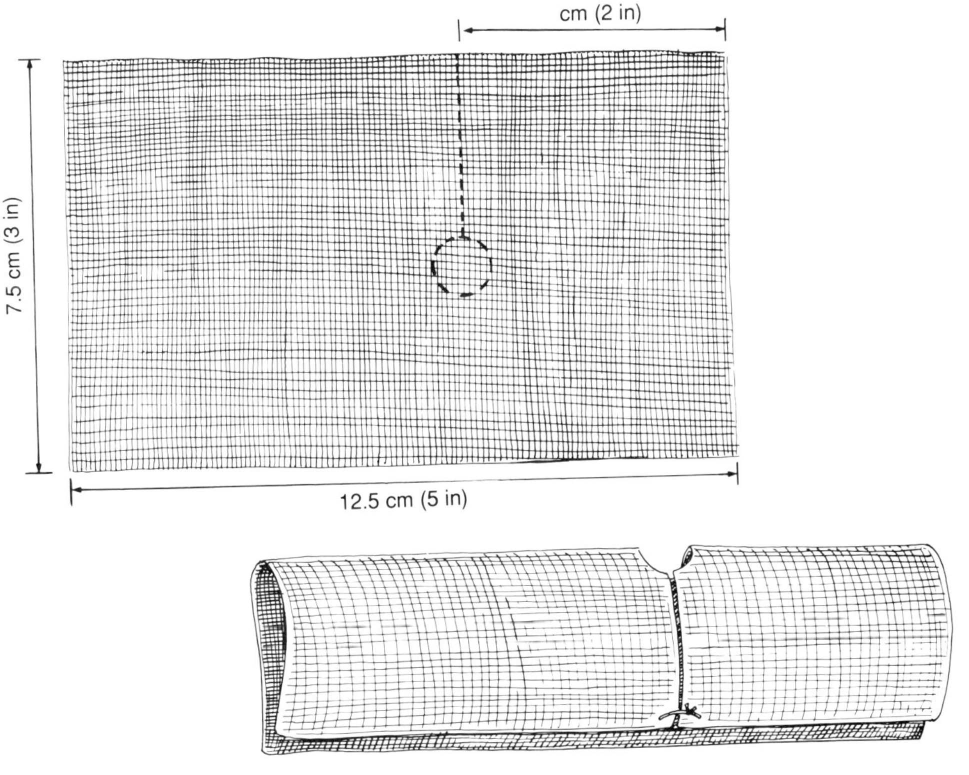

Figure 42.2: Cutting and preparing the mesh for placement.

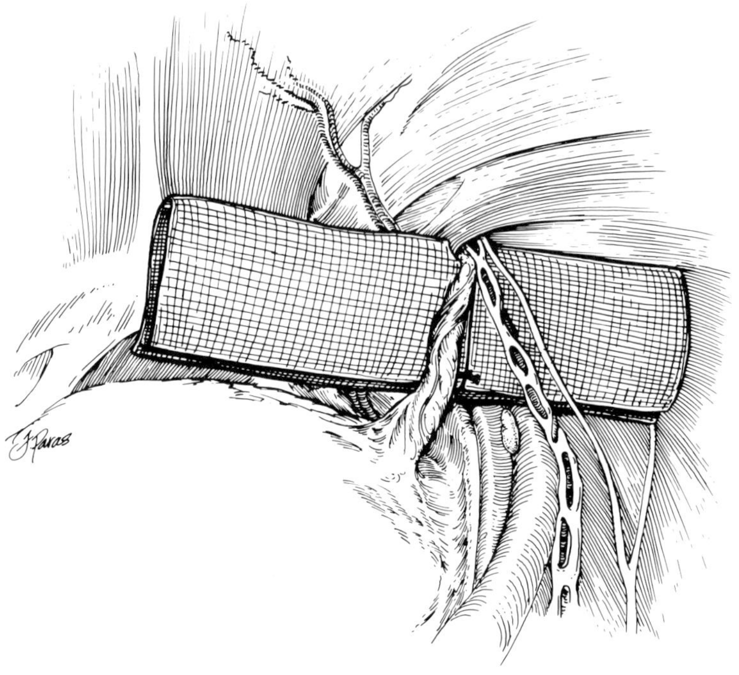

Figure 42.3: Placement of prosthesis, showing the cord structures passing through the 1 cm opening in the mesh.

Results and advantages of laparoscopic extraperitoneal prosthetic repair procedure

In the almost 200 procedures we have performed, operative time for our laparoscopic extraperitoneal approach has averaged approximately one hour and is similar to that of traditional open inguinal hernia repair operations. Postoperative recovery has been uneventful for most patients with no need for injectable analgesics. Almost all of our patients were discharged on the day of surgery, and all returned to normal activities, including strenuous physical exertion, within seven days. Complications have been few and have consisted of one patient with postoperative orchitis that resolved without development of testicular atrophy and one patient who developed bleeding after the inferior epigastric vessel was inadvertently severed. Two other surgical teams have used an extraperitoneal operation for repair of an inguinal defect: Phillips and Carroll in the USA[9] and Dulucq in France[10]. Collectively, over 500 inguinal defects have been repaired using a laparoscopic extraperitoneal approach, and to date no recurrences have been reported.

To repair effectively direct or indirect inguinal hernias using our laparoscopic procedure, it is imperative that the surgeon remain in the preperitoneal space. By working directly at the level of the defect, the surgeon can clearly identify the type and extent of the defect and can also reinforce the weak tissues at the proper plane of the hernia origin. The preperitoneal approach has been advocated for recurrent hernias because it allows the surgeon to circumvent adhesions and scar tissue resulting from previous operations and to dissect through fresh, unscarred tissue. This approach has also been advocated for femoral and complicated hernias (e.g. sliding or incarcerated hernias or bilateral defects) because of the greater visibility it affords of the inguinal region and because of the relatively greater ease of effecting difficult repairs.

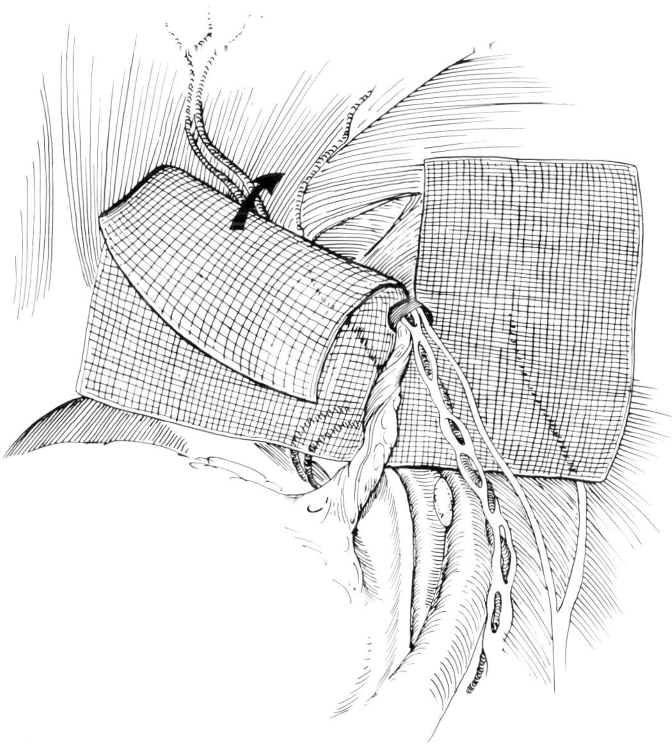

Figure 42.4: Lifting mesh into position after severing of stay sutures.

By operating outside of the peritoneum, there is a higher probability of preventing side-effects associated with severance of the superficial inguinal nerves, such as testicular atrophy and neuralgia. Nevertheless, the surgeon using our laparoscopic procedure must exercise considerable care, during dissection and severance of an indirect hernia and in placement of the staples used to secure the prosthetic mesh, not to compromise or injure the cord structures.

Our laparoscopic extraperitoneal inguinal hernia repair procedure also shares the benefits associated with other surgical laparoscopic techniques, namely small incisions, minimal postoperative discomfort and pain, shorter hospitalization and quicker return to normal activities. Moreover, our procedure has the added benefit of fortifying the inguinal defect with an overlay prosthetic buttress.

For the above reasons, the laparoscopic extraperitoneal prosthetic repair has become the procedure of choice for our patients with recurrent as well as bilateral inguinal hernias. Furthermore, we consider this laparoscopic extraperitoneal procedure for active, postpubertal patients with primary inguinal defects because of the increased speed of recovery and diminished pain associated with this and other laparoscopic procedures. The only absolute contraindication is an inability to tolerate general anaesthesia.

Summary

We have successfully used our laparoscopic extraperitoneal prosthetic repair technique to treat indirect or direct inguinal hernias, including several bilateral or recurrent defects. In our approach, a piece of polypropylene mesh, placed extraperitoneally, is used to reinforce or replace the

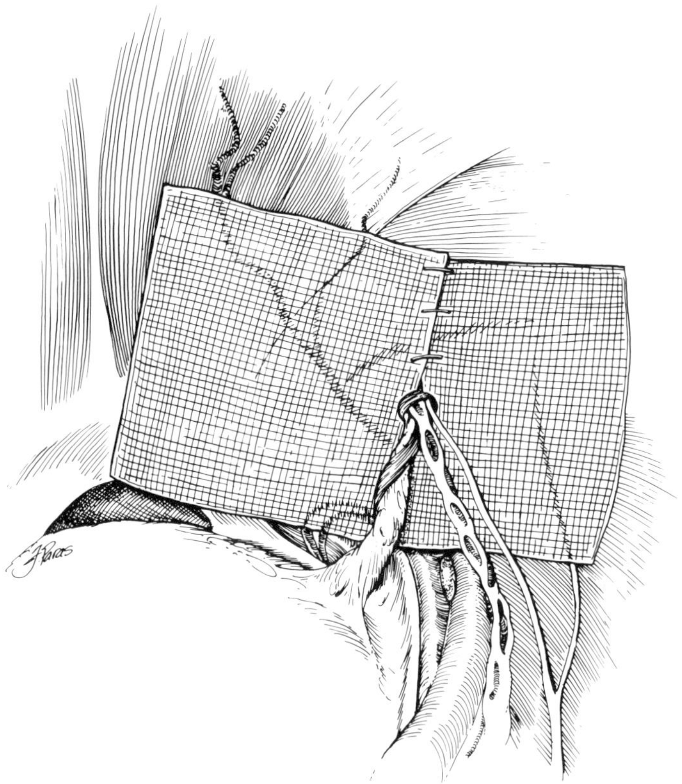

Figure 42.5: Cut in mesh stapled together.

transversalis fascia. Operative time for our laparoscopic repair is similar to that for traditional open procedures. Notably, most patients are able to be discharged on the day of surgery and all have returned to normal activities with seven days, with no patient experiencing recurrent herniation.

In performing our laparoscopic extraperitoneal inguinal hernia repair procedure, it is imperative that certain guidelines be followed. These include dexterity in endoscopic bimanual surgery, facility with the use of angled scopes and, perhaps most importantly, an intimate knowledge of the region's anatomy.

References

1. Vayda E, Mindell WR, Rutkow IM. A decade of surgery in Canada, England, and the United States. *Arch Surg* 1982; **117**: 846.
2. Bassini E. *Nuovo metodo per la cura radical dellerna inguinale.* Padua: R Stabilmento Prosperini, 1889.
3. Cheatle GL. An operation for the radical cure of inguinal and femoral hernias. *BMJ* 1920; **2**: 168.
4. Nyhus LM, Condon RE, Harkins HN. Clinical experiences with preperitoneal hernial repair for all types of hernia of the groin with particular emphasis to the importance of transversalis fascia analogues. *Am J Surg* 1960; **100**: 234.
5. Stoppa R, Petit J, Henry X. Unsutured Dacron prosthesis in groin hernias. *Int Surg* 1975; **60**: 411.
6. Stoppa RE, Warlaumont CR. The preperitoneal approach and prosthetic repair of groin hernia. In: Nyhus LM, Condon RE, eds. *Hernia*, 3rd ed. Philadelphia: JB Lippincott, 1989: 199.

7. McKernan JB, Laws HL. Laparoscopic preperitoneal prosthetic repair of inguinal hernias. *Surg Rounds* 1992; **July**: 597.

8. Adams JG, Weigelt JA, Poulos E. Usefulness of preoperative laboratory assessment of patients undergoing elective herniorrhaphy. *Arch Surg* 1992; **127**: 801–5.

9. Phillips EH, Carroll BJ. Laparoscopic inguinal hernia repair. *Gastrointest Endosc Clin North Am* (in press).

10. Dulucq JL. Treatment of inguinal hernias by placing a sub-peritoneal prosthetic patch under retroperitoneoscopy. In: *Third World Congress of Endoscopic Surgery*, Bordeaux, France, June 18–20, 1992. Session 4/9 Abstract.

43

Laparoscopic Treatment of Inguinal Hernia

JL DULUCQ AND JACQUES M HIMPENS

The laparoscopic treatment of inguinal hernia is a step forward provided it represents a safe and reliable alternative to open surgery. This chapter describes our technique, as we have developed it since 1990, and the results achieved over the past three and a half years.

The technique is based on the work by Stoppa, who proved the efficacy of hernia treatment with a large prosthesis introduced by a strictly extraperitoneal approach. The working space and placement area in our endoscopic technique are exactly the same.

Indications

Initially only small hernias were treated, but at the present time all types of adult hernias, except for very large scrotal hernias, are treated. A history of an inferior laparotomy is not considered a contraindication for the procedure.

Technique

General anaesthesia is induced using tracheal intubation. An indwelling urinary catheter is inserted. The operation table has a 10° reversed Trendelenburg. The surgeon is placed at the opposite side of the hernia. The TV monitor is located at the patient's feet. A Verres needle is inserted suprapubically and directed dorsally until it perforates the rectum muscle fascia. One litre of CO_2 is then insufflated in Retzius' space. This insufflation facilitates the subsequent dissection, which is carried out from an infraumbilical position. To do so, a small incision is done and a reusable 10 mm trocar is introduced subcutaneously over 5 cm. It is then inserted caudally and distally at a 45° angle, the rectus fascia is perforated and the Retzius space is reached. A 0°, 10 mm laparoscope is then placed through the trocar. The preperitoneal fatty tissue is dissected, under direct vision, by the laparoscope itself, using careful sweeping movements, until the pubic bone is reached, which can readily be felt and seen.

Lateral movements of the laparoscopic increase the retropubic space and a second 5 mm trocar is then introduced suprapubically under direct vision. A dissecting instrument is passed in this latter trocar and blunt dissection is initiated laterally. The first anatomical landmark is the epigastric vessels, located anteriorly. Locating these vessels can be rather difficult with a direct hernia. If this is the case, reduction of the hernia must first be carried out. Dissection of the epigastric vessels downwards gives access to the superior edge of the (indirect) hernia sac. The hernia sac is now pushed down posteriorly and the space lateral to the sac is entered; the peritoneum can now be reclined away from the abdominal wall, on both the median and the lateral side of the hernia sac.

A third trocar can now be placed at the level of the anterior superior iliac spine and dissection can be performed with the two-handed technique, forceps in one hand and scissors in the other. The hernia sac is carefully grasped and dissected away from the neighbouring structures. Once the sac is completely free, it is left alone and not resected nor ligated. Thorough dissection of the sac will have caused a satisfactory parietalization of the elements of the cord. The psoas muscle and the iliac vessels are now liberated in order to prepare the space in which to place the prosthesis.

We use a 7 × 12 cm polypropylene prosthesis (Ethicon, Neuilly, France). The prosthesis is introduced through the 10 mm working trocar, carefully rolled like a cigarette. A Vicryl stitch, which has been placed on the short side of the mesh, gives a good orientation for placement. Once unrolled, the prosthesis is stapled on Cooper's ligament medially and on the psoas muscle laterally. The magnified endoscopic view provides sufficient guarantee for the surgeon so as not to injure the nerves in that muscle. The staple on the psoas muscle are placed parallel with the muscle and nerve fibres. The way it is fixed, the patch now bridges the iliac vessels and the elements of the cord, which can now be reclined posteriorly thanks to dissection of the sac.

No other staples are used. The pneumoperitoneum is released and one can watch the patch being squished between the abdominal wall and the peritoneum. No drains are used. The trocar openings are closed and the Foley catheter removed. The patients are allowed to walk and to eat the same day.

Results

Between June 1990 and February 1993, 210 hernias were treated with our technique: 130 were indirect, 26 were direct and 30 were of combined nature (Pantaloon hernias); 12 were bilateral hernias. There were 195 male and three female patients; their average age was 52 years. The average stay in hospital was two days.

There were eight conversions to open treatment, early in our experience. On one occasion preperitoneoscopy could not be performed, and 'classic; laparoscopic treatment was done. Perioperative morbidity included one early recurrence (on the table), treated by open surgery, and one case of excruciating neuralgic pain caused by the psoas staple and necessitating immediate removal via the endoscope.

Postoperatively, 14 patients presented with an inguinal haematoma. One of those had to be drained surgically. Twelve patients presented an impressive subcutaneous emphysema, without physiological implications. There was no mortality.

At follow up (median 14 months), no other recurrences were noted. There were no long-term neuralgic problems and no cases of postoperative small bowel obstruction.

Conclusions

The endoscopic treatment of inguinal hernias makes sense, because it does not damage the abdominal wall, as occurs when exposing the tissues in the classic repair. It is probably the most logical approach because it is based on a very reliable technique in open surgery[1].

McKernan[2] and E Phillips use a similar method. They prefer to do an 'open' properitoneoscopy, however. The open properitoneoscopy is cumbersome to our opinion, and can be avoided by using CO_2 insufflation in Retzius' space as a first step. We have not encountered any problem with our technique. The presence of the Foley catheter provides adequate protection to the bladder.

The transperitoneal route seems less acceptable. Small bowel adhesions can be caused by the intraperitoneal manipulations and by inadequate closure of the peritoneum[3]. Adequate peritoneal closure is mandatory in this technique, but can not always be performed[4]. Intraperitoenal onlay of a prosthesis is even less attractive in our opinion; others[4], however, report good results. It is obvious that long-term results have to be awaited, especially here, because there is no feedback with an open technique.

The choice of the mesh material is obviously an important one. We decided in favour of polypropylene mesh. Its biocompatibility is good, and its handling in laparoscopic procedures has proven to be adequate[5]. It is, however, necessary to fix the prosthesis as in open surgery[6]. Stapling has to be selective so as not to injure any nerves. Good dissection provides an excellent view of the nerve structures over the psoas muscle, so they can be avoided quite easily. Because staples are not used on the abdominal wall, ilioinguinal neuralgia has not been a problem.

Summary

The routine use of laparoscopy and its reliability make its use in more common procedures such as hernioplasty acceptable. The preperitoneoscopic technique is simple and efficacious, and carries a low morbidity and a recurrence rate that appears to be close to zero. Longer follow up has to be awaited but the future looks bright for this technique.

References

1. Stoppa RE, Rives JL, Warlaumont CR. The use of Dacron in the repair of hernias of the groin. *Surg Clin North Am* 1984; **64**: 269–85.
2. McKernan BJ, Laws HL. Laparoscopic repair of inguinal hernias using a totally extraperitoneal prosthetic approach. *Surg Endosc* 1993; **7**: 26–8.
3. Himpens J. Laparoscopic inguinal hernioplasty. *Surg Endosc* 1993; **7**: 315–18.
4. Toy FK, Smoot RT. Toy–Smoot hernioplasty. *Surg Laparosc Endosc* 1991; **1**: 151–5.
5. Stoppa RE, Warlaumont CR. The preperitoneal approach and prosthetic repair of groin hernia. In: Nyhus LM, Condon RE, eds. *Hernia*, 3rd ed. Philadelphia: JB Lippincott, 1989: 199–255.
6. Arregui M, Davis C, Yucel O, Nagan R. Laparoscopic mesh repair of inguinal hernia using a preperitoneal approach: a preliminary report. *Surg Laparosc Endosc* 1992; **2**: 53–8.

44

Complications of Laparoscopic Hernia Repair

NAMIR KATKHOUDA

Complications of laparoscopic hernia repairs are usually related to errors in:

- the indications
- the choice of procedures
- the technique.

Complications related to incorrect indications

Several mistakes can be made, but among the most frequent are the following.

An operation performed on *cardiac patients* under general anaesthesia and with a CO_2 pneumoperitoneum. Obviously, there is a high risk of cardiac decompensation and myocardial infarction. Indeed, the few mortalities reported from around the world are usually related to myocardial infarction. The best approach is probably a conventional anterior approach (Shouldice, Lichtenstein or McVay) (Figure 44.1) under local anaesthesia. *Incarcerated sliding scrotal hernias*[1,2] containing small bowel are

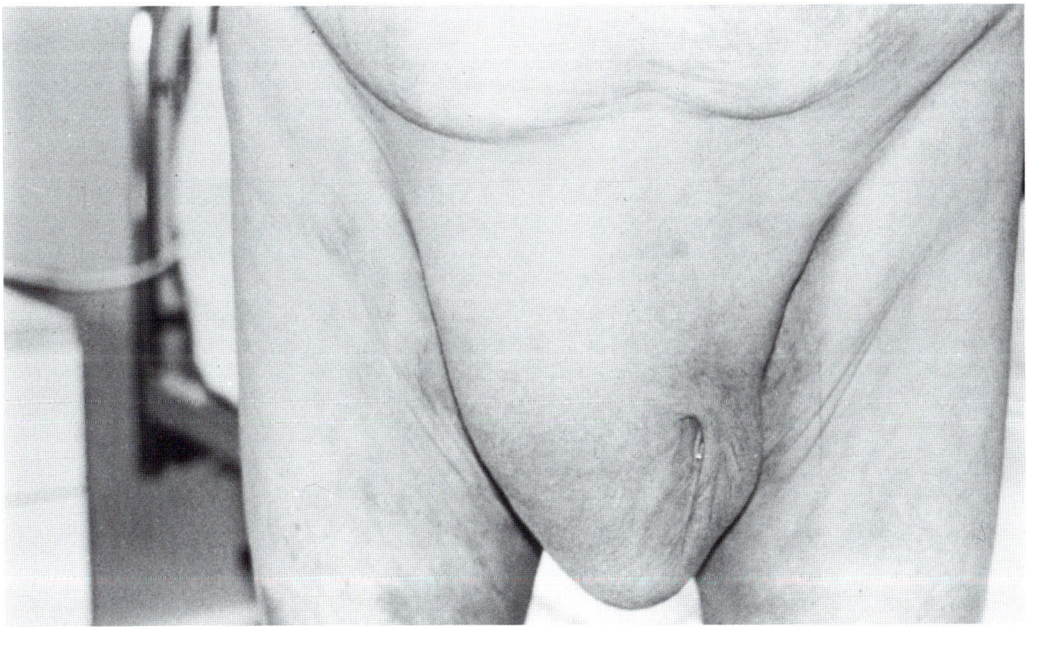

Figure 44.1: Incarcerated scrotal hernia.

also a bad indication for laparoscopy. During the dissection there is a significant risk of colonic lesion which can go unrecognized, leading to major postoperative problems. The best approach for treating these hernias is a simpler anterior approach with an inguinal incision.

Paediatric hernias (Nyhus type 1) are best treated simply by a high ligation sac. There is no need to endanger babies by using a CO_2 pneumoperitoneum and a major intra-abdominal operation. If there is some doubt about the presence of an incarceration, a diagnostic laparoscopy should be considered and a laparoscopic high ligation of the sac may be necessary. Otherwise, we do not see any justification for treating hernias in babies and infants using a laparoscope.

A *recent history of infection* should represent a major contraindication to the use of mesh. One should wait for an infection-free period of more than one year before inserting a mesh when repairing a hernia.

Complications related to incorrect procedures

In benign and recurring disease, reliable and simple laparoscopic procedures for hernia repair should be performed. The use of complicated techniques or procedures have often proved to have disastrous results leading to immediate recurrences. Among them is the stuffing of mesh, sometimes of several layers, leading to a migration in the scrotum felt by the patient, and also to an early recurrence (Figure 44.2).

Closure of the internal ring for a type 3 hernia with a defect in the posterior wall, whether direct, indirect or femoral (or a type 4 recurrent hernia), can also lead to an early recurrence. Even when staples or sutures are used, this will not prevent recurrences, as the posterior inguinal wall will not have been repaired.

An intraperitoneal onlay mesh for direct or femoral hernias has not, in the past, proved to be efficient. However several teams (Spaw, Zucker, Franklin) are using this technique and reporting good results[3,4].

Finally, a high ligation of the sac alone, without any repair of the internal ring and the posterior wall, is not sufficient and usually leads to recurrences.

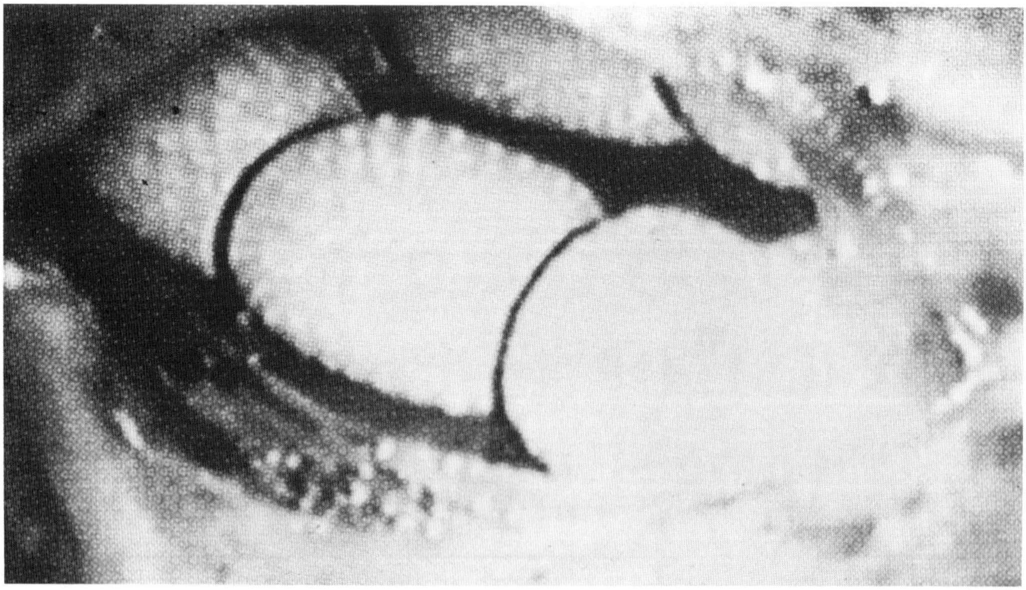

Figure 44.2: Stuffing of mesh is an inappropriate procedure.

Complications related to technical problems

It is technical problems that usually lead to recurrence and postoperative problems.

During the CO_2 insufflation in total extraperitoneal mesh repair, there is a risk of hypercarbia and a high blood diffusion of CO_2. This can at first be controlled by an anaesthesiologist and requires a change in the mechanical ventilatory control parameters. A serious sign is the presence of subcutaneous emphysema; most surgeons do no consider this to be significant, but in the author's experience it is an early sign of problems leading to serious cardiac disorders.

When using total extraperitoneal mesh repair, the presence of a hole in the peritoneum during the dissection can lead to a valve system, making dissection very difficult[5–7].

There is possibility to enlarge the hole, to equilibrate the pressures between the preperitoneal space and the intra-abdominal cavity, but the hole has to be sutured at the end of the operation, which is very difficult in the preperitoneal approach.

Low insertion of the trocars limits the lateral dissection, as the instruments are usually long. Low insertion of the trocar in the thin patient can endanger the iliac vessels. Such incidents have been reported elsewhere.

Insertion of a urinary catheter can be responsible for postoperative bladder infection. It is better for the patients to urinate before the operation, therefore avoiding the need for a urinary catheter.

A thin peritoneal flap, when using a transabdominal preperitoneal repair, can be difficult to close. In order to have a good amount of tissue, the flap should be made at the superior aspect of the internal ring.

The use of non-isolated instruments out of the view of the telescope can cause burns of the small bowel; these may go unnoticed and lead to postoperative complications.

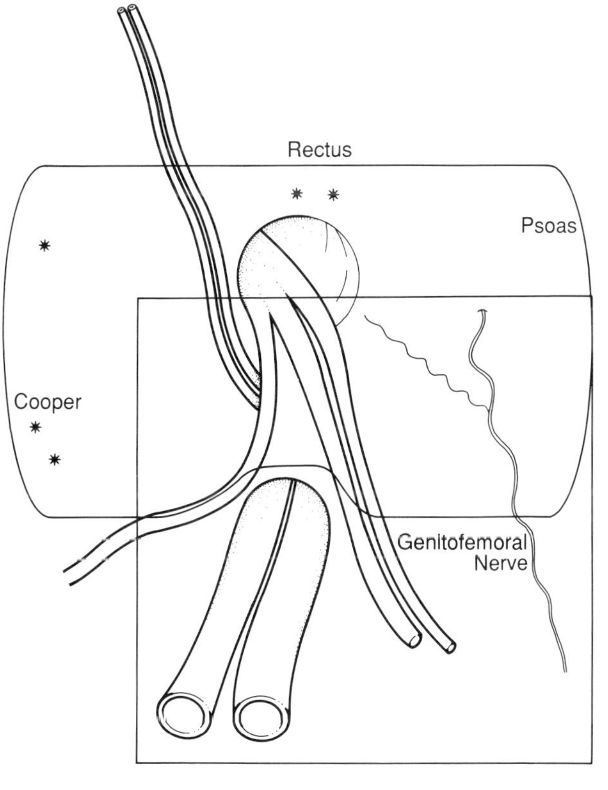

Figure 44.3: Square of doom.

Injury to the vas or spermatic vessels during the operation can lead to scrotal or pelvic haematomas, an epididymitis and even testicular ischaemia.

During total extraperitoneal mesh repair, the dissection behind the rectus muscle can lead to severe haematomas under the anterior abdominal wall.

Closure of the peritoneal flap is of critical importance: it has to be performed ideally in an overlap fashion if staples are used, or using sutures. Indeed, an incomplete closure leading to windows in the peritoneum can provoke adhesions of bowel to the mesh, and therefore obstructions. A traumatic dissection of a large flap can also theoretically induce a peritoneal ischaemia and a new one of a flap leading also to small bowel adhesions although this has not been yet reported. Therefore, this closure has to be performed very carefully and precisely and should not be considered as a minor step in the procedure.

Complications related to the use of mesh

The choice of material has to be precisely assessed. Indeed, one should avoid using polypropylene or Marlex non-resorbable mesh in the intraperitoneal onlay mesh technique, because they lead to adhesions or small bowel obstructions. The use of PTFE or Interceed in the intraperitoneal onlay mesh technique is currently under evaluation. It is known that PTFE causes no adhesions with contact to small bowel and therefore should be the recommended material when using the intraperitoneal technique[8–10].

Incomplete coverage of the hernia spaces leads to immediate recurrence. Therefore, anatomical dissection of the area revealing the solid landmarks (Cooper's, rectus muscle and psoas muscle) is mandatory[11].

The piece of mesh has to be tailored perfectly and the shape must follow the general configuration of the pelvic inlet[12].

When placing the mesh, one should avoid wrinkles in the mesh. These wrinkles have frequently been found when reoperating on patients for infection or recurrence. A good way to prevent such folds and wrinkles is to cut the tails of the mesh in a circular fashion.

Fixation of the mesh has to follow very precise rules. One should have a stapler available and 0-sutures[11].

Fixation to solid landmarks of the area is mandatory (Cooper, rectus muscle). There is no need to use more than five staples for the mesh to be kept in place.

An important fact is the enlargement of the concept of the 'triangle of doom' to the 'square of doom' (Figure 44.3). The triangle of doom described initially by Spaw consists of a triangle between the vas deferens and the spermatic arteries and veins. There are iliac vessels in this space and Spaw recommended avoiding placing any staples or suturing material in this triangle. This triangle has to be enlarged to the square of doom as described recently by the author. The borders of the square are the vas and the iliopubic tract. In this square the genitofemoral nerve runs along the psoas before its division into the genital branch and the femoral nerve branch. Lateral stapling in this square of doom can injure the nerve leading to compression and early ischaemia. Clinically, the patient will present with hypoaesthesia of the groin, transient pain and even a neuroma that would necessitate removal of the staple.

Parietalization of the cord

This very important concept was initially described by Stoppa and Rives. It consists of an atraumatic dissection and separation of the vas deferens and spermatic vessels from the peritoneum. The elements of the spermatic cord can then be pushed laterally on to the pelvic wall, and the mesh, with the help of intra-abdominal hydrostatic pressure, can be positioned perfectly and kept in place[12].

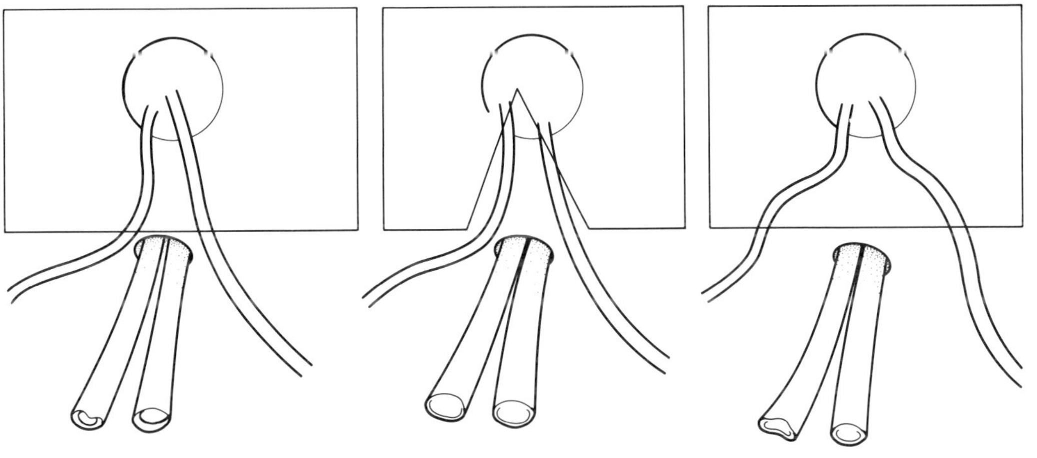

Figure 44.4: Parietalization of the cord.

This parietalization means that it is not necessary to put slits in the mesh for the passage of the cord. This is advantageous as these slits can cause weakness in the mesh.

When the cord is parietalized, the risk of inferior recurrence above the iliac vessels is eliminated. This site is known as the major site of recurrences (Figure 44.4).

Conclusion

Complications can be prevented by identifying *high-risk patients* (cardiac patients) and by adopting the technique using the Nyhus classification. The paediatric type 1 patient needs a ligation of the sac. A Nyhus type 2 in the young adult with a strong posterior wall and a large internal ring can be treated by closure of the ring and avoiding the use of a mesh. Mesh should be used only when there is a posterior wall defect (type III and IV)[13].

The operation should be kept simple and the use of complicated unproven techniques avoided.

Finally, the suppression of CO_2 and general anaesthesia, and the concept of gasless laparoscopic hernia repair under regional anaesthesia, described elsewhere in this book, could help solve the major problems in hernia repair (cost, general anaesthesia), and prove to be a better procedure.

References

1. Griffith GA. The Marcy repair of indirect inguinal hernia: 1870 to present. In: Nyhus LM, Condon RE, eds. *Hernia*, 3rd ed. Philadelphia: JB Lippincott; 1989: 106–18.
2. Lichtenstein IL, Shulman AG, Amid PK, Montlor MM. The tension-free hernioplasty. *Am J Surg* 1989; **157**: 188–93.
3. Spaw AT, Ennis BW, Spaw L. Laparoscopic hernia repair: the anatomic basis. *J Laparoendosc Surg* 1991; **5**: 269–77.
4. Franklin Jr ME. Personal communication. *Laparosc Focus* 1992; **1**: 1–12.
5. Katkhouda, N, Mouiel J. Traitement laparoscopique des hernies de l'aine de l'adulte. *Chir Endoscop* 1992; **3**: 7–10.

6. McKernan JB. Laparoscopic repair of inguinal hernias using a totally extraperitoneal prosthetic approach. *Surg Endosc* 1983; **7**: 26–8

7. Arregui ME, Davis CJ, Yucel O, Nagan RF. Laparoscopic mesh repair of inguinal hernia using a preperitoneal approach: a preliminary report. *Surg Laparosc Endosc* 1992; **2**: 53–58.

8. Salerno GM, Fitzgibbons Jr RJ, Filipi CJ. Laparoscopic inguinal hernia repair. In: Zucker KA, ed. *Surgical laparoscopy*. St Louis: Quality Medical Publ; 1991: 281–93.

9. Corbitt Jr JD. Laparoscopic herniorrhaphy. *Surg Laparosc Endosc* 1991; **1**: 23–5.

10. Schultz L, Graber J, Pietraffittas J, Hickok D. Laser laparoscopic herniorrhaphy: a clinical trial. Preliminary results. *J Laparoendosc Surg* 1991; **1**: 41–5.

11. Katkhouda N, Mouiel J. Traitement laparoscopique. In: Mouiel J (ed.) Actualitiés digestives médico-chirurgicales, Paris: Masson; 1993: 115–21.

12. Stoppa RE, Warlaumont CR. The preperitoneal approach and prosthetic repair of groin hernia. In: Nyhus LM, Condon RE, eds. *Hernia*, 3rd ed. Philadelphia: JB Lippincott; 1989: 236–52.

13. Nyhus LM, Pollack R, Bombeck TC, Donahue PE. The preperitoneal approach and prosthetic buttress repair for recurrent hernia. *Ann Surg* 1988; **208**: 733–7.

Shearburn EW, Myers RN. Shouldice repair of inguinal hernia. *Surgery* 1969; **66**: 450–9.

Ger R, Monroe K, Duvivier R, Mishrick A. Management of the sac. *Am J Surg* 1990; **159**: 370–3.

Ger R. The laparoscopic management of groin hernias. *Contemp Surg* 1991; **39**: 15–19.

Laparoscopic Surgery: The international experience. Indianapolis, Ind. May 20–22 1991.

Toy FK, Smoot RT. Toy–Smoot laparoscopic hernioplasty. *Surg Laparosc Endosc* 1991; **3**: 151–5.

45

Transabdominal Preperitoneal Laparoscopic Herniorrhaphy: Method, Complications and Re-explorations

JOHN D CORBITT Jr

The transabdominal preperitoneal tension-free laparoscopic herniorrhaphy (TAPP) method of hernia repair is used for all groin hernias including direct, indirect, femoral and recurrent hernias. The major indications for this repair are the recurrent hernia because of the preservation of anatomy through this approach and the bilateral hernia because of decreased postoperative pain.

Method

For this repair a long-acting prophylactic antibiotic is given when preoperative medication is administered. Following induction of general anaesthesia a Foley catheter is inserted and the patient is placed in the Trendelenburg position. A 12 mm umbilical incision is made and an insufflation needle is used to insufflate the abdomen to a pressure of 15 mmHg. Another puncture site is used if the patient has had previous abdominal surgery in the area of the umbilicus. A 12 mm port is placed through the umbilical incision and a 10 mm 30° laparoscope is utilized to observe the placement of secondary ports, lateral to the rectus sheath at about the level of the umbilicus. The secondary ports may vary 2.5 cm superior or inferior to this umbilical line. The secondary ports are placed at an angle pointing towards the hernia to be repaired, or in the case of the bilateral hernia, towards the symptomatic or larger hernia. This angled placement of the ports will prevent the need for postoperative suturing of the fascia in the secondary port incisions. The secondary ports are usually 10 mm; however, if a request is made for minimal scaring, 5 mm ports may be used as secondary ports, which will require the use of a 5 mm laparoscope during the stapling procedure.

All hernias are repaired from the left side of the patient. The laparoscope remains in the umbilical port throughout the dissection of the pelvis and placement of the graft. The initial incision of the peritoneum is carried transversely from the umbilical ligament, medially to the anterior superior iliac spine laterally, across the top of the direct and/or indirect space. The anterior superior iliac spine area is identified by exterior palpation of the abdominal wall. All direct sacs are reduced into the abdominal cavity with the dissection of the posterior peritoneum. If a large indirect sac exists, it is excised from the parietal peritoneum with a 350° circumferential incision made around the inside of the neck of the hernia. The indirect sac is allowed to retract distally and remain intact. Leaving this sac in place will not cause a hydrocele. The sac is not removed in the case of the indirect hernia because of the possibility of damage to the posteriorly located cord structures and genitofemoral nerve during this dissection.

The preperitoneal space is exposed by reflecting the posterior flap initially, using traction and counter-traction. Cooper's ligament is exposed medially and the iliopubic tract is exposed laterally. Dissection extends posteriorly below the iliopubic tract. The 'triangle of doom' consisting of the

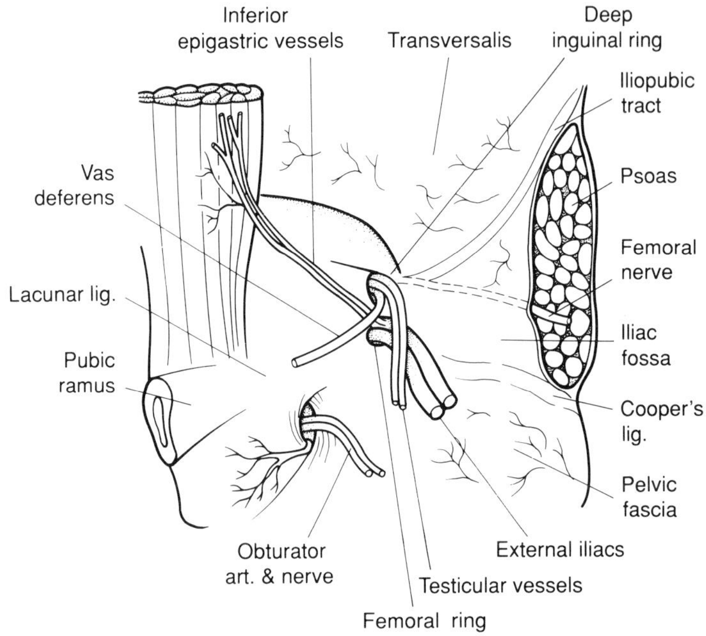

Figure 45.1: See in text.

spermatic vessels, the vas deferens and the iliac vessels lying below these structures is dissected cautiously to prevent injury to these major structures.

After complete exposure of the posterior area the anterior flap of peritoneum is dissected, special consideration being given to the inferior epigastric vessels anteriorly. All fatty tissue and areolar tissue is removed from the entire pelvic floor. Initial exposure of the pubis and Cooper's ligament will reveal loose areolar tissue or fatty tissue in this area. These structures are most easily identified initially by palpation with a dissecting instrument, after which they must be cleared of this fatty material (Figure 45.1).

A 7.5 × 12.5 cm (3 × 5 inch) polypropylene mesh is then forced through the 10 mm secondary port or, if 5 mm secondary ports are being used, the mesh must be placed blindly through the 12 mm umbilical port. In either case, the laparoscope is replaced into the umbilical port and the secondary ports are used to place the mesh over the pelvic floor. This prosthesis must overlap the hernia defect by at least 3–4 cm. In the presence of a direct hernia the mesh will extend slightly more medially, and in the presence of an indirect hernia the mesh will extend slightly more laterally. The ingrowth of fibrous tissue into this mesh will account for the permanent repair of the hernia, so positioning is extremely important.

With the mesh in the proper position (Figure 45.2), the laparoscope is removed from the umbilical port and placed into the port on the contralateral side of the hernia. The ipsilateral secondary port is used to hold the mesh in position and the hernia stapler is passed through the 12 mm umbilical port.

An anterior row of staples is first inserted. Tension is then placed on the mesh posteriorly and the lateral and medial row of staples are placed with the mesh on tension. The 4.8 mm United (USSC) staples are used for all of the fascial attachments to the mesh. The 4.0 mm (USSC) staple is used to secure the mesh to Cooper's ligament and the inguinal ligament. In the mid-portion of the mesh staples are not placed over the triangle of doom, to prevent injury to the cord structures and iliac vessels lying superficial to the mesh. Laterally the staples are not placed below the iliopubic

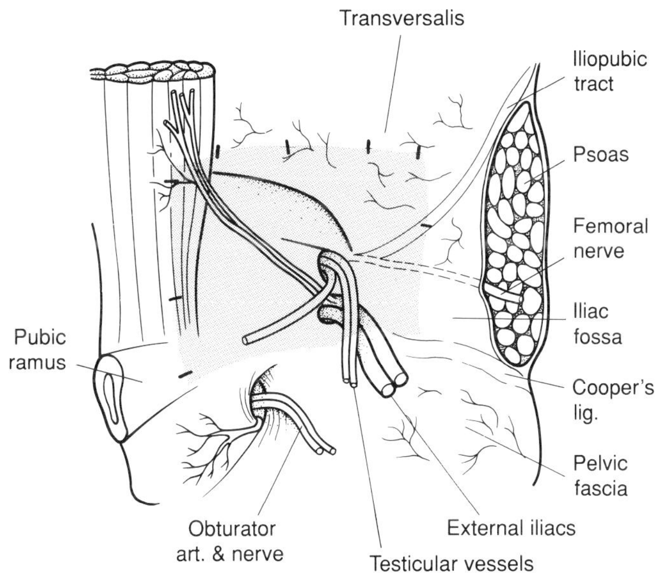

Figure 45.2: Mesh in place.

tract. The iliopubic tract is identified by anterior compression of the abdominal wall. If the hernia stapler can be palpated and the abdominal wall can be seen to indent, it will be safe to place staples in this area. The staples are not placed posterior to the iliopubic tract in order to prevent injury to the lateral femoral cutaneous nerve.

After securing the prosthesis in place, the CO_2 pressure is reduced to 8 mmHG and a corresponding amount of CO_2 is allowed to escape from the abdominal cavity. The peritoneum is approximated with the graspers and stapled using the hernia stapler to cover the mesh securely with the peritoneum. These staples should be placed approximately 1 cm apart to prevent incarceration of small bowel between the peritoneum and the mesh.

All blood and irrigation fluid is removed from the pelvis. The fascia of the 12 mm umbilical incision is closed with an absorbable suture and all skin incisions are closed with a subcuticular absorbable suture and sterile adhesive strips. The patient is discharged on the day of the procedure and is allowed to return to normal activity in 48 hours.

Complications

In this personal series there have been no major complications. The complications that have occurred are as follows.

Scrotal emphysema

Scrotal emphysema has occurred in approximately 5% of the cases but has now markedly been reduced by leaving the indirect sacs in place. If scrotal emphysema occurs, it is removed by gentle compression of the scrotum with the patient still under anaesthesia. By the time the patient is discharged from the hospital, the majority of this emphysema has been reabsorbed.

Haematoma or seroma

Haematomas or seromas of the area have been noted in 7% of the patients, and are manifested by a bulge on examination of the patient one week postoperatively. This bulge does not respond to the Valsalva manoeuvre or cough, and is therefore determined not to be a recurrent hernia. If this area is examined three months postoperatively, the bulge will have disappeared.

Nerve injury

Injury to the lateral femoral cutaneous nerve has occurred in 1% of the patients early in the series. The notation of the nerve posterior to the iliopubic tract and discontinuation of the use of staples in this area has eliminated the complication.

Recurrence

The recurrence rate now is less than 1% and consists of a recurrence following the repair of an indirect inguinal hernia. The recurrence was caused by the lack of substantial fixation of the mesh posteriorly. This has been corrected by placing more staples medially and laterally to ensure that the mesh stays in place. A single staple may be placed in the posterior lateral corner to hold the mesh in place while the peritoneum is allowed to cover the mesh with desufflation of the abdominal cavity. This posteriorly placed staple should be into the fatty tissue only and should not be forced through the fascia, to prevent the possibility of injury to the lateral femoral cutaneous nerve.

Complications in other series

In a series of 3000 herniorrhaphies presented at Berkeley, California, in March 1993, by the University of Southern California, additional complications not seen by this author were noted.

- *Deaths* during herniorrhaphies were examined and were usually found to have been due to the initial insertion of the umbilical trocar and were thus a complication of laparoscopy rather than of herniorrhaphy.
- *Injury to the iliac vessels* is a life-threatening complication and is corrected by immediate abdominal laparotomy. This complication is prevented by thorough knowledge of the anatomy of the pelvis.
- *Small bowel incarceration* between the peritoneum and the mesh is due to failure of substantial closure of the peritoneum at the termination of the procedure.
- *Bladder injuries* may be the result of carrying the medial dissection beyond the umbilical ligament and failure to identify properly the bladder in that area. This complication is rare.
- *Injury to the genitofemoral and lateral cutaneous nerve* still remains a very high rate of 2% due to the placement of the staples below the iliopubic tract laterally.
- *Injury to the genitofemoral nerve and cord structures* has been associated with removal of the indirect sac. This is avoided by leaving this sac in place. If it is necessary or the preference of the surgeon to remove this sac, it should be done with care to prevent injury to these structures.
- The *recurrence* rate nationally for the transabdominal preperitoneal (TAPP) repair and the extraperitoneal repair remains below 1%.

Re-exploration

Major indications for re-exploration following a laparoscopic herniorrhaphy are those for a recurrent hernia and for injury to the lateral femoral cutaneous nerve. Fortunately, recurrent hernias are rare following laparoscopic repair, with the exception of the plug-and-patch method which originally resulted in a high recurrence rate. Most of the experience for re-exploration was a previous plug-and-patch repair. After dissection of the preperitoneal space, whether the surgery is done transabdominally or limited to the extraperitoneal space, re-exploration is extremely difficult. The mesh and overlying tissues bond securely and are extremely difficult to dissect. Whilst these recurrent hernias may be repaired laparoscopically, the amount of time and tissue damage involved does not warrant re-exploration of the recurrent laparoscopic hernia. It is suggest that a transgroin approach be attempted for the recurrent laparoscopic hernia. The exception to this would be the patient who has had multiple recurrences, in which case a second laparoscopic approach may be of benefit.

The other major indication for re-exploration is that of entrapment of the lateral femoral cutaneous nerve of the thigh. If the patient has pain or numbness along the distribution of this nerve immediately postoperatively, the patient should be re-explored immediately and the offending staple removed. This staple will lie posterior to the iliopubic tract and is located laterally in the repair. If the onset of the pain and numbness occurs a week or more following the repair, these paraesthesias will subside spontaneously. Injection of steroids may hasten the resolution of this problem but it is not necessary to re-explore this patient.

If the patient is seen several months after the initial laparoscopic hernia repair, complaining of pain and numbness that had their onset immediately postoperatively, re-exploration is extremely difficult and cannot be done laparoscopically but rather through a transgroin approach. In this case a CT guided needle similar to breast biopsies in cases of calcifications of the breast may be of assistance in locating the staple causing nerve entrapment. Removal of this staple is performed only after conservative steroid injections. The removal of the staple even several months after the initial injury has produced excellent results in relief of pain and numbness due to this entrapment.

A patient presenting with small bowel obstruction shortly after herniorrhaphy should be re-explored laparoscopically for incarceration of small bowel through the peritoneal closure. This is easily reduced laparoscopically and additionally staples are used to close the peritoneal defect.

Laparoscopic herniorrhaphy is, as described, an excellent approach to hernia repairs, with a recurrence rate of less than 1%. The complications are a direct result of the learning curve and are similar to that of the transgroin approach to hernia repair. The major indication for laparoscopic herniorrhaphy is that of the recurrent and bilateral hernia; however, there is a progressive increase in the number of requests to repair all groin hernias using this approach.

46

Laparoscopic Inguinal Herniorrhaphy: Complications and Pitfalls

BRUCE V MACFADYEN Jr

Inguinal herniorrhaphy is the second most common surgical procedure performed in the USA. Some 500 000–600 000 operations are performed each year[1]. There have been reports indicating low morbidity, mortality and recurrence rates with the use of polypropylene mesh placed through an anterior approach[2,3]. Stoppa *et al.*[4] reported similar results with a low recurrence rate of 2.2% when a large prosthetic mesh was placed in the preperitoneal space. It appears that the primary defect in an inguinal hernia is in the transversus abdominis aponeurosis and transversalis fascia in the inguinal region called the myopectineal orifice. This anatomical space is defined as the transversus abdominis arch superiorly, the lateral border of the rectus sheath medially, Cooper's ligament inferiorly, and laterally the anterior iliac spine (Figure 46.1).

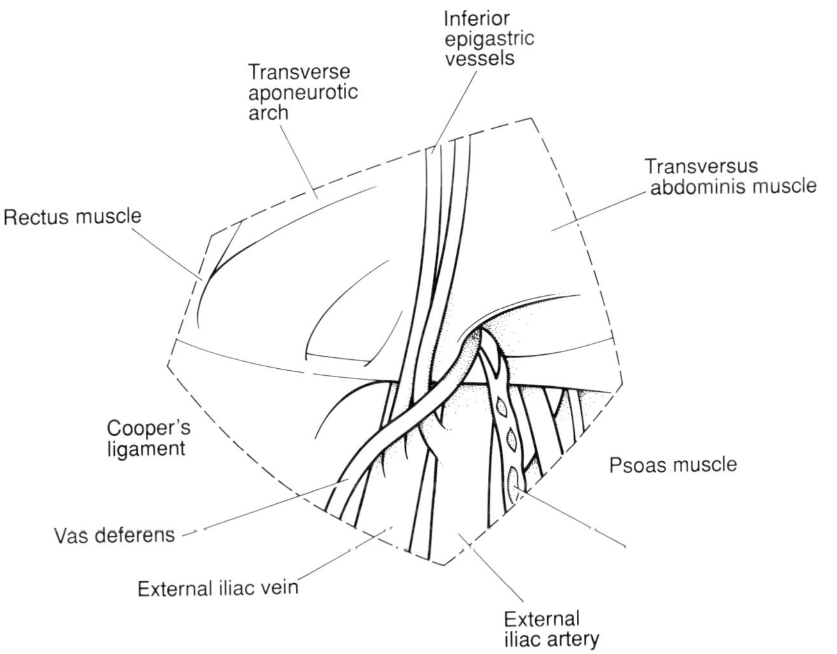

Figure 46.1: Laparoscopic view of the myopectineal orifice. Reprinted with permission of publisher from Filipi CJ, Fitzgibbons Jr RJ, Salerno GM, Hart RO. Laparoscopic herniorrhaphy. *In* Laparoscopy for the General Surgeon. *Surg Clin North Am* 1992; **72**: 1109–24.

With the success of laparoscopic techniques in general surgery, such as in laparoscopic cholecystectomy, they have been applied to inguinal hernia repair as advocated by several investigators[5–8]. The laparoscopic inguinal hernia technique has evolved from the simple stapling of the internal ring to the placement of a plug and a patch of the internal ring, and to the repair of the hernia defect by suturing the transversus abdominis muscle and aponeurosis to either the iliopubic tract or Cooper's ligament. A recent development has been the placement of a very large piece of synthetic mesh in the preperitoneal space over the entire myopectineal orifice[6]. It appears that, in an inguinal hernia repair, it is important to strengthen the transverse abdominis aponeurosis and fascia in the myopectineal orifice. Whether the hernia sac is or is not removed and decreasing the internal ring size do not appear to be critical factors.

Several other issues, however, need to be addressed in the laparoscopic management of all inguinal hernias: management of the hernia sac itself, hernia recurrence, intra-abdominal adhesions, complications that are unique to the laparoscopic procedure, to repair or not repair bilateral inguinal hernias, the issue of when the patient can return to work, the length of hospitalization and the type of anaesthesia. Because laparoscopic inguinal herniorrhaphy has been performed for only three to four years, length of follow up is an important consideration when evaluating any surgical results. The study reported here was undertaken to address some of these issues in several large surgery centres in order to determine the operative results in a short follow-up period ranging from five to seven months.

Methods and material

In this analysis, 16 surgeons reported on 762 patients with 841 inguinal hernias. Four types of inguinal hernia repairs were determined:

1 Simple closure of the internal inguinal ring and hernia sac[9]

2 Plugging the internal inguinal ring and patching this area with a small piece of polypropylene mesh[8]

3 Laparoscopic transperitoneal suture repair of the transversalis fascia to the iliopubic tract or Cooper's ligament[10]

4 Transabdominal preperitoneal repair using a synthetic prosthesis.

Within this fourth group, there were three types of repair. In subgroup A, polypropylene mesh covered with Interceed (Ethicon, Inc., Cincinnati, Ohio)[6] or polytetrafluoroethylene (PTFE; Gore-Tex, Flagstaff, Arizona)[11] was transabdominally placed as an onlay prosthesis on the peritoneum overlying the myopectineal orifice. Subgroup B included patients who had transperitoneal placement of a polypropylene mesh into retroperitoneal space overlying the myopectineal orifice[6]. In subgroup C, the mesh was placed extraperitoneally and covered the myopectineal orifice[12].

In group 1, there were 87 patients with 89 hernias and the average follow-up was 24 months. Group 2 consisted of 76 patients with 87 hernias, with an average follow-up of eight months. In group 3, there were 28 patients with 30 hernias, with an average follow-up of less than six months. In group 4, there was a total of 563 patients with 635 hernias. Within the fourth group, the first subgroup included 182 patients with 186 hernias, with an average follow-up less than five months. In the second subgroup there were 328 patients with 359 hernias, with an average follow-up of five months. The third subgroup comprised 53 patients with 90 hernias, with an average follow-up of seven months. In all of these patients in group 4, a large piece of mesh, measuring 8–10 × 10–15 cm, was placed in the preperitoneal space and covered the entire myopectineal orifice such that the potential direct, indirect and femoral hernia areas were completely covered with the prosthesis.

Results

The results from simple closure of the internal inguinal ring and hernia sac in group 1 patients was associated with a 2.2% recurrence rate and had a 2.2% incidence of testicular pain (Table 46.1). Group 2 patients with the plug and patch technique had a 6.8% recurrence rate and morbidity included a palpable mesh, bladder injury and mesh migration in several patients (Table 46.1). The laparoscopic transperitoneal suture repair of the transversalis fascia to the iliopubic tract or Cooper's ligament (Group 3) was associated with a 6.6% recurrence rate, and conversion to an open procedure occurred in 6.6%. Other complications included inability to visualize the iliopubic tract (3.3%), postoperative hydrocele (3.3%), and bladder injury (3.3%).

In patients with transperitoneal onlay prosthesis there was a recurrence rate of 3.2%. In this group, two hernias were considered to be retained hernias and may have been related to redundancy of the mesh rather than secondary to an inadequate repair of the hernia. Scrotal hydrocele, bladder injury, abdominal bloating, urinary retention, thigh pain and pelvic osteitis were also noted.

With the transabdominal preperitoneal prosthesis repair, the follow up in this series was five months with a recurrence rate of 0.84%. Two of these hernias were considered questionable and may have been due to redundant prosthesis. Haematomas were also noted in the scrotal region, trocar insertion site, and in the preperitoneal space. Thigh pain, emphysema of the scrotum, and urinary retention were also observed.

With the extraperitoneal repair, patients had an average follow up of seven months with a recurrence rate of 0%. Haematomas were noted in the inguinal canal and in the intra-abdominal wall, and testicular pain was noted as well.

A summary of group 4 patients using prosthesis to cover the entire myopectineal orifice is given as sub-group D. It is noted that the average follow up was 5.6 months with an overall recurrence rate of 1.4%.

The recurrences in group 4 patients included five direct and four indirect inguinal hernias, and it was noted that the causes of recurrence were related to either a small prosthesis or inadequate fixation of the mesh.

Anterior or lateral thigh pain was noted in several patients who had stapling of the mesh. It was observed that this complication most probably resulted from staple injury to the lateral femoral cutaneous nerve of the thigh or the femoral branch of the genitofemoral nerve. Once staples were removed, this pain often decreased.

Conclusions

It is apparent from this study that there has been an evolution in the development of the technique of laparoscopic inguinal herniorrhaphy. It has progressed from simple closure of the internal ring to the placement of a large prosthesis over the myopectineal orifice. As to which type of prosthesis is best, there is general agreement that the PTFE prosthesis is the choice when placing a transabdominal onlay prosthesis over the peritoneum covering the myopectineal orifice. When the mesh is to be located preperitoneally, Vicryl mesh, polypropylene, polyester fibre and Dacron have been employed although polypropylene is the most frequently used. One of the advantages of this type of mesh is its ability to create an inflammatory response which increases the fixation of the mesh to the tissue. This fixation prevents future migration and enhances the strength of the myopectineal orifice.

One of the other complications that was noted in this series and in another report[13] was the development of pain in the upper anterior and lateral thigh. This pain appeared to be related to the placement of sutures or staples laterally and inferiorly in the myopectineal orifice region or around the femoral vessels, thus causing injury to the lateral femoral cutaneous nerve or the femoral branch of the genital femoral nerve. It is now recommended that staples not be placed in these regions but

Table 46.1: Complications of laparoscopic inguinal hernia repair

	Patients/ Hernias	*Age (years)*	*Follow up*	*No – Complications – %*
1 Closure of internal inguinal ring and hernia sac	87/89	av. < 50	1–64 mo. av. 24 mo.	2 – Recurrences – 2.2 2 – Testicular pain – 2.2
2 Plug and patch of internal ring	74/87	av. < 50	1–15 mo. av. 8 mo.	6 – Recurrences – 6.8 3 – Palpable mesh – 3.4 1 – Bladder injury – 1.1 (recognized and repaired) 1 – Mesh migration into scrotum – 1.1 1 – Hydrocele of scrotum – 1.1
3 Laparoscopic transperitoneal suture repair of transversalis fascia to iliopubic tract or Cooper's ligament	28/30	av. < 55	< 6 mo.	2 – Recurrences – 6.6 2 – Laparoscopic procedure converted to open procedure – 6.6 1 – Unable to visualize iliopubic tract – 3.3 1 – Bladder injury – 3.3 1 – Hydrocele – 3.3; treated with aspiration [× 3 resolved] 1 – Bladder injury – 3.3

Table continues over

rather allow fixation of the tissue to occur on its own by the inflammatory reaction with sutures placed in the other three quadrants of the myopectineal orifice.

Mesh size has changed greatly since the beginning of laparoscopic inguinal herniorrhaphy. Initially a 3 × 5 cm patch was used to cover the internal ring, particularly in small indirect inguinal hernias[8]. However, the mesh size was often found to be too small and has now increased to approximately 8–12 × 10–15 cm. It is important that the entire myopectineal orifice be covered because of its anatomical significance with regard to direct, indirect and femoral hernia formation. Because it is difficult to assess visually the strength of the transversus abdominis aponeurosis and transversalis fascia at the time of surgery, it is important that all of these areas be strengthened with the use of the prosthesis at the initial procedure.

Although anterior inguinal herniorrhaphy and the preperitoneal approach are the 'gold standards' by which laparoscopic hernia repair should be judged, several conclusions can be reached from this study. The first conclusion is that the overall complication rate is low when a large prosthesis is placed over the entire myopectineal orifice. Secondly, simple closure of the internal ring is not adequate for long-term repair although it may be useful in patients who have type 1 hernias. The plug and patch technique of the internal ring is not an adequate repair as it addresses only an indirect inguinal hernia. Because it is difficult to assess the strength of the remaining portion of the transversus abdominis aponeurosis and fascia, it is important that the entire myopectineal orifice be covered.

Another conclusion is that direct recurrences were more common in this series although not statistically significant. Recurrences occurred more frequently in the early experience of the surgeon, emphasizing the importance of a learning curve, as suggested by Fitzgibbons *et al.*[14]. The reason for hernia recurrences in this series was primarily related to a small prosthesis and inadequate fixation of the prosthesis. The removal of the indirect hernia sac was noted as having no significance, and it may have actually increased the potential for testicular and scrotal pain following the procedure. However, most investigators in this series removed a direct hernia sac and this technical feature

Table 46.1 *continued*

	Patients/ Hernias	*Age* (years)	*Follow up*	*No – Complications – %*
4 Repair of inguinal hernia with a large prosthesis				
A Transperitoneal onlay prosthesis	182/186	13–78 av. 48	3–52 wk av. < 5 mo.	6 – Recurrences – 3.2 (2 retained hernias) 3 – Scrotal hydrocele – 1.6 resolved with aspiration 2 – Bladder injury – 1.0 1 – Abdominal bloating – 0.5 1 – Urinary retention – 0.5 1 – Thigh pain – 0.5 1 – Pelvic osteitis – 0.5
B Transabdominal preperitoneal repair with prosthesis	328/359	32–84 av. 52.5	13–104 wk av. 5 mo.	3 – Recurrence – 0.84 (2 = questionable) 11 – Haematomas – 3.0 7 – Scrotal 2 – Trocar insertion site 2 – Inguinal preperitoneal space 8 – Thigh pain – 2.2% 8 – Emphysema of scrotum – 2.2 7 – Urinary retention – 1.1
C Extra peritoneal repair using video	53/90	27–75 av. 45	3–40 wk av. 7 mo.	0 – Recurrence – 0 6 – Haematomas – 6.6 5 – Inguinal canal 1 – Anterior abdominal wall 1 – Testicular pain – 1.1
D *Summary*: repair of inguinal hernia with a large prosthesis	563/635	13–84 av. 48.5	3–104 wk av. 5.6 mo.	9 – Recurrences – 1.4 17 – Haematomas – 2.6 9 – Thigh pain – 1.4 8 – Emphysema of scrotum – 1.2 8 – Urinary retention – 1.2 3 – Scrotal hydrocele – 0.4 2 – Bladder injury – 0.3 1 – Pelvic osteitis – 0.15 1 – Abdominal bloating – 0.15 1 – Testicular pain – 0.15

Reprinted, with permission, from Jensen SL, Olsen D, Ferrers A: *Textbook of Videoscopic Surgery*, Berlin: Springer-Verlag, 1993

created redundant peritoneum and allowed for easier closure of the peritoneum. This decreased the chance of contact of the intestine against the prosthesis and subsequent development of small bowel obstruction. In addition, haematomas occasionally developed in the inguinal canal or the scrotum after removal of an indirect inguinal hernia sac. They occurred most frequently when the sac extended down into the scrotum.

So-called retained hernias that developed after a procedure were often asymptomatic and were most probably related to either inadequate fixation of the mesh or redundancy of the mesh. Thus intra-abdominal pressure tended to cause protrusion of the mesh material until fixation of the mesh occurred.

Although intra-abdominal adhesions were not noted in this study, subsequent reports have indicated a small incidence of small bowel obstruction, especially when the peritoneum over the mesh was not closed completely, thus allowing contact of the small bowel to the prosthesis.

Summary

It appears, therefore, that the best repair at the present time is the placement of a prosthesis over the entire myopectineal orifice, and this mesh can be positioned either transabdominally or extraperitoneally. Over all, the complication rate of laparoscopic herniorrhaphy is low and, as clinical experience increases, the learning curve and potential complications will decrease. It appears that laparoscopic inguinal herniorrhaphy will become the procedure of choice, for the complication rate is low and postoperative pain is significantly reduced compared to anterior inguinal herniorrhaphy.

References

1. American College of Surgeons. Sections B–L. In: Polister P, Cunico E, eds. *Socio-economic factbook for surgery*. Chicago: American College of Surgeons, 1989: 25–42.
2. Barnes JP. Inguinal hernia repair with routine use of Marlex mesh. *Surg Gynecol Obstet* 1987; **165**: 33–7.
3. Lichtenstein IL, Shulman AG, Amid PK, *et al.* The tension-free hernioplasty. *Am J Surg* 1989; **157**: 188–92.
4. Stoppa RE, Rives JL, Warlaumont CR, *et al.* The use of Dacron in the repair of hernias of the groin. *Surg Clin North Am* 1984; **64**: 269–85.
5. Corbitt JD. Laparoscopic herniorrhaphy. *Surg Laparosc Endosc* 1991; **1**: 23–5.
6. Fitzgibbons Jr RJ, Salerno GM, Filipi CJ, Hart RO. A laparoscopic intraperitoneal onlay mesh technique for repair of an indirect inguinal hernia (intraperitoneal onlay mesh procedure). *Am Surg*, in press
7. Popp LW. Improvement in endoscopic hernioplasty: transcutaneous aquadissection of the musculofascial defect and preperitoneal endoscopic patch repair. *J Laparoendosc Surg* 1991; **1**: 83–90.
8. Shultz L, Graber J, Pietraffita J, Hickok D. Laser laparoscopic herniorrhaphy: a clinical trial preliminary results. *J Laparoendosc Surg* 1990; **1**: 41.
9. Ger R. The management of certain abdominal hernias by intraabdominal closure of the sac. *Ann R Coll Engl* 1982; **64**: 342–4.
10. Gazareli MM. Anatomical laparoscopic hernia repair of direct or indirect inguinal hernias using the transversalis fascia and iliopubic tract. *Surg Laparosc Endosc* 1992; **2**: 49–52.
11. Toy FK, Smoot Jr RT. (1991) Toy–Smoot laparoscopic hernioplasty. *Surg Laparosc Endosc* 1991; **1**: 151–5.
12. McKernan JB, Laws HL. Laparoscopic repair of inguinal hernias using a totally extraperitoneal prosthetic approach. *Surg Endosc* 1993; **7**: 26–8.
13. Starling JR, Harm BA. Diagnosis and treatment of genitofemoral and ilioinguinal neuralgia. *World J Surg* 1989; **13**: 586–91.
14. Fitzgibbons Jr RJ, Annibali R, Litke B, Filipi C, Salerno G, Cornet D. A multicentered clinical trial on laparoscopic inguinal hernia repair: preliminary results. *Surg Endosc* 1993; **7**: 115.

15. Ger R, Monroe R, Duvivier R, *et al.* Management of indirect inguinal hernias by a laproscopic closure of the neck of the sac. *Am J Surg* 1990; **159**: 370.

16. Nyhus LM, Pollack R, Bombeck CT, Donahue PE. The preperitoneal approach and prosthetic buttress repair for recurrent hernia. *Ann Surg* 1988; **179**: 567.

17. Rignault DP. Properitoneal prosthetic inguinal hernioplasty through a Pfannenstiel approach. *Surg Gynecol Obstet* 1986; **163**: 465.

18. Salerno GM, Fitzgibbons Jr RJ, Hart RO, Corbitt Jr RD, Fillipi CJ. Laparoscopic herniorrhaphy. In: Zucker KA, ed. *Surgical Laparoscopy Update.* St Louis: Quality Medical Publishing, 1992: 373–94.

47

Reasons for Recurrence following Laparoscopic Hernioplasty

EDWARD H PHILLIPS, BRENDAN J CARROLL, MOSES J FALLAS, MAURICE E ARREGUI, JOHN CORBITT Jr, ROBERT J FITZGIBBONS Jr, JOSEPH PIETRAFITA, ROBERT W SEWELL, ARNOLD S SEID, LEONARD S SCHULTZ, FREDERICK K TOY AND ROBERT L WADDELL

The incidence and reasons for recurrence following laparoscopic hernioplasty have not been studied. Because the incidence is small and follow up has been short, a multi-institutional study was performed among the pioneers in the field. Additional individual cases were accepted by the principal author when all the data could be reviewed.

Method

The incidence figures were obtained by a survey of surgeons who were selected because they had significant experience (over 100 cases) and kept concurrent records. The data on recurrences included some but not all cases in this survey. The information on recurrences included cases referred to the participants and cases submitted to the principal author.

Results

Fifty-four recurrences (1.7%) occurred after 3229 laparoscopic hernia repairs. There were 1944 transabdominal preperitoneal (TAPP) repairs with 19 recurrences (1%) and 578 preperitoneal repairs with no recurrences. There were 345 intraperitoneal onlay mesh (IPOM) repairs with seven recurrences (2%) and 286 plug and patch repairs with 26 recurrences (9%). Simple closures were performed 76 times with two recurrences (2.6%).

Fifty-seven patients had 60 recurrent hernias. Their average age was 49 years, and five patients (9%) had significant co-morbid illness. The recurrences were noted, on average, 5.1 months postoperatively (range 0–30 months).

There were 71 primary hernias present in these 57 patients. They were repaired as listed in Table 47.1.

There were 28 direct recurrent hernias. The number of primary techniques employed and the reasons for recurrence are listed in Table 47.2.

There were 32 indirect recurrent hernias. The number of primary techniques employed and the reasons for recurrence are listed in Table 47.3.

Twenty-six recurrences were repaired most commonly by traditional anterior approaches with mesh. However, three were repaired without mesh. Ten were repaired by the TAPP technique and two by IPOM. One each were repaired by the preperitoneal and the plug and patch techniques.

Table 47.1: Repair of 71 primary hernias in 57 patients

Direct Hernias	29	*Indirect hernias*	42
TAPP:	10	TAPP	19
IPOM:	7	IPOM	3
Plug and patch	12	Plug and patch	19
		Simple closure	1

Table 47.2: Primary techniques employed and reasons for recurrence of direct hernia

Technique	*Reason for recurrence*	
TAPP: 8	Mesh too small	6
	Clips pulled through	2
	Never stapled	1
	Other	2
IPOM: 7	Mesh too small	5
	Clips pulled through	1
	Other	1
Plug and patch: 12	Mesh too small Hernia never repaired	8
	Never stapled	4
Simple closure: 1	Never repaired	1

Table 47.3: Primary techniques employed and reasons for recurrence of indirect hernia

Technique	*Reason for recurrence*	
TAPP: 15	Never stapled	6
	Mesh too small	5
	Clips pulled through	3
	Hernia never repaired	1
	Other	3
IPOM: 2	Unknown because neither repaired yet	
Plug/patch: 15	Mesh too small	12
	Never stapled	8
	Never repaired	3
	Other	2

The most common reason for recurrence was that the mesh was too small – 36 (60%).

The mesh was never stapled in 19 instances (32%) and the hernia was never repaired in 3 cases (20%). The clips pulled through the tissue in six cases (8%) and in 10 cases (15%) the repair has not yet been undertaken or the aetiology was unclear. There was more than one reason in 19 patients.

The reasons for direct recurrences were similar to those in indirect recurrences.

Table 47.4: Reasons for recurrences: direct and indirect

Reasons for recurrences	*Direct*	*Indirect*
Mesh too small	19	17
Never stapled	5	14
Hernia never repaired	9	4
Clips pulled through	3	2
Other	3	7

Conclusions

Technical factors were responsible for nearly all early recurrences. The most common reason for recurrence following laparoscopic hernioplasty was an undersized mesh patch. The next most common cause was that the mesh was not stapled because of the unavailability of staplers early in the development of laparoscopic hernioplasty. The third most common reason was that the hernia was not repaired at the initial procedure and the least common was that the clips pulled through the tissue. Consequently, it is recommended that the largest possible piece of mesh is used and that it be stapled securely. It is also important to cover both the indirect and direct portions of the inguinal floor in all cases.

Acknowledgements

Special thanks to Arthur Kahn and Harvey Kalan for submitting case material, and to Emma Matt and Lizabeth Knight for help in preparing this document.

48

Transabdominal Preperitoneal Laparoscopic Inguinal Herniorrhaphy: Lessons Learned and Modifications

LEONARD S SCHULTZ, JOHN N GRABER AND DAVID F HICKOK

Transabdominal preperitoneal inguinal hernia repair is a technique that has evolved over a four-year period based upon analysis of outcome data. The results serve as the substance of this chapter.

In the initial series, dating back to 22 December 1989[1], the repair was based on the concept that two things cannot occupy the same space at the same time; that is, if we filled the inguinal defect with mesh plugs which were then covered over with a patch, abdominal contents could no longer herniate through the abdominal wall. This method, known as the 'plug and patch' technique, worked. To this day, with a 98%, 3½-year follow up, not one of these has recurred. However, there was a flaw to the thinking: we failed to realize that the rest of the inguinal area represented potential defects that also needed primary attention. As experience taught us, even with direct visual examination offered with laparoscopy, we could not adequately assess present or future integrity of the tissue surrounding the obvious hernia defect. Furthermore, the length of the plug was critical, as too long a plug resulted in extension beyond the external inguinal ring with pressure on the pubic bone causing significant discomfort in some patients.

From this experience, we shifted to the use of a more parachute-like plug which patients did not feel. We put it down the trocar, into the canal and then covered it over with another small patch of mesh. The peritoneal edges were then reapproximated over the mesh with Hulka clips, which were later replaced with haemostatic clips as they became available in 1990 (Figure 48.1).

Whether direct or indirect, the technique for hernia repair remained the same. Each was treated as an independent entity, and we fixed only what we visualized as a hernial defect. When we had the opportunity laparoscopically to reoperate a recurrence (in the unprotected area) we examined the mesh plugs. What we found was that they usually did not cause the effect we anticipated, notably a contraction of the tissue of the canal onto the plug. Rather, the plug appeared to condense into a fibrosed mass with minimal circumferential narrowing of tissue around it.

At the end of one year, we analysed our first 25 cases and noted eight recurrences with the failure always occurring in the unprotected portion of inguinal area. So we decided it was time to change our methods, which we did as of 18 October 1990. Based upon the observations discussed above, we started to make a peritoneal flap spanning the entire length of the inguinal area with an inferolateral extension so that one could visualize Cooper's ligament which defined the inferior extent of the dissection. The peritoneal sacs were dissected out and left attached to the flap whenever possible, to help provide the redundancy necessary to cover over the polypropylene mesh more easily. Although our favoured dissection tool at that time was the Nd:YAG laser with contoured tip 1000 μm quartz fibre, the high cost of using lasers forced conversion to electrosurgical energy when bipolar cutting–coagulation instrumentation became available (Figure 48.2). We have consistently avoided

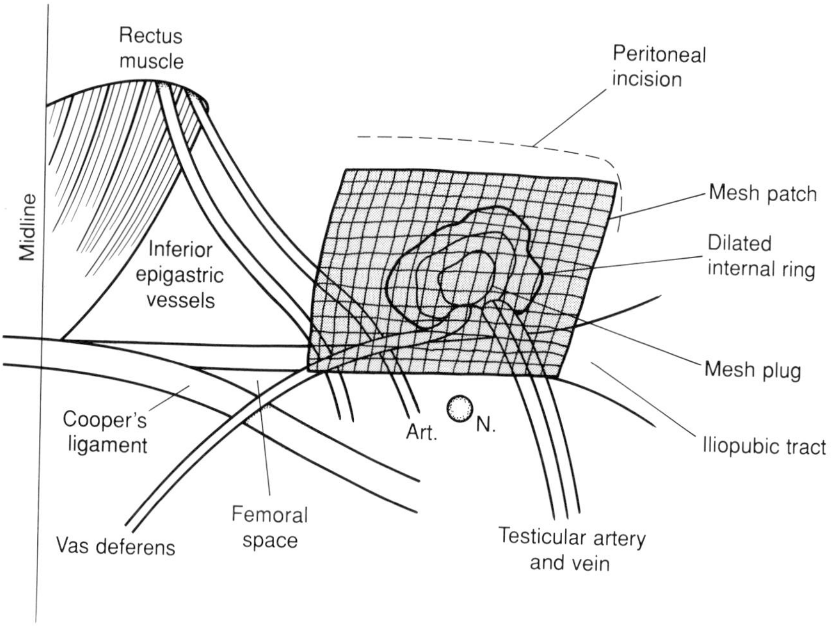

Figure 48.1: Diagrammatic representation of a plug and patch mesh hernia repair of a right indirect inguinal hernia.

the use of monopolar cautery which represents a distinct potential surgical hazard because of capacitative coupling and/or surface burns.

Once the inguinal area was dissected completely, the area was covered with an ever-increasing size of polypropylene mesh (Marlex, C.R. Bard Inc.) which now measures 14 × 11 cm. The mesh was rolled up tightly and placed within a 10 mm reducing sleeve which was then passed down a 10/11 mm trocar. Alternatively, the mesh can simply be pulled through the trocar and placed into the defect. Of course, pneumoperitoneum is sacrificed with this manoeuvre. Coverage extended from the line of Douglas just past the midline, over Cooper's ligament and lateral to the internal ring. In the initial series, before fixation devices were available, the mesh was placed superficial to the inferior epigastric vessels. Despite concern that the mesh might cause rupture or scarification of the vessels, in over three years of follow up it has never proved to be a problem. When fixation with staples became available in late 1991, the mesh was placed directly over the vessels, which no longer had to serve as a fixation technique.

Before the advent of staples, with simple placement of a large-sized prosthesis into the preperitoneal space, was tried for the correction of large scrotal hernias, including 'sliders'. Three failures followed, usually on the third or fourth postoperative day after a strong cough. Reoperation revealed that the mesh served as the leading edge of the herniation, which protruded through the external inguinal ring. It was soon realized that in 'sliders', where there is no internal ring and almost no intact transversalis fascia, the only structure preventing migration of the mesh was the external ring. The introduction of staplers prevented the migration of mesh and allowed the use of laparoscopic technique for all sizes and types of inguinal hernias. Staples attached the mesh into Cooper's ligament and transversalis fascia below the line of Douglas and into the midline fascia. The mesh extended

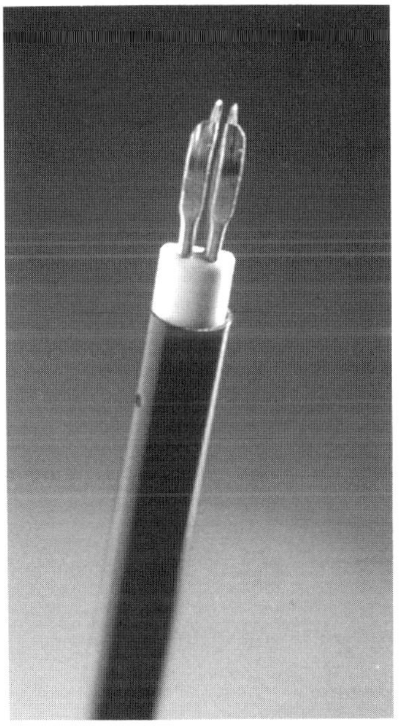

Figure 48.2: This bipolar probe (Everest Medical Inc., Minneapolis, Minnesota) replaced Nd:YAG laser dissection of the inguinal region. It has the capabilities of both incision and coagulation.

beyond the midline to offer support and to prevent recurrence through the suprapubic space. The same holds true for the femoral space which is also covered over by the mesh.

Just as there are areas that are stapled, there is one that we are reluctant to put staples into, and that is lateral and inferior to the internal inguinal ring. The policy has been followed for a long time because of the possibilities of nerve entrapment which can present in either of two ways. In the first type, there is immediate pain secondary to nerve impingement by the staple. This is not likely to resolve with time and pain medications. The other type is transient and usually manifests itself seven to ten days after the operative procedure. These cases are treated with heat and anti-inflammatories and they usually abate within a month, although the longest case that I known of took five months to resolve. Anatomically, the nerves involved are the lateral femoral cutaneous and the femoral branch of the genitofemoral nerve, which are parallel nerves located posterior to the mid point and just lateral to the internal inguinal ring in an anteroposterior orientation, after which they pierce muscle to continue over the anterior thigh (Figure 48.3).

It may not always be possible to avoid placing staples in this area, as in the case of large scrotal hernias where additional mesh fixation is desired. In such cases, lift up the iliopubic tract with an instrument, thus separating it from the femoral nerve below to prevent injury to this important structure. Furthermore, remember that staples need only a light touch, to provide fixation of mesh to the immediately adjacent transversalis fascia.

Finally, to complete the procedure, the peritoneal edges are reapproximated with closely placed staples so as to prevent the possible occurrence of small bowel obstruction. In our series, we have had four such occurrences: two in association with disruption of peritoneal closures done with haemoclips and two in patients with staple closures that were placed too far apart. In each case, the small bowel became adherent to the mesh from which is could be surgically separated. If this occurs, the night after surgery patients will complain of unremitting nausea which should not occur with this operation. Because of this experience, it is suggested that the staples be placed close together for peritoneal closure.

Our experience over the past three and a half years has identified three major requirements for success with this method for inguinal hernia repair.

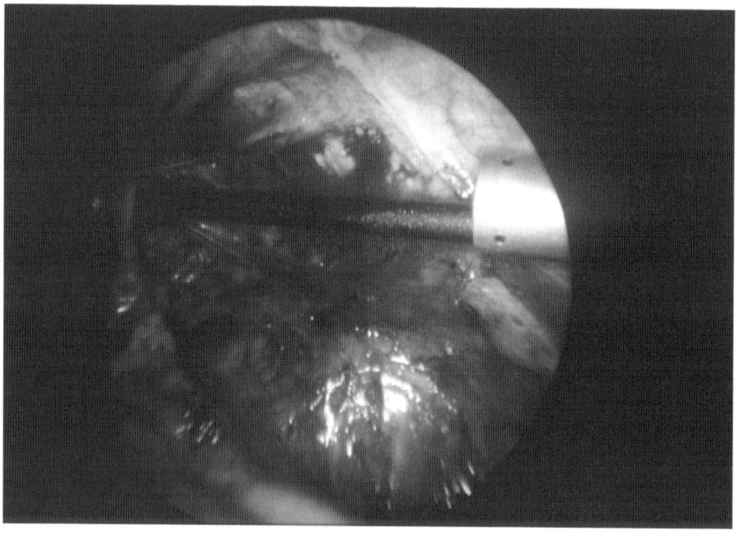

Figure 48.3: The lateral femoral cutaneous and femoral branch of the genitofemoral nerve. Not that the nerves run parallel to each other and pierce muscle at the lateral aspect of the mid internal inguinal ring.

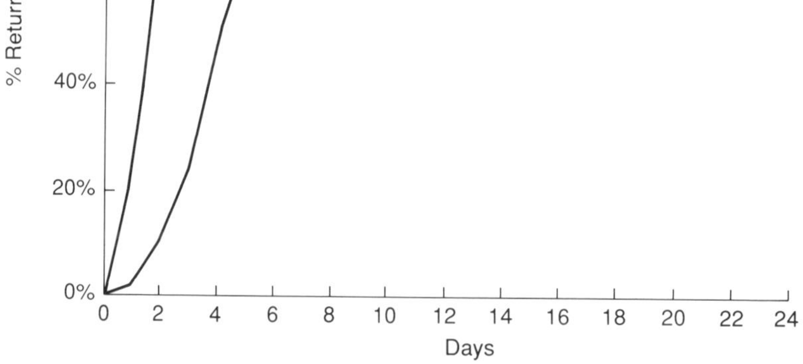

Figure 48.4: Return to activities of daily living (ADL) and work after operation. Data indicate a return to unrestricted activity in 80% of patients within five to seven days.

Table 48.1: Characteristics of the four groups (200 patients, 238 hernias)

Group	*Number of hernias*	*Definition*
I	58	Small mesh without fixation
II	120	Large mesh without fixation
III	10	Small mesh with staple fixation
IV	50	Large mesh with staple fixation

Table 48.2: Recurrence rates

Group	*Length of follow-up* (weeks)	*Rate of recurrence* (%)
I	128	26
II	88	0.7
III	46	20
IV	50	0

- Need for a size of polypropylene mesh that more than covers the entire inguinal area.
- The mesh requires staple fixation to allow use of this technique for all types of inguinal hernia.
- Staples for peritoneal closure must be placed close together to avoid bowel entrapment.

It has taken time to learn these things. During that period of learning, we were roundly criticized – as one would anticipate when introducing new techniques. But now, outcome data strongly suggest a successful method that deserves thoughtful consideration by the surgical community.

Results

We have studied our first 250 patients who had 311 inguinal hernias repaired laparoscopically. The average age was 46 years reflecting self-referrals by patients who sought out this procedure that promised a quick return to unrestricted activity. Their enthusiasm became infectious, especially after the difference in the degree of discomfort and shortened convalesence was compared with that of patients who had also experienced an earlier anterior repair (Figure 48.4).

Minor complications have included trocar site bleeding, urinary retention and shoulder-strap pain. Protocol revisions have corrected these problems. Postoperative neuralgias were a more serious concern not seen prior to the advent of staple fixation of the prosthesis. Again, technical changes with avoidance of staple placement lateral and inferior to the internal ring have done much to eliminate this complication.

The most important part of this discussion of results is the rate of recurrence. Fortunately, the evolving technique that was developed resulted in four groups of patients (Table 48.1), an examination of which reveals the parameters that are critical for a successful operation.

Group I, our earliest group, had a plug and patch repair of the visualized defect. The high recurrence rate (26%) led us to use an extended patch over the entire inguinal area, which resulted in the recurrence rate dropping to 0.7% (group II). The introduction of staples (group III), did not improve the plug and patch technique (20%) but as part of our standard technique (group IV), staple fixation has led to complete elimination of recurrence since its inception in 1991 (Table 48.2).

Conclusion

It is safe to conclude from these data that excellent results can be expected with transabdominal preperitoneal inguinal herniorrhaphy with polypropylene mesh when the principles developed during its evolutionary changes are upheld.

References

1. Schultz LS, Coraber JN, Pietrafitta J, *et al.* Laser laparoscopic herniorrhaphy: a clinical trial. Preliminary results. *J Laparosc Surg* 1990; **1**: 41–5.

2. Henry AK. Operation for femoral hernia by a midline extraperiton approach. *Lancet* 1936; **1**: 531–3.

Further Reading

Nyhus LM, *et al.* Preperitoneal herniorrhaphy. A preliminary report in 50 patients. *West J Surg* 1959; **67**: 48–53.

Stoppa R, Petit J, Henry X. Unsutured Dacron prosthesis in groin hernias. *Int Surg* 1975; **60**: 411–15.

Lichtenstein IL, Shulman AG. Ambulatory outpatient hernia surgery including a new concept, introducing tension free repair. *Int Surg* 1986; **71**: 1–6.

McKernan JB. Laws HL. Laparoscopic preperitoneal prosthetic repair of inguinal hernias. *Surg Rounds* 1992; **7**: 597–610.

Ger R, *et al.* Management of indirect inguinal hernia by laparoscopic closure of the neck of the sac. *Am J Surg* 1990; **159**: 371–3.

Schultz LS, *et al.* Laser laparoscopic herniorrhaphy: a clinical trial. Preliminary results. *J Laparosc Surg* 1990; **1**: 41–5.

49

Laparoscopic Repair of Recurrent Hernias – the German Experience

THOMAS NEUFANG, ARMIN BRÜGGEMANN, F-E LÜDTKE AND G LEPSIEN

Controversy regarding laparoscopic hernia surgery has aroused increasing interest in the methods and results of groin hernia repair in Germany. Conventional and laparoscopic techniques were the main topic of discussion at the annual meeting of German surgeons in Munich, in April 1993.

A study by Schumpelick, based on questionnaires, indicates that about 105 000 primary and 15 000 recurrent hernias are repaired in Germany every year[1]. These figures imply that overall about 14% of primary hernia repairs recur. Most primary and recurrent hernias are repaired using the Shouldice or Bassini techniques. The posterior approach and repairs using mesh are not common in Germany; laparoscopic methods are still in their infancy. The Shouldice repair seems to be the 'gold standard', low recurrence rates and the possibility of performing the procedure under local anaesthesia have been cited as the main advantage. Table 49.1 summarizes some recent results of groin hernia surgery in Germany.

Schumpelick from Aachen, perhaps the German surgeon most experienced in the Shouldice technique, and Ulrich from Dusseldorf report low recurrence rates for primary and recurrent hernias.

Willmen from Grevenbroich is one of the few surgeons using other techniques. He combines a Bassini repair with a so-called 'Vicryl cushion', consisting of a large block of Vicryl, which is shaped like a cushion. He placed this block on the posterior inguinal wall before tightening his Bassini sutures. His results may be the best achieved in Germany in recent years (Table 49.2)[1].

In contrast to the achievements of these experienced surgeons, are the preliminary results of a quality-control study, performed by Seidel from Sindelfingen, including nearly all hospitals in Baden-Wurttemberg (one of the smaller states in Germany). Evaluation of about 4100 patients showed a recurrence rate of 8.1% in primary and up to 36% in recurrent hernias (Table 49.3)[1].

Table 49.1: Groin hernia surgery in Germany

Number of operations per year		
Infants	28 000	
Adults:		
primary	105 000	
recurrent	15 000	
Techniques used		
	Primary	*Recurrent*
Bassini	39%	32%
Shouldice	48%	59%
Laparoscopic	6%	?

Numbers are based on answers received on 1656 questionnaires (evaluation was possible in 50.4%)[1]

Table 49.2: Some results using conventional techniques in Germany[1]

	Primary hernias		*Recurrent hernias*		*Follow up*	
	n	*Recurred*	*n*	*Recurred*	*%*	*Time*
Schumpelick (Shouldice)	1217	1.4%	532	2.8%	89	1 years
	460	1.0%	197	3.1%	85	5 years
Ulrich (Shouldice)	421	2.9%	73	5.9%	84	2 years
Willmen (Bassini + Vicryl 'cushion')	828	1.0%	189	1.7%	90	4 years

Table 49.3: Preliminary results of a quality control study in Baden-Württemberg, included 93 hospitals using Shouldice, Bassini and other techniques[1]

Primary hernias		*Recurrent hernias*		
n	*Recurred*	*n*	*Recurred*	*Follow up period*
4095	8.1%	516	36.2%	3–4 years

In summary, experienced surgeons may obtain excellent results but, in general, results are unsatisfactory, especially with recurrent hernias.

Few results of laparoscopic hernias repair have been published. Kunz and Beger from Ulm performed a laparoscopic preperitoneal mesh repair in 73 hernias. The recurrence rate with absorbable mesh was 25%; with non-absorbable material there were no recurrences. They operated on only two recurrent hernias[2]. Meyer reported a technique using a special needle (awl) to close the hernia defect by a transcutaneous stitch under laparoscopic control[3]. This technique had to be abandoned because of high recurrence rates and complications reported by other surgeons trying the method[4]. Despite this, many surgeons expect laparoscopic repair to improve results, especially in recurrent hernias.

Procedure

We started with laparoscopic hernia surgery in December 1990, using a plug and patch technique for 101 primary and recurrent hernias in 88 patients[5]. Absorbable material (polyglactin/polydioxanon) was used in 23 cases, non-absorbable polypropylene in 101 hernias.

In February 1992 we changed to a transabdominal preperitoneal mesh repair, using a piece of polypropylene mesh of 8 × 5 cm which was stapled to the posterior abdominal wall, overlying epigastric vessels and cord[6].

As we became more familiar with the laparoscopic technique and the preperitoneal view of the anatomy of the groin, we modified our methods, performing a more complete dissection of the posterior abdominal wall (Table 49.4). Indirect as well as direct defects are now closed using suturing, in an attempt to create a flat surface for placement of the mesh, which prevents the incarceration of the mesh into the defect. Creating tension with sutures is avoided. Posterior wall reinforcement is achieved by using a large (> 12 × 9 cm) polypropylene mesh. The mesh is cut at its anterior edge, and so can be placed between epigastric vessels and posterior abdominal wall, surrounding the cord posteriorly. The mesh is fixed with staples. The gap in the mesh is carefully closed with staples, using the underlying interfoveolar ligament for secure anchorage. Sometimes additional sutures are required. Laterally to the epigastric vessels no staples are placed below the iliopubic tract in order to prevent nerve injuries. The procedure is performed in the same way in primary as well as in recurrent hernias. A few cases of recurrent hernias following plug and patch have been successfully repaired with the same technique.

Table 49.4: Principal steps of laparoscopic preperitoneal mesh repair[1]

1 Incision of the peritoneum
2 Isolation of epigastric vessels
3 Mobilization of the cord; removal of lipoma
4 Suturing larger defects of posterior inguinal wall, laterally as well as medially
5 Mesh insertion (polypropylene < 12 × 9 cm):
 – between epigastric vessels and posterior inguinal wall
 – deep to the cord
6 Mesh fixation with staples
7 Closure of the peritoneum with sutures

Table 49.5: Results of 259 laparoscopic hernia repairs from December 1990 to 1993

	Primary hernias (n = 209)		*Recurrent hernias* (n = 50)		*Follow up*	
	n	*Recurred*	n	*Recurred*	%	*Time*
Plug and patch:						
absorbable	18	6 (30%)	5	2 (40%)	75	< 3 years
non-absorbable	67	7 (10.4%)	11	–		
Large preperitoneal patch, non-absorbable	124	2 (1.6%)	34	–	85	< 1 year

Results (Table 49.5)

The plug and patch technique resulted in high recurrence rates in primary hernias, especially when absorbable material was used. Fortunately, we did only a few cases using absorbable material. In contrast, results in recurrent hernias were better.

Laparoscopic reoperation of six patients with recurrent hernia following a plug and patch repair with absorbable (polyglactin/polydioxanon) mesh showed no macroscopic evidence of fibrous tissue induction; the material seemed to be completely absorbed without leaving any scars (these cases are not included in Table 49.4).

Preperitoneal repair with polypropylene mesh achieved good results in primary and recurrent hernias. The outcome is expected to be improved further by using suture closure of the defect(s) and improved mesh placement. Our two recurrencies occurred in the early series of transabdominal preperitoneal repair in which quite a small piece of mesh had been used, placed as a simple overlay on epigastric vessels and cord. Although these patients have not yet been operated on again, follow-up with ultrasound examination showed the reason for reccurrence: probably a new sac had developed, accompanying the cord structures and passing below the posterior edge of the mesh, which seemed to be lifted upwards. Similar ultrasound findings were obtained in a few patients with small pieces of mesh, which have so far shown no clinical evidence of recurrence. Figure 49.1 shows the incidence of recurrences in our series. Most of the recurrences occurred in the first year after surgery.

A brief overview of complications is given in Table 49.6. Both small bowel obstruction and postoperative bleeding were related to the lateral 12 mm trocar incisions. We now close any 12 mm incision carefully with sutures, using laparoscopic control. Cord injury occurred in one of our early patients, who suffered from pain in the lower right abdomen following an appendectomy. He needed adhesiolysis in addition to repair of his groin hernia. Cord injury occurred as a result of misinterpretation of the anatomy, which was confused by strong adhesions masking the normal inner aspect of the groin.

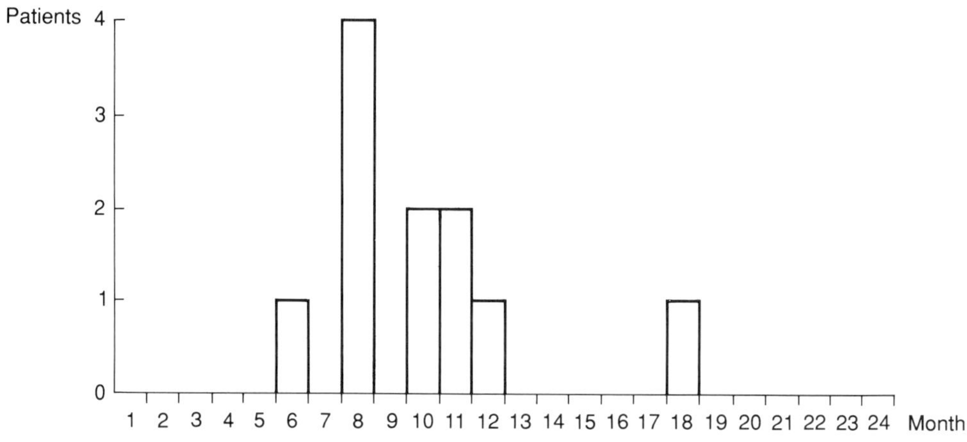

Figure 49.1: Incidence of recurrence.

Table 49.6: Major complications in 259 laparoscopic hernia repair

Dislocation (plug)	1
Injury of ductus deferens	1
Infection	1
Small bowel obstruction	1
Postoperative bleeding	1

Conclusions

- Results achieved with conventional techniques in the treatment of recurrent hernias are disappointing, especially those undertaken in non-specialized hospitals.
- The laparoscopic plug and patch technique with non-absorbable material produces acceptable recurrence rates in procedures repairing recurrent hernias, but has been abandoned because of high recurrence rates in primary hernias and other disadvantages.
- The laparoscopic transabdominal preperitoneal approach using polypropylene mesh is very suitable for recurrent hernias. Technique, rate of complications and results are the same as for primary hernias.
- Advances in operative technique (suture closure of the defect, larger mesh with better placement and fixation) should further improve the outcome.

Special considerations in recurrent hernias

- We repaired 16 recurrent hernias with plug and patch and 34 with preperitoneal mesh (*see* Table 49.5 for results). All of these recurrences had previously undergone Shouldice or Bassini repair.
- Preperitoneal dissection allowed precise anatomical identification of the type of recurrent defect (*see* Figure 49.2). Most of them – 68% – were found medially as direct hernias. We also observed three formal hernias.
- In most of our cases, recurrences presented three characteristic findings using a laparoscopic view (*see* Table 49.7): Recurrent defects seem to be localized commonly in the most medial corner

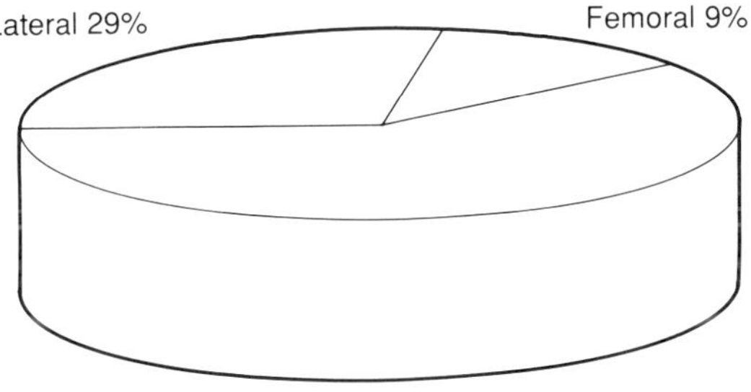

Figure 49.2: Recurrent hernias.

Table 49.7: Typical findings in direct recurrent hernias

Defect localized in the medial corner of Hesselbach's triangle
Iliopubic tract stretched upwards, resulting in opening of the femoral ring
Cord/internal ring pulled laterally

of Hesselbach's triangle, formed by the iliopubic tract and the origin of the rectus muscle at the public tubercle. In this area, tension created by the sutures used in classic methods of hernia repair are maximal[7]. This tension cannot disperse into surrounding soft tissue because there is none. The pubic tubercle, origin of rectus muscle together with 'conjoined tendon' as well as the iliopubic tract are hardly elastic structures, so they cannot be approximated by sutures without causing tension. Thus, transversalis fascia is overstreched when the suture is tightened, leading to recurrence from intra-abdominal pressure later.

References

1. Schumpelick V, Seidel W, Ulrich B, Willmen HR. *110. Kongress der Deutschen Gesellschaft für Chirurgie*, Hernia Session. Munich, Germany 13–17 April 1993.

2. Kunz R, Schütze F, Beger HG. Laparoskopischer Bruchpfortenverschluβ der Leistenhernie. *Chirurg* 1993; **64**: 341–5.

3. Meyer HJ. Die laparoskopisch kontrollierte Herniorrhaphie direkter und indirekter Leistenbrüche. *Chirurg* 1992; **63**: 353–6.

4. Wilker DK. Unsere Erfahrungen mit dem laparoskopisch kontrollierten perkutanen Hernienverschluss. 3. Workshop Laparoskopische Operationen. *Hernie – Colon: Trend '9e3*. Göttingen, Germany, 25–26 June 1993.

5. Schultz L, Graber J, Pietraffitta J, Hickok D. Laser laparoscopic herniorrhaphy: a clinical trial. Preliminary results. *J Laparoendosc Surg* 1990; **1**: 41–5.

6. Arregui ME, Chad JD, Osman Y, Nagan RF. Laparoscopic mesh repair of inguinal hernia using a preperitoneal approach: a preliminary report. *Surg Laparosc Endosc* 1992; **1**: 1–6.

7. Read RC, McLeod PC. Influence of a relaxing incision on suture tension in Bassini's and McVay's repairs. *Arch Surg* 1981; **116**: 440–5.

50

Bursting Strength Evaluation: Comparison of 0-Prolene Sutures and Endoscopic Staples in an Experimental Prosthetic Patch Repair of Abdominal Wall Defect*

YVES-MARIE DION, JAMAL CHARARA AND ROBERT GUIDOIN

The repair of groin hernias is classically divided into two broad categories[1]. One is the herniorrhaphic repair, which uses sutures to approximate tissue[2–4]. The other is the hernioplastic type of repair, in which a mesh is used to cover the defect. A giant mesh (20 × 30 cm) placed in the preperitoneal space is immobilized by the intra-abdominal pressure[5–8]; a relatively small mesh (7 × 12 cm) must be fixed in place by sutures to prevent displacement or deformation, leading to recurrence[5,9–12].

How well fixed to the surrounding healthy musculoaponeurotic layer this small prothesis should be is an unsettled issue. Staples were recently designed to fix the mesh laparoscopically. We compared in an *ex vivo* abdominal wall defect model the force needed to disrupt (bursting strength (BS)) the defect repaired with Prolene mesh attached to tissue using 0-Prolene suture, the Endopath EMS stapler or the Endo Hernia stapler. These two staplers were tested because they were the only ones of clinical interest. In the second part of the study, mechanical testing of sutures and staples were performed.

The study

For the first part of the experiment (the *ex vivo* study), we used 16 35-kg female piglets of the same age (12–13 weeks) and breed. A xyphopubic incision was performed under general anaesthesia. The skin, subcutaneous tissue and peritoneum were removed so that only the musculoaponeurotic layers of the abdominal wall remained. Two 3.5 × 6 cm elliptic incisions were then made, one on each side of the abdominal wall. A Prolene mesh (Ethicon Endo-Surgery, Cincinnati, Ohio) measuring 5 × 8 cm was placed on the inner surface of each defect and maintained in place on one side of the abdomen with interrupted 0-Prolene sutures (Ethicon Endo-Surgery) tied with at least four knots, and on the other side with Endopath EMS staples (Ethicon Endo-Surgery) (group 1, 8 piglets), or with Endo Hernia staples (Auto Suture, Norwalk, Connecticut) (group 2, 8 piglets) (Figures 50.1 and 50.2). Sutures and staples were evenly distributed around the defect site. An average of 17 0-Prolene sutures was sufficient to achieve an adequate repair. For this study, 20 staples were applied through the mesh into healthy muscle parallel to this acute defect. The stapling technique is similar to that used clinically.

*This chapter is reproduced with the kind permission of Springer-Verlag, New York, and has been accepted for publication in *Surgical Endoscopy*.

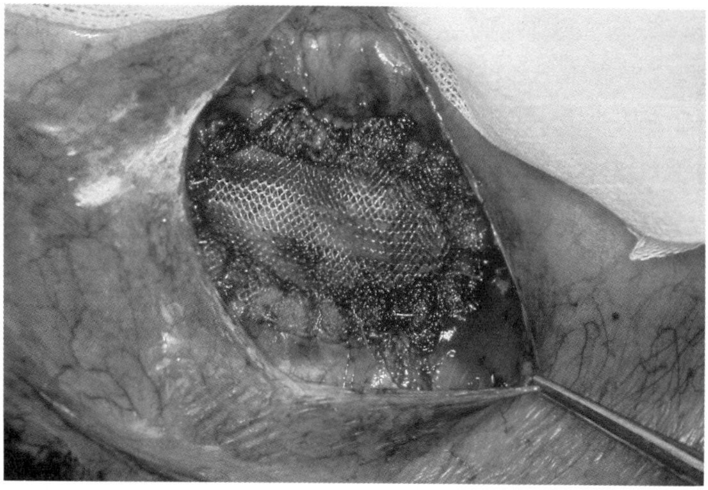

Figure 50.1: Porcine abdominal wall defect model. After a midline laparotomy, preperitoneal fixation of a Prolene mesh is performed with 0-Prolene sutures, as in this case, or with staples.

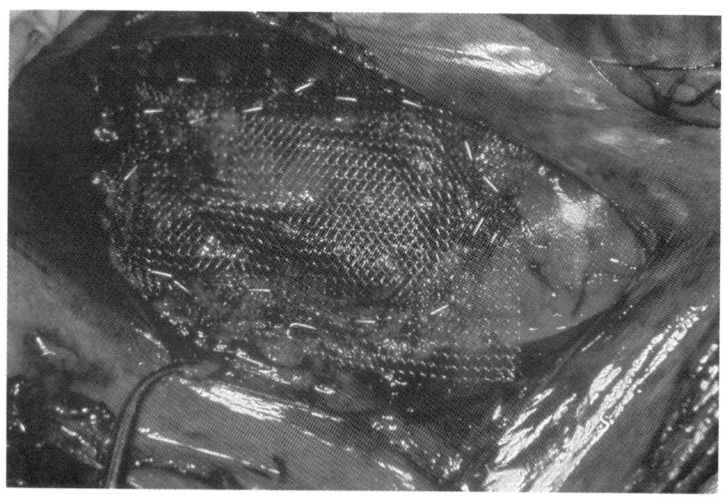

Figure 50.2: Porcine abdominal wall defect model: preperitoneal fixation of a Prolene mesh with staples. This photograph was taken during a preliminary study; one can see that the mesh is too small, does not cover adequately the defect and the clips are not evenly distributed. Appropriate corrections were made for the present study.

A large portion of the abdominal wall was then removed and placed in 0.9% saline solution at 4 °C until BS measurements were performed (within four hours).

Measurement of the BS of the abdominal wall defect model was carried out with a well-known device for testing materials, an Instron tester, model 1122, fitted with a compression cell (5000 N load cell, crosshead speed 200 mm/min), a specially designed cylindrical probe with a spherical tip (7.62 cm in diameter) and a special holder for circular specimens (10 cm diameter) (Figure 50.3). The force was recorded in newtons and converted to millimetres of mercury by dividing by the area of the specimen supporting the applied load. The Instron tester is basically a device that records the force applied on the specimen by a moving probe (Figure 50.3). Photographs of the specimens were taken before and after the bursting test for macroscopic evaluation.

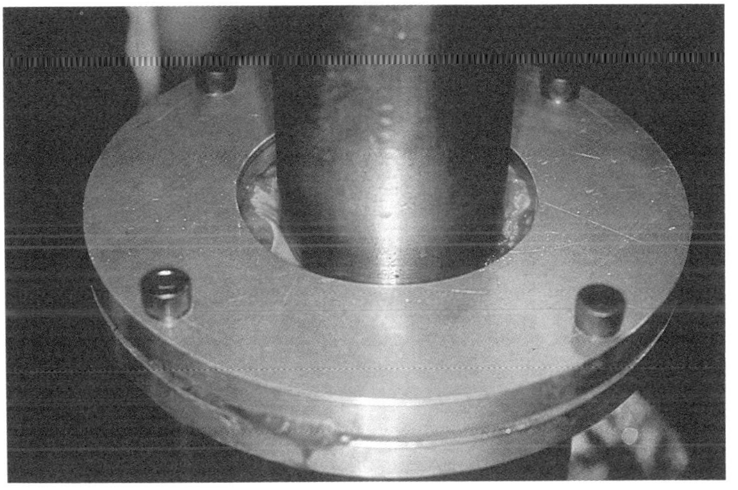

Figure 50.3: Specimen during the bursting strength test. Note the advancing cylindrical probe applying the load on the tissue.

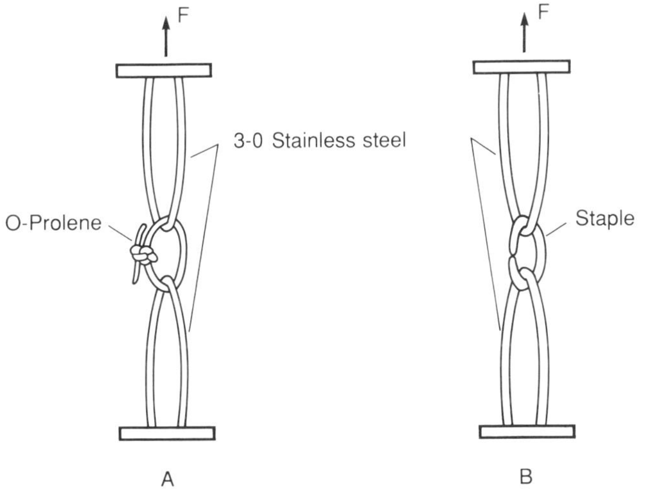

Figure 50.4: Schematic illustration of the model used for the tensile strength test evaluating 0-Prolene sutures and staples.

In the second part of this experiment (the mechanical tests), we performed the mechanical characterization of the 0-Prolene suture and the surgical staples. The longitudinal tensile strength test was performed first on five 0-Prolene sutures (Figure 50.4). A surgical knot was made and two stainless steel wires were passed through the suture. The strength test was then performed using the Instron model 1130 tensile tester (500 N load cell, crosshead speed 100 mm/min). Five staples of each group were also similarly tested.

Then One-Way Analysis of Variance and the Newman–Keuls Multiple Comparison Test were used for statistical evaluation of the data.

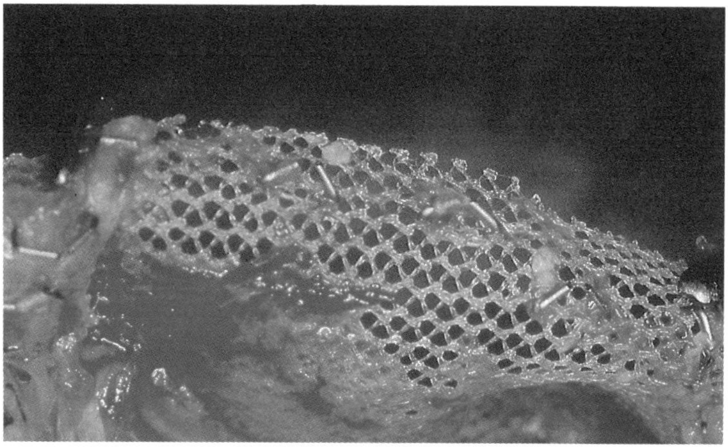

Figure 50.5: Specimen maintained in the holder prior to bursting strength testing.

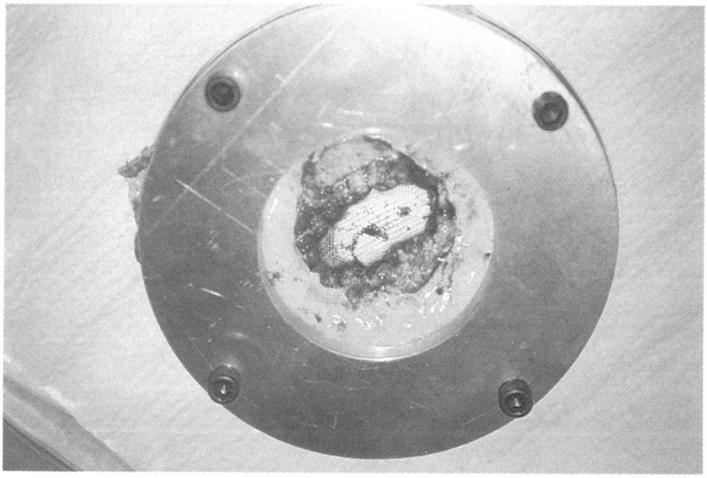

Figure 50.6: Typical appearance of the specimen after bursting (view from the undersurface of the mesh). Disruption has occurred at the site of fixation of the mesh to the tissue. Staples can be observed still fixed to the mesh at sites of disruption.

Results

Figure 50.5 shows a specimen maintained in the holder prior to BS testing with the Instron machine, while Figure 50.3 shows the specimen during the bursting test. Bursting was mostly due to tissue failure at the prosthesis muscle interface (Figure 50.6). Two of the 16 meshes fixed with 0-Prolene sutures tore with no evidence of tissue disruption at the site of fixation. In the other 14 repairs, tissue failed. The mean BS of the mesh attached with 0-Prolene was 1461.1 mmHg (s.d. 127.4) in the eight piglets whose other side was treated with EMS staples and 1462.2 mmHg (s.d. 217.5) in the piglets whose other side was fixed with the Endo Hernia staples ($p = 0.988$), confirming the homogeneity of the population studied.

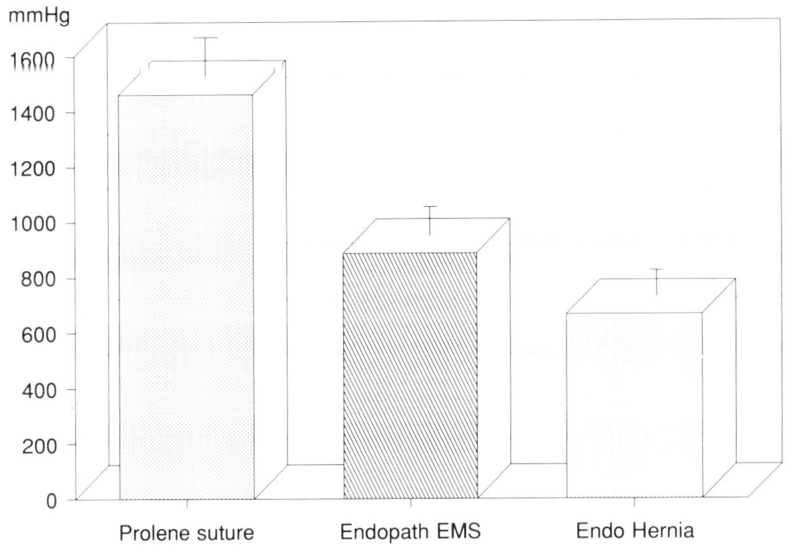

Figure 50.7: Bursting strength of a mesh fixed with 0-Prolene sutures, Endopath EMS and Endo Hernia staples. Significant difference is noted between each group ($p < 0.05$).

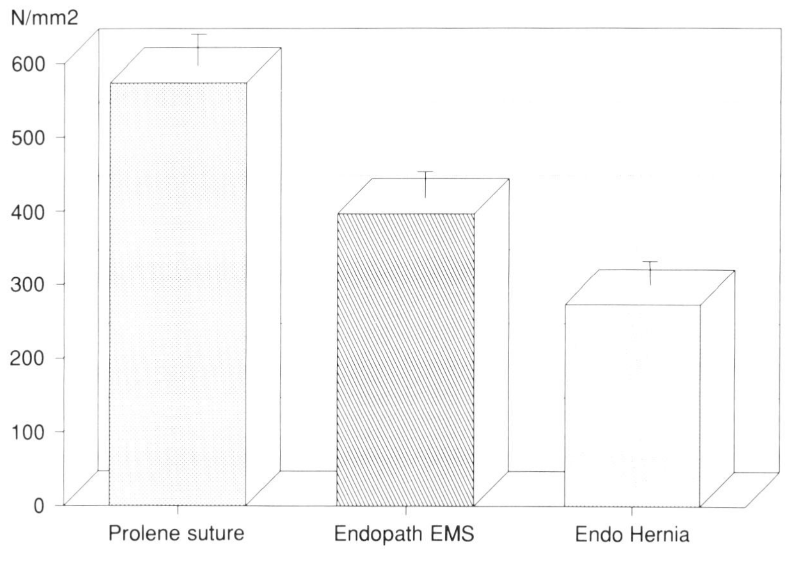

Figure 50.8: Tensile strength test results. Significant difference ($p < 0.05$) is noted between each type of suture material, the strongest being the 0-Prolene suture and the weakest the Endo Hernia staple.

The mean BS of the mesh fixed with the Endopath EMS staples was 885.6 mmHg (s.d. 121.4) and that of the mesh fixed with Endo Hernia staples was 665.4 mmHg (s.d. 122.9). The difference between the BSs of the mesh fixed with 0-Prolene sutures and both types of staples was statistically significant ($p < 0.05$) (Figure 50.7). The difference between the BSs of the mesh fixed with the Endopath EMS staples and the Endo Hernia staples was also significant ($p < 0.05$) (Figure 50.7).

The tensile strength test results of the different suture types tested are shown in Figure 50.8. It can be seen that the force needed to break a 0-Prolene suture (573.86 N/mm^2, s.d. 55.18) is significantly higher than that necessary to open the staples ($p < 0.05$). Endopath EMS staples (396.42 N/mm^2, s.d. 29.55) are stronger than their Endo Hernia (272.73 N/mm^2, s.d. 34.77) counterparts ($p < 0.05$).

Conclusions

Tension on the repair is identified as an important factor causing recurrent herniation[5,13]. A variety of studies have evaluated the acute rise in the intra-abdominal pressure following different activities[14–16]. It is noticeable that coughing or straining causes a greater increase than lifting 25 kg or jogging[17]. Maximum intra-abdominal pressure noted in a human while coughing is 220 mmHg, and while straining is 150 mmHg[15]. Because these two activities occur early in the postoperative period, stress is delivered to the repair well before fibrocyte infiltration of the mesh takes place. In our model, the slow speed of the probe used during measurements (200 mm/min) (*see* Figure 50.3) could simulate straining rather than coughing. Although maximal intra-abdominal pressure encountered in human seems far lower than pressures needed to disrupt the repair of our animal model, one cannot conclude that the three repairs performed in our experiment are equally effective, as the reported values of intra-abdominal pressure were obtained from different studies. Our animal abdominal wall defect model is not similar to the human groin defect.

Factors known to influence the development of human groin hernias are summarized by Stoppa[18,19].

- Anatomical factors may weaken the inguinal region: presence of two orifices, the inguinal and the femoral; conformation of the pelvis: a male pelvis, deep and narrow, would allow for a wider musculopectineal orifice (corresponding to the posterior wall and the two orifices) than a female pelvis which is shallow and wide, explaining the decreased frequency of inguinal hernias in the female who also has the rather small round ligament in lieu of the large cord of the male.
- Anomaly of collagen synthesis; fatty degeneration, disorganization, fissure formation and decreased elasticity of aponeurotic fibres[20,21].
- A dynamic factor other than the intra-abdominal pressure already alluded to is the protective (shutter) mechanism of the posterior wall, which may become deficient either because of anatomical muscular variation or the effect of ageing. The erect position opens and weakens the groin region.

Summing up on these factors involved in the development of recurrence of groin hernias, Stoppa wrote: 'The fact of musculofascial weakness having taken the lead over the saccular hernia theory has important consequences in the choice of repairs available to the surgeon. Prosthetic repairs benefit by their logic and radical aim.'[22].

Stoppa believes that 'the principle of the giant bilateral prosthesis (the immediate and definitive stability of the prosthesis owing to Pascal's hydrostatic principle) is different from those of all classical herniorrhaphies and hernioplasties using prosthetic patches (small meshes)'[11].

Stoppa[12,23], Rives[9,10], Bendavid[24] and Nyhus[25], among others, consider that when a relatively small mesh (7 × 12 cm) is used for the treatment of groin hernias, it must be fixed to surrounding structures. Giving further support to the concept of adequte fixation of the patch, Neufang[26] has noted, following laparoscopic and ultrasonic evaluation, cases of recurrent herniation associated with contraction of the patch attributed to the process of incorporation.

What should be considered sufficient fixation of a patch (small mesh)? Our study was not designed to answer this question but rather to evaluate the respective merits of each type of suture.

The abdominal wall of piglets is composed of the same three muscles and fascias encountered in humans[27]. Individual muscles measure approximately 2.5 mm in thickness except the transversus abdominis which is thinner, averaging 1.0 mm. 0-Prolene sutures penetrated all layers without difficulty, whilst staples reached the internal oblique.

The difference in results between the 0-Prolene sutures and staples as well as between the staples themselves can be explained by the fact that the staple penetrates less tissue than a suture (5–7 mm). The former can therefore be dislodged with less force than the latter. We measured the leg length of fired staples and found that they were 1.5–1.7 mm for the Endopath EMS staple and 0.95–1.2 mm for the Endo Hernia stapler.

The strength of the different suture materials was different, as demonstrated by the tensile strength tests. These tests evaluated in newtons per square millimetre the point at which a 0-Prolene sutures breaks and staples open or break. Figure 50.8 shows a significant difference between the sutures and the staples ($p < 0.05$). This test also shows that Endopath EMS staples are significantly stronger ($p < 0.05$) than the Endo Hernia staples. The reason is that the Endo Hernia staple is square when looked at in cross-section, whilst the Endopath EMS is circular. This difference in staple geometry is important because the mechanical stress applied on the clip is force divided by the area on which this force is applied (the Endopath EMS staples provides more surface in cross-section than the Endo Hernia staple). Therefore, more mechanical stress is sustained by the Endo Hernia staple than by the Endopath EMS staple when a similar force is applied. The engineer explains the phenomenon in terms unfamiliar to the surgeon: 'since the cross-section of the Endo Hernia staple is square, the force during loading is applied to the front area of the staple, which is 0.40 mm thick as measured by a micrometric device. In the case of the Endopath EMS staple, which has a circular cross-section, the load is applied to the front half perimeter area, which is 0.82 mm ($\pi \times 0.52/2$, where the diameter is 0.52 mm). Therefore, the shape of the Endopath EMS staple has the advantage of reducing the applied stress.' The longitudinal strength test was performed to compare the mechanical resistance of each type of suture. We did not intend to relate these results to the bursting strength test.

Summary

Our *ex vivo* study was designed to evaluate the maximal stress (BS) that a repair performed with 0-Prolene suture or staples can bear. Although our results obtained from animal studies cannot be directly translated to humans, they allow for comparison between 0-Prolene sutures, which are frequently used for various hernia repairs, and the two types of staples. This study shows that repair of an abdominal wall defect with a mesh fixed with 0-Prolene is stronger than one fixed with staples. Stapling with the Endopath EMS stapler produces a significantly higher BS than stapling with the Endo Hernia. The mechanical experiment confirmed that, of the three suture materials used, 0-Prolene was the strongest. The Endopath EMS staple was significantly stronger than the Endo Hernia staple.

References

1. Rignault DP. Properitoneal prosthetic inguinal hernioplasty through a Pfannenstiel approach. *Surg Gynecol Obstet* 1986; **163**: 465–8.
2. Bassini E. *Nuovo metodo per la cura radicale dellernia inguinale*. Padua: Prosperini, 1889.
3. Lazorthes F, Browne AF. Cure de hernie inguinale selon la technique de Shouldice. *J Chir (Paris)* 1984; **121**: 765–70.
4. McVay CB, Chapp JD. Inguinal and femoral hernioplasty: evaluation of a basic concept. *Ann Surg* 1958; **148**: 499–512.
5. Nyhus LM, Klein MS, Rogers FB. Inguinal hernia. *Curr Probl Surg* 1991; **28**: 401–450.

6. Stoppa R. The treatment of complicated groin and incisional hernias. *World J Surg* 1989; **13**: 545–54.
7. Stoppa R, Petit J, Abourachid H, *et al.* Procédé original de plastie des hernies de l'aine: l'interposition sans fixation d'une prothèse en tulle de Dacron par voie médiane sous péritonéale. *Chirurgie* 1973; **99**: 119–24.
8. Stoppa R, Petit J, Henry X. Unsutured Dacron prosthesis in groin hernias. *Int Surg* 1975; **60**: 411–12.
9. Rives J, Fortesa F, Drouard J, Hibon J, Flament JB. La voie d'abord abdominale sous-péritonéale dans le traitement des hernies de l'aine. *Ann Chir* 1976; **32**: 245–53.
10. Rives J, Lardennois B, Flament JB, Convers G. La pièce en tulle de Dacron, traitement de choix des hernies de l'aine de l'adulte. *Chirurgie* 1973; **99**: 564–75.
11. Stoppa R. Groin hernia repair. In Arregui M and Nagan RF, eds. *Inguinal hernia: advances or controversies?* Oxford: Radcliffe Medical Press, 1994.
12. Stoppa R, Warlaumont C, Verhaeghe P, Henry X. Tulle de Dacron et cure chirurgicale des hernies de l'aine. *Chirurgie* 1983; **109**: 847–54.
13. Lichtenstein IL, Shulman AG, Amid PK, Montllor MM. The tension free hernioplasty. *Am J Surg* 1989; **157**: 188–93.
14. Grew ND. Intraabdominal pressure response to loads applied to the torso in normal subjects. *Spine* 1980; **5**: 149–54.
15. Hemborg B, Moritz U, Hamberg J, Holmstrom E, Lowing H, Akesson I. Intra-abdominal pressure trunk muscle activity during lifting. *Scand J Rehabil Med* 1985; **17**: 15–24.
16. Nachemson AL, Andersson GBJ, Schultz AB. Valsalva maneuver biomechanics. Effects on lumbar trunk loads of elevated intraabdominal pressures. *Spine* 1986; **11**: 476–9..
17. Twardowski ZJ, Khanna R, Nolph KD, *et al.* Intraabdominal pressures during natural activities in patients treated with continuous ambulatory peritoneal dialysis. *Nephron* 1986; **44**: 129–35.
18. Stoppa R, Verhaeghe P, Marasse E. Mécanisme des hernies de l'aine. *J Chir (Paris)* 1987; **124**: 125–31.
19. Stoppa R, Warlaumont C, Verhaeghe P. Comment se constitue une hernie de l'aine? *Revue du Praticien* 1987; **37**: 2337–742.
20. Peacock EE. Biology of hernia. In: Peacock EE *Hernia*, 2nd ed. Philadelphia: JB Lippincott, 1978: 79–93.
21. Read RC. Preperitoneal exposure of inguinal herniation. *Am J Surg* 1968; **116**: 653–8.
22. Stoppa R. Groin hernia repair. In Arregui M and Nagan RF, eds. *Inguinal hernia: advances or controversies?* Oxford: Radcliffe Medical Press 1994.
23. Stoppa R, Henry X, Verhaeghe P, Odimba BBK. La place des prothèses réticulées non résorbables dans le traitement chirurgical des hernies de l'aine. *Chirurgie.* 1981; **107**: 333–41.
24. Bendavid R. New techniques in hernia repair. *World J Surg* 1989; **13**: 522–31.
25. Nyhus LM. The recurrent groin hernia: therapeutic solutions. *World J Surg* 1989; **13**: 541–4.
26. Neufang T. Laparoscopic repair of recurrent hernias – the German experience. In Arregui M, Nagan RF, eds. *Inguinal Hernia: advances or controversies?* Oxford: Radcliffe Medical Press, 1994.
27. Odlaug TO. *Laboratory anatomy of the fetal pig*, 3rd ed. 1966: Dubuque, Iowa: WMC Brown, 8–19.

Part IV: Selected studies on hernia repair

Diagnosis of inguinal hernias
Classification of inguinal hernias
Open repair of inguinal hernias
Laparoscopic repair of inguinal hernias
- Transabdominal preperitoneal repair of inguinal hernias
- Transabdominal preperitoneal repair of recurrent hernias
- Totally extraperitoneal repair of inguinal hernias using mesh
- Intraperitoneal repair of inguinal hernias with mesh
- Laparoscopic repair of inguinal hernias with high ligation

Technical modifications in laparoscopic hernia repairs
Complications in laparoscopic hernia repairs
Mesh considerations in hernia repairs
Repair of ventral hernias

51

The Role of Herniography In Undiagnosed Groin Pain

MOHAMMED BADRUDDOJA, IRVING M BUSH, GABRIEL ANGRES,
SHAHID AZIZ ANSARI, MICHAEL P SCHWARTZ AND KENNETH P SULLIVAN

Unilateral or bilateral, persistent, undiagnosed groin pain is a challenge to urologists, gynaecologists and general surgeons, as well as to family physicians. This is especially true if symptoms are work related without physical signs of groin hernia. Various techniques are currently available to establish the diagnosis of undiagnosed groin pain (Table 51.1). Some of these techniques are unreliable, others are expensive, and some are expensive and invasive.

Herniography is of great value in the diagnostic procedures for undiagnosed groin pain due to occult groin hernia. The presence of hernia is very frequently found by herniography and such occult hernia is the cause of groin pain[1]. Some reports in the surgical literature have mentioned that small peritoneal protrusions represent early hernia and can only be diagnosed by herniography[2]. The role of herniography in detecting occult groin hernias causing groin pain is well documented[3]. However, this simple, inexpensive and minimally invasive technique has not been used. Instead, expensive invasive investigations have been used to diagnose this ailment[4]. The most recent report shows that, during laparoscopy, one can find dilated ring or syndrome of broad and deep fossae in about 35% of the cases[5]. Such patients do not have any symptoms and this indicates that laparoscopic evaluation of inguinal ring is not an appropriate investigation of groin pain due to groin hernia. The purpose of this chapter is to describe the simple technique of herniography, and its role in the diagnosis of occult groin hernia causing persistent groin pain.

The patients

We have studied a highly select group of 26 patients over a period of 18 months. Each of these patients had persistent, long-standing groin pain for a period of six months to two years. They had been treated as cases of either urological disorder in males or pelvic problems in females (Table 51.2).

Table 51.1: Methods available for diagnosis

Physical examination
Ultrasonography
Computed tomography
Diagnostic laparoscopy
Herniography:
Indirect
Direct
Herniography with femoral venography (Gullomo)

Table 51.2: Clinical diagnosis

Urological disorders	20
Levator syndrome	3
Pelvic pathology	2
Pelvic fasciitis	1

These patients obtained no relief of the symptoms by conservative treatment. There were no physical signs of groin hernias.

There were 24 males and two females. The median age was 49 years, ranging form 24 to 75 years. The groin pain was experienced on strain in 30% of the patients, and 70% had nagging, persistent groin pain requiring intermittent use of oral analgesic and muscle relaxant. Herniography was performed in all 26 patients.

Herniography technique

The technique used was similar to that of Gullomo[6], with some modification as proposed by Bush, Badruddoja and Angres. The patient was placed supine on an X-ray table in the radiology department. Adequate preparation and draping of the lower abdomen on the left and midline from umbilicus to symphysis pubis was carried out. The midpoint of the lateral border of left rectus muscle was identified. 5 ml of 1% Xylocaine was used to anaesthetize the abdominal wall in this area, and a tiny skin incision was made. Originally a Verres peritoneal needle was used. Recently, a 16-gauge radio-opaque FEP Teflon Catheter (B-D IV; Dupont) with a 19-gauge inner needle was introduced into the peritoneal cavity in an oblique direction toward the pelvis. When the peritoneum was penetrated, the patient felt some discomfort and the operator also felt something 'give away' – indicating that the needle had entered into the peritoneal cavity. The inner needle was removed from the catheter and the catheter was introduced further into the pelvis over the descending and sigmoid colon, and it slid over easily.

A test dose of 5 ml of dye was injected under fluoroscopic control to be sure that there was no extravasation of dye into the abdominal wall or that it was not injected into mesentery or in any solid or hollow viscus in the abdomen. (If the needle is in the pelvis, the dye will flow immediately into the pouch of Douglas. If the catheter is not in the proper position, the catheter is withdrawn under fluoroscopic control to achieve the proper position.) Once the catheter was in the proper position, 100 ml of non-ionic dye (Omnipaque) was injected and the catheter removed. X-rays were taken in supine, prone, standing and oblique positions while the patients was in the Trendelenburg position. The patient continued to do Valsalva manoeuvre during the whole procedure.

The patient was monitored in the recovery room for one-half hour after the procedure, to be sure that no untoward reaction occurred as a result of the procedure.

Results

It was possible to establish a diagnosis of persistent groin pain in these 26 patients following herniography (Figures 51.1–51.4). The results of this study are highly encouraging (Table 51.3). Herniography was positive in 24 patients (92%). Contralateral asymptomatic hernia was discovered in five patients (19%) in the process of investigation of symptomatic side. We found nine (35%) indirect inguinal hernias: seven (78%) on the left side and two (22%) on the right side. There were fourteen (54%) direct hernias: ten (71%) on the right side and four (29%) on the left side. One (3.8%) hernia was a 'nice knuckle' hernia. Ten (38%) hernias were bilateral.

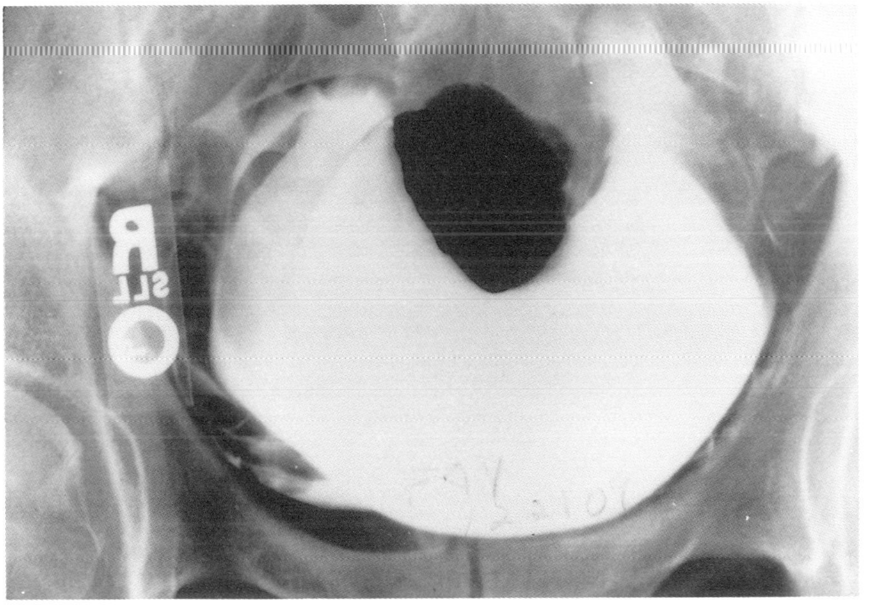

Figure 51.1: Normal herniogram, which shows well-defined pouch of Douglas without any abnormal filling defect.

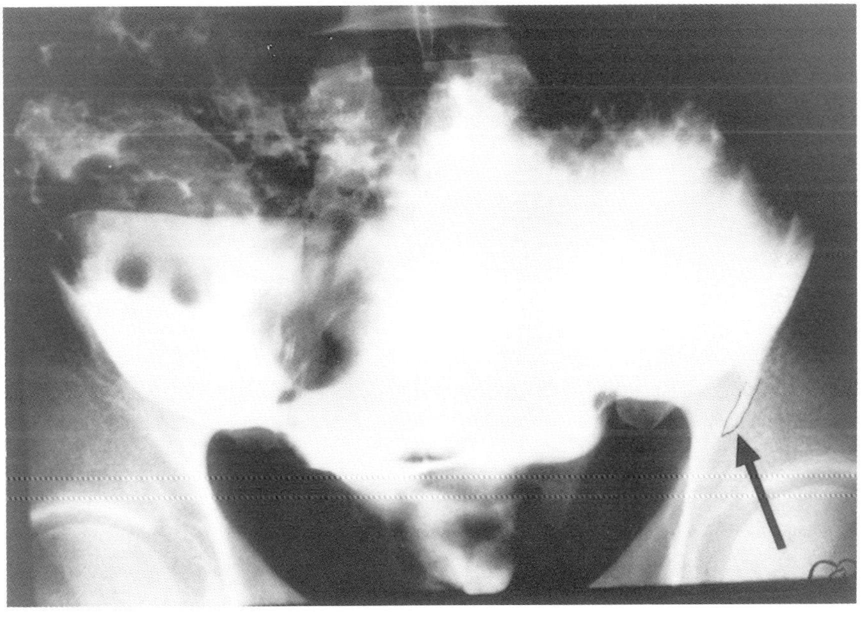

Figure 51.2: Small direct left inguinal hernia – without any physical finding. The patient had persistent groin pain. Laparoscopy confirmed the herniographic finding. Repair was done via laparoscopy. The patient is now asymptomatic.

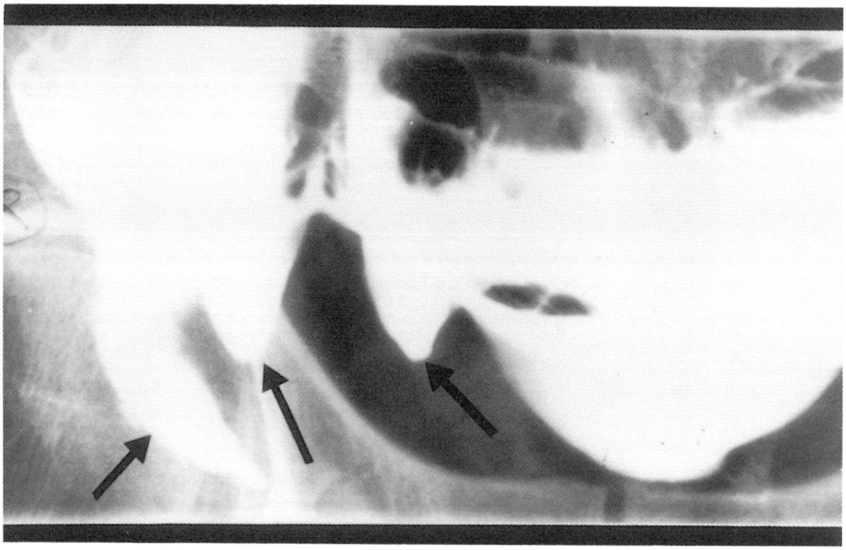

Figure 51.3: Persistent right groin pain. Physical examination was normal. The herniogram revealed multiple direct and single indirect hernias.

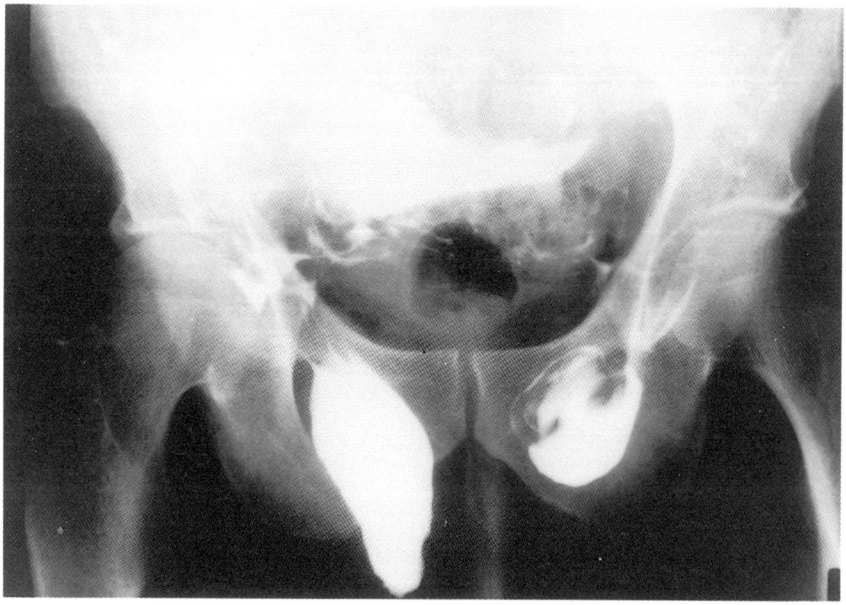

Figure 51.4: Bilateral large indirect hernia. The physical examination was normal. Laparoscopic repair was done.

Table 51.3: Herniographic findings in 26 patients

Indirect hernia:	9
Left side	7
Right side	2
Direct hernia:	14
Right side	10
Left side	4
Contralateral asymptomatic hernia	5
'Nice knuckle' hernia	1
Bilateral hernia	10
Normal	2

Table 51.4: Symptomatology

Long-standing groin pain	22
Low pelvic pain simulating pelvic disease, in female	2

Table 51.5: Working diagnosis of patients

Urological disorder: 20
Levator syndrome: 3
Pelvic pathology: 2
Pelvic fasciitis: 1

Table 51.6: Operative findings

Indirect hernia	9
Direct hernia	21
'Nice knuckle' hernia	1
Bilateral hernia	10

Asymptomatic hernias were not operated on.

The symptomatology of these 26 patients is shown in Table 51.4. It is clear that almost 90% of the patients were seen by us because of persistent long-standing groin pain prior to herniography. The working diagnosis of these 26 patients is shown in Table 51.5. Our initial working diagnosis was urological disorder in 90% of the patients, and they were treated accordingly prior to herniography without any substantial relief of symptoms. It is possible that some of these patients obtained some minor relief of symptoms because there may be some urological disorder, such as prostatitis, seminal vesiculitis, levator syndrome or pelvic fasciitis concomitant with symptomatic occult hernia.

Two patients had a positive herniogram on the side contralateral to the pain. They were not operated on, but the other 22 patients with groin pain, bilateral or unilateral, were operated on as they had positive herniography (Table 51.6). Of these 22 patients, eight underwent laparoscopic herniorrhaphy with Marlex mesh using the Ethicon Endoclip. The rest of the patients had undergone tension-free hernioplasty of Lichtenstein with pre-cut keyhole Marlex mesh. Our follow-up period is six months to one year. All of our patients have had satisfactory results.

Discussion

By definition, herniography is peritoneography used for evaluation of the inguinal region and pelvic floor. The procedure begins and ends with evaluation of the pouch of Douglas[7]. Herniography is not a new technique for the diagnosis of occult symptomatic hernia in general. Its usefulness is well documented for the diagnosis of all varieties of occult symptomatic hernia, including the syndrome of broad-base fossae[8].

There are two types of herniography: direct and indirect. *Indirect herniography* consists of injecting dye into a hollow viscus, such as the bowel or genitourinary tract, as described by Allen and Condon[9]. The position of this dye-filled viscus compared with that of a normal one is used to determine occult hernia. Allen and Condon described lateral protrusion of the urinary bladder (bladder ear) into the deep inguinal ring in 9% of 406 intravenous pyelographies and cystograms. Laurell[10] first published a report regarding the possibility of indirect herniography for diagnosis of occult groin hernia as early as 1929. Subsequently, there were several reports of indirect herniography for the diagnosis of occult groin hernia as a cause of persistent groin pain[11–13]. *Direct herniography* was performed by injecting contrast media in animals and was first described by Sternhill and Schwarz in 1961[14]. Clinical herniography was first performed by Ducharme[15] in infants. Gullomo[16] and others reported extensive series using herniography with femoral phlebography in both adults and children as early as 1957 for investigating undiagnosed groin pain due to occult groin hernias. The combination of herniography and femoral vein phlebography can establish the diagnosis of occult femoral hernia. Herniography is thus a well-accepted, minimally invasive investigation for undiagnosed groin pain due to occult groin hernia.

Very careful clinical evaluation of a patient is essential for the diagnosis of undiagnosed groin pain due to occult groin hernia. There are various causes of groin pain, and groin hernia is only one of them (*see* Table 51.7). In our series, we have treated 18 patients as urological disorders, which

Table 51.7: Causes of groin pain

Urological
Levator syndrome
Pelvic fasciitis
Gynaecological pathology
Groin hernia(s)
Syndrome of broad and deep fossae
Musculoskeletal

include prostatitis and seminal vesiculitis; two cases have been treated as pelvic fascitis, three as levator syndrome, and two female cases as pelvic inflammatory disease. None of these patients obtained relief of their symptoms. Physical examination in these groups of patients was normal. Because hernias are not palpable even though they may be of considerable size, it is doubtful whether physical examination would have been productive even in experienced hands. Therefore, the result of herniography was of considerable importance because the patients became symptom-free after surgical intervention.

Knowledge of the radiological anatomy of the groin is very important when interpreting a herniogram for the diagnosis of groin pain (Figure 51.5). The inguinal fossa is divided into medial and lateral parts by the epigastric fold containing the inferior epigastric artery coming from the femoral artery. This ligament has a fixed position, and is displaced in either direction in groin hernia, depending on the type of hernia. The area lateral to the epigastric fold is called the lateral inguinal fossa, and is the site of the deep inguinal ring as well as the site of indirect hernia. The area medial to the epigastric fold is called the medial inguinal fossa, and is the site of direct hernia. The medial fossa is again divided into medial and lateral parts by the lateral umbilical fold containing obliterated

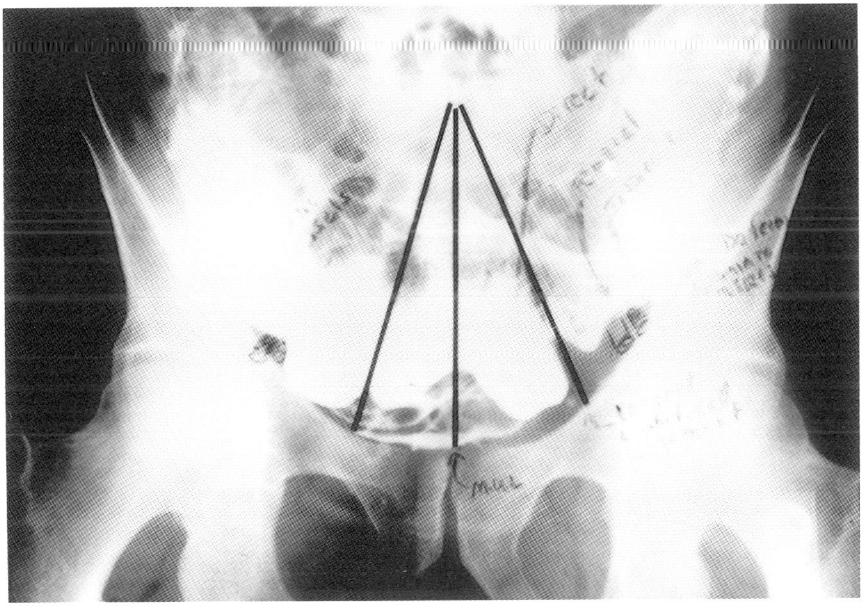

Figure 51.5: Radiological anatomy of a normal herniogram. Well-defined median, lateral and epigastric fold.

umbilical artery. It is quite possible that single or multiple direct hernia can occur on both sides of the lateral umbilical fold (*see* Figure 51.4). Such hernias can be detected only on herniogram preoperatively and can be treated appropriately. The surgeon can miss such hernias during surgery without herniography. So preoperative herniography will prevent so-called 'recurrence' and, in fact, these are really 'missed hernias' during surgery. The midline ligament is called the median umbilical ligament containing urachus. A detailed description of inguinal fossae on herniogram has been given by Okeberg and Kesek[17].

Herniography is a very safe and minimally invasive diagnostic procedure with a high degree of accuracy[18]. Some minor findings on herniogram, such as bulging of inguinal fossae or dilated deep inguinal ring, are of no significance if the patient does not have symptoms and therefore herniorrhaphy is not required[17]. However, Smedberg[19] observed that asymptomatic open processus vaginalis, detected on herniography, may develop into true hernia. So any abnormality of the inguinal fossae discovered by herniography should be followed very closely. There is an increasing demand for non-operative methods to avoid unnecessary exploration of the groin for undiagnosed groin pain. Herniography reduces such unnecessary exploration.

Positive herniographic results do not mean that the patient's symptoms are due to hernia. Smedberg and colleagues[20] have therefore advocated further investigations to exclude other causes of groin pain. However, our personal experience in this small, highly selective group of cases indicates that there is no need for further investigation with positive herniography, as these patients have already undergone all kinds of investigations and treatment with the diagnoses of various other causes of groin pain, excluding groin hernia. It is possible that in a highly selective group of cases positive results of herniography may reach as high as 90%. Among the cases of symptomatic non-palpable hernia, the incidence of direct hernia is as high as 80% because it is very difficult to feel a direct hernia. Again, herniography is the best non-operative method to detect symptomatic, non-palpable direct hernia. Symptomatic, non-palpable direct hernia is a common cause of groin pain. Another indication for herniography is questionable recurrent hernia.

Table 51.8: Complications of herniogram

Intramural bowel haematoma
Haematoma in rectus sheath
Intramesenteric haematoma: 2
Puncture of hollow viscus
Penetration through posterior abdominal wall
Extraperitoneal extravasation: 1
Reflux phenomena from hernial sac
Chemical irritation causing pain: 2

The complication rate of this minimally invasive procedure is negligible (Table 51.7). Only one case has been reported of intramural haematoma in the bowel caused by infection of the bowel and requiring bowel resection[21]. Other complications, such as haematoma in the rectus sheath, puncture of bowel lumen, injection into the mesentery and intra-abdominal wall are very minor and are of no significance. There were no significant, serious complications in our series.

Another important phenomenon noted during herniogram is called 'reflux phenomenon'. This occurs in a very small sac where dye regurgitates into the peritoneal cavity and the patient experiences shooting pain in the groin after straining. We have used intraherniographic intravenous sedation to avoid this complication.

Addendum

Since writing this paper, the author has 50 more herniograms with successful outcomes both preoperatively and postoperatively.

Conclusions

Undiagnosed groin pain is a challenging problem for general surgeons, urologists and gynaecologists. Direct herniography is of great value in the diagnosis of occult symptomatic groin hernia. Herniography is a simple, minimally invasive and inexpensive technique with minimal morbidity. Herniography should be considered in all undiagnosed groin pain.

References

1. Ekberg O. Inguinal herniorrhaphy in adults. *Radiology* 1981; **138**: 31.
2. Smedberg SG, Broome AE, Elmer O, Gullomo A. Herniography in diagnosis of obscure groin pain. *Acta Chir Scand* 1981; **151**: 663.
3. Gullomo A. Positive contrast herniography combined with study of pelvic floor and the pouch of Douglas. Paper read at the XIVth International Congress of Radiology, Rio de Janeiro, 1977. Book of Abstract, p. 376.
4. Nyhus L. Role of laparoscopy in diagnosis of undiagnosed groin pain. Personal communication, January 1993.
5. *Nashville Group Laparoscopist in General Surgery* (a monthly surgical newsletter). May 1993.
6. Gullomo A. On herniography. *Proc Swed Soc Radiol* 1973; **2**: 19.
7. Gullomo A. Om herniografti (in Swedish). *Swed Soc Med Radiol* 1973; **2**: 19.
8. Gullomo A. Herniography. *Acta Radiol Suppl* 1980; **361**: 5.
9. Alen RP, Condon RV. Transistory extraperitoneal hernia in infants. *Radiology* 1969; **75**: 668.

10. Laurell PG. Uber Die Rortgenuntersuchung von Bruchen, insbesondere klinisch schwer zu diagnostizierender formen. *Acta Radiol* 1929; **10**: 462.

11. Read PC. Observation on etiology of speigelian hernia. *Ann Surg* 1960; **152**: 10004.

12. Bryk D. Spiegelian hernia containing sigmoid colon. *Am J Roentgenol* 1967; **99**: 17.

13. Holder LE, Schneider HJ. Spiegelian hernia anatomy and roentgenographic manifestation. *Radiology* 1974; **112**: 309.

14. Sternhill B, Schwartz S. Effect of Hypaque on mouse peritoneum. *Radiology* 1960; **75**: 81.

15. Ducharme JC, Bertrand R, Chachar R. Is it possible to diagnose inguinal hernia by X-ray? *Can Assoc Radiol J* 1967; **18**: 448.

16. Gullomo A. The strain obstruction syndrome of femoral vein. *Acta Radiol* 1957; **47**: 119.

17. Okeberg O, Kesek P. Herniographic appearance of lateral inguinal fossae. *Acta Radiol* 1987; **28**: 563.

18. Okeberg O. Complications after herniography in adults. *Am J Roentgenol* 1983; **140**: 491.

19. Smedberg S. Herniography and Hernial Surgery. Thesis. Lund, 1981.

20. Smedberg S, Broome AEA, Elmer O, Gullomo A. herniography in diagnosis of obscure groin pain. *Acta Chir Scand* 1985; **151**: 663.

21. Butsch JL, Kulm JP. Intramural hematoma of small bowel. A possible lethal complication of herniography surgery. 1978; **83**: 121.

52

Obturator Hernia Diagnosed by Herniography

TAKESHI NAGAHAMA, AKIRA NAKASHIMA, TOSHIHISA ASHIKAWA, NORIHIDE SUGANO, TORU KAWAMURA, SATORU OOTAWA, YASUSHI SATO AND MITSUO ENDO

Obturator hernia is a rare but well-known pelvic condition, first reported by Arnaud de Ronsil in 1724. About 500 cases of obturator hernia have been reported in the English literature; in Japan about 350 cases have been reported. Preoperative diagnosis is difficult and most cases are diagnosed at laparotomy investigating intestinal obstruction of origin unknown. The frequency of intestinal resection is up to 50% and mortality is 20%.

Clinical problems related to obturator hernia

- Pain in the anterior medial thigh radiating from the hip or groin lesion (the Howship-Romberg sign). It is caused by the compression of the obturator nerve. However, it is usually noticed only retrospectively.
- Most obturator hernias occur in thin women in their 70's. Their preoperative condition tends to be poor.
- A narrow obturator canal often results in necrosis of the herniated intestine, so the mortality rate is higher than with other groin herniae.

In Japan, about 350 cases of obturator hernias have been reported in the literature. As mentioned above, preoperative diagnosis is usually made during laparotomy, but recently some cases have been diagnosed preoperatively using CT scan, ultrasonography, magnetic resonance imaging (MRI) and herniography.

Herniography

Positive contrast peritoneography was first performed experimentally by Tanaka in 1951, using aborted foetuses. Clinically herniography was first used by Ducharme to demonstrate occult contralateral hernia in paediatric patients in 1967. But it was not widely accepted because of complications related to the puncturing of the peritoneal cavity, problems with contrast medium and unnecessary radiation exposures. However, Ekberg and his colleagues reported the usefulness of herniography in diagnosing groin hernia among adults.

We have been using herniography since December 1988. About 400 patients with clinical or subclinical hernias and obscure groin pain have been evaluated using herniography. Contraindications are infancy, pregnancy, intestinal obstruction and allergy to contrast medium.

Technique

Puncturing the peritoneum and injecting contrast medium are performed under local anaesthesia using a plastic venous infusion needle, with the patient supine. When the needle enters the peritoneal cavity, the loss of resistance is felt; 50 ml water-soluble, non-ionized contrast medium is then injected into the peritoneal cavity under fluoroscopic observation. The upper part of the patient's body is then raised and the radiographic study is performed. Radiographic study should include frontal and oblique views from both sides in the prone position and a frontal view in the supine position. We usually perform herniographies in the outpatient clinic.

Advantages of herniography

- By analysing the shape, type and size of the hernia, it is possible to determine whether it is subclinical and coexisting, contralateral or recurrent.
- Determining the type of hernia is important in planning suitable treatment. Under radiographic diagnosis, we choose which operation and operating procedures to use.
- As a follow-up study.

Interpretation

In normal cases there are five pelvic peritoneal folds in the groin. They originate from the epigastric vessels (lateral umbilical fold) (Figures 52.1 and 52.2), obstructed umbilical artery (medial umbilical fold) and obstructed urachus (median umbilical fold). Each side of the pelvic cavity is divided into three fossae (supravesical, medial umbilical and lateral umbilical). By radiographic study each type of hernia can be interpreted by its shape, its relation to the fold and fossa and the direction of the protrusion.

Typical herniographic findings are as follows:

- an indirect hernia protrudes medially from the lateral inguinal fossa lateral to the lateral inguinal fold
- a direct hernia protrudes anteriorly from the medial (most often) or median umbilical fossa

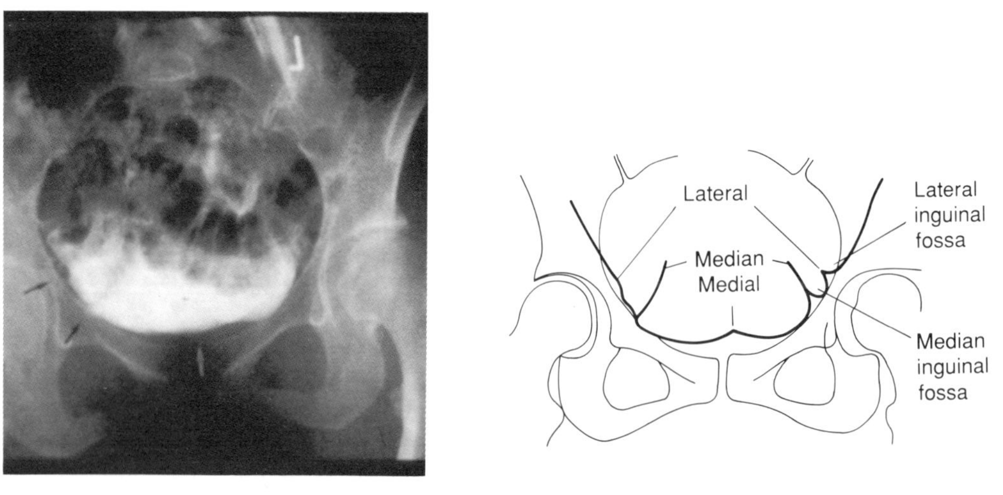

Figure 52.1: Normal case herniography. The arrow shows each umbilical fold.

- a femoral hernia usually protrudes laterally from the median umbilical fossa over the pubic bone. Radiography typically shows femoral obturator hernias to be pear-shaped with a narrow neck
- an obturator hernia protrudes downward anteriorly through the obturator foramen beneath the pubic bone. The typical shape of an obturator hernia is very similar to that of the femoral hernia so radiographic examination is important in differentiating between them.

Case reports

We describe here three cases of obturator hernia: one with intestinal obstruction, one with a history of operation for inguinal hernia on the same side and one that was diagnosed coincidentally.

Case one

An 88-year-old female suffered from intestinal obstruction. On admission she complained of pain in the medial anterior thigh on the right side. We considered obturator hernia and a CT scan was performed. The CT scan showed an incarcerated hernia mass between the internal and external obturator muscles (Figure 52.3). Operation was performed by the inguinal approach. In this case, the small intestine was perforated and direct closure was performed. Postoperative herniography revealed the presence of a contralateral obturator hernia and a coexisting femoral hernia.

Case two

A 51-year-old female had suffered from right inguinal pain for three months before admission to hospital. Operation for a right inguinal hernia had been performed two months previously, but her pain had not improved. Herniography revealed a small but definite obturator hernia on the right side (Figure 52.4). After surgery, her inguinal pain improved. She was discharged seven days postoperatively.

Case three

An 84-year-old female had noticed a protrusion in the groin on the right side several years previously. Herniography revealed a large direct inguinal hernia on the right side, coexisting bilateral obturator

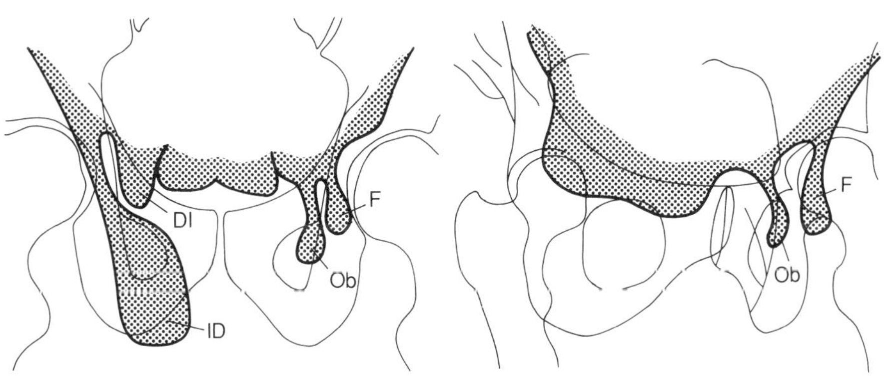

DI	:	Direct hernia	ID	:	Indirect hernia
F	:	Femoral hernia	Ob	:	Obturator hernia

Figure 52.2: A hernia in the groin lesion: a typical radiographic finding.

hernias and a femoral hernia on the left side. As in the case, obturator hernia usually exists bilaterally (Figure 52.5) and often complicates other types of groin hernia, especially femoral hernia.

Operative procedure

The inguinal approach to the obturator foramen is as follows:

The procedure is performed with a longer skin incision and usual treatment of the inguinal canal, then transverse fascia is incised. With retraction and dissection of the preperitoneal fat tissue along

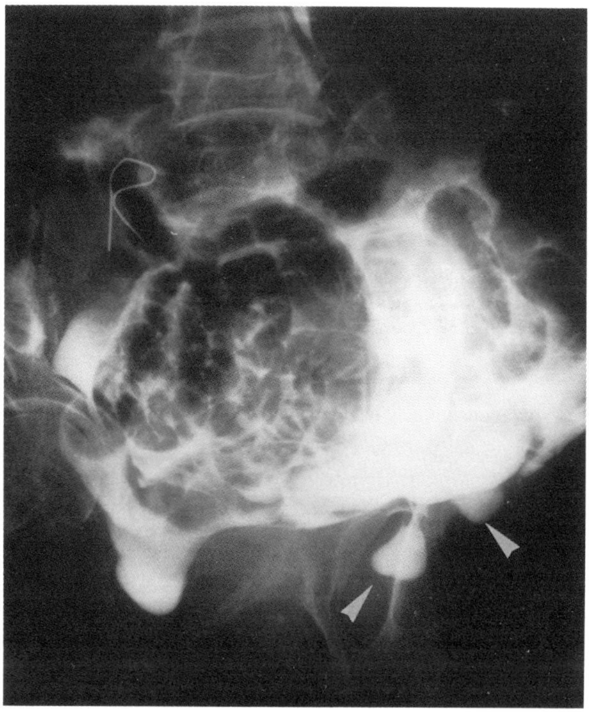

Figure 52.3: A CT scan showing an incarcerated hernia mass.

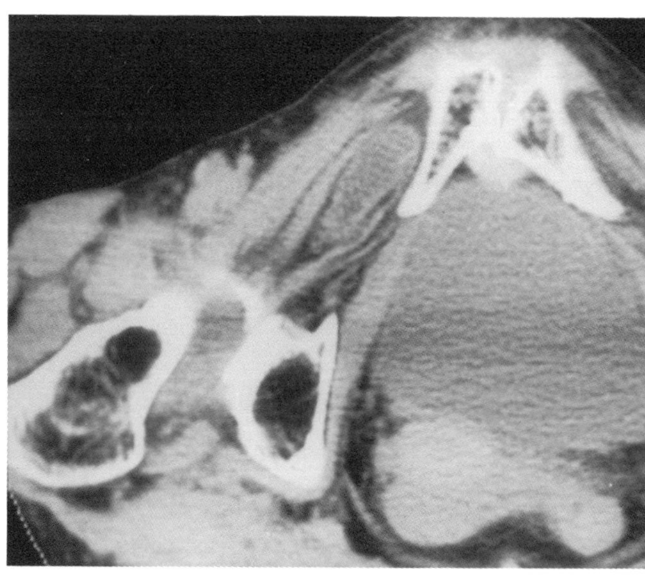

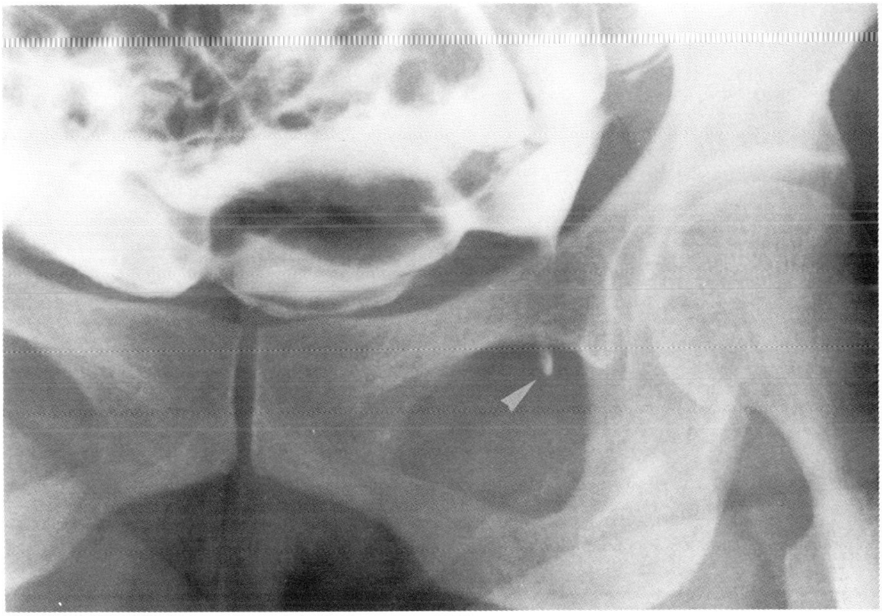

Figure 52.4: Herniography revealed a small but definite obturator hernia on the right side.

the pubic bone, the obturator foramen and hernia content are visualized (Figure 52.6). After reduction and resection of the hernia sac, repair of the obturator foramen is performed by applying one suture, avoiding obturator vessels and nerve.

All our 13 patients, (22 sides) with obturator hernias had them successfully repaired with direct closure. In two cases we repaired the obturator foramen via a preperitoneal approach because of previous operations. Repair or resection of non-viable intestine could easily be performed by the inguinal approach. To prevent postoperative infection, thorough irrigation is recommended. This inguinal approach can be applied to any case of obturator hernia diagnosed preoperatively except when there is peritonitis.

Results

Since 1988, we have treated 14 cases of obturator hernia: 10 female and four male. Seven were symptomatic (e.g. abdominal pain). Surprisingly, ten cases were bilateral and only four cases were unilateral.

Five patients had a history of operation for a previous inguinal hernia on the same side. Six patients had coexisting femoral hernia and five had an inguinal hernia on the same side. In 11 cases, operation was performed via the inguinal approach and two cases via the preperitoneal approach

We did not need to perform an intestinal resection nor did our patients experience postoperative complications.

Conclusions

The clinically serious problem of obturator hernia is the difficulty in it s diagnosis. The hernia sac is never visible and rarely palpable. The Howship-Romberg symptom is known to be a specific

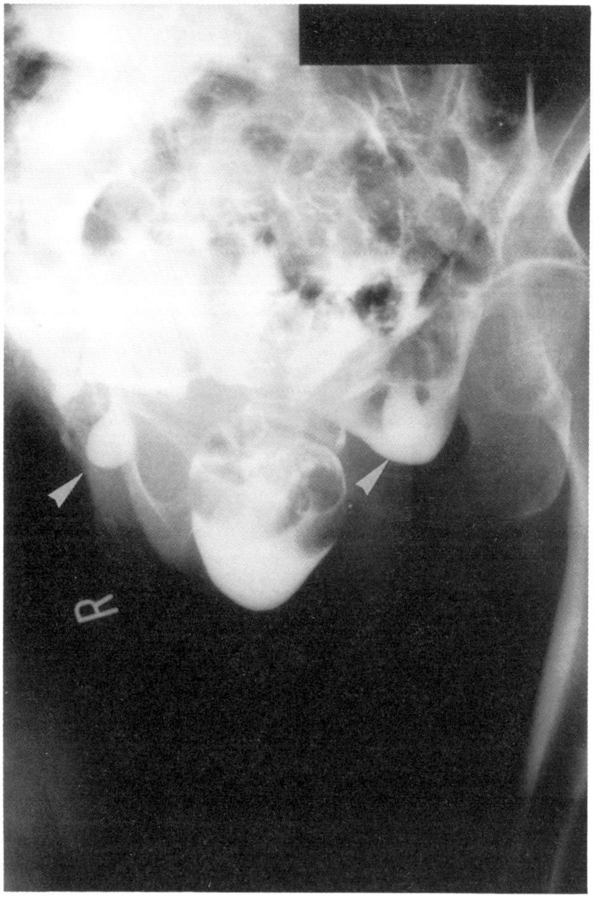

Figure 52.5: Herniography revealed a large direct inguinal hernia on the right side, coexisting bilateral obturator hernias and a formal hernia on the left side.

physical finding but it is usually noticed only postoperatively. Recently, CT scan and ultrasonography has been reported to be useful in diagnosing incarcerated obturator hernia; however, they are useful only in cases of incarceration. Detailed study of their course reveals that some of them have experienced intermittent intestinal obstruction and spontaneous remission. In the remission or asymptomatic obturator hernia, CT scan and ultrasonography give us no information. We consider the merits of herniography to be as follows:

- it can be performed without general anaesthesia, at an outpatient clinic
- false negative and false positive cases are very rare
- herniographic study shows us the whole hernie and provides information on its orifice, size, laterality, shape and content

Previously, obturator hernia was thought to be a rare pelvic disease. Therefore, no consideration was given to its possible relation to other groin hernias. According to our study, using herniography could reveal new findings as follows:

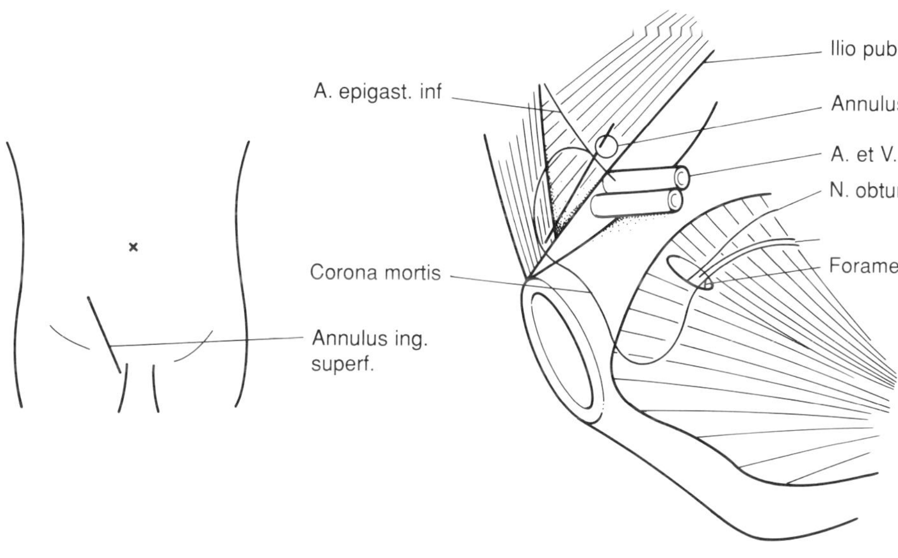

Figure 52.6: With retraction and dissection of the preperioneal fat tissue along the pubic bone, the obturator foramen and hernia content are vizualized.

Bilateral obturator hernia is very common

Diagnosis of obturator hernia has previously been made during laparotomy. In such cases, most were complicated by incarceration, and evaluation of the contralateral side of the obturator foramen from the peritoneal cavity is rather difficult. Our study indicates that the frequency of bilateral obturator hernia is about 71%.

Most cases of obturator hernia are associated with other types of hernia in the groin.

In our 14 cases of obturator hernia, ten were associated with other types of groin hernia. These ten cases included six of femoral hernia, three of direct inguinal hernia and three of indirect inguinal hernia. Two patients complaining of a femoral groin lesion were misdiagnosed as having inguinal hernia, and the obturator hernia was missed at the first operation (Table 52.1).

Laparoscopic herniography will become more popular in the future. During laparoscopic procedure, careful observation of the obturator foramen is strongly recommended.

Obturator hernia is much more common than had previously been thought

We have performed herniography in 396 patients, mainly in an outpatient clinic. Seven cases were diagnosed as symptomatic obturator hernia and another seven as associated obturator hernia. The frequency (3.5%) is much higher than that given in earlier reports.

We have no experience of laparoscopic observation of obturator hernia, and so it is difficult to compare herniography with laparoscopic observation. This is one of our future aims.

We have operated on 13 patients with obturator hernia. In 12 cases (20 sides), the operation was performed via the inguinal approach, by which a direct view of the obturator foramen was easily obtained. With a better view of the obturator foramen, treatment avoiding the obturator vessels and obturator nerve is performed more easily than via the transperitoneal approach.

In two patients (two sides) operation was performed via the preperitoneal approach because of a previous operation for another groin hernia in the same side. With this manoeuvre, the obturator foramen was felt to be relatively distant. We now apply this manoeuvre in cases of single obturator hernias.

Table 52.1: 14 cases of obturator hernia diagnosed by herniography

Age:	51–88 years (average 72.7 years)	
Sex:	male: 4, female: 10	
Complaint	intestinal obstruction	5
	groin pain	2
	no complaint	7
Laterality	unilateral	4 (right 3, left 1)
	bilateral	10
Associated other hernia		10
	inguinal hernia	4
	femoral hernia	5
	complicated hernia	1
Previous operation for groin hernia on the same side		
	guinal hernia	3
	femoral hernia	2
Operative approach	inguinal	12 (20 sides)
	preperitoneal	2 (2 sides)
Intestinal resection		0
Complication after operation		0
Stay in hospital after operation		7–14 days

We consider the problem of the obturator hernia to be the difficulty of diagnosing the preincarcerated condition. Therefore, we believe that an operation for obturator hernia should be performed whether it is symptomatic or not. Study of the natural course and evaluation of the risk for incarceration is needed, and the indications for the operation may well change.

Bibliography

1. Bjork KJ, Mucha P, Cahill DR. Obturator hernia. *Surg Gynecol Obstet* 1988; **167**: 217–22
2. Ekberg O. Inguinal herniography in adults: technique, normal anatomy, and diagnostic criteria for hernias. *Radiology* 1981; **138**: 31–6.
3. Ekberg O. Herniography of femoral, obturator and perineal hernias. Fortschr Röntgenstr 1985; **143**: 193–9.
4. Gullmo Å. Herniography. The diagnosis of hernia in the groin and incompetence of the pouch of Douglas and pelvic floor. *Acta Radiol Suppl* 1980; **361**: 1–76.
5. Megibow AJ, Wagner AG. Obturator hernia. *J Comput Assist Tomogr* 1983; **7**: 350–2.
6. Meziane MA, Fishman EK, Siegelman SS. Computed tomographic diagnosis of obturator foramen hernia. *Gastrointest Radiol* 1983; **8**: 375–7.
7. Nakashima A, Sugano N, Nagahama T. Herniography in 3 case of obturator hernia. *Clin Surg* 1990; **45**: 393–6 (in Japanese).
8. Persson NH, Bergqvist D, Ekberg O. Obturator hernia – clinical significance of radiologic diagnosis. *Acta Chir Scand* 1987; **153**: 361–4.

9. Skandalakis JK, Gray SW. Strangulated obturator hernia. In: Nyhus LM, Condon RE, eds. *Hernia*, 3rd ed. Philadelphia: JB Lippincott, 1989: 416–31.

10. Smedberg SG, Broomé AE. Herniography. In: Nyhus LM, Condon RE, eds. *Hernia*, 3rd ed. Philadelphia: JB Lippincott, 1989: 531–40.

11. Sugano N, Nakashima A, Nagahama T. The usefulness of herniography in diagnosis of the adult groin hernias. *J Jap Clin Surg* 1991: **52**: 760–4 (abstract in English).

12. Tanaka H. Studies on the inguinal anatomy of the Japanese, with special reference to the inguinal hernia. *J Jap Surg* 1953; **54**: 772–85 (abstract in English).

53

The TSD Classification: A Nomenclature for Groin Hernias

ROBERT BENDAVID

The classification of any surgical condition is a must, if communication is to be established with an audience. Beyond classification, the accurate definition of that condition with reference to site, extent and size permits a reliable expectation of treatment results. Most important, once the lesion is correctly identified, the optimal available therapy may be logically instituted. Examples of classifications that have been rewarding are the TNM (Tumour, lymph Nodes, Metastases) system in staging breast cancer[1] and the Duke classification of colon cancer[2]. Such a classification for groin hernias has remained elusive.

'Classification' implies the possibility of observing, analysing and cataloguing hundreds, preferably thousands, of individual situations, looking for common factors and features that would constitute distinct groups. The Shouldice Hospital provides an ideal setting for such an endeavour. Every year, about 7500 operations are performed on all types of abdominal wall hernias. Each patient's chart includes a statistical sheet that accurately defines the nature of the hernia, its extent and the treatment instituted. These charts have provided the information which led to the TSD classification proposed here (T = type, S = staging, D = dimension). Each hernia will be identified in those terms. The inguinal ligament, as will be discussed later, demarcates the anterior from the posterior aspect of the myopectineal orifice.

Type

Five types of groin hernias can be observed, according to their location (Figures 53.1 and 53.2):

Type I Anterolateral (*formerly* indirect)

Type II Anteromedial (*formerly* direct)

Type III Posteromedial (*formerly* femoral)

Type IV Posterolateral (*formerly* prevascular)

Type V Anteroposterior (*formerly* inguinofemoral)

Statistically and anatomically, serendipity has allowed types I to IV to have a clockwise direction on the right (counterclockwise on the left) and a descending order of incidence. Type V differs in being a combined type of hernia, ie a combination of types II and III.

The percentages shown on Table 53.1 are based on the 1989 statistics of the Shouldice Hospital, when 7529 abdominal wall hernia operations were carried out, 7085 (94%) of which were groin hernias. The remaining 444 (6%) were incisional, umbilical, epigastric and the rare types of hernias.

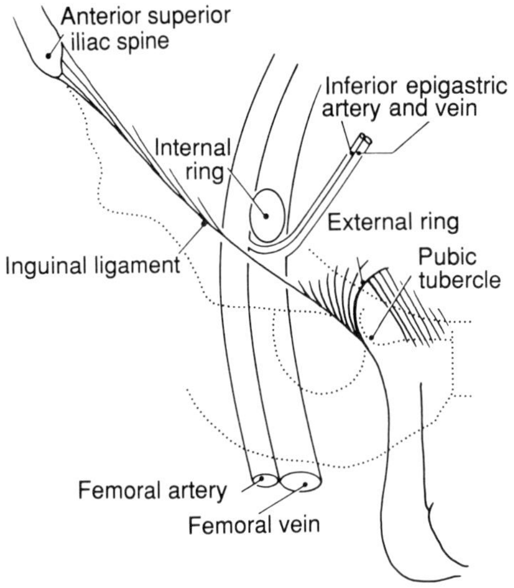

Figure 53.1: Anatomy of the groin as displayed in the chart of classification (*see* Figure 53.3).

Staging

Each type will be characterized by three stages (Figure 53.3), which will denote the extent of the herniation, anatomically.

Type I

Stage 1: The anterolateral hernia extends from the deep inguinal ring to the superficial inguinal ring.

Stage 2: The anterolateral hernia extends from the deep inguinal ring beyond the superficial inguinal ring but not into the scrotum.

Stage 3: The anterolateral hernia extends from the deep inguinal ring to the scrotum.

Type II

Stage 1: The anteromedial hernia remains within the confines of the inguinal canal.

Stage 2: The anteromedial hernia extends beyond the superficial inguinal ring but not into the scrotum.

Stage 3: The anteromedial hernia extends beyond the superficial inguinal ring into the scrotum.

Type III

Stage 1: The neck of the posteromedial hernia occupies a portion of the distance between the femoral vein and the lacunar ligament.

Stage 2: The neck of the posteromedial hernia occupies the entire distance between the femoral vein and the lacunar ligament.

Stage 3: The neck of the posteromedial hernia extends from the femoral vein to the pubic tubercle (recurrences, destruction of lacunar ligament).

Type IV

The posterolateral hernias represent the rarest types of hernias. The established term of 'prevascular' hernia is grossly inaccurate, as these hernias can appear anterior, posterior and lateral to the femoral

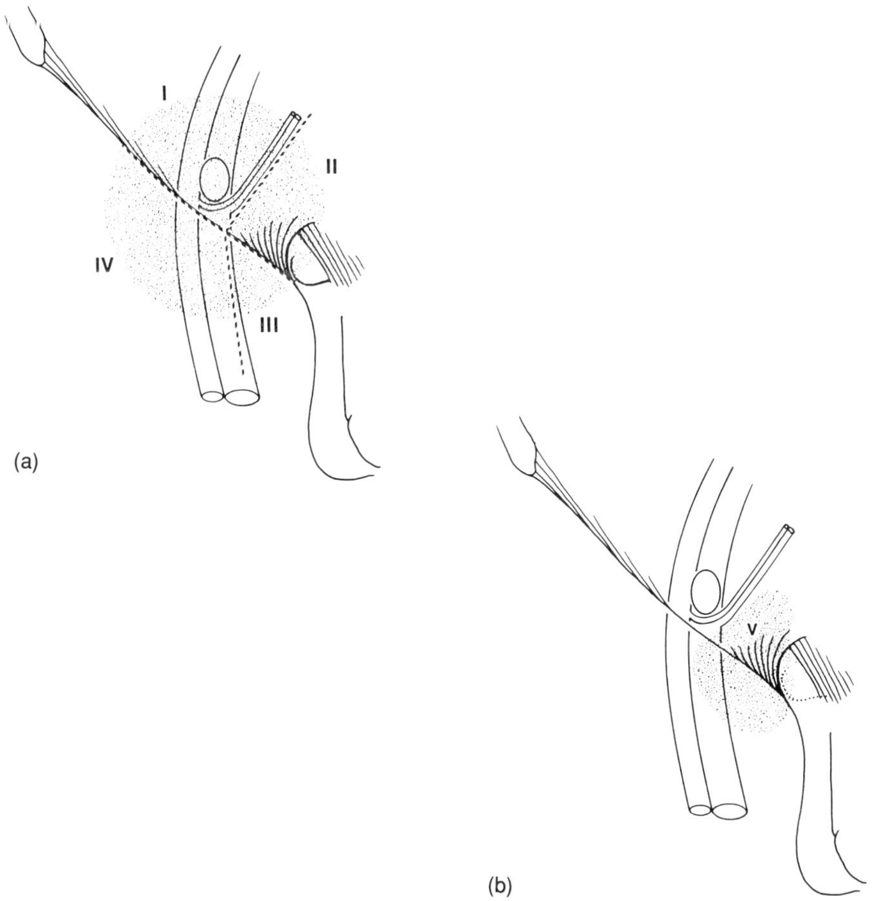

Figure 53.2: (a) Types I, II, III and IV, and their areas of emergence; (b) type V and its area of emergence.

Table 53.1: The incidence of the various 'types' of hernias

Type I (anterolateral)	56.80%
Type II (anteromedial)	40.80%
Type III (posteromedial)	2.03%
Type IV (posterolateral)	0.05%
Type V (anteroposterior)	0.32%

vessels. These rare forms can be classified into three groups (herein called 'stages' to facilitate their classification; no progression of the lesion is implied). In this group of hernias will be included the Cloquet hernia (posteromedial hernia emerging through the pectineus fascia) and the Laugier hernia (through the lacunar ligament). These two varieties are included in type IV because of their rarity and their parafemoral position.

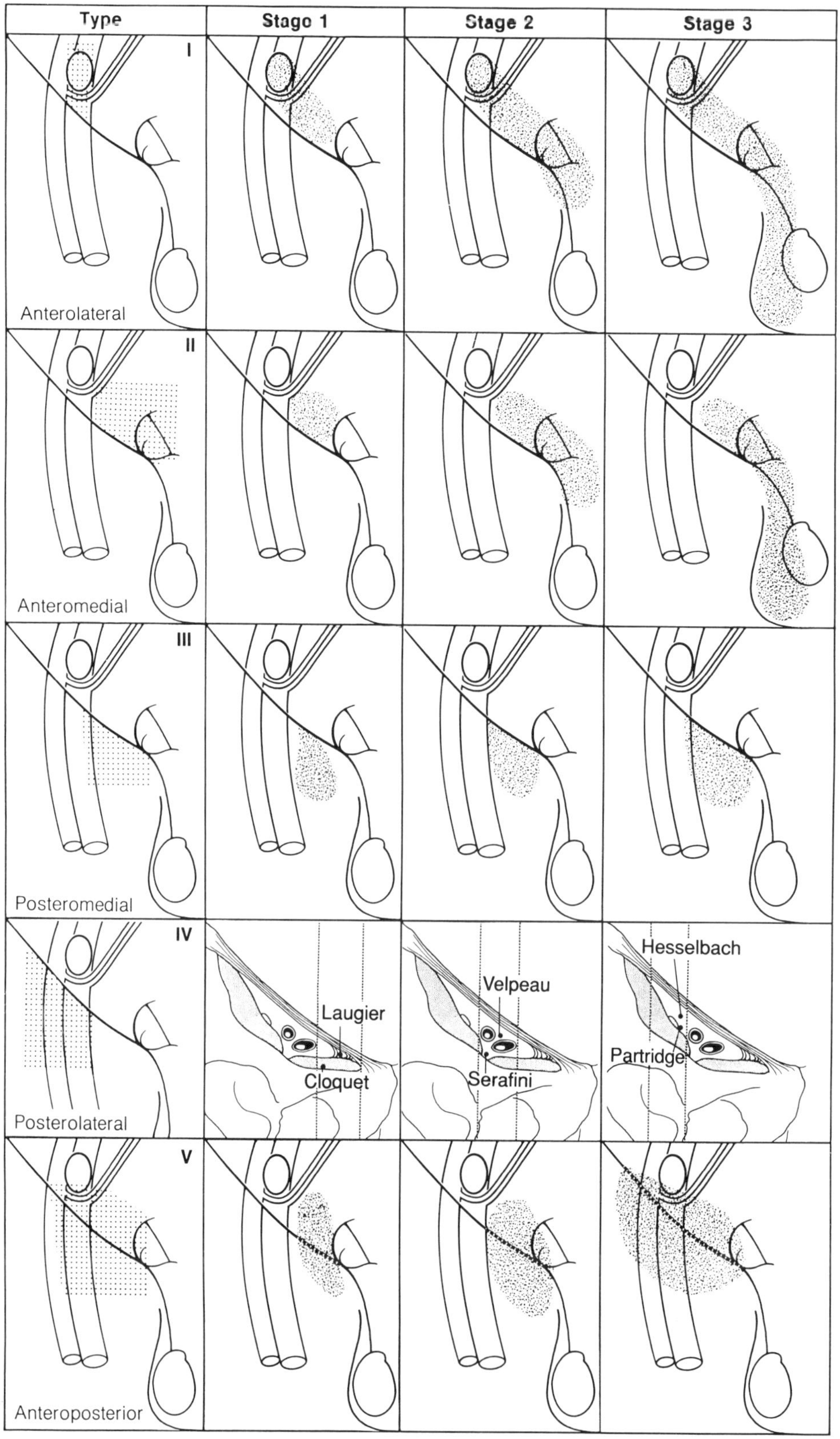

Figure 53.3: Chart of classification.

Stage 1: The hernias located medial to the femoral vein: Cloquet and Laugier hernias.

Stage 2: The hernias at the level of the femoral vessels: Velpeau (the true prevascular, hernia and Serafini (retrovascular) hernia (rare).

Stage 3: The hernias lateral to the femoral vessels: Hesselbach's hernia through the cribriform fascia and Partridge's hernia lateral to the femoral artery.

Type V

The anteroposterior hernias represent a combination of anteromedial and posteromedial hernias.

Stage 1: The anteroposterior hernia originates as an anteromedial hernia which has lifted or destroyed a portion of the inguinal ligament between the pubic crest and the femoral vein.

Stage 2: The anteroposterior hernia originates as an anteromedial hernia which has lifted or destroyed the inguinal ligament from the pubic crest to the femoral vein.

Stage 3: The anteroposterior hernia originates as an anteromedial hernia which has destroyed the inguinal ligament from the pubic crest to a point lateral to the femoral vein (the most difficult type to correct).

Dimension

The size of a hernia must be identified accurately for it has a bearing on treatment and prognosis. Such terms as 'small', 'medium', 'large', 'moderately small', 'moderately large', 'giant' and 'massive' must be eliminated. These are relative terms and do not convey a true picture. Accurate determination of size will suggest whether a simple herniorrhaphy may be carried out or if prostheses are to be called upon as well as promoting comparative studies of analogous hernias from different centres. 'D' will therefore refer to the diameter of the hernial defect at the level of the abdominal wall. Where a defect is not circular but ovoid or elliptical, the widest laterolateral measurement should be recorded in centimetres. This dimension reflects the defect that is to be corrected. The wider the defect, the more the tension and, hence, the more likely a prosthesis is to be used. The best example would be seen in a type II hernia through the entire floor of the inguinal canal, when the laterolateral measurement would reflect the distance between the transversus arch and the inguinal ligament.

Subclassification

For more detailed identification in the case of type II hernias (anteromedial hernias), small letters 'm', 'l', 'c' and 'e' will denote whether a defect is located, respectively, through the medial, lateral, central or entire portion of the posterior wall of the inguinal canal. An anteromedial hernia, near the pubis, 2 cm in diameter would be labelled: 'Type II, stage 1 (m), D2'. An anterolateral hernia with a deep inguinal ring measuring 4 cm and extending into the scrotum would be labelled: 'Type I, stage 3, D4'.

Where a hernia has failed twice, this may be indicated as 2R ('R' for recurrence) and noted after the type; for example, a second recurrence at an anterolateral hernia extending to the superficial inguinal ring and with a diameter at the internal ring of 5 cm would be labelled: 'Type I (2R), stage 1, D5'. When a portion of a viscus contributes to a sliding hernia (eg the urinary bladder), the letter 'S' (for slider) will be noted after the type and recurrence; for example, a first recurrence of an anteromedial hernia through the entire floor of the canal (7 cm lateral measurement), containing a portion of the urinary bladder but remaining within the inguinal canal (not beyond the superficial ring) would be labelled: 'Type II (1R) (S), stage 1 (e), D7'.

If incarceration or necrosis of a viscus has occurred, the letters 'I' or 'N' would be noted, also after the type. When the herniating component consists of adipose tissue only (the properitoneal lipomas, fatty hernias), the letter 'L' (for lipoma) would be noted after the type and given all the characteristics of a hernia; for example, a properitoneal lipoma 4 cm long and 3 cm at the base through the internal ring would be labelled: 'Type I (L), stage 1, D3'.

Some surgical purists may question how to classify the so-called interstitial hernia composed of fatty tissue dissecting through the transversus and internal oblique fibres near the deep inguinal ring (superiorly or laterally). These fatty hernias, once reduced, are still 'fatty anterolateral hernias' – type I (L). Missed (overlooked) hernias would be labelled 'M' after type and 'R', because they always present early following a previous operation. If more than one hernia is present, each hernia is described individually.

Discussion

The challenge of classifying groin hernias has never been met entirely or satisfactorily. Each attempt will have shortcomings, invariably because of the unusual and rare cases or the uncommonly large hernias that are no longer the rule but the exception. The classifications put forth by Casten[3], Gilbert[4] and Nyhus[5] unfortunately have drawbacks. They include:

- all types of hernias are not clearly identified,
- dimensions are not accurately assessed
- the extent of tissue destruction can only be guessed
- which categories are likely to require mesh is not ascertained
- anatomical delineation of the lesion is not obvious.

These classifications will not allow one to picture a lesion to the extent that it can be visualized by a detached reader.

The hallowed tradition of describing hernias must now be called into question. Is there any value in determining whether a hernia is type I or type II when examining a patient? Certainly all of us have been wrong in the past and will be again. At the Shouldice Hospital, admitting diagnoses never differentiate between these two most common hernias. Type III hernias also are beset by erroneous diagnoses, from 2% to 25%[6–9]. The concept of direct and indirect inguinal hernias also betrays the surgical tendency to follow the beaten path. There is nothing in the 'indirect' hernia that is indirect, except for the path of least resistance along the obliquity of the inguinal canal. All surgeons have seen 'direct' inguinal hernias emerging through the superficial ring, in the same manner as the 'indirect' hernia. Both types of hernias are, in fact, anterior hernias, anatomically speaking, for that is the direction of the herniation.

Astley Cooper may well have been the earliest author to have recognized that the deep and superficial rings were not superimposed[10]. It was not until his second publication[11], however, that he differentiated between 'direct' and 'indirect' hernias in those terms. Hesselbach had used the terms 'external' and 'internal' hernias, with the inferior epigastric vessels as the reference point[12]. Here again, there is nothing 'external' or 'internal' about an 'indirect' or 'direct' hernia.

To rationalize and facilitate the understanding of the present classification, one must refer to Fruchaud[13]. His textbook on the anatomy of the groin stands out as a classic reference which, unfortunately, has never been translated into English. Fruchaud looks at the groin as a 'myopectineal opening' with potential areas of weakness. Each type of weakness, and hence herniation, is determined by the nature, quality and layering of the various muscular and ligamentous structures, as one proceeds from the preperitoneal space to the subcutaneous space. His anatomical description defines the four areas that represent the hernias I have labelled types I, II, III and IV, type V being a combination of types II and III and a real clinical entity.

The groin is seen, therefore, as having an anterior and a posterior area, the division being the inguinal ligament; each area has a medial and lateral aspect – the anterior areas being demarcated by the inferior epigastric vessels, the posterior areas by the femoral vein.

Conclusion

'Tradition', 'precedent' and 'trend' are words that govern and express our ways of thinking, transcending language and national barriers. Time-honoured practices linger, though a rationale for that practice may be missing. So it has been with groin hernias. In the age of computers, storage and retrieval of countless facts and statistics become a simple matter. The data, however, must be clearly and accurately identified, preferably on the basis of our most stable, reliable and tangible of sciences – anatomy and its language.

References

1. Sabiston D, ed. *Davis-Christopher: Textbook of Surgery*, 10th ed. Philadelphia, London, Toronto: WB Saunders, 1972: 591–3.
2. Sabiston D, ed. *Davis-Christopher: Textbook of Surgery*, 10th ed. Philadelphia, London, Toronto: WB Saunders, 1972: 971–2.
3. Casten DF. Functional anatomy of the groin area as related to the classification and treatment of groin hernias. *Am J Surg*, 1967; **114**: 894–9.
4. Gilbert AI. An anatomic and functional classification for the diagnosis and treatment of inguinal hernia. *Am J Surg*, 1989; **157**: 331–3.
5. Nyhus LM, Klein MS, Rodgers FB. Inguinal hernia. *Curr Probl Surg*, 1991; **28**: 417–19.
6. David T. Strangulated femoral hernia. *Med J Aust* 1967; **1**: 258–61.
7. Ponka JL, Brush BE. The problem of femoral hernia. *Arch Surg* 1971; **102**: 417–23.
8. Butters AG. A review of femoral hernias with special reference to recurrence rate of low operation. *BMJ* 1948; **2**: 743–5.
9. McClure RD, Fallis LS. Femoral hernia. Report of 90 operations. *Ann Surg* 1939; **109**: 987–1000.
10. Cooper A. *The Anatomy and Surgical Treatment of Inguinal Congenital Hernia*. London: T Cox, 1804.
11. Cooper A. *Anatomy and Surgical Treatment of Abdominal Hernia*, 1st US ed, from 2nd UK ed. Philadelphia: Lea and Blanchard, 1844.
12. Marcy HO. *The Anatomy and Surgical Treatment of Hernia*. New York: D Appleton, 1982.
13. Fruchaud H. *Anatomie chirurgicale des hernies de l'aine*. Paris: Editions Doin, 1956: 322–55.

54

An Expanded PTFE Soft Tissue Patch as an Inlay Graft for Inguinal Hernia

STANLEY D BERLINER

Halsted recognized, a century ago, that a tension-free hernioplasty is essential. A sound approach to the repair of inguinal hernias rests on an evaluation of the integrity of the posterior wall and on the status of the internal inguinal ring.

In 15% of primary hernias and in 18% of recurrent hernias I found it necessary to use mesh as an inlay graft to reconstruct the posterior wall and deep ring.

The procedures are performed under local anaesthesia in an outpatient (ambulatory) facility. Total operating room time is one hour, and the patient is discharged home an hour later.

Proper exposure is essential. The genital branch of the genitofemoral nerve is divided along with the accompanying external spermatic vessels. The internal ring and posterior wall are exposed by liberally incising the muscular arch of the internal oblique and excising all red muscle of internal oblique and cremaster. The posterior wall is incised and a flap dissected superiorly to the rectus

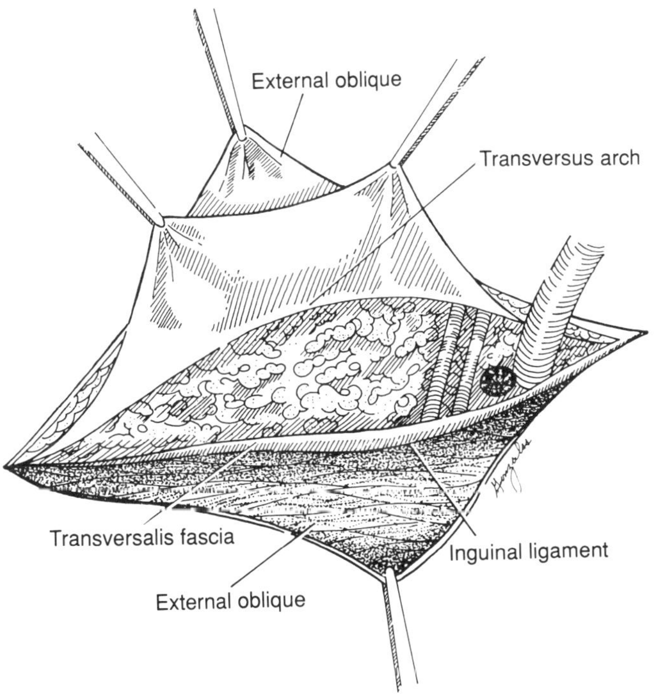

Figure 54.1: The posterior wall is incised and a flap dissected superiorly to the white line of the transversus arch. At the completion of the dissection, the inferior epigastric vessels retract into the preperitoneal space.

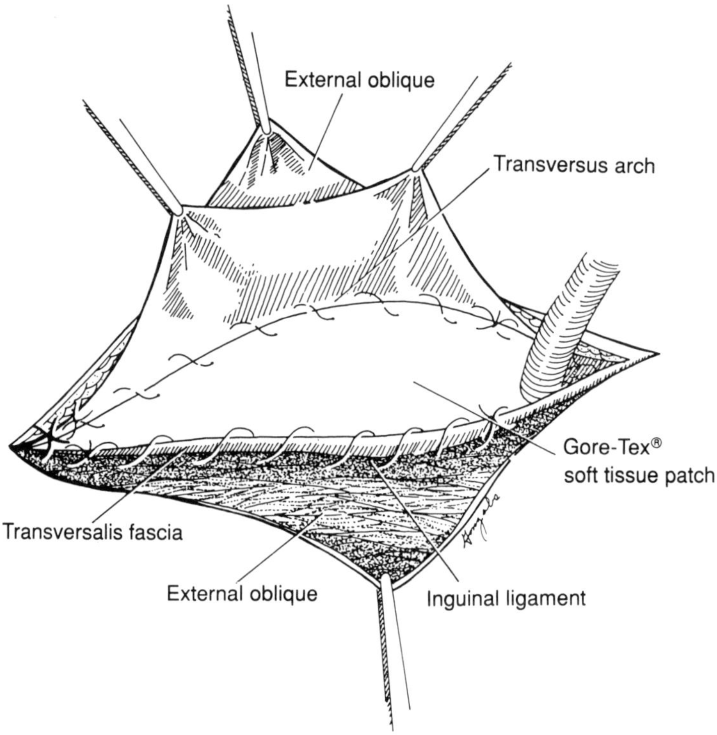

Figure 54.2: The soft-tissue patch is securely fixed to the pubis with a figure-of-eight 0 monofilament. The mesh is fixed to the transversus arch above and to both transversalis fascia and inguinal ligament below with continuous sutures of a 3–0 monofilament. This repairs the anatomical defect in the posterior wall without tension and establishes a new internal ring lateral to the epigastric vessels.

margin, which allows the inferior epigastric vessels to retract into the preperitoneal space (Figure 54.1). The femoral cone is carefully explored and a mesh plug inserted if indicated.

A 5 × 10 cm Gore-Tex soft tissue patch 1 mm in thickness is fashioned to fit the defect and is sutured to the pubis with a figure-of-eight zero monofilament (Figure 54.2). The biomaterial is fixed to the transversus arch above with a continuous suture of a 3–0 monofilament, and to both transversalis fascia and inguinal ligament below with a similar suture. The patient tests the repair by straining vigorously. An additional layer of a 3–0 monofilament approximates the superior cut edge of the posterior wall to the undersurface of the inguinal ligament adjacent to the previous suture line. A total of 350 cases were performed, with a mean follow-up time of 53.83 months plus or minus 17.14 months; 91% were followed by personal examination. The failure rate is 1.1%.

55

Stapled Mesh Herniorrhaphy

BRENDAN J CARROLL AND CHESTER J SEMEL

The use of staples to replace conventional sutures in surgery dates back to the turn of the century, and today staples have replaced sutures in many procedures[1]. Since May 1991 we have successfully employed a technique of herniorrhaphy that relies on stapled mesh placed through a 5 cm anterior incision as the sole basis of the repair. In this chapter we describe the technique and our early clinical experience with it.

Operative technique

For inguinal hernias, a 5 cm incision is made transversely over the internal ring. Marcaine 0.25% is used for local anaesthesia. The external oblique aponeurosis is divided, and the cord structures are dissected free and retracted. The ilioinguinal and iliohypogastric nerves are identified and protected. If an indirect sac is present it is dissected out, and high ligation is performed in the usual fashion using a Vicryl suture.

Polypropylene mesh is then stapled to the floor of the inguinal canal, covering any direct or sliding components. We currently use the Ethicon EMS Stapler, which is inconveniently long but is being redesigned for this application. If a large direct sac is present, it may be inverted with one or two sutures of Vicryl to facilitate placement of the mesh. The mesh is securely fastened to the shelving portion of Poupart's ligament laterally, and to the lacunar ligament, transverse aponeurosis and rectus fascia, forming a multilayer repair. Some 20–25 staples are placed throughout the body of the Prolene mesh, rather than just at its edges. This affords increased cohesion between the mesh and the fascia, which may promote early fibrous ingrowth.

The cord is brought through a slit in the mesh laterally. The aperture for the cord is created, leaving a 1 cm opening for the cord structures, by overlapping the tails of mesh and securing them in position with additional staples laterally. The external oblique aponeurosis is closed over the cord structures using a running Vicryl suture, and the skin is closed with subcuticular Vicryl stitches or surgical clips.

For femoral hernias the direct floor is opened, and the mesh is tacked to Cooper's ligament. In ventral hernias the mesh is stapled as an onlay patch over the hernia defect.

Results

Forty-nine hernia repairs were performed in 47 patients, ranging in age from 15 to 91 years. There was no attempt to exclude difficult hernias from this study, ie recurrent, sliding, bilateral or incarcerated. Patients were given the choice of conventional herniorrhaphy or laparoscopic herniorrhaphy. There were 38 inguinal hernias, nine ventral or umbilical hernias and two femoral hernias. Seven of the hernias were recurrent and two were bilateral.

All patients underwent a repeat physical examination for the purpose of this study between one and 24 months after surgery. All patients were treated as outpatients, and released within two to three hours after surgery, except for one female with a small bowel obstruction secondary to an incarcerated ventral hernia, who was hospitalized for three days. The average operative time was 33 minutes for inguinal hernias. Most patients were able to return to work and/or normal physical activities within one week of surgery. There were no restrictions placed on normal physical activities after the seventh postoperative day.

There were no recurrent hernias, nerve injuries, orchitis or wound infections. Four patients had minor wound seromas or haematomas, and one patient required needle aspiration twice. Follow up was performed between one and 24 months postoperatively. All patients were followed and re-examined specifically for the purpose of this study.

Conclusions

Anterior stapled herniorrhaphy with polypropylene mesh is safe and effective. Studies in the porcine model have demonstrated that mesh can be firmly attached to tissue with staples, and that intra-abdominal pressures do not exceed the strength of the stapled fixation[2]. We have confirmed the security of the mesh in humans during the Valsalva manoeuvre and cough, using fluoroscopy in the early postoperative period. We have observed no early recurrences, which suggests that there is no conceptual flaw to the technique. We anticipate that long-term recurrence rates will be no higher than other mesh repairs with[3] or without[4] sutures.

Stapled mesh herniorrhaphy offers many advantages over other methods. It is a simple procedure that is easy to learn and to perform. The use of multiple small staples placed atraumatically throughout the mesh into the fascia has advantages over sutured repairs. Multiple areas of the floor can be incorporated into the repair with speed, ease and precision, providing an effective and seemingly reliable repair that incorporates multiple fascial layers in one step. The avoidance of deep biting sutures reduces tissue manipulation and trauma, thereby reducing postoperative pain. This probably accounts for some of the reduced pain noted in the laparoscopic technique of herniorrhaphy. Staples are less reactive than commonly used suture materials, thereby reducing the chance of granuloma or stitch abscess. Additionally, the use of interrupted staples has theoretical advantages over continuous sutures in the avoidance of nerve compression or entrapment.

The procedure also lends itself to better cosmetic results, when this is desired, because of the ease of properly securing the mesh through a skin incision that is smaller than would be possible in sutured repairs. Because multiple points of fixation throughout the body of the mesh allow for a secure repair without the need for deep biting and accurately placed running sutures, less dissection is required. Operative time can be reduced to approximately 20 minutes for routine inguinal herniorrhaphy, and postoperative discomfort is reduced.

Summary

Anterior stapled mesh herniorrhaphy is a valuable option, with many potential advantages over other repairs. It may become the procedure of choice for inguinal herniorrhaphy. Staples may replace sutures, as they have in many other areas of surgery.

References

1. Ravitch MM, Steichen FM. Staples and staplers. *Adv Surg* 1984; **17**: 214–79.
2. Dion YM, Charara J, Guidoin R. Bursting strength evaluation of an experimental hernia repair using Prolene mesh attached to tissue with EMS Stapler or with US Surgical Endopath. Scientific presentation, SAGES Annual Meeting, Phoenix, Arizona, April 1993.
3. Lichtenstein IL, Shulman A, Amid P. The tension-free hernioplasty. *Am J Surg* 1989; **157**: 188–93.
4. Gilbert A. Sutureless repair of inguinal hernia. *Am J Surg* 1992; **163**: 331–5.

56

Laparoscopic Hernia Repair: a Rural Perspective

RODERICK B BROWN

The feasibility of repairing hernias laparoscopically has been demonstrated by Ger[1], Popp[2], Schultz[3,4], Corbett[5] and Toy[6] in their reported series. There continues to be considerable speculation and debate as to the practicality and value of the laparoscopic hernia repair.

Operative procedure

Between March 1991 and April 1993, 76 patients from Minnesota had 106 hernias repaired laparoscopically at one of five rural hospitals having 30 or fewer beds. All of the patients were treated by the author.

Informed consent was obtained from all patients preoperatively. The patients were advised that laparoscopic hernia repair is still an investigational procedure, as we do not have long-term (five- to ten-year) follow-up results on patients who have had their hernias repaired with the laparoscopic technique. The patients were further advised that the laparoscopic procedure requires general anaesthesia, whereas the standard open hernia repair can be done with a general, regional or local anaesthetic. All patients were also advised that they could resume unrestricted activity as soon postoperatively as they desired (except baths or swimming for one week) with the laparoscopic repair; however, there would be six to eight weeks of activity restrictions after the standard open repair.

General anaesthesia with tracheal intubation provided by the local certified registered nurse anaesthetist was used. All patients received a preoperative dose of intravenous antibiotics, usually 1 g of ceftriaxone sodium. All patients had an indwelling Foley catheter, which was inserted at the time of surgery and removed at the end of the procedure. Male patients had the genitalia as well as the groin area and abdomen prepared in the sterile field. Three trocar sites were used for the procedure. A 0° 10 mm video laparoscope was placed through the umbilicus via a 10 mm disposable trocar sleeve with a retractable safety shield. A reusable 11 mm trocar was placed lateral to the rectus muscle on the same side as the hernia, and a 5 mm trocar was placed lateral to the rectus muscle on the opposite side, both at about the level of the umbilicus. The placement of the trocars for the repair of the umbilical, incisional and ventral hernias was determined by the location of the hernia. Abdominal insufflation pressure of 14 mmHg was used and maintained throughout the procedure.

A unique method of dissecting an indirect hernia sac in male patients was developed. The first step is to grasp the apex of the hernia sac and invert it by pulling the apex of the hernia sac back into the peritoneal cavity. One must be careful to grasp only the peritoneum with this manoeuvre. While maintaining traction on the apex of the hernia sac, the surgeon then grasps the ipsilateral testicle and cord structures, which will have been pulled high into the scrotum. By applying firm, steady downward traction to the spermatic cord, you can often quickly and cleanly strip the hernia sac away from the cord structures. Once the sac has been dissected free, the remainder of the dissection is relatively easy.

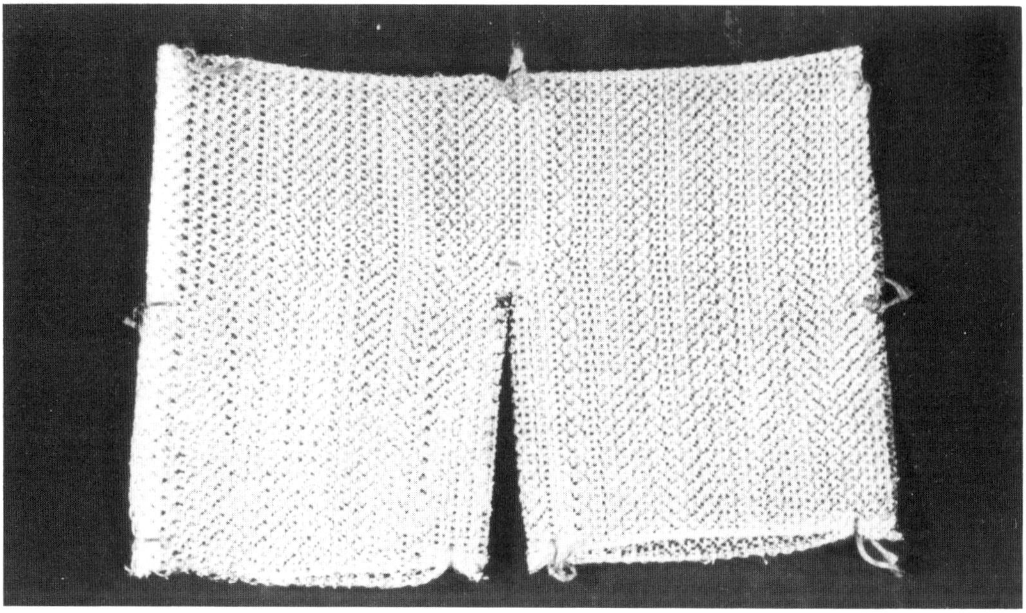

Figure 56.1: Prosthetic hernia patch made with folded piece of woven polypropylene mesh that is sutured at the corners and at the middle of each edge. Two sutures are placed at the middle of the unfolded edge, between which a slit is made to the centre of the patch to accommodate the inferior epigastric vessels.

An Nd:YAG contact laser was used for the peritoneal incision, which was made transversely from anterolateral to the indirect space to the umbilical fold medially. Using the contact laser in conjunction with blunt dissection, the peritoneal flap and hernia sac were dissected down and away from the hernia defect and surrounding fascia. The inferior epigastric vessels were isolated and preserved.

The prosthetic patch used was made from a piece of woven polypropylene mesh which was folded to make a double layer of mesh. This was then sutured at the corners and at the middle of each edge, two sutures being placed near the middle of the unfolded edge with a slit cut between these sutures and extending to the centre of the patch to accommodate the inferior epigastric vessels. This patch design provides better tensile strength and allows for a smaller sized patch to be used without compromising the repair (Figure 56.1).

The incisional hernia and one ventral hernia were repaired with a preperitoneal mesh, whereas the umbilical hernia and two of the ventral hernias were closed with intracorporeal suturing without mesh. The patches were made at the time of surgery and were approximately 9 × 6 cm. The mesh was introduced into the peritoneal cavity by rolling it and inserting it into a hollow 10 mm trocar sleeve that was then introduced via the 11 mm trocar. The mesh was then placed anterior to and around the inferior epigastric vessels. The mesh was placed in such a way as to cover both the direct and the indirect spaces (Figure 56.2).

In selected cases, a piece of mesh shaped like a bow tie was placed partially into the hernia defect. This was made by using a piece of woven polypropylene about 8 × 3 cm tied about the middle with a suture (Figure 56.3). A 2–0 polyglactin suture was used for making the patch and 'bow tie'.

For the larger hernias it was determined that securing the hernia patch to the underlying fascia with sutures or staples resulted in stronger repair. The peritoneum was closed over the patch with 2–0 polyglactin suture so that the entire piece of mesh was covered. The fascial defects from the 10 mm and the 11 mm trocars were closed with a 0 polyglactin suture.

When irrigation fluid was required, a mixtures of normal saline with 5000 units of heparin per litre and 1 g of cefazolin sodium per litre (if the patient was not allergic) was used. All the irrigation

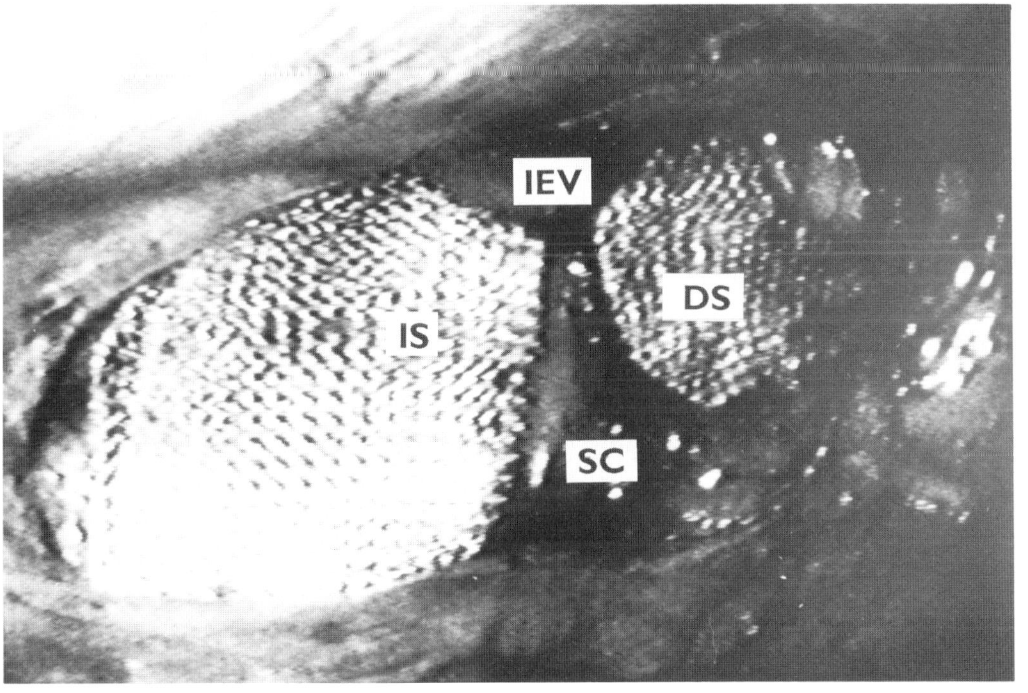

Figure 56.2: Prosthetic hernia patch in a left-sided repair. DS, direct hernia space; IEV, inferior epigastric vessels; IS indirect hernia space; SC, spermatic cord structures.

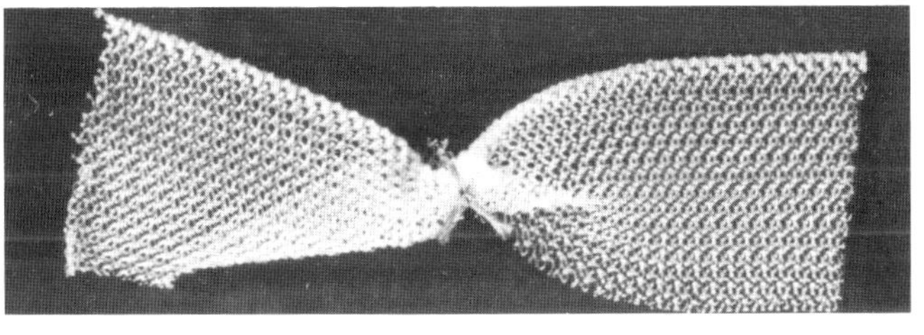

Figure 56.3: Polypropylene woven mesh 'bow tie' used in selected cases to obliterate the hernia defect prior to placement of the prosthetic patch.

fluid was removed by suctioning at the end of the procedure. The stab incisions were infiltrated with 0.25% bupivacaine hydrochloride with adrenaline (epinephrine) 1 : 200 000 and closed with a 3–0 polyglactin subcuticular suture and steri strips. Patients were routinely given 60 mg of ketorolac tromethamine via intramuscular injection at the conclusion of the procedure.

Results

In this series 76 patients (67 male and nine female) had a total of 106 hernias repaired: 59 were indirect hernias, with 20 on the right side, 21 on the left side and nine bilateral; 23 were direct hernias, with 14 on the right side and nine on the left. There were no bilateral direct hernias. There were 13 double (pantaloon) hernias, of which nine were on the right side and four on the left, including a direct/femoral hernia. There were also three ventral, one umbilical and one incisional hernia. Thirty-one patients had additional procedures performed at the time of their laparoscopic hernia repair: five had laparoscopic cholecystectomy, 20 had adhesiolysis, two had hydrocelectomy, one had a tubal transection, one a vasectomy, one a laparoscopic hysterectomy and there was one closure of a small bowel perforation that occurred during adhesiolysis.

A distinct advantage that the laparoscopic approach has over the conventional open method is the ability to diagnose other, unsuspected, intraperitoneal pathology. In this series of patients, there was a 21% incidence of previously undiagnosed inguinal hernias, which were repaired. The average operating time for unilateral hernias without additional procedures was 70 minutes, and for bilateral hernias was 110 minutes. The age range was 12–80 years , the average age being 55 years and the median age 61 years. Thirty of the patients were farmers (39.47%). Patients were interviewed 1–24 months after their operation and reported the following results. The average number of days to return to full activity was seven. The average length of hospital stay was 15 hours. Most of the patients who had their surgery in the afternoon stayed until the following morning. There were three recurrences, a rate for this series of 2.8%. Of the three patients with recurrence, two elected to have them repaired laparoscopically, and have had no further problems. The third patient has indicated that he is going to have his recurrent hernia repaired laparoscopically again.

There was one complication, an abdominal wall haematoma which resolved without treatment. There were no infections or problems with urinary retention or neuralgias or nerve injuries in this series of patients. Three patients experienced a subsequent pubitis and all three resolved after a local injection of betamethasone.

Patients were questioned about the degree of postoperative pain they experienced. Eleven patients (14%) reported no pain after surgery, 52 (68%) reported mild postoperative pain, 12 (16%) reported moderate pain and one patient said he experienced severe pain. Twenty-four patients (32%) did not require any pain medication postoperatively.

Patients were questioned about their level of satisfaction with their laparoscopic hernia repair, and 60 (79%) reported they were completely satisfied with the procedure and the results. Thirteen (17%) said they were somewhat satisfied, two patients were somewhat dissatisfied and one patient was completely dissatisfied. Not surprisingly, the patients who were dissatisfied were those who experienced a recurrence of their hernia. The two patients who had their recurrent hernias repaired laparoscopically a second time expressed complete satisfaction with the procedure after the subsequent repair. Eleven patients (14.5%) had previously experienced a standard 'open' herniorrhaphy and all of these preferred the laparoscopic procedure to the 'open' procedure. They all cited less postoperative pain and a quicker recovery and return to full activity as the reasons for their preference.

All 76 patients (100%) said they would choose the laparoscopic procedure again should they need another hernia repaired in the future.

Conclusions

Laparoscopic hernioplasty appears to be an attractive alternative to the standard 'open' hernia repairs. It will take a few more years of follow up on the patients who have undergone laparoscopic hernioplasty before we will be able to determine the long-term efficacy of this procedure. We can conclude at this time from our limited experience that it is the procedure that our patients clearly prefer. The early results compare favourably with open herniorrhaphy with regard to recurrence rate. With the continued development of new laparoscopic modalities and additional experience, I believe we can reduce the recurrence rate even further. The procedure may cost more than standard hernia repair but, as is the case with laparoscopic cholecystectomy, the rapid recovery and return to work may offset the additional operating room costs.

In this series, 21% of the patients were found to have an inguinal hernia that had not been previously diagnosed and was repaired. The laparoscopic approach saved those patients an additional subsequent procedure and the associated costs, disability, time off from work or school, etc.

Patients experience less pain after this procedure than after an open hernia repair, and it is hard to put a price tag on the value of this benefit of the procedure.

Another area where substantial savings can be realized relates to patients who develop their hernia with work-related activities, as was the case with several patients in our series. The shortened recovery time and quicker return to unrestricted work activities resulted in significant savings in workers compensation costs.

I have been as pleased and as impressed as my patients with the results of this procedure. I believe that continued evaluation of this exciting and promising new procedure is warranted. Over the next decade the laparoscopic approach to hernia repair, driven by patient demand and supported by good clinical outcomes, will evolve as the procedure of choice for this age-old problem.

References

1. Ger R, Monroe R, Duvier R, *et al.* Management of indirect inguinal hernia by laparoscopic closure of the neck of the sac. *Am J Surg* 1990; **159**: 370.
2. Popp LW. Endoscopic patch repair of inguinal hernia in a female patient. *Surg Endosc* 1990; **4**: 10.
3. Schultz L, Graber J, Pietrafitta J, Hickok D. Laser laparoscopic herniorrhaphy: a clinical trial – Preliminary results. *J Laparoendosc Surg* 1990; **1**: 41.
4. Schultz L, Graber J, Pietrafitta J, Hickok D. Laser laparoscopic inguinal herniorrhaphy. *Lasers Surg Med* 1991; suppl 3: 26.
5. Corbitt JD. Laparoscopic herniorrhaphy. *South Med J* 1991; **84**: 25101.
6. Toy FK, Smoot RT. Laparoscopic hernioplasty. *Surg Laparosc Endosc* 1991; **1**: 151.

57

Laparoscopic Inguinal Herniorrhaphy with the Mushroom Plug: Outcome and Classification

ABDELKADER HAWASLI

Since the introduction of laparoscopic inguinal herniorrhaphy by Ger[1], Schultz[2] and others[3,4], various modifications have been made to this technique in order to achieve the lowest recurrence rate possible. The transabdominal preperitoneal approach, being the most commonly used technique, has progressed from placement of cylindrical plugs and screen[2] to screen alone. In the early stages, when hernia clips were not available, we developed the Mushroom Plug[5] to decrease the chance of the plug migrating into the inguinal canal (in the indirect hernia) or the subcutaneous tissue (in the direct hernia). Later, when hernia clips became available we continued to use the Mushroom Plug and screen technique with placement of a few clips to stabilize the mesh.

We introduced a laparoscopic classification[6] of these hernias to be able to evaluate the results of these different methods in a more scientific way.

Operative technique

The patients

Between March 1991 and December 1992, 318 hernias were repaired by the author in 253 patients using the transabdominal preperitoneal approach. There were 240 males and 13 females; the average age was 56 years (range 18–82 years) and an average weight of 82 kg (range 43–137 kg) (average 180 lb, range 96–302 lb).

There were 277 (87%) primary hernias and 41 (13%) recurrent hernias. Sixty patients (24%) had bilateral hernias, and there were 154 hernias on the right side and 164 on the left side. Two patients with femoral hernias are not included.

These hernias were classified into five different types based on the site of the defect (direct or indirect), the size of the defect and whether the hernia was primary or recurrent (Table 57.1). There were 145 (45.6%) indirect hernias; 66 (45.5%) of them were (type IB) (ie indirect hernia with dilated internal ring greater than 2 cm). Direct hernias totalled 100 (31.4%); 50 of them were (type IIC) (ie direct hernia with defect greater than 2 cm). Twenty-four (7.5%) were pantaloon hernias; 12 (50%) of them were (type III–IIC) (ie the major component of the hernia was a direct defect greater than 2 cm). Eight hernias (2.5%) were scrotal and 41 (12.9%) were recurrent. Three of the recurrent hernias were failed laparoscopic repairs that were repaired again laparoscopically at the patient's request (Table 57.2).

A computerized chart is created for each hernia and the patients are followed up six-monthly.

Candidates for this repair were all adults, able to tolerate general anaesthesia and had no bleeding diatheses. Patients who were pregnant or had a giant hernia were excluded. Previous lower abdominal surgery was not considered a contraindication to this approach.

Table 57.1: Classification of hernias

Type I: Indirect
A Dilated internal ring < 2 cm
B Dilated internal ring > 2 cm
Type II: Direct
A Weakness with no fascia defect
B Fascia defect < 2 cm
C Fascia defect > 2 cm
Type III: Pantaloon
Subdivided into I or II depending on the major component of the defect
Type IV: Scrotal
A Dilated internal ring < 2 cm
B Dilated internal ring > 2 cm
Type V: Recurrent
Subdivided into I or II depending on the recurrence site

Table 57.2: Classification of 318 hernias

Type	*Subtype*		*Total*
Type I	A	79	
	B	66	145
Type II	A	15	
	B	35	
	C	50	100
Type III	IA	2	
	IB	3	
	IIB	7	
	IIC	12	24
Type IV	A	2	
	B	6	8
Type V	IA	7	
	IB	3	
	IA	1 (LIH)*	
	IB	2 (LIH)*	
	IIB	16	
	IIC	12	41

* LIH: recurrent after laparoscopic repair, were repaired laparoscopically again

The technique

The operation is performed under general anaesthesia as previously described by the author[6]. The patient's arms are placed to his side. A Foley catheter and an oral gastric tube are inserted during the operation and removed at the end of the procedure. The pneumoperitoneum is created via an infraumbilical incision under 15 mmHg pressure. A 10 mm trocar is placed in the infraumbilical position for the 10 mm 0° laparoscope.

A video monitor is placed at the foot of the table. The hernia site is inspected as well as the rest of the abdomen. The operator stands opposite to the hernia. A 12 mm trocar is placed opposite to the hernia (for the introduction of the hernia clip device) and a 10 mm trocar is placed at the side of the hernia (unless the patient has bilateral hernias, in which case both trocars are 12 mm). The lateral trocars are placed at the level of the umbilicus at the edge of the rectus muscle to prevent injury to the inferior epigastric vessels.

Using a two-handed technique, the peritoneum is incised cephalad to the internal ring, laterally to medially, stopping at the medial umbilical ligament. Dissection in the preperitoneal space is performed, avoiding injury to the inferior epigastric vessels.

With an indirect hernia, the hernia sac is removed from the inguinal canal after dissecting the cord structures. The sac is everted to the abdominal cavity without transection. However, with a scrotal hernia, the sac is dissected as far as possible distally and transected, leaving the distal part of the sac in the patient. The direct space is dissected, exposing Cooper's ligament.

A polypropylene Mushroom Plug is placed in the dilated internal ring after taking a still picture and measuring the defect. One or more of this plug is used to obliterate the dilated internal ring. Two hernia clips are used to fix the mesh to the anterior and lateral abdominal wall. A mesh screen 6 × 9 cm is placed over both direct and indirect spaces. The screen is secured to the abdominal wall and Cooper's ligament with few clips (Figure 57.1). Care must be taken not to clip inferior to the inguinal ligament laterally, to prevent injury to the lateral femoral cutaneous nerve and the femoral branch of the genitofemoral nerve.

With a direct hernia, the dissection is performed in a similar fashion. The defect in the direct space is obliterated with one or more Mushroom Plugs after measuring its size. The stem of the plug is shortened to 1 cm. These plugs are fixed to the edges of the defect with few clips. A mesh screen 6 × 9 cm is placed over both direct and indirect space as described above (Figures 57.2 and 57.3).

The abdominal pressure is decreased to 6 mmHg to facilitate approximation of the peritoneal edges. Regular clips are used to close the peritoneum. The fascia at the trocar sites is closed to prevent future incisional hernias.

Recurrent hernias are repaired in a similar way according to the site of recurrence.

Results

Three different groups can be identified during the study period of 21 months. The first group of patients had acylindrical plugs and screen as described by Schultz: 37 repairs were done with this method from March 1991 to July 1991. The second group of patients had the Mushroom Plug and screen from July 1991 to November 1991, with total of 53 repairs. The third group of patients had additional placement of hernia clips to the Mushroom Plug and screen repairs, 228 hernias being repaired between November 1991 and December 1992. Two hernias were converted to conventional repair because of incarceration that could not be managed laparoscopically.

There were three recurrences in the *first group*, a recurrence rate of 8.1%). All recurrences occurred within the first nine months (two, five and nine months, respectively). The total follow up was 18–21 months. The first two recurrences were in indirect hernias with dilated internal rings greater than 2 cm (type IB). The third recurrence was also in an indirect hernia but with a dilated internal ring less than 2 cm (type IA).

There were no recurrences in the *second group* in whom the Mushroom Plug was used. This group has had a total follow up of 11–18 months.

Two recurrences occurred in the *third group*, which has had a follow up of 1–14 months. The first recurrence occurred after eight months in an indirect hernia with a dilated internal ring of 4 cm (type IB). This recurrence was repaired conventionally. The second recurrence was after conventional

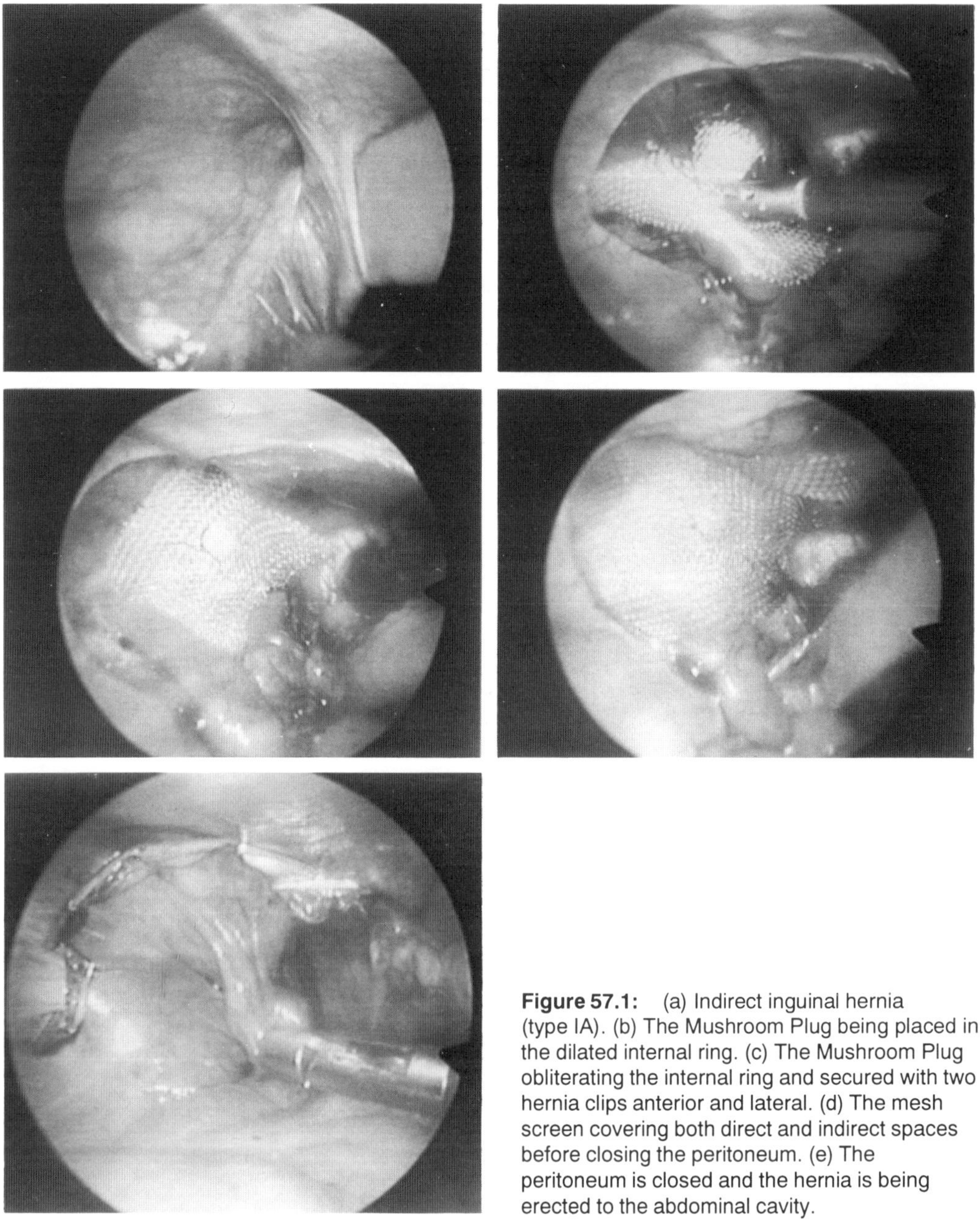

Figure 57.1: (a) Indirect inguinal hernia (type IA). (b) The Mushroom Plug being placed in the dilated internal ring. (c) The Mushroom Plug obliterating the internal ring and secured with two hernia clips anterior and lateral. (d) The mesh screen covering both direct and indirect spaces before closing the peritoneum. (e) The peritoneum is closed and the hernia is being erected to the abdominal cavity.

repair; the patient had a direct defect of 1.5 cm (type V–IIB). The recurrence after the laparoscopic repair was noticed in the first month of follow up. The overall recurrence rate with the Mushroom Plug and screen (groups two and three) was 0.7% in 281 hernia repairs.

All but 11 patients were discharged the same day of surgery. Ten patients were admitted owing to urinary retention and one patient was admitted because of a scrotal haematoma.

Pain was limited to the first two to three days; it was easily controlled with oral analgesics. Patients returned to normal activity and work within one to two weeks.

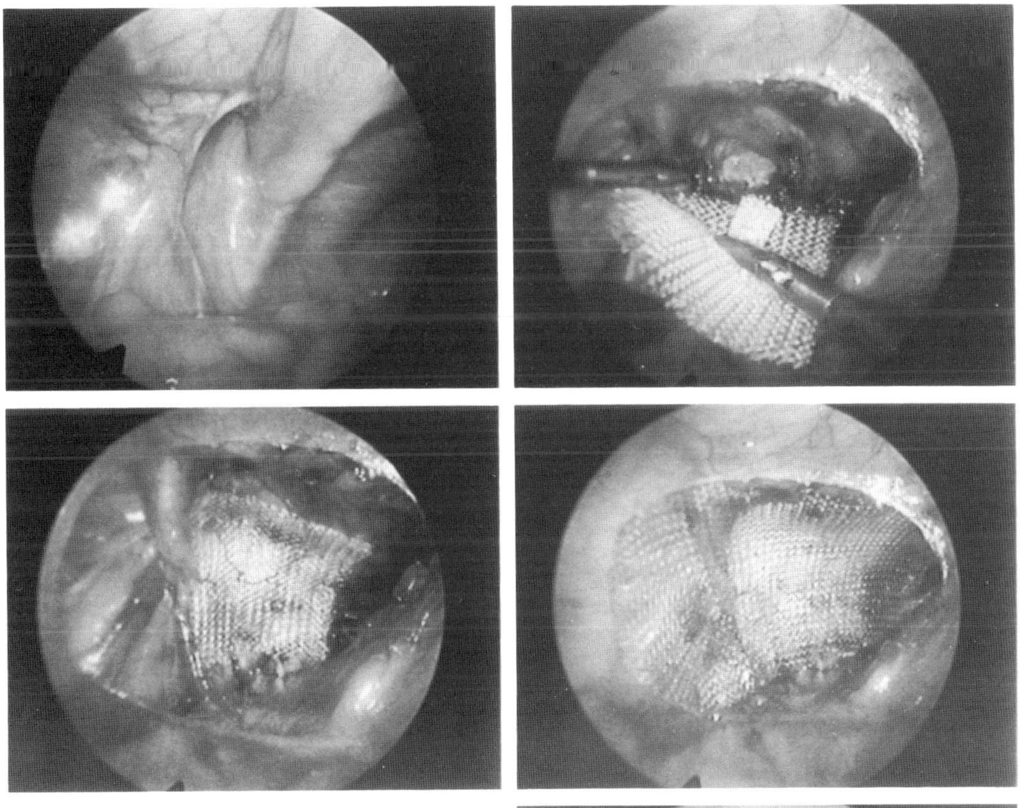

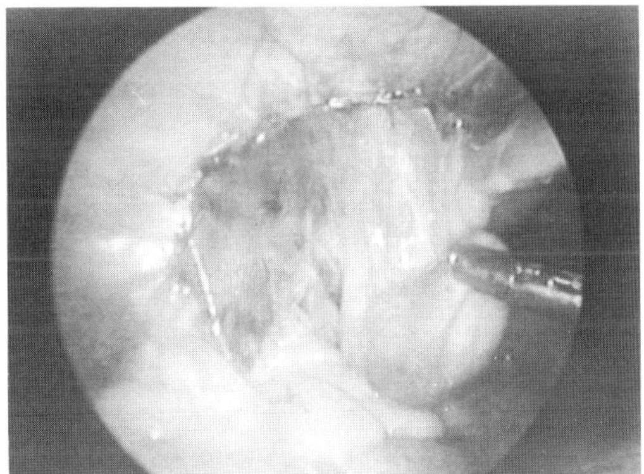

Figure 57.2: (a) Direct inguinal hernia (type IIB). (b) The Mushroom Plug being placed in the direct defect (the stem has been shortened). (c) The Mushroom Plug is placed in the direct defect and secured to the edges with a few hernia clips. (d) The mesh screen covering both direct and indirect spaces before closing the peritoneum. (e) The peritoneum is closed.

Complications

Of the 318 repairs, 40 (12.6%) developed complications. Two of these (0.6%) were considered major complications. One patient had scrotal haematoma; he was admitted for observation without blood transfusion. The second patient developed epididymitis and was treated with antibiotics on an out-patient basis.

The remaining 38 (12%) were minor complications. The most common complications were seroma (16) and haematoma (12). These were treated by aspiration as an out-patient procedure. The remaining ten complications (3%) were urinary retention requiring hospitalization.

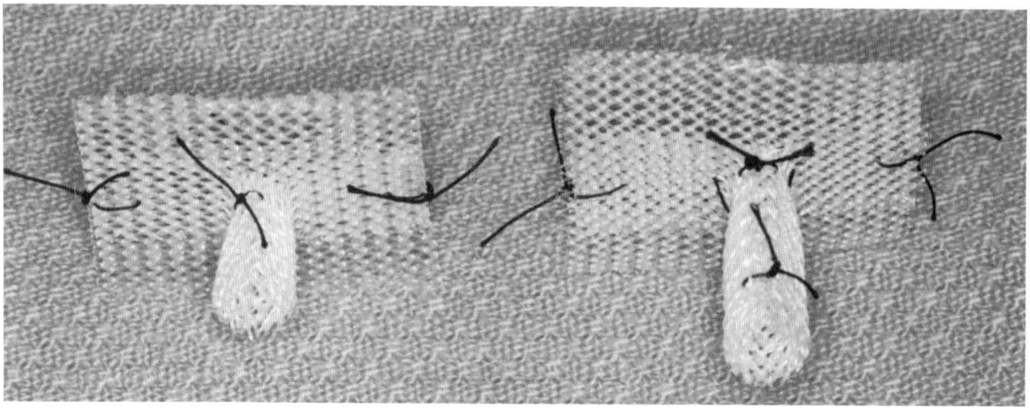

Figure 57.3: The Mushroom Plug. *Left*: for direct hernia (short stem). *Right*: for indirect hernia (long stem).

Even though this technique requires general anaesthesia and converts an extra-abdominal procedure to an intra-abdominal one, there has been no anaesthesia-related complication or abdominal complication due to adhesions or trocar insertion.

Conclusions

The modern principles of conventional repair of inguinal hernias were introduced by Bassini[7] in 1884 when he emphasized the need to repair the floor of the inguinal canal to achieve a recurrence rate under 10%. Marcy, in 1869, also emphasized the need for high ligation of the sac. Since then, several different modifications have been attempted to reach the perfect repair with low recurrence rate. More recently, Nyhus[8] regenerated interest in Cheatle's[9] preperitoneal approach for repairing recurrent inguinal hernias. However, the lowest recurrence rate is reported by Lichtenstein[10] using a tension-free repair with synthetic material.

The laparoscopic transabdominal preperitoneal repair of inguinal hernias using the Mushroom Plug and screen follows the principles of conventional repair mentioned above. It is a tension-free repair, using synthetic material through a preperitoneal approach. The mesh is placed against the fascia of the floor and the defect is plugged after removal of the sac. The flat top of the Mushroom Plug seems to prevent the plug from migrating into the inguinal canal or the subcutaneous tissue. In addition, the use of hernia clips seems to provide additional security to prevent migration of both the plug and the screen.

The use of the laparoscopic hernia classification will allow us to better evaluate the results of this repair in terms of recurrence and complications, as well as comparing different types of repairs for the same type of hernia. In addition, it may be used to qualify or disqualify patients for this technique.

Our early results with this repair (although with, as yet, a short follow up), with a recurrence rate of 0.7% in 281 repairs using the Mushroom Plug and screen, compare well with other reports of recurrence following conventional preperitoneal repairs such as Read[11] (6.6%) in 1186 repairs) and Stoppa[12] (1.4% in 604 repairs). It also compares favourably with Lichtenstein's[13] 0.7% in 6321 tension-free repairs.

Summary

Laparoscopic inguinal herniorrhaphy is emerging as an attractive alternative to conventional repair. It adheres to the principle of the conventional technique with preperitoneal approach and a tension-free repair. It has the advantage of decreasing postoperative pain, recovery time and disability. It allow patients to walk in an erect posture postoperatively, with excellent cosmetic results. It avoids two operations in patients with bilateral inguinal hernias, while maintaining the same short recovery time. In addition, it has the advantage, in recurrent inguinal hernias, of avoiding dissection through scar tissue from the previous conventional repair, thus minimizing cord structure injury.

Our short-term results with the Mushroom Plug and screen repair are encouraging and a long-term follow-up is planned.

References

1. Schultz L, Graber J, Pietrafitta J, Hickok D. Laser laparoscopic herniorrhaphy: a clinical trial. Preliminary results. *J Laparoendosc Surg* 1990; **1**: 41–5.
2. Ger R, Monroe K, Duvivier R, Mishrick A. Management of indirect inguinal hernias by laparoscopic closure of the neck of the sac. *Am J Surg* 1990; **159**: 370–3.
3. Corbitt Jr J. Laparoscopic herniorrhaphy. *Surg Laparosc Endosc* 1991; **1**: 23–5.
4. Toy F, Smoot Jr R. Toy–Smoot laparoscopic hernioplasty. *Surg Laparosc Endosc* 1991; **1**: 151–5.
5. Hawasli A. Laparoscopic inguinal herniorrhaphy: 'the mushroom plug repair'. *Surg Laparosc Endosc* 1992; **2**: 111–16.
6. Hawasli A. Laparoscopic inguinal herniorrhaphy: classification and 1 year experience. *J Laparoendosc Surg* 1992; **2**: 137–43.
7. Bassini E. *Nuovo metodo per la cura radicale dellerna inguinale.* Padua: R Sabilimento Prosperini, 1889.
8. Nyhus LM, Condon RE, Harkins HN. Clinical experience with preperitoneal hernia repair for all types of hernia of the groin. *Am J Surg* 1960; **100**: 234–44.
9. Cheatle GL. An operation for the radical cure of inguinal and femoral hernia. *BMJ* 1920; **2**: 168.
10. Lichtenstein IL, Shulman AG, Amid PK, Montllor MM. The tension-free hernioplasty. *Am J Surg* 1989; **157**: 188–93.
11. Read RC. Recurrence after preperitoneal herniorrhaphy in the adult. *Arch Surg* 1975; **110**: 666–71.
12. Stoppa RA, Warlaumont CR, Verhaeghe PJ, Ropmero ER, M'Balla-N'-Di CJ. Prosthetic repair in the treatment of groin hernia. *Int Surg* 1986; **71**: 154–8.
13. Lichtenstein IL. Herniorrhaphy. A personal experience with 6,321 cases. *Am J Surg* 1987; **153**: 553–9.

58

Laparoscopic Herniorrhaphy: the Veterans General Hospital–Taipei Experience

SHING-MOO HUANG AND WING-YIU LUI

A definitive preperitoneal procedure for inguinal hernia repair was first described by Cheatle in 1920[1] and was popularized by Nyhus and colleagues[2] in the 1960s. It has been advocated for recurrent hernias because it avoids scar tissue from previous operations, and for femoral and complicated hernias (eg sliding or incarcerated inguinal hernias or bilateral groin defects) because of the greater visualization of the region it afford compared with the anterior approach.

An additional distinction between the various hernia repair techniques is whether the posterior lamina of the transversalis fascia is re-established with the use of sutures or prosthetic materials. Prostheses in hernia repair were first described by Usher and associates in 1958[3]. In 1975, Stoppa and associates introduced the application of a large unsutured polyester prosthesis placed preperitoneally for inguinal hernia repair[4]. Stoppa and Warlaumont[5] and Nyhus[6] have reported a preperitoneal approach using prosthetic material to cover the inguinal floor, with an extremely low recurrence rate of 1.4% and 1.7% (in 572 and 203 repairs). Traditional groin hernia repair disables the patients for one to two weeks, with significant discomfort and complications such as neuroma, orchitis, epididymitis and permanent neuralgia. Laparoscopic herniorrhaphy has developed from recent advances in operative laparoscopy to offer the advantages of less postoperative pain and reduced hospitalization and recuperation periods.

Inguinal hernia repair is one of the most common operative procedures, with about 500 000 operations performed annually in the USA alone[7]. The surgical treatment of inguinofemoral hernia can be broadly divided into two categories: those using a posterior approach to the inguinal region (via the preperitoneal or transabdominal plane) and those approaching it via the groin (anterior). In 1884, Bassini first described a technique for reconstruction of the inguinal floor anteriorly in the treatment of primary direct and indirect inguinal hernias[8]. Depending on the literature, this repair has a recurrence rate as high as 1.5%–10%, thought to be a result of placing tension on tissues that are not normally in apposition to each other.

The first laparoscopic repair of inguinal hernia dates back in 1980s when Ger performed laparoscopic stapling closure of the hernia sac neck in beagle dogs and later in human patients[9]. Corbitt used a plug and patch method for laparoscopic hernia repair with Endo-GIA to achieve high ligation in 1989[10]. After following these patients for two years, a recurrence rate greater than 15% became evident. The rationale for preperitoneal mesh repair in laparoscopic treatment for inguinal hernia became widely accepted by pioneers such as Schultz[11], McKernan[12] and Rodriguez[13]. The five types of laparoscopic herniorrhaphy available at present are listed in Table 58.1.

The purpose of this chapter is to evaluate the efficacy and complications of preperitoneal mesh repair in the laparoscopic treatment of direct, indirect, bilateral and recurrent inguinal hernias.

Table 58.1: The five types of laparoscopic herniorrhaphy currently available

1 Stapling closure of neck of hernia sac (Ger, 1980s)
2 Plug and patch method (Corbitt, 1989)
3 Preperitoneal approach:
 a Defect filling technique (Schultz, 1990)
 b Extraperitoneal mesh technique (McKernan, 1990)
4 Intraperitoneal approach:
 a Lateral suture repair and onlay patch technique (Spaw, 1991)
 b Intraperitoneal onlay mesh (IPOM) technique (Fitzgibbons, 1990)
5 Transabdominal preperitoneal mesh repair (TAPP):
 a Without butterfly cut or slit in mesh
 b Preperitoneal butterfly mesh technique (Rodriguez, 1991)

The patients

From May 1992 to December 1992, 25 patients with 30 inguinal hernias underwent laparoscopic herniorrhaphy in Veterans General Hospital–Taipei. There were no conversions.

All the patients were male veterans. Their mean age was 66.1 years, with a range from 62 to 72 years. There were 15 groin hernias on the right side, four on the left and five were bilateral. Eighteen of the hernias were indirect type and twelve were direct type; there was one recurrent inguinal hernia.

Ten patients had undergone previous operations: appendectomy (three), contralateral inguinal herniorrhaphy (two), ipsilateral inguinal herniorrhaphy (one), laparoscopic cholecystectomy (one) cholecystectomy plus splenectomy plus bilateral truncal vagotomy plus pyloroplasty (one), transurethral resection of prostate (TURP) (one) and nephrolithotomy (one).

Operative technique

Techniques of laparoscopic herniorrhaphy

One patient underwent plug and match method as described by Corbitt. The patient had postoperative fever up to 38.5°C for two days, thought to have resulted from foreign body reaction. He was discharged on the fifth postoperative day. This procedure was then abandoned.

Transabdominal preperitoneal mesh repairs (TAPP) were used for the other laparoscopic herniorrhaphy, with minor variations. Twenty-two procedures were performed using the TAPP technique and no slit in mesh was made to accommodate the vas deferens or the inferior epigastric vessels. seven procedures used the Rodriguez technique with a butterfly cut in the mesh to lay anterior to inferior epigastric vessels. All 30 procedures were successful, without a single conversion.

Results

Postoperative pain was minimal and no patient required intramuscular analgesics. Oral analgesics were all that were needed. Average postoperative hospital stay was 1.5 days. 90% of patients had returned to normal activity or work within one to three days after operation.

Recurrence

There was one recurrence in the follow-up period, which ranged from three to 11½ months postoperatively. The recurrence was a bilateral direct inguinal hernia which was repaired using the TAPP technique with a Mersilene mesh. The patient was discharged on the day after the operation. He had a clinical cough that was not well controlled. Three months after operation, in a vigorous bout of coughing, the left inguinal hernia recurred. At reoperation six months after the first operation, the bilateral pieces of Mersilene mesh had slipped off the transversus abdominis muscle arch and shrunken at Cooper's ligament region. Recurrent inguinal hernial sac was found on the left side, while the mesh was stacked at the inguinal canal to deep ring on the right side, obliterating the defect, thus preventing a clinical recurrence. Reoperation of bilateral mesh repair was performed using a higher arch dissection and stapling. The patient was followed up three months after reoperation: no recurrence was found.

There was no major complication nor mortality. However, there were three minor complications (10%): prolonged postoperative fever (two) and preperitoneal haematoma (one). No wound infection was found. The postoperative fever in the first patient was thought to have resulted from foreign body reaction caused by the Marlex plugs. The other postoperative fever was caused by an acute attack of gouty arthritis of the left elbow. The postoperative preperitoneal haematoma presented at follow-up seven days postoperatively. It was confirmed by ultrasonography of the inguinal region. The haematoma resolved spontaneously four weeks later.

Conclusions

Initial experience from 25 cases comprising 30 procedures of laparoscopic herniorrhaphy were presented here. Mersilene mesh plug was not recommended due to foreign reaction and fever[4]. High recurrence rate was also reported in other series: up to 15% in two years' follow-up.

Laparoscopic herniorrhaphy using preperitoneal mesh and stapling was recommended because of ease of performance, low complication rate and low short-term recurrence rate (3.3%). Less postoperative pain, faster recuperation (one to three days), shorter hospital stay (one and a half days), and better wound cosmesis were found compared with the traditional approach.

The present disadvantages associated with laparoscopic herniorrhaphy using preperitoneal mesh repair are the lack of long-term follow-up periods for recurrence and potential risk for intestinal adhesions. At least five to ten years of follow-up are needed before any firm conclusion can be drawn for laparoscopic herniorrhaphy.

References

1. Cheatle GL. An operation for the radical cure of inguinal and femoral hernias. *BMJ* 1920; **2**: 168.
2. Nyhus LM, Condon RE, Harkins HN. Clinical experiences with preperitoneal hernia repair for all types of hernia of the groin. *Am J Surg* 1960; **100**: 234.
3. Usher FC, Ochsner J, Tuttle LL. Use of Marlex mesh in the repair of incision hernias. *Am Surg* 1958; **24**: 969.
4. Stoppa RE, Petit J, Henry X. Unsutured Dacron prosthesis in groin hernias. *Int Surg* 1975; **60**: 411.
5. Stoppa RE, Warlaumont CR. The pre-peritoneal approach and prosthetic repair of groin hernia. In: Nyhus LM, Condon RE, eds. *Hernia*, 3rd ed. Philadelphia, PA: JB Lippincott, 1989: 199–225.
6. Nyhus LM, Pollak R, Rombeck TC, Donahue DE. The preperitoneal approach and prosthetic buttress repair for recurrent hernia. *Am Surg* 1988; **208**: 733–7.
7. Vayda E, Mindell WR, Rutkow ZM. A decade of surgery in Canada, England and the United States. *Arch Surg* 1982; **117**: 846.
8. Bassini E. *Nuovo metodo per la cura radicale dell ernia inguinale*. Padua: R. stabilimento Prosperini, 1889.
9. Ger R, Monroe K, Duvivier R, Mishrick A. Management of indirect hernias by laparoscopic closure of the neck of the sac. *Am J Surg* 1990; **159**: 370.

10. Corbitt Jr JD. Laparoscopic herniorrhaphy. *Laparosc Endosc Surg* 1991; **11**: 23–5.

11. Schultz L, Graber J, Pietrafitta J, Hickok D. Laser laparoscopic herniorrhaphy: a clinical trial preliminary results. *J Laparoendosc Surg* 1990; **1**: 41–5.

12. McKernan JB, Laws HL. Laparoscopic repair of inguinal hernias using a totally extraperitoneal prosthetic approach. *Surg Endosc* 1993; 7: 26–8.

13. Lauderdale RA, Rodriguez RP. Laparoscopic (laser) inguinal herniorrhaphy – a preliminary report. Presented before the Northern Texas Chapter of America College of Surgeons, 1–2 March 1991.

59

Laparoscopic Inguinal Hernia Repair in a Rural Community Hospital

JOHN A MORRISON

The James Paton Memorial Hospital is located in the town of Gander, Newfoundland, the most easterly Province of Canada. The town itself boasts a population of some 12 000 people, and provides regional surgical services to a population of approximately 125 000 people. Prior to the introduction of advanced laparoscopic procedures, and government budgetary restraints, we had a total of 60 active surgical beds; however, with the reduction of hospital stay and lack of government funding, our surgical beds have been reduced to 30. At the present time our beds are divided between general surgery, orthopaedics, gynaecology and ophthalmology. The institution has three fully equipped operating rooms but no surgical intensive care unit.

Given the above statistics, an interested observer might well ask what a small place such as this is doing in the realm of laparoscopic surgery. To answer this question one must examine several facets of the equation; when all are considered, it will become obvious why it is not merely necessary but vital for hospitals in similar locations, with similar demographics, to become involved in this type of surgery. In this chapter, one surgical procedure in particular – inguinal hernia repair – is considered, and from this the whole field of minimal access surgery can be divined.

Demographics

The town of Gander is situated in the central portion of the island of Newfoundland. The total population of Newfoundland and Labrador is approximately 500 000 people, divided among 600 communities, over a land mass of 400 000 km^2 and 12 000 km of coastline – over three times the size of New York State.

St John's, the capital, is located at the most easterly point of the island, and boasts all the amenities of a small city, including Memorial University, and the only tertiary care institutions in the Province. The city of St John's is almost four hours by road from Gander, or 45 minutes by air. The town of Gander, by virtue of its location, provides regional laparoscopic surgical services to a population of 125 000 people. Considering the geographical distribution of the population, patients may be required to travel up to seven hours at times of inclement weather, to avail themselves of laparoscopic surgery. During the winter, it is not unusual for an ice-breaker to be employed to clear a passage so that patients can come from outlying islands. Therefore, it most important to these patients to have a procedure carried out that:

- carries as little discomfort as possible considering the distances they must travel
- provides the shortest possible hospital stay
- allows the resumption of normal work as soon as possible.

The laparoscopic inguinal hernia repair represents an excellent example of such a procedure.

Procedure

The pneumoperitoneum is established, and a 10-mm trocar is inserted in the periumbilical area. A 12-mm trocar is introduced on the ipsilateral side of the hernia, and a 5-mm trocar on the contralateral side. Both these trocars are placed lateral to the rectus sheath, and no lower than the level of the umbilicus.

The peritoneum along the superior border of the sac is incised, and the sac approached from its superior aspect, preperitoneally. The sac is then traced distally until the apex is reached, and, with gentle dissection, the sac is prolapsed back into the abdominal cavity. In the case of a large sac, an incision may be made in the superior portion of the sac to permit adequate retraction and definition of the anatomy. Extreme care must be taken when dissecting along the medial border of the sac in the case of an indirect hernia, or the lateral border in the case of a direct hernia, so as to prevent damage to the vas deferens, or the spermatic vessels posteriorly. Electrocautery or laser is used only when absolutely required. No dissection is carried out lateral to the lateral margin of the internal inguinal ring, for fear of damage to the ilioinguinal and genitofemoral nerves.

Once the hernia sac has been prolapsed into the abdominal cavity, the inguinal canal is ready to receive the mesh.

Mesh: material, size and shape

In our repairs, Marlex has been used exclusively. It is important that the mesh lies flat without buckling, so as to reduce possible seroma formation and to provide as much contact as possible with the surrounding tissues to promote fibrous ingrowth. In order to achieve this, it is necessary to shape the mesh. Initially, the ends of a rectangular piece of Marlex, at least 13 cm × 6 cm, are rounded until the rectangle has become egg shaped. At this point, a series of radial incisions are made around the circumference of the mesh. These incisions are placed about every 1.5–2 cm apart, and about the same length radially. These incisions form a series of tabs, which help the flat, rather rigid, mesh conform to the contours of the inguinal area. Once the mesh is positioned, two staples are placed – one in the area of the posterior rectus sheath, medially, and the other in the iliopubic tract, laterally. Another staple may be placed in 12 o'clock position if necessary. Under no circumstances should staples be placed below the iliopubic tract, for fear of entrapping the groin nerves or damaging the iliac vessels. No attempt is made to mobilize the spermatic cord, nor to close the internal inguinal ring. Areolar adhesions within the inguinal canal are left undisturbed for the most part. The floor of the inguinal canal is otherwise left undisturbed.

Reperitonealization

It is mandatory that precise closure of the peritoneal defect be carried out, so as to reperitonealize the mesh. If this is not done, the patient risks the occurrence of adhesions forming between the bowel and mesh, or herniation of the bowel into the preperitoneal space and possible obstruction. In order to close the peritoneum comfortably over the mesh, a flap of peritoneum, based inferiorly, is fashioned from the sac. This is swung up to cover the mesh, and stapled in place; any excess sac is removed through the 12-mm trocar. Using the hernia sac to reperitonealize also has the advantage of maintaining the pneumoperitoneum so that there is adequate vision.

Operating time ranged from 16 to 95 minutes, averaging 38 minutes.

Results

From September 1991 to March 1993 a total of 64 laparoscopic hernia repairs were carried out. Of these, 36 were indirect, 15 direct, two bilateral, six recurrent, two incarcerated and three sliding. A total of 12 patients were found to be medically unfit for general anaesthesia, and so were excluded from the study.

All patients with recurrences had undergone previous open repair. The series was made up of 61 males and one female. Ages ranged from 17 to 83 years, with a mean of 55 years. There has been a recurrence of one hernia in the series. Follow-up time has ranged from 15 months to one month, with a mean of 9.4 months.

Initially, the first 30 patients in the series were treated by a plug and patch method. In follow up of these patients, there were very few complications, although one patient complained of a palpable plug and another complained of some bulging following direct inguinal hernia repair. At the present time, no plugs are used and the mesh is stapled in place.

All patients in the series returned to their normal occupation within ten days of surgery. This includes patients whose normal occupations consisted of commercial fishing, lumberjacking and general labouring. Office workers usually returned to work within one week.

Complications

In this series, there were no infections. One patient suffered a recurrence of the groin hernia within one month of repair. One patient complained of some ipsilateral bulging following direct inguinal hernia repair, and there was a single instance of a small scrotal haematoma.

Analgesics

All patients in the series were managed on pentazocine (Talwin) 50 mg orally. Only two patients required intramuscular analgesia postoperatively. Under previous open surgery, virtually all patients required at least one dose of intramuscular analgesia.

Length of stay

Prior to the commencement of laparoscopic inguinal hernia repair, the average length of hospital stay was 3.8 days. This has now been reduced to approximately seven hours.

Conclusions

Laparoscopic repair is now the operation of choice for groin hernia for most patients in our institution. This method provides the patient with an operation that is relatively comfortable, safe and allows return to full activity much earlier than with open procedures.

With increased use of outpatient surgical procedures, it has been necessary to increase the quality and quantity of patient education preoperatively. A preoperative anaesthesia clinic, where patients are assessed prior to surgery, has also been established. This system has been designed so that the patient is in the optimum condition possible for the outpatient procedure. Postoperatively, we are establishing a number of 'self-care' beds, where patients may spend the night with a very minimum of supervision.

Laparoscopic hernia repair is an operation that allows most patients to be treated on an outpatient basis in a very rural setting. In an institution such as ours, where surgical beds are at a premium, the increasing use of minimal access surgical techniques combined with decreasing hospital funding, has had a severe impact on our hospital demographics. In our case, 50% of the beds shared by all surgical specialties have been closed, with the resulting lay-offs in nursing and support staff. Some of the beds which have been closed to active treatment patients, have been converted to an enlarged day surgery unit and self-care beds.

In a small rural institution advanced laparoscopic procedures can be carried out just as easily and safely as those in the larger tertiary care centres. By providing these types of laparoscopic services, the rural hospital can provide a complete range of modern treatment to common surgical problems, without the necessity of referring the patient to an institution often far removed from the patient's own community and surroundings.

60

Laparoscopic Herniorrhaphy – a Review of our First 200 Cases

LUCIAN NEWMAN Jr III, W STEVE EUBANKS, EDWARD MASON AND TITUS DUNCAN

The laparoscopic approach to inguinal herniorrhaphy has become a satisfactory alternative to traditional open herniorrhaphy in many cases. The laparoscopic repair may be accomplished using several technical modifications of the traditional open preperitoneal approach. The authors in this study utilize a transperitoneal anatomical approach with mesh placement in all repairs. We have analysed our first 200 repairs and report the results.

Approximately 500 000 hernia repairs are performed in the USA each year. Many surgeons have acquired a great deal of experience with laparoscopy and have used this technique to repair hernia defects. The primary approaches include the transabdominal preperitoneal repair (TAPP), the totally extraperitoneal hernia repair and the intraperitoneal onlay mesh repair employing a large sheet of mesh within the peritoneal cavity.

The operation for the repair of groin hernia has been in continuous evolution since the ancient truss was used circa 1500 BC[1,2]. Modern herniorrhaphy continued to evolve, from suture reconstruction of the weakened inguinal floor to replacement of this weakened floor with prosthetic mesh. The value of prosthetic mesh was demonstrated by Nyhus in 1960 when he used a prosthetic patch in his preperitoneal hernia repair[3,4]. Stoppa described the repair of groin hernia with a giant mesh prosthesis through a midline preperitoneal approach as early as 1973[5–7]. The value of preperitoneal mesh reinforcement of the posterior inguinal wall has been demonstrated by these authors. The liberal application of prosthesis in groin hernia has been used by Lichtenstein and others with great success[8]. The laparoscopic approach seems to be able to achieve a repair similar to that of the open techniques but with much smaller incisions and less wound morbidity[9].

The evolution of laparoscopic hernia repair is traced back to Ger, who, in 1991, published the results of 24 cases in human subjects[10]. Gynaecologists, including Bogajavelensky and Popp, described different techniques for repairs of abdominal wall hernias in the late 1980s[12]. In 1991, Schultz published the first series of patients whose hernias were repaired with the patch and plug technique[13]. The vast majority of interest today centres on two approaches, namely the transabdominal preperitoneal and the totally extraperitoneal approach. Both of these repairs employ mesh in virtually all patients.

Concerns have been expressed about the liberal application of intra-abdominal or preperitoneal mesh materials. The potential for adhesions and fistula formation seems real but remains undefined. Many authors have published reports of large series using prosthetic material with negligible infection rates and complications, a result which will, ideally, be duplicated by laparoscopic hernia repair[8].

Materials and methods

The first 200 consecutive unselected laparoscopic hernia repairs serve as the basis for our review. A standardized worksheet was maintained for prospective data collection and retrospective review.

Table 60.1: Complications

Early recurrence	2
Myalgia paraesthetica	4
Scrotal haematoma	2
Flank haematoma	2
Richter's hernia at lateral port site, necessitating reoperation	1
Laryngospasm after extubation, requiring reintubation	1
Bladder injury	1

All procedures were performed at Georgia Baptist Medical Center in Atlanta, Georgia. General anaesthetic was used in all of these first 200 cases. The transversus aponeurotic arch, Cooper's ligament and the iliopubic tract were identified in all patients and served as the framework to which polypropylene mesh was affixed.

Operative technique

All patients underwent laparoscopic herniorrhaphy using a tension-free technique employing a synthetic mesh to the posterior inguinal wall over the defect. The patients were placed in the lithotomy position, and a single monitor was placed between the legs. Trocar placement included one umbilical trocar and two lower quadrant trocars, one on each side of the abdomen.
The peritoneum was incised with a flap, exposing the posterior inguinal wall. The flap was begun on the lateral aspect of the obliterated umbilical vessels and carried laterally over the top of the internal ring. The hernia defect was repaired by approximating a synthetic mesh graft to the fascia of Cooper's ligament and iliopubic tract as well as the transverse aponeurotic arch superiorly. The hernia sac of indirect defects was handled, depending on the size and depth of the sac. Small shallow sacs were everted and removed as part of the peritoneal flap. Deeper sacs were left *in situ* by incising around the opening of the internal ring. After the mesh was firmly secured to the fascial structures, the peritoneal flap was used to cover the mesh. The abdomen was completely desufflated and the incisions were primarily closed.

Results

In our first 200 cases, 169 patients underwent this repair; 31 repairs were bilateral. The series includes patients enrolled between April 1991 and January 1993. The overall operative time average 85 minutes; however, the first 50 repairs were performed in an average of 70 minutes. In all, 65% of the hernias were indirect and 35% were direct; 12% of the repairs were done for recurrent hernia from previous open repairs. The average age of the patients was 48 years (range 22–84 years), and 93% of the patients were male. In 92% of the cases the repairs were done as outpatient procedures. The complications are listed in Table 60.1.

Satisfaction with the operation was judged as excellent by over 90% of the patients polled. A visual analog pain scale was maintained and ascertained from the patients. Pain was reported as minimal to moderate in 82% of the patients at 24 hours after operation. The pain was judged minimal to none in 96% of the patients one week after the repair. The patients returned to full activity in an average of nine days following the repair.

Summary

A number of authors have demonstrated the satisfactory application of laparoscopy to hernia repair. We have included an honest report of complications of laparoscopic herniorrhaphy in our series. We believe that these rates of complications are similar in pattern and nature to open herniorrhaphy. Our postoperative results have indicated a significant reduction in pain and morbidity in the laparoscopic hernia group. We believe that laparoscopic herniorrhaphy may be used successfully in selected patients.

References

1. Read RC. The development of inguinal herniorrhaphy. *Surg Clin North Am* 1984; **64**: 185
2. Bassini E. *Nuovo Metodo per la Cura Radicale Dell' Ernia Inguinale.* Padua, R. Stabilimento Prosperin, 1889.
3. Nyhus LM, Condon RE, Harkins HN. Clinical experience with preperitoneal hernial repair for all types of hernias of the groin, with particular reference to the importance of the transversalis fascia analogues. *Am J Surg* 1960; **100**: 234.
4. Nyhus LM, Pollak R, Bombeck CT *et al.* The preperitoneal approach and prosthetic buttress repair for recurrent hernia, the evolution of a technique. *Ann Surg* 1988; **208**: 733.
5. Stoppa R, Petit J, Abourachid H *et al.* Procede original de plastie des hernies de l'aine: l'Interposition sans fixation d'une prothese en tulle de dacron par voie mediane sous-peritoneale. *Chirurgie* 1973; **99**: 119–23.
6. Stoppa R, Warlaumont C, Verhaeghe P *et al.* Preperitoneal placement of Dacron mesh in the repair of groin hernias. *Surg Rounds* 1983; **6** (4): 38–51.
7. Stoppa R, Rives J, Warlaumont C *et al.* The use of Dacron in the repair of hernias of the groin. *Surg Clin North Am* 1984; **64** (2): 269–85.
8. Lichtenstein IL, Shulman AG, Amid PK *et al.* The tension free hernioplasty. *Am J Surg* 1989; **157**: 188.
9. Newman L, Eubanks WS, Mason E, Duncan T. Its laparoscopic herniorrhaphy an effective alternative to open hernia repair? *J Laparoendosc Surg* 1993; **3** (2): 121–8.
10. Ger R. The laparoscopic management of groin hernias. *Contemp Surg* 1991; **39**: 15.
11. Toy FK, Smoot RT. Toy-Smoot laparoscopic hernioplasty. *Surg Laparosc Endosc* 1991; **1**: 51.
12. Popp LW. Hernioscopic stuffing of direct inguinal hernia in female patients using resorbable mesh. *Surg Endosc* 1993; **7**: 22–5.
13. Schultz LS, Graber J, Pietrafitta J *et al.* Laser laparoscopic herniorrhaphy: A clinical trial – Preliminary results. *J Laparoendosc Surg* 1990; **1**: 41.

61

Laparoscopic Herniorrhaphy – Transabdominal Preperitoneal Floor Repair

HOWARD OLGIN, ARNOLD S SEID AND TENNISON DONG

Between December 1990 and April 1993 we performed 300 laparoscopic inguinal hernia repairs in 262 patients – 259 males and three females, ranging in age from 20 to 82 years. follow-up was from one to 28 months. All patients had transabdominal preperitoneal tension-free repair of the entire floor. In all but the first 50 cases, a double-buttress technique was employed. Polypropylene mesh was stapled securely to cover the entire floor, direct, indirect and femoral spaces in all these patients. Patients returned to normal activity within three days to four weeks.

There have been four recurrences to date, with only one recurrence since using staples to anchor the mesh. Other complications include wound seromas (6), superficial wound infection (trocar sites 4), trocar site hernia (1) and nerve injury (4). nerve injuries to the ileoinguinal, lateral cutaneous nerve of the thigh and genital femoral nerves have been described (Table 61.1). All these cases were self-limiting and further operations were unnecessary.

Table 6.1: Complications

Seromas	6
Wound infection (trocar sites)	4
Trocar hernias	1
Neuralgias	4 (early)
Cardiac	2
Urinary retention	3
'Meshomas'	3 (early)

The authors concluded that transabdominal preperitoneal floor repair for laparoscopic herniorrhaphy appears to be an excellent technique with acceptable early recurrent rates using the double-buttress technique. In addition, the nerves of the groin are vulnerable to injury during laparoscopic herniorrhaphy. A complete understanding to the course and anatomy of these nerves is necessary to avoid compromise during laparoscopic repair.

62

A Randomized Prospective Comparison between the Laparoscopic, Preperitoneal and the Anterior 'Tension-free' Repair of Inguinal Herniation with Mesh

JOHN H PAYNE Jr, LISA M GRININGER, MARK T IZAWA, EILEEN F PODOLL AND PAULA J LINDAHL

The repair of an inguinal hernia is one of the most frequently performed surgical procedures. Over 500 000 are done in the USA annually[1–3]. At Kaiser Foundation Hospital in Honolulu, over 200 patients have one or more inguinal hernias repaired each year. The procedure is relatively safe and seldom requires more than local anaesthesia with supplementary sedation[4–6]. Several techniques have been described and each has its cadre of loyal supporters[2,3,7–22]. The patients usually go home the same day. Their return to work will vary with the amount of dissection required, the nature of their job, the extent of disability coverage and other factors. It may take four to six weeks before full activity can be comfortably resumed after traditional repairs[1,2,6]. The economic impact of such disability is enormous[1,20].

Following the experience with laparoscopic cholecystectomy, where patients are frequently back to full activity within a week, there has been growing interest in applying the technique to hernia repair. Many reports have described a particular method of laparoscopic repair for a limited number of patients. While the number of patients in a few series has grown steadily, the short follow up has limited the assessment of both the morbidity and the ultimate recurrence rate. The role of the instrument manufacturers in the development and dissemination of the approach has been criticized[23].

Despite the well-recognized need for such a study[4,24], there has not been a randomized prospective trial comparing the short-term and long-term results of any of the proposed laparoscopic procedures with standard techniques. Once a surgeon establishes a reputation as a 'laparoscopic herniorrhaphist', patients motivated by the reportedly shorter recovery are likely to be referred preferentially. As a result, there may be a sample bias which would make a randomized trial even more difficult for these surgeons to conduct. This initial report covers the first nine months of such a randomized, prospective comparison. Although only 52 of the intended 100 patients are included, statistical significance has been achieved in two important parameters. The results for all 100 patients will be published in due course.

Characteristics of patients

From September 1992 to May 1993, 71 patients were referred to the General Surgery Service at the Hawai'i Permanente Medical Group with symptomatic inguinal hernias. Otherwise healthy patients between 20 and 70 years of age were considered eligible if they were suitable for general anaesthesia and could tolerate a pneumoperitoneum. Direct, indirect, femoral, recurrent and bilateral hernias were acceptable for inclusion. Because of the additional risks and extensive dissection that

Table 62.1: Characteristics of the patients in the study (52 of 71 available)

	Open	*Laparoscopic*
Number	26	24
Age	49	49
M/F	25/1	24/0
Direct/Indirect	12/14	8/16
Bilateral	4	1
Recurrent	2	1

Table 62.2: Performance assessment

Measured:
- Preoperatively
- Postoperatively at 1 week and at 1 month

Supervised by a registered kinesiotherapist

Warm-up: 4 minutes on a stationary bicycle
Straight-leg raises
Curled partial sit-ups
Work Evaluation System Technology (WEST): Lift a weighted bar, ground to 122 cm (48 in)
Exercise just to mild fatigue or pain

may be required, patients with incarcerated hernias were excluded. While the prior removal of a non-perforated appendix was acceptable, any other pelvic surgery excluded the patient from participation. Of the 71 patients, 52 met the above criteria and agreed to be randomly assigned to either a laparoscopic or an open repair. No patients withdrew from the study after randomization. The characteristics of these patients are summarized in Table 62.1. At the completion of the initial phase of the study, 50 patients will have been randomized into each group.

Study parameters

All patients are to be followed by direct examination at one week; at one, three and six months; and annually for five years after their surgery. Operative times and costs, recurrence rates and early as well as late complications, including adhesion formation and bowel obstruction, are among the parameters considered. As 'return to work' may vary with a patient's motivation and disability coverage[24] as much as surgical morbidity, recovery was also assessed using a panel of exercises (Table 62.2). Performance was measured preoperatively, and one week and one month postoperatively, allowing each patient to serve as his or her own control.

The unique nature of our health maintenance organization (HMO) practice, with a unified chart and relative economic and geographic isolation, should ensure the identification of recurrences even if the patient does not return to the initial surgeon.

Operative procedures

Surgeons entering patients in this study have completed an 'Advanced Laparoscopy' course covering the techniques of laparoscopic herniorrhaphy. They also have repaired at least ten hernias with each of the study techniques prior to their participation. Most of the repairs were performed by a single surgeon (JHP). All patients received 1 g cephazolin (cefazolin) i.v. just before the procedure. No special prophylaxis for deep vein thrombosis was employed.

Group I patients had their hernias repaired via an anterior approach to the inguinal canal. The repair involves the implantation of a Surgipro mesh prosthesis (7.5 × 12.5 cm; 3 × 5 in) in a 'tension-free' manner similar to that described by Lichtenstein[1,5]. Most were performed under local anaesthesia with sedation. Spinal or general anaesthesia was used if requested by the patient. Skin incisions were 6 cm or less. The genitofemoral nerve was not divided. While indirect sacs were excised, direct ones were inverted. The mesh was overlapped onto the pubic bone and secured with interrupted sutures.

Group II patients had their repairs done under general anaesthesia by a laparoscopic transabdominal preperitoneal (TAPP) technique described by several investigators[2,7,8]. A nasogastric tube and Foley catheter were used in each patient. Nitrous oxide was avoided. Following the elevation of peritoneal flaps with monopolar electrosurgical scissors (Weck), indirect sacs were detached and left in place. Surgipro mesh (7.5 × 12.5 cm; 3 × 5 in) was stapled in place with the US Surgical Endo Hernia instrument to cover potential sites of femoral, direct and indirect herniation. Special effort was made to secure the mesh to Cooper's ligament and to avoid placement of lateral staples below the inguinal ligament. At the completion of the repair, the pneumoperitoneum was reduced to 6–8 mmHg and the peritoneum closed over the mesh with additional staples.

Patients in group II converted to an open procedure were repaired as in group I.

Results

Thirty hernias in 26 patients were repaired by the open, 'tension-free', technique; 25 hernias in 24 patients were repaired laparoscopically. Mean operative times were not significantly different between the two techniques. They were 63 minutes for open and 69 minutes for laparoscopic repairs. Four open repairs and one laparoscopic repair were done on patients with bilateral hernias. Mean operative times were 95 and 85 minutes, respectively. Two open and one laparoscopic repair of recurrent hernias were included in the first 50 patients. Mean operative times were 65 and 72 minutes, respectively. Two laparoscopic patients had their repairs converted to an open procedure. Mean time to discharge for patients with unilateral primary repairs was not significantly different. Patients left hospital an average of six hours after open and seven hours after laparoscopic repair. Urinary retention in three open and one laparoscopic patient resulted in an overnight stay. Two of these open repairs were performed with spinal anaesthesia.

Those patients having primary open repairs of unilateral hernias returned to work after an average of 13 days. Following laparoscopic repair, the average was nine days (Figure 62.1). Multiple regression analysis, controlling for the intensity of the job, found this difference to be significant at $p < 0.008$. When the patients were stratified according to job types, these differences persisted (Figure 62.2). However, there were not enough patients in each group to be significant. Although there was also a marked difference for patients having bilateral and recurrent hernias repaired (bilateral: 26 days = open *vs* 9 = laparoscopic; recurrent: 25 days = open *vs* 13 = laparoscopic), there were too few patients in these groups to achieve statistical significance.

Among the panel of exercises in the performance assessment profile, the straight-leg raising (SLR) and curled sit-ups (CSU) were the most helpful. Following unilateral repairs, 21% of the open and 52% of the laparoscopic patients had returned to their baseline number of SLR by one week. For the CSU, 26% of the open and 52% of the laparoscopic patients had returned to baseline at one week. By one month, however, nearly 70% of patients in both groups were at or above baseline in SLR and nearly 90% had exceeded baseline for CSU. The single patient having bilateral laparoscopic repair exceeded baseline for both exercises by one week. None of the four with open repairs of bilateral hernias regained this level for SLR by one month; they did, however, return to baseline

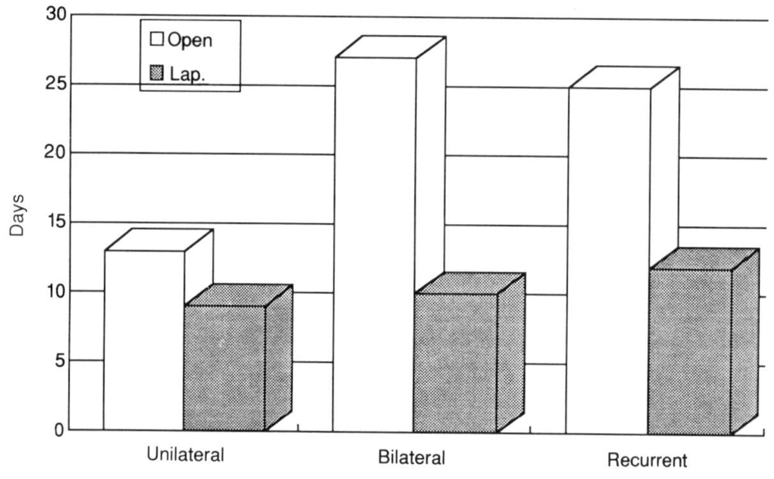

Figure 62.1: Time to return to work after hernia repair.

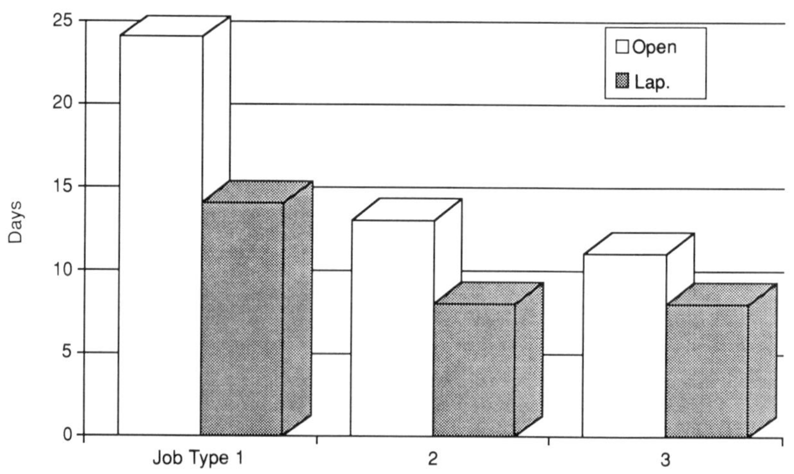

Figure 62.2: Time to return to work after hernia repair, according to job type.

for CSU by one month after operation. These differences in patients having bilateral repairs were not significant because of sample size.

Urinary retention kept three patients in hospital overnight after open repair and after one laparoscopic procedure. Two of these open cases were done with spinal anaesthesia. Bleeding led to a scrotal haematoma in one laparoscopic case; it resolved spontaneously. Two laparoscopic procedures were converted to open. One, the second case in the series, involved very complicated anatomy in a recurrent hernia. After an hour of non-productive dissection, an open repair with mesh was performed. The second conversion was required to deal with haemorrhage from an aberrant obturator artery. It arose from the inferior epigastric and arched directly across the femoral triangle and Cooper's ligament. Following suture ligation of the vessel, an open repair was performed. Ten days after a laparoscopic repair another patient returned, complaining of inguinal pain and a mass was

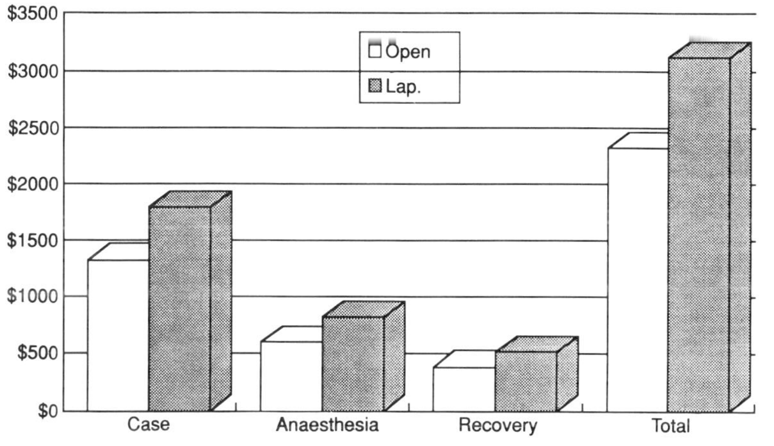

Figure 62.3: Costs of unilateral procedures.

detected. Ultrasound revealed a 'complex mass' and the patient underwent laparoscopy again. Omentum had become incarcerated between the clips used to close the peritoneum over the mesh. This was reduced without difficulty. As the mesh was firmly adherent to the pelvis, a small patch of PTFE was used to close the peritoneal defect. There has been no incidence of entrapment of the lateral femoral nerve. With a median follow up of six months and 100% compliance, there have been no recurrences noted.

The mean total charge for unilateral procedures was $2386 for open and $3132 for laparoscopic repair (Figure 62.3). The difference was significant at $p < 0.0001$. These figures include supplies, operating room time and personnel, anaesthesia and the recovery room. Professional fees were not included. These charges represent the amount for which the patient would have been billed if he was not a member of our Health Plan. There was little difference between the groups in the charges for bilateral repairs.

Conclusions

This chapter presents the very early results of the first 50 patients in one of the few randomized prospective comparisons of laparoscopic and open hernia repairs. We chose the TAPP procedure for the laparoscopic repair because it seems to have accumulated the most experience in the literature[2,7–9,15,19,22,25]. It has also been adopted by the Mayo Clinic[1], and is reportedly easier to learn than the totally extraperitoneal repair[8,10,17,26]. Concerns about the secure and precise fixation of the prosthetic as well as the desire to use the same material as in the open repair eliminated the intraperitoneal onlay mesh with PTFE[20,27]. We chose to begin the randomization after performing ten laparoscopic repairs. Although waiting until we had greater experience may have prevented some of the problems, we wanted to approximate the situation that the average surgeon might face when first learning this procedure.

The 'tension-free' approach was chosen as our control procedure to have both repairs employ mesh. We have used it selectively for many years and were confident that it would provide a rigourous test of the purported advantages of laparoscopic over open repairs. An Australian study which is underway is using the Shouldice repair as the control[16]. This is an important study and we are eager to review the results. The decision to leave indirect sacs in place rather than dissect them was based on the concern about increased ischaemic orchitis following sac dissection[8]. This may need to be balanced against the risk of hydrocele formation when very large sacs remain. Additional data will be required to settle this point.

We must be very cautious about reaching any conclusions at this stage of the investigation. The following observations do seem to be supported by the data collected so far:

- Laparoscopic hernia repair by the TAPP method can be accomplished with operative and hospitalization times that are not significantly different from the open 'tension-free' procedure. The use of general anaesthesia did not significantly delay discharge.
- Recovery and 'return to work' seem to be faster after laparoscopic repair. The differences are, in some instances, statistically significant. Whether they are clinically significant remains to be seen. Additional data and analysis will be necessary to determine whether any of the panel of exercises is of value in evaluating recovery from the two procedures.
- There is a definite 'learning curve' to be negotiated for laparoscopic hernia repair[28]. The anatomy of the inguinal area has always been the source of debate[29,30]. When it is viewed from the inside, it can become even more confusing. The pioneering work of Skandalakis[31,32], Spaw[27] and others should be carefully reviewed by all surgeons planning to perform laparoscopic inguinal hernia repair. Many of the complications that can occur after laparoscopic hernia repair have just been reported[28]. We would also strongly encourage additional training which includes animal experience. Wherever possible, assisting and being assisted by an experienced laparoscopic surgeon for the first few cases will shorten the learning process considerably.
- The laparoscopic procedure is more costly than the open one. Some of the difference is due to the longer operative time, even though this difference is not statistically significant. At $20–25 per minute, this can be one of the most expensive factors. The other major factor in the increased cost is the additional supplies required. While most of the major capital equipment costs will have been incurred and offset by laparoscopic cholecystectomy, there are no hospital costs to offset the staplers, mesh and other equipment currently required for the laparoscopic repair. Whether the apparent savings in disability will make these higher costs more acceptable remains to be seen. Certainly, operative experience, improved instruments and other modifications in technique may also reduce these expenses.

Additional investigation will be necessary to determine the recurrence rates for the many published techniques of laparoscopic repair. The patients in this study will be followed for at least five years and examined by at least two of us. As we have a 'unit chart', any patient who is found to have a recurrent hernia will be identified, whether or not he or she returns to the original surgeon. Because seeking care outside our Health Plan would be at the patient's expense, we believe that our follow up will approach 100%.

The appropriate indications, the 'best' technique, recurrence rates and safety of laparoscopic hernia repair remain the topics of intense interest. Through trials such as this, the answers to these questions should become clear[22,27].

References

1. Litin SC. Laparoscopic herniorrhaphy. *Mayo Clin Update* 1993; **9**: 1–3.
2. Newman, L, Eubanks S, Mason E, Duncan TD. Is laparoscopic herniorrhaphy an effective alternative to open hernia repair. *J Laparoendosc Surg* 1993; **3**: 121–7.
3. Schultz L, Graber J, Pietrafitta J, Hickok D. Laser laparoscopic herniorrhaphy: a clinical trial preliminary results. *J Laparoendosc Surg* 1990; **1**: 41–5.
4. Amid PK, Rutkow IM, Arregui ME, Wantz GE, Rosser JC. Opinion survey – laparoscopic hernia repair. *Gen Surg Lap News* 1993; **Feb**: 5.

5. Amid PK, Shulman AG, Lichtenstein IL. Critical scrutiny of the open 'tension-free' hernioplasty. *Am J Surg* 1993; **165**: 369–75.

6. Lichtenstein IL, Shulman AG, Amid PK, Montilor MM. The tension-free hernioplasty. *Am J Surg* 1989; **157**: 188–93.

7. ·Arregui ME, Davis CJ, Yucel O, Nagan RF. Laparoscopic mesh repair of inguinal hernia using a preperitoneal approach: a preliminary report. *Surg Laparosc Endosc* 1993; **2**: 53–8.

8. Corbitt Jr JD. Laparoscopic herniorrhaphy. *Surg Laparosc Endosc* 1991; **1**: 23–5.

9. Felix EL, Michas C. Double-buttress laparoscopic herniorrhaphy. *J Laparoendosc Surg* 1993; **3**: 1–7.

10. Ferzli GS, Massad A, Albert P. Extraperitoneal endoscopic inguinal hernia repair. *J Laparoendosc Surg* 1992; **2**: 281–6.

11. Gazayerli MM. Anatomic laparoscopic hernia repair of direct or indirect inguinal hernias using the transversalis fascia and iliopubic tract. *Surg Laparosc Endosc* 1992; **2**: 49–52.

12. Ger R, Mishrick A, Hurwitz J, Romero C, Oddsen R. Management of groin hernias by laparoscopy. *World J Surg* 1993; **17**: 46–50.

13. Ger R, Monroe K, Duvivier R, Mishrick A. Management of indirect inguinal hernias by laparoscopic closure of the neck of the sac. *Am J Surg* 1990; **159**: 370–3.

14. Himpens JM. Laparoscopic hernioplasty using a self-expandable (umbrella-like) prosthetic patch. *Surg Laparosc Endosc* 1992; **2**: 312–16.

15. Kavic MS. Laparoscopic hernia repair. *Surg Endosc* 1993; **7**: 163–7.

16. Nathanson L. Personal communication.

17. Phillips EH, Carroll BJ, Fallas MJ. Laparoscopic preperitoneal inguinal hernia repair without peritoneal incision. *Surg Endosc* 1993; **7**: 159–62.

18. Popp LW. Endoscopic patch repair of inguinal hernia in a female patient. *Surg Endosc* 1990; **4**: 10–12.

19. Seid AS, Deutsch H, Jacobson A. Laparoscopic herniorrhaphy. *Surg Laparosc Endosc* 1992; **2**: 59–60.

20. Toy FK, Smoot Jr RT. Toy–Smoot laparoscopic hernioplasty. *J Laparoendosc Surg* 1991; **1**: 151–5.

21. Toy FK, Smoot Jr RT. Laparoscopic hernioplasty update. *J Laparoendosc Surg* 1992; **2**: 197–205.

22. Voeller Gr, Mangiante EC, Britk LG. Preliminary evaluation of laparoscopic herniorrhaphy. *Surg Laparosc Endosc* 1993; **3**: 100–5.

23. Rutkow IM. Laparoscopic hernia repair the socioeconomic tyranny of surgical technology. *Arch Surg* 1992; **127**: 1271.

24. Wexner SD. Laparoscopic hernia repair: a plea for statistics. *Surg Endosc* 1993; **7**: 150–1.

25. Hawasli A. Laparoscopic inguinal herniorrhaphy: classification and 1 year experience. *J Laparoendosc Surg* 1992; **2**: 137–43.

26. McKernan JB, Laws HL. Laparoscopic repair of inguinal hernias using a totally extraperitoneal prosthetic approach. *Surg Endosc* 1993; **7**: 26–8.

27. Spaw AT, Ennis BW, Spaw LP. Laparoscopic hernia repair: the anatomic basis. *J Laparoendosc Surg* 1991; **1**: 269–77.

28. MacFadyen BV, Arregui ME, Corbitt Jr JD, *et al.* Complications of laparoscopic herniorrhaphy. *Surg Endosc* 1993; **7**: 155–8.

29. Condon RE. The anatomy of the inguinal region and its relation to groin hernia. In Nyhus LM, Condon RE, eds. *Hernia* Philadelphia: JB Lippincott, 1978: 18–60.

30. Lichtenstein IL, Amid PK, Shulman AG. The iliopubic tract. Is it important in groin herniorrhaphy? *Contemp Surg* 1992; **40**: 22–4.

31. Skandalakis JE, Colborn GL, Gray SW, Skandalakis LJ, Pemberton LB. The surgical anatomy of the inguinal area. *Contemp Surg* 1991; **38**: 20–34.

32. Skandalakis JE, Gray SW, Skandalakis LJ, Pemberton LB. Surgical anatomy of the inguinal area. *World J Surg* 1989; **13**: 490–8.

63

The Driving Force Behind Laparoscopic Hernia Repair

LUIS REYES, PRASANTA RAJ AND STEPHEN G REMINE

The surgical repair of the inguinal hernia is a dynamic subject with a number of variations and advances. Even the classic techniques such as the Cooper ligament repair or the Shouldice repair are still challenged by continuous changes and trials[1,2]. In the quest to find a better approach to repairing this anatomical disorder, the field of laparoscopic repair has emerged as a result of progressive and ingenious minds[3–6].

The conventional way to visualize the inguinal region from the outside has changed to visualizing it from within the abdominal cavity. Terminology such as the Hesselbach triangle has shifted to focusing on the 'triangle of Doom'[7]. The fear of injuring the ilioinguinal nerve has changed to concern about injuring the femorocutaneous nerve[8].

The purpose of inguinal repair remains the same, which is to offer the best care for our patients, to use the best technique and to take advantage of the latest technology. The absence of lengthy follow up for laparoscopic hernia repair has left some unanswered questions. How long do we have to wait to determine the recurrence rate with this technique? How does it compare with other techniques with regard to recovery time, missed work days and pain? How cost effective is this procedure? Although debatable, the fact remains that there is a drive to perform laparoscopic hernia repair.

Methods

A retrospective study, using a chart review and follow-up questionnaire, was completed on 45 laparoscopic herniorrhaphies performed in a nine-month period. Follow-up questionnaires were completed on 25 cases; 16 people could not be contacted. Data obtained from the questionnaire included the reason for preference for this type of surgery, degree of pain and discomfort, length of hospital stay and resumption of normal activities. In addition, patients were asked to compare previous hernia repair to laparoscopic hernia repair, and to choose which procedure they would consider for a recurrent hernia.

Results

Between February 1992 and October 1992, 41 patients underwent laparoscopic herniorrhaphies. A transabdominal preperitoneal procedure with Prolene mesh placement, as described by Filipi[9], was performed on the patients. All of the patients were male between ages of 19 and 65. Of the hernias that were repaired, ten were direct, 30 were indirect and five were recurrent. Of these hernias, four were bilateral. One patient underwent two repairs, one on the right side and one on the left side, within a three-month period. Twenty-two patients had same-day surgery, 15 patients were discharged after an overnight stay and four patients stayed in the hospital for longer than one day.

One complication noted was an intrascrotal haematoma, and one patient experienced a recurrence after laparoscopy.

Eleven patients chose the laparoscopic procedure because of a short recovery period, and five chose it because it was less painful. Six chose the procedure because of a short recovery period and because it was less painful. Three chose the laparoscopic herniorrhaphy based on their physician's advice.

Pain and discomfort following the procedure was also evaluated. Two patients experienced moderate pain, six experienced mild pain without requiring an analgesic, two patients experienced 'gas' pain after surgery and one patient experience rib cage discomfort. Three patients felt a burning sensation in the medial area of the leg on the same side of the repair.

Patients were asked if they would consider the laparoscopic procedure again. Twenty-one would have it again, one would consider the regular surgical procedure, and three would follow their physician's decision. Patients resumed their normal activities in one day (mean) following the procedure and returned to work within three weeks. All of the patients were satisfied with the decision to have a laparoscopic herniorrhaphy instead of conventional hernia repair. Five patients who had undergone both types of hernia repair felt that they would not consider conventional hernia repair in the future in the event of recurrence.

Conclusions

Laparoscopic hernia repair remains controversial. This may be because of the lack of controlled trials and long-term follow-up, massive advertising campaigns with weak arguments, the misuse of words such as 'minimally invasive', short-term learning sessions, and a number of well-established procedures that have been successfully tested[10,11].

The controversies surrounding laparoscopic repair of inguinal hernias are now a common topic when discussing this disorder. There are several factors to take into consideration. Some of the complications may be due to the learning curve of the surgeon performing the operation. In our series, there was an imagined recurrence of a hernia due to the inadvertent identification of a direct hernia on the same side. Even though there are centres reporting all operations performed, there are numerous cases not reported. It is interesting that, in our study, 40% of the patients could not be located during a period of nine months that the study was being conducted. This indicates that the criteria for selecting patients who choose this procedure should include their availability and compliance for the appropriate follow-up. All our patients knew about laparoscopic herniorrhaphy at the time of the preoperative visit. The procedures were explained by the surgeon, leaving the patient to decide about the procedure – although three patients felt that the surgeons advised the laparoscopic procedure.

The public's awareness of the procedure has placed pressure on the surgeon to be current with the latest techniques and to be able to present patients with several options available and be able to perform them. Our patients were aware of the less painful operation and the quicker recovery period with laparoscopic hernia repair.

In our study we were able to assess that the recovery time is as good, but not better than, with some of the conventional herniorrhaphies. What was enlightening was the fact that the patients experienced less discomfort with the laparoscopic repair. The patients who had previously undergone the conventional type of repair concurred that the laparoscopic technique was a less painful procedure.

There is also controversy about the type of hernia repairs that benefit from this procedure. In the Nyhus classification of inguinal hernias, types I and II are definitely not benefiting from the laparoscopic procedure. Type III is the area of great controversy, and type IV, or recurrent inguinal hernia, seems to be the group that benefited more from this surgery[12]. This may be due to the lack of avoiding the dissection of the region that is already scarred, with the result that there is a great possibility that the nerves and cord structures will be injured.

Although the trend is to provide cost-effective health-care, in our institution, laparoscopic repair is about twice as expensive as conventional hernia repair. We are responsible for educating our patients. We are responsible for obtaining appropriate training before performing this type of procedure single-handed. Our patients are responsible for choosing the type of surgery to be performed, and the manufacturing industry has to be responsible for lowering the cost of the procedure. Over all there is a drive to perform laparoscopic repair of inguinal hernias. At our institution the advice is to perform this in selected adult patients placed in a protocol with appropriate follow-up.

Acknowledgements

The author thanks Ms Emilia Leone for her continuous and outstanding assistance in the preparation of this manuscript, and to Dr Mark Petricevic for his assistance.

References

1. Welsh DRJ, Alexander MAJ. The Shouldice repair. *The Surgical Clinics of North America*. Hernia Surgery (451). WB Saunders Company. June 1993.
2. Rutledge RH. The Cooper ligament repair. *The Surgical Clinics of North America*. Hernia Surgery (471). WB Saunders Company. June 1993.
3. Schultz L, Graber J, Pietrafitta J, Hickok D. Laser laparoscopic herniorrhaphy: A clinical trial. preliminary results. *J Laparoendosc Surg* 1990; **1**: 41–5.
4. Popp LW. Improvement in endoscopic hernioplasty: transcutaneous aquadissection of the musculo-fascial defect and preperitoneal endoscopic patch repair. *J Laparendosc Surg* 1991; **1**: 83–9.
5. Dion YM, Morin J. Laparoscopic inguinal herniorrhaphy. *Can J Surg* 1992; **35**: 209–12.
6. Rutkow IM. Laparoscopic hernia repair. *Arch Surg* 1992; **127**: 1271.
7. Spaw AT, Ennis BW, Spaw LP. Laparoscopic hernia repair: the anatomic basis. *J Laparoendosc Surg* 1991; **1**: 269–77.
8. Arregui ME, Navarrete J, David CJ, Castro D, Nagan RF. Laparoscopic inguinal herniorrhaphy: techniques and controversies. *The Surgical Clinics of North America*. Hernia Surgery (531). WB Saunders Company. June 1993.
9. Filipi CJ, Fitzgibbons RJ, Salerno GM, Hart RO. Laparoscopic herniorrhaphy. *Surg Clin North Am* 1992; **72**: 1109–24.
10. Moossa AR. Random thoughts on laparoscopic cholecystectomy: is it an advance of a gimmick? *Ann Surg* 1991; **214**:
11. Pories WJ. Tunnel vision through the laparoscope. *Curr Surg* 1992; **49**: 333.
12. Nyhus LM, Condon RE, eds. *Hernia* 3rd ed. Philadelphia: JB Lippincott, 1989.

64

Outpatient Laparoscopic Herniorrhaphy

JACK K RINER AND RAMA JAGER

Most surgeons are now comfortable with laparoscopic procedures. They have been quick to accept the advantage of this in advancing the patient's interest in biliary tract surgery. Even though similar improvements from the patient's viewpoint are available in repairing inguinal hernias, there has been a reluctance to convert from accepted procedures using local anaesthesia to one requiring both general anaesthesia and entry into the abdominal cavity, thus being more invasive. Also, there is no long-term follow up to determine the recurrence rates. However, the procedures now available offer clear improvement for the patient and, best of all, can be achieved virtually free from hospital admission and with very comparable operative risk.

In the autumn of 1991, we answered patients' requests and began conducting laparoscopic inguinal hernia repair in the outpatient setting of a 'free-standing' surgery centre. The technical ease of performance of the procedures varies greatly, and the time required to perform laparoscopic inguinal herniorrhaphy in the outpatient setting does not appear to alter the outcome. This chapter reviews our methods of patient processing and compares two sets of patients matched by age and sex who were operated upon by the classic anterior or the laparoscopic techniques.

Operative methods

Patients' options

Patients appearing for surgical correction of inguinal hernias at the Hernia Center Plus of Indianapolis, Indiana, were informed of two approaches available – the classic and the laparoscopic – and each was discussed fully. Returning home promptly following their operation was the same after either approach. The patients were told to expect the discomfort experienced from the laparoscopic operation to be remarkably reduced compared to the classic method. Furthermore, they would return to work much earlier, perhaps in two to ten days after surgery. It was emphasizes that conversion to the classic open groin approach would be required if there was any problem with the laparoscopic approach technically or with the administration of general anaesthesia. They were always carefully informed of possible major intra-abdominal injuries as a result of the laparoscopy itself, and 'informed consent' was obtained.

Case selection

Case selection for outpatient laparoscopic procedures was strongly influenced by the patient's suitability for major elective outpatient surgery and general anaesthesia. Overweight patients and the elderly probably are more appropriately scheduled in the hospital, where admission may be accomplished readily if it becomes advisable.

Patient preparation

Preoperative preparation was standard as in most hernia operations. Colon evacuation was not required of any patient. After general anaesthesia was administered, a Foley urinary catheter was anchored, but a nasogastric tube was not.

Laparoscopic equipment

Laparoscopic equipment used to perform the procedures was standard and widely available. The synthetic prosthesis used laparoscopically was polypropylene mesh (Prolene) as its properties include flexibility, memory of shape and Velcro-like adherence to tissue. All prostheses were soaked in a solution of neomycin (Neosporin) antibiotic before use. Standard electrocautery units were used and laser was not.

Techniques

The classic approach used by us was the 'tension-free' repair of Lichtenstein[1]. This was done using field block and local anaesthesia, supplemented by intravenous medication for conscious sedation. The repair was reinforced by a Marlex mesh prosthesis secured by continuous suture. The laparoscopic approach depended upon the principle designed by Stoppa[2] and supported by the Nyhus[3] concepts. This proposed the use of alloplastic materials, placed intra-abdominally in the preperitoneum, and secured to surrounding structures, to cover and buttress fascial defects. There was no other tissue rearrangement or reconstruction. We closed all fascial defects at the trocar sites that could be reached beneath the subcutaneous fat with suture, and closed the skin by subcuticular suturing. Inflation pressures and all standard laparoscopic precautions were observed.

Going home

Postoperative care included fully instructing patients verbally and in writing. They were sent home when fully awake from the anaesthesia. They were told to return to work when the reduction of discomfort of their trocar stab wounds permitted, usually in one to five days.

Results

Laparoscopy group

A total of 53 patients elected laparoscopy. The distribution of patients included 51 males and two females. Their ages ranged from 18 to 63 years. Eight patients had bilateral inguinal hernias and 45 had unilateral hernias. Of all hernias, 35 were indirect and 38 direct types. There were 11 patients with recurrent hernias. No femoral hernias were found. Herniorrhaphy was successful in every case, by laparoscopy in most, but a few were converted to the 'open' procedure. No patient required hospitalization. There was no intraoperative nor significant postoperative complication. Of the first 53 cases started laparoscopically, five required completion by open groin techniques. When a problem was not readily correctable, conversion to the open classic approach seemed to be a minor sacrifice in achieving a safe conclusion to the operative repair.

The operative time varied from 380 minutes for a bilateral preperitoneal (McKernan technique[4]) in an early case to 80 minutes for a unilateral TAPP. (The length of time consumed in the learning curve was threatening, but the patients were only impressed with their decreased pain and early functional return. Most were asked to do a deep knee bend at their first follow-up visit and did so with ease.) When the laparoscopy approach was abandoned and a groin incision had to be placed, it was feared that there would be greater morbidity and more complications. However, those patients experienced the usual postoperative pain and discomfort of a standard groin repair, with no additional complication due to the trocar stab sites and the intra-abdominal procedure. They recovered with no discernible problems, except for disappointment.

Postoperative pain invariably was reported as minimal. Some patients were comfortable using only non-narcotic analgesics. No hospital admission was required. Return to normal activity occurred quickly for the laparoscopic group. Temporary scrotal inflammation had resolved quickly, and no haematomas, seromas, urinary retention or spermatic cord or testicular problems were noted. Nausea and vomiting occasionally occurred in this general anaesthesia group at times before they were released from the recovery room. In our series, 14 patients reported nausea and vomiting. Vomiting occurs with some regularity in any series of patients receiving general anaesthesia. Codeine is known to cause nausea and vomiting in some patients, but was administered to all except for a few. Those given codeine were also given a prescription for six or eight tablets of prochlorperazine (Compazine) 10 mg. The average number of doses of narcotics was very low. Only 1.6 were taken, and only during two days on the average. No one reported a temperature greater than 37.7 °C (100 °F). This was probably achieved by patients adhering to the activity instructions in both groups. None received additional antibiotics. No infection has been observed. It is anticipated that laparoscopic procedures will have no overall increase in the rate of infection. The rate may even be reduced by avoiding the inguinal and scrotal areas.

Urinary tract symptoms occurred occasionally. This was attributed to the use of an indwelling catheter during surgery. Abdominal distension did occur but was reported as difficulty in obtaining a bowel movement. It was rarely mentioned on the first visit unless the patient was questioned. The return to work interval after surgery was short. The questionnaire returns indicated the average of 4.1 as the usual day of return to work. Listed as reasons for not returning promptly to work included instructions by the foreman to remain off two weeks so that workman's compensations insurance would begin paying benefits, or a vacation was due and therefore taken.

Groin incision group

The review of 53 similar cases undergoing the classic incisional herniorrhaphy is as follows. There were 49 males and four females, ranging in age from 18 to 62 years. No patient required hospital admission. There were eight patients with recurrent and 45 with primary hernias: eight patients with bilateral inguinal hernias, 45 with unilateral. Of all hernias, 29 were direct and 31 were indirect. No femoral hernia was found. The operative time for 'tension-free' repair varied from 160 minutes for a bilateral repair to 45 minutes for unilateral repair. There was no nausea and vomiting reported. Pain usually developed some hours after reaching home. Pain was experienced in every case, of several days' duration, incapacitating and requiring a consistent intake of narcotics. The average requirement was 9.7 tablets, reported by survey. There was no report of fever, infection, genitourinary symptoms, nausea or vomiting. Return to work was an average of 10.8 days after surgery. Return to heavy work was encouraged after three to six weeks.

Recurrence rate

No recurrent hernia has been reported or found in either group. We hope that our results will reach the high standards established by the Lichtenstein group.

Conclusion

From the very favourable responses of patients because of the reduced pain, an earlier return to work and the apparent minimal morbidity, we believe that patients will, in rapidly increasing numbers, demand repair of their groin hernias by laparoscopic techniques. We believe it will be done routinely without hospital admission and with no increase in mortality or complications. We see no reason why the recurrence rate will exceed that achieved by the 'tension-free' repair, and it could conceivably achieve a lower rate as there is no dependence on suturing any structures together. Patients quickly grasp the advantages of the procedure for them, but they must also understand the as yet undetermined recurrence rate.

From the technical viewpoint, the intraperitoneal (TAPP) is faster than the extraperitoneal (PP) approach. It is good for recurrent and ideal for identifying and repairing bilateral hernias. We believe that the intraperitoneal approach (TAPP) will become the most commonly used. Also, it is no great threat technically to the capabilities of any well-trained general surgeon today. We believe that it will be the new 'gold standard' for inguinal hernia repair in a large percentage of patients needing repair and early return to work with minimal suffering.

References

1. Lichtenstein IL. 'Tension-free' hernia repair. *Am J Surg* 1987; **153**: 553–9.
2. Stoppa RE, Warlaumont CR. The preperitoneal approach and prosthetic repair of groin hernia. In Nyhus LM, Condon RE, eds. *Hernia*. Philadelphia: JB Lippincott, 1989: 199–225.
3. Nyhus LM, Pollack R, Bombeck TC, Donahue PE. The preperitoneal approach and prosthetic buttress repair for recurrent hernia. *Ann Surg* 1988; **208**: 733–7.
4. McKernan JB, Laws HL. Laparoscopic preperitoneal prosthetic repair of inguinal hernias. *Surg Rounds* 1992; **July**: 597–610.
5. Schultz L, Graber J, Pietrafittas J, Hickok D. Lasar laparoscopic herniorrhaphy: a clinical trial. Preliminary results. *J Laparoendosc Surg* 1991; 1: 41–5.
6. Corbit JD Jr. Laparoscopic herniorrhaphy. *Surg Laparosc Endosc* 1991; 1: 23–5.

65

The Evolution of Laparoscopic Hernia Surgery

ROBERT W SEWELL AND ROBERT L WADDELL

During the last few years the development of laparoscopic general surgical procedures has been truly explosive. Led by laparoscopic cholecystectomy, many new techniques have become widely adopted throughout the world. However, the use of the laparoscopic approach for the repair of inguinal hernias has been embraced less than enthusiastically[1]. Perhaps the most significant reason for this lies in the fact that the preperitoneal approach remains foreign to most surgeons. Moreover, the initial laparoscopic techniques were seemingly inadequate and therefore were quickly rejected by most surgeons as laparoscopic gimmicks. The clinical experience presented here reflects the authors' efforts to develop an adequate technique to repair inguinal hernias laparoscopically. Whilst the most recent product of this evolutionary process is laparoscopic transperitoneal hernioplasty, an explanation of each of the earlier techniques is included to provide a better understanding of how this procedure developed in a private practice setting.

In an editorial in 1966 in the journal *Surgery, Gynecology and Obstetrics*, Chester McVay severely criticized preperitoneal hernia repairs being performed by Nyhus and others at that time. However, in his opening statement, McVay may have actually provided the most compelling argument for repairing hernias through a posterior approach. He said, 'For a proper understanding of the normal and pathologic anatomy of the inguinal region, it is necessary for the surgeon to visualize the hernia in the groin from behind, even though he uses the conventional anterior approach.' This statement remains true today. Very frequently, it is impossible or impractical to identify all the important structures of the inguinal floor from the anterior approach. The laparoscopic approach allows for an improved view of the inguinal anatomy, and therefore should lead to a more anatomically correct repair.

Methods and materials

From October 1990 to April 1993, 329 laparoscopic hernia repairs were performed on 268 patients with a wide variety of inguinal hernias. Four different techniques were used over this 31-month period as the procedure evolved. These operations included high ligations of the sac (HLS), plug and patch (PAP), a laparoscopically assisted preperitoneal herniorrhaphy (LAPH) and laparoscopic transperitoneal hernioplasty (LTH).

High ligation of the sac (HLS)

Laparoscopic high ligation of the sac was limited to ten patients with a total of 12 hernias. Nine of the ten patients were female, and all patients had small to moderate sized indirect defects. The procedure consisted of simple inversion of the direct sac followed by ligation of the base of the sac using an Endoloop or Endo-GIA. No effort was made to close the fascial defect during this type of repair and no prosthetic mesh was used. There were no complications noted in this group, but these procedures were performed only on patients with small indirect hernias which were largely asymptomatic and typically were incidental findings during other laparoscopic procedures.

Plug and patch (PAP)

This procedure has been thoroughly described by several authors[2,3]. Briefly, our technique involved an initial excision of the hernia sac in nearly all indirect defects. For direct and femoral defects the peritoneum was simply incised anterior to the hernia, allowing exposure of the fascial defect in the inguinal floor. The defect was filled with one to three rolled pieces of polypropylene mesh, to obliterate the space and promote the ultimate closure by scarification. The defect was then covered by a sheet of polypropylene mesh, not directly attached by any method other than the closure of the peritoneum, typically accomplished with metal clips.

For the first few days, the stability of the mesh placement relies solely on the intra-abdominal pressure pushing it against the fascia. The mesh eventually becomes adherent to the surrounding tissues due to fibrous ingrowth through its interstices.

This procedure was used to repair 51 hernias in 49 patients (47 males and two females). There were three early recurrences in this group, secondary to inadequate sized pieces of mesh or early migration of the unattached mesh patch. There were two instances of plug migration into the scrotum, whilst one patient developed a hydrocele of the cord, and one patient suffered an intraoperative bladder injury.

Laparoscopically assisted preperitoneal herniorrhaphy (LAPH)

This procedure was used as an alternative to the plug and patch method. LAPH was devised in an effort to work round the lack of laparoscopic mesh fixation while still offering the minimally invasive advantages of the laparoscopic technique.

Performing LAPH involved the initial laparoscopic dissection of the inguinal floor, similar to that described for the PAP repair. After exposing the defect, a small (4–5 cm) vertical incision was made in the suprapubic midline and the abdominal cavity entered. The abdominal wall was manually elevated with a Deaver retractor, allowing continued visualization of the inguinal region laparoscopically despite the loss of pneumoperitoneum. Aided by laparoscopic visualization, conventional sutures were used, via the small midline opening, to effect primary closure of the fascial defect. In some cases, prosthetic mesh reinforcement was added by suturing a small sheet of mesh over the defect. The peritoneum was closed with a running absorbable suture.

This technique was essentially a preperitoneal herniorrhaphy and therefore was accompanied by tension at the point where the edges of the defect were approximated. It was used to repair 16 hernias in 14 patients, (13 male and one female). There were two early recurrences, presumed to have been secondary to either excessive tension on the repair or failure to identify and repair all areas of fascial weakness. One of the recurrences had mesh placed whilst the other had suture closure only. One patient developed a postoperative hydrocele.

Laparoscopic transperitoneal inguinal hernioplasty (LTH)

Since the introduction of laparoscopic staplers in 1991, LTH has become our laparoscopic technique of choice for repairing inguinal hernias. This procedure combines the advantages of a tension-free repair, with the security of firmly attaching the prosthetic mesh material to substantial, normal structures that surrounded the defect.

When repairing small, indirect defects, the hernia sac is dissected away from the cord structures and removed. If the sac is more than a few centimetres in length, the base of the sac is merely incised cirumferentially and the residual sac is left in the inguinal canal. Extensive dissection along the cord is avoided to minimize the risk of injury to the cord structures. In cases of direct or femoral hernias the sac is never removed.

Regardless of what type of hernia is present, the entire inguinal floor is routinely exposed. The peritoneum over the floor is incised sharply from well lateral to the internal inguinal ring to at least the medial umbilical ligament medially. However, because this latter structure is quite variable in location, it cannot be used as a reliable landmark. The peritoneal incision must be extended far enough medially to allow for complete exposure of the floor. Because the urinary bladder is near the medial edge of the dissection, a Foley catheter is used in every case to ensure complete decompression, and sharp dissection is limited to the peritoneum only.

The preperitoneal fatty tissue must be swept off the fascia with the plane of dissection directly on the transversalis fascia. Not infrequently, unsuspected defects are identified either in the region of Hasselbach's triangle or in the femoral space, and significant lipomas of the cord are often found in conjunction with direct or femoral hernias. Such lipomas of the cord are frequently encountered at the internal inguinal ring, and can extend a considerable distance down the inguinal canal. These elongated lobules of preperitoneal fat are only loosely attached to the cord, and are easily removed without disturbing the cord structures. Because such lipomas are commonly the source of significant inguinal pain, they have been uniformly removed.

The lateral margin of the rectus muscle, the iliopubic tract and Cooper's ligament are all identified in the medial aspect of the inguinal floor. The medial margin of the iliac vein is also identified, but no effort is made to expose this structure further. Dissecting lateral to the inferior epigastric vessels exposes the margins of the internal inguinal ring. This opening is bounded superiorly and laterally by the arching fibres of the transversus abdominis aponeurosis and medially by Hasselbach's ligament which lies just anterior to the inferior epigastric vessels. The inferior margin of the internal inguinal ring is the iliopubic tract. It is identified as it emerges from behind the spermatic cord structures and is followed laterally well beyond the actual ring. The iliac artery, the femoral nerve and the genitofemoral nerve all course beneath the iliopubic tract and can potentially be injured by indiscriminate dissection below this structure.

Once the fascia of the inguinal floor has been exposed, the inferior epigastric vessels are carefully dissected away from the underlying fascia. These vessels are not sacrificed unless they become injured, causing troublesome bleeding. This complication has not occurred thus far in our series.

A sheet of polypropylene mesh is then cut to match the area of dissection, overlapping onto the surrounding normal fascia well beyond any fascial defects. It should be noted that the piece of mesh has become progressively larger as experience has been gained with this procedure. The mesh is passed anterior to the inferior epigastric vessels and positioned to completely cover the myopectineal orifice, lying in direct contact with the transversalis fascia. Placing the mesh anterior to the vessels not only ensures continuous contact with the transversalis fascia but also the vessels actually help hold the mesh in approximate position prior to securing it with staples. Multiple staples are used to attach the mesh to Cooper's ligament from near the iliac vein to the pubic tubercle. Superiorly, staples are placed into the posterior aspect of the rectus muscle and around to Hasselbach's ligament immediately anterior to the inferior epigastric vessels. Two or three additional staples are placed into the iliopubic tract medial to the iliac vessels, ensuring that the mesh remains in direct contact with the fascia across the entire floor.

Lateral to the inferior epigastric vessels, the mesh is secured to the transversus abdominis aponeurosis superior and lateral to the internal inguinal ring. Finally, the mesh is secured to the iliopubic tract lateral to the cord structures, paying particular attention not to place any staples below the iliopubic tract. Injuries to the femoral and genitofemoral nerves in this area have been reported. Likewise, it is important not to stretch the mesh too tightly across the cord structures because this could potentially compromise venous return from the testicle.

When the repair is complete, the peritoneum is reapproximated to completely cover the mesh. Closing this layer has been accomplished by several different techniques, including metal or absorbable clips and the stapler. Laparoscopic suturing has recently become the preferred method for closing the peritoneum but requires considerable practice to attain proficiency.

The lateral laparoscopic ports are removed under direct visualization, and the fascia of each puncture site is closed with an absorbable suture. The skin incisions are closed with subcuticular sutures and sterile tapes, and the area around each puncture site is infiltrated with a long-acting local anaesthetic. All patients receive a single prophylactic dose of a cephalosporin antibiotic preoperatively, but generally no additional antibiotics are used postoperatively. Patients are routinely dismissed from the hospital within eight hours and are given a prescription for an oral analgesic.

For the first 10–14 days following LTH, patients are instructed to avoid lifting any weight in excess of 4.5 kg (10 lb) or engaging in vigorous sports or other strenuous activities. After this initial period they are uniformly allowed to resume totally unrestricted activity. An examination is performed on all patients by the operating surgeon five to ten days after surgery. Subsequent examinations are done as needed for any lingering symptoms, and each patient is contacted at three-month intervals thereafter.

A total of 195 patients, with 250 hernias (229 males and 21 females), underwent LTH. The mean age for this group was 48 years, ranging from 15 years to 97 years. All types of inguinal hernias were repaired, including 104 indirect defects (41.6%), 110 direct defects (44%), 29 recurrent defects (11.6%) and seven femoral defects (2.8%).

An attempt was made to quantify the subjective issue of patient discomfort by recording how many 'pain pills' each patient took. The average was 6.5 oral analgesic tablets per patient. Several patients related not having their prescriptions filled, while a few required more than 30 tablets. This is obviously only an approximation of the relative degree of discomfort and has no statistical significance. However, in the opinion of the authors, patient complaints following the LTH were dramatically decreased, compared with patients undergoing the conventional herniorrhaphy repairs used previously (i.e. Bassini and McVay).

The average recovery time following LTH, as measured by days lost to employment, was 9.85 days. Because many of our patients were 'worker's compensation' cases, this measurement may be somewhat misleading. In several instances, patients were physically able to return to work but elected not to do so until they had taken full advantage of their allotted disability.

Conclusions

There can be no doubt that the impact of laparoscopy on the practice of general surgery is unparalleled in modern times. Ultimately, the role of this new modality will depend not only on the particular procedures being performed but also on the technical expertise of each surgeon. The complete dissection of all important anatomical structures has always been essential to the proper performance of any surgical procedure, and for the repair of inguinal hernias it is paramount. The laparoscopic approach to inguinal hernias makes it possible to identify the entire inguinal anatomy in a way not feasible through any conventional incision. Any and all fascial defects of this region can be identified and repaired as the surrounding supporting structures are more completely understood and visualized by this posterior approach.

Our current procedure, laparoscopic transperitoneal hernioplasty, has rapidly become a viable alternative to open, conventional surgical techniques. Whether or not any individual surgeon elects to perform a laparoscopic hernia repair, it is clear that this method of visualizing the inguinal area from the inside leads to a more complete understanding of the problem of inguinal hernia. Therefore, as suggested by McVay, all those who study this approach will ultimately become better hernia surgeons regardless of what approach they employ.

References

1. Nyhus LM. Laparoscopic hernia repair: a point of view. *Arch Surg* 1990; **127**: 137.
2. Schultz L, Graber J, Pietrafitta J, Hickok D. Laser laparoscopic herniorrhaphy: a clinical trial preliminary results. *J Laparoendosc Surg* 1990; **1**: 41.
3. Spaw AT, Ennis BW, Spaw LP. Laparoscopic hernia repair: the anatomic basis. *J Laparoendosc Surg* 1990; **1**: 269.

66

Improved Patient Well-being following Laparoscopic Inguinal Hernia Repair – the St George's Experience

ROBERT S TAYLOR, PW LEOPOLD AND A LOH

Some differences in hernia surgery between the UK and America

In the UK, Between 80 000 and 100 000 hernia operations are carried out each year. Surprisingly, some 45% of hernias are never actually referred for surgery, a large number of trusses are still being prescribed. Techniques used for repair are very different. While the Shouldice operation appears to be the 'gold standard' in North America, a survey in the UK[1] has shown that it is employed regularly by only about 20% of surgeons. Approximately 25% use a modified Bassini operation, which covers a multitude of sins and does not usually involve incising the inguinal floor. Of greater concern is the fact that 35% of surgeons still use a nylon darn despite the fact that if has been shown to be an inferior technique.

The incidence of recurrence has been estimated to be in the region of 15–20% and the overall American figure is probably not dissimilar if follow up is continued for long enough. Yet where do these patients come from? It is a rare surgeon who does not feel that his current technique for hernia repair is satisfactory, with a minimal recurrence rate.

Perhaps more surprisingly, while over 70% of patients in the USA are treated as day cases, the figure for the UK is under 10%. The average length of hospital stay is three days and the average time off work is between six and eight weeks[2]. The relative unpopularity of day-case repair in the UK may be explained by a recent report from Oxford suggesting that 'surgeon satisfaction' may be greater than 'patient satisfaction'[3].

The St George's experience

Impressed with our experience of laparoscopic cholecystectomy, in April 1991 we decided to carry out a pilot study of laparoscopic hernia repair. The specific aim of the project was to evaluate postoperative well-being by assessing the severity and duration of pain, the length of convalescence and the rapidity of return to normal activities, including work. This chapter details the learning curve of one surgeon and represents only part of our overall experience of laparoscopic hernia repair at St George's Hospital, London.

Between May 1991 and December 1992, 107 laparoscopic inguinal hernia repairs were carried out in 100 patients. Seven patients had bilateral hernias repaired at the same time. Twenty-one had recurrent hernias, two of these having had four and one patient five previous repairs. A standardized questionnaire covering all aspects of recovery was sent to all patients and they were reviewed in the outpatient department at one, six and 12 weeks after the operation, and thereafter at six-monthly intervals. Follow-up, therefore, varies between six and 24 months.

Technique

The operative technique was similar to that now used by most laparoscopic surgeons. A mesh plug was employed for the first eight patients but subsequently all the hernias were repaired by insertion of one or occasionally two preperitoneal Prolene patches (Surgipro Mesh, Auto Suture Ltd, Ascot, Berkshire). Our earlier transperitoneal approach has now been largely replaced by an extraperitoneal technique which may prove to be superior[4].

For direct hernias the margins of the defects were clearly defined and the sac usually reduced, but for indirect hernias the sac was circumcised around the neck. Initially we used no fixation, but, following two recurrences, sutures are now placed in Cooper's ligament and at one or two other points. No fixation is used inferolaterally below the iliopubic tract. We neither like nor can we afford staples, and the peritoneum is closed with a continuous Prolene purse-string suture, taking care to make sure that the lower edge of the mesh is not pulled upwards.

There are three modifications to the technique which we have found useful. For the transperitoneal approach a blunt rod (5 mm diameter, 20 cm long; code no. BN320, Aesculap Ltd, Sheffield) is used to dissect the upper peritoneal flap under direct vision before incising the peritoneum[5]. This is very helpful in expediting the dissection, particularly in younger, muscular men whose abdominal wall remains flat. If access is impaired by a fatty umbilical ligament, this can be retracted medially with ratcheted grasping forceps inserted through an additional 5-mm port in the opposite groin. Correct orientation and fixation of the mesh is facilitated by passing a 2.0 Prolene suture through the patch close to the inferomedial margin while it is still outside the abdomen. The needle is then inserted through the 12-mm port, a firm bite is taken of Cooper's ligament, the needle extracted and the patch slid down into position by parachuting along the stitch which is then tied externally.

Results

Most patients were discharged the next day, only five requiring a longer hospital stay. These included one who was on long-term anticoagulation for a previous pulmonary embolus and three who developed acute retention of urine, two of whom subsequently required a transurethral resection of the prostate. There have been no more cases of retention since we stopped using urinary catheters. (One further patient stayed in for five days because he had nowhere to go!) There were five recurrences, all early, and all underwent successful repeat laparoscopic repair. In one patient with a recurrent hernia, an unfixed mesh plug had been used and at re-operation was found to have dislodged and was lying under the peritoneum. We replaced it, suturing this time to the margins of the defect, and the repair remains intact nearly two years later. Two of the recurrences occurred with unfixed patches and another two were related to an inadequate size of mesh patch in large pantaloon hernias.

Other complications included six small cord and two abdominal wall haematomas, all of which settled without surgical intervention. Cord haematomas can be prevented by circumcising large indirect sacs rather than dissecting them out. Five patients experienced significant neuralgic pain, lasting approximately two weeks. However, these were all early in the study during a period when we were using a non-disposable stapler in the region of the iliopsoas muscle. In common with everyone else, we have now stopped doing this. There were no instances of haemorrhage, bowel obstruction, wound infection, epididymitis, or bladder or testicular damage.

Eleven patients had no discomfort after 24 hours and more than half were pain free within three days. Only 14 reported any discomfort after two weeks. Normal activities had been resumed by 73% within one week, and 89% within two weeks; consistent with this, more than half of the 54 employed patients had returned to work by one week and 77% by two weeks. All but three patients who were employed had returned to work by four weeks. Of course, we have to remember that motivation plays an important part in this regard and not everyone is in a hurry to return to work! The 33 patients who had undergone a previous hernia repair, either on the same or on the other side, much preferred the laparoscopic technique, and all said they would choose it if they developed another hernia.

Conclusions

The laparoscopic insertion of a large preperitoneal patch for hernia repair is not so much a new operation as a new way of doing an old and well-established operation. The results of open preperitoneal mesh repair for primary inguinal hernia are excellent, recurrence rates of under 2% comparing well with rates of between 2 and 21% for sutured repair[6]. When mesh is used for conventional repair of recurrent hernias the recurrence rate[7,8] is only 2–3%, compared with up to 33% for sutured repairs[9]. It seems unlikely that the results of a comparable laparoscopic repair will be inferior, but clearly this still remains to be proven.

This small series represents the learning curve of one consultant surgeon who was already experienced in other laparoscopic techniques. In developing any new technique, it is inevitable that problems will arise, and we feel that this accounts for our relatively high early recurrence rate. In fact, these should not be regarded as true recurrences but as technical failures. We feel strongly that the size of the patch must be tailored to the individual patient and that the widely available 10×7.5 cm mesh may not be an adequate size for the larger defects. Since the establishment of a more definitive technique, there have been no further recurrences and only a few minor complications in another 82 patients. In this regard, it is worth remembering that even the Shouldice Clinic reported early recurrence rates of 17% in 1945, falling to 1% in 1950. All of our patients with recurrences elected to have a second laparoscopic repair, which must surely say something for the technique.

Of course, it is important to remember that recurrence is only one of the many factors by which a technique for hernia repair should be judged. Our preliminary results suggests that the most significant advantages of laparoscopic primary hernia repair relate to the minimal discomfort and the more rapid recovery and return to normal life and work, compared with the conventional operation. These benefits are even more apparent for the repair of recurrent and bilateral hernias. With careful selection and increasing experience, we believe that most patients can be treated as day cases and return to even heavy work within three to seven days. The incidence of complications is probably less than with conventional repair[10], and with experience most can be avoided.

A factor that emerged very clearly from our survey was the need to supply better and, preferably, written information to the patients, to the nursing staff and to the general practitioners. Our failure to emphasize this was undoubtedly the cause of some patients delaying their return to work and sometimes receiving contradictory advice.

As a result of our very positive findings we have now embarked on a prospective randomized trail comparing all aspects of laparoscopic and conventional hernia repair, including costs. Unless such a trial is carried out soon, it may become impossible as public demand is accelerating the adoption of laparoscopic hernia repair as has happened already with cholecystectomy.

Acknowledgements

The authors thank Aesculap Ltd, Sheffield, for their assistance in this project.

References

1. Morgan M, Swan AV, Reynolds A, Beech R. Are current techniques of inguinal hernia repair optimal? A survey in the United Kingdom. *Ann R Coll Surg Engl* 1991; 73: 341–5.

2. Robertson GSM, Burton PR, Haynes IG. How long do patients convalesce after inguinal herniorrhaphy? Current principles and practice. *Ann R Coll Surg Engl* 1992; 75: 30–3.

3. Michaels JA, Reece-Smith H, Faber RG. Case-control study of patient satisfaction with day-case and inpatient inguinal hernia repair. *J R Coll Surg Endinb* 1992; **37**: 99–100.

4. Dulucq JL. The treatment of inguinal hernias by insertion of mesh through retroperitoneoscopy. *Postgrad Gen Surg* 1992; **4**: 173–4.

5. Taylor RS, Loh A. A simplified technique for peritoneal dissection during laparoscopic hernia repair. *Surg Laparosc Endosc*, in press.

6. Shulman AG, Amid PK, Lichtenstein IL. The safety of mesh repair for primary inguinal hernias. Results of 3,019 operations from five diverse surgical sources. *Am Surg* 1992; **58**: 255–7.

7. Mozingo DW, Walters MJ, Otchy DP, Rosenthal D. Properitoneal synthetic mesh repair of recurrent inguinal hernias. *Surg Gynecol Obstet* 1992; **171**: 33–5.

8. Nyhus LM, Pollak R, Bombeck CT, Donahue PE. The pre-peritoneal approach and prosthetic buttress repair for recurrent hernia. *Ann Surg* 1988; **208**: 733–7.

9. Ijzermans JNM, de Wilt H, Hop WCJ, Jeekel H. Recurrent inguinal hernia treated by classic hernioplasty. *Arch Surg* 1991; **126**: 1097–100.

10. Wantz GE. Complications of inguinal hernial repair. *Surg Clin North Am* 1984; **64**: 287–97.

67

Laparoscopic Herniorrhaphy: Transabdominal Preperitoneal Repair of Inguinofemoral Hernia Recurrences

FRANCO FAVRETTI, S VALLETTA, A DA ROLD, M BONENTI, E BURIGO AND L DE LAZZER

Since the development of video-endoscopy, the application of a preperitoneal non-reabsorbable mesh (the Rives–Stoppa method) has been proved to be a valid approach in the treatment of inguinofemoral hernia recurrences[1–4].

The authors have been using basically the same operation, performed laparoscopically, in the treatment of bilateral inguinofemoral hernia recurrences[1,5]. Their experience is reported below. The series comprised 32 patients (30 males, 2 females), their ages ranging from 37 to 73 years.

Operative technique

A total of 48 hernias were repaired by 'open' laparoscopy using general anaesthesia. The hernias were located lateral to the epigastric vessels in 31 patients, medial in 15 and in the femoral triangle in two; 21 were recurrences and 27 primary but bilateral (Table 67.1).

The peritoneal defect as well as the key anatomical landmarks are identified. The peritoneal covering at the top of Hasselbach's triangle, lateral to the umbilical ligament, is incised. This is continued on the other side above and lateral to the internal inguinal ring (Figure 67.1).

Once two peritoneal flaps are created, landmarks are re-identified and the defect is reassessed. The hernia sac is pulled into the intra-abdominal cavity and the peritoneum inverted. The entire inguinofemoral region is covered by a mesh of 7.5 × 12.5 cm (Marlex and SurgiPro).

The graft is large enough to overlap all the inguinofemoral weak points. The mesh is stapled (Multifire Endo-Hernia) to Cooper's ligament and to the lateral aspect of the posterior rectus aponeurosis, above and lateral to the spermatic cord (Figure 67.2).

Table 67.1: Patients undergoing laparoscopic herniorrhaphy

Number of patients	59 (M 55, F 4)
Mean age (years)	51 (27–75)
Hernia repaired	89
Recurrences	38
Primary (bilateral)	46
Localization	
Indirect	57
Direct	22
Femoral	5

The peritoneal flaps are brought together and stapled with the Multifire Endo-Hernia stapler (Figure 67.3).

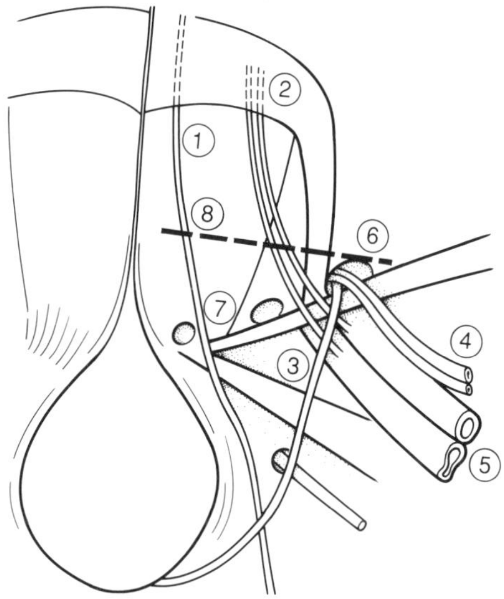

Figure 67.1: Laparoscopic view of the right male inguinofemoral region. 1, umbilical ligament; 2, epigastric vessels; 3, vas deferens; 4, spermatic vessels; 5, external iliac vessels; 6, internal inguinal ring; 7, Cooper's ligament; 8, line of peritoneal incision.

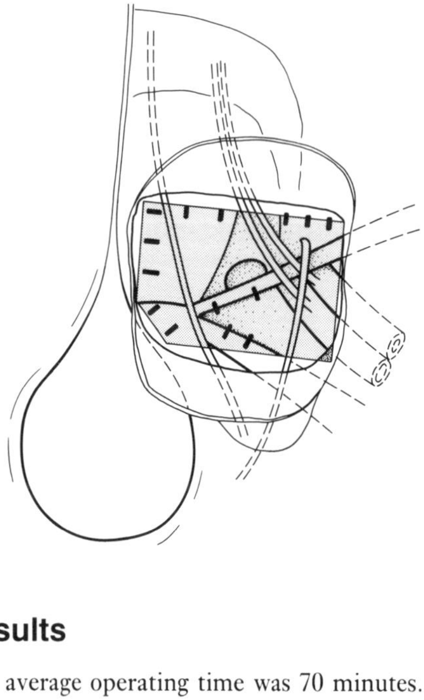

Figure 67.2: Peritoneal flaps developed and mesh placed and stapled on the right inguinofemoral region.

Results

The average operating time was 70 minutes. With regard to postoperative morbidity, two patients complained of pain in the inguinal area and one experienced a haematoma in the epigastric vessels. All the other patients were discharged on the second day after the operation.

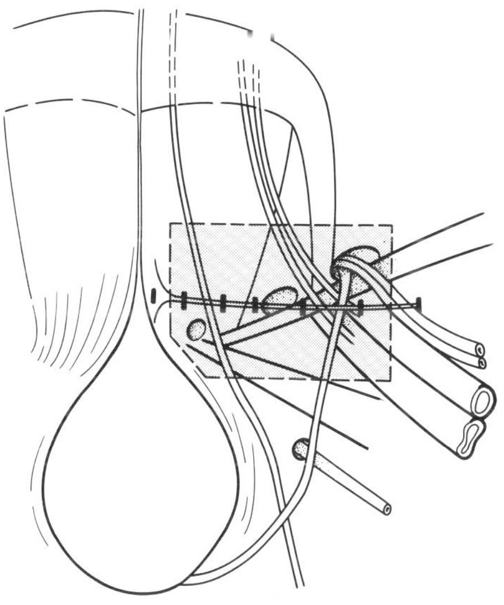

Figure 67.3: Peritoneal flaps stapled together to cover the mesh.

Table 67.2: Results of laparoscopic herniorrhaphy

Early morbidity:	
Postoperative pain	2 patients (3.4%)
Epigastric vessel haematoma	1 patient (3.4%)
Late morbidity	Nil
Operative time:	
Mean	70 minutes
range	60–150 minutes
Follow-up:	
Average	10 months
Range	10 days to 20 months

Table 67.3: Conclusions reached about the value of laparoscopic herniorrhaphy for recurrences and bilateral hernias

Different approach but otherwise same as the Rives–Stoppa operation
Same indications as for Rives–Stoppa
Security of mesh together with the advantages of laparoscopic surgery
Prospective multicentre trials

Late morbidity seems, so far, to be insignificant and no further recurrences were detected. Nevertheless, the follow-up period is as yet limited: an average of six months (Table 67.2).

Conclusions

Even though our results are encouraging and the above technique is routinely performed in our department, laparoscopic methods for hernia recurrences repair have not yet been proved superior to open surgery procedures in the long term. The postoperative benefit to the patient is the most likely argument for using these procedures[3,4] (Table 67.3).

Long-term follow-up and comparative studies with other techniques will establish the value of the method.

References

1. Filipi CJ, Fitzgibbons RJ, Salerno GM, *et al.* Laparoscopic herniorrhaphy. *Surg Clin North Am* 1992; 72: 1109.

2. Lichtenstein IL. *Hernia Repair Without Disability*. St Louis: Ishiyaku Euramerica, 1986: 9–17.

3. Stoppa RE, Rives JL, Warlaumont CR, *et al.* The use of Dacron in the repair of hernias of the groin. *Surg Clin North Am* 1984; **64**: 269–85.

4. Stoppa RE, Warlaumont CR. The preperitoneal approach and prosthetic repair of groin hernia. In: Nyhus LM, Condon RE, eds. *Hernia*, 3rd ed. Philadelphia: JB Lippincott, 1989: 199–225.

5. Fitzgibbons RJ. Laparoscopic groin hernia repair: preliminary results from a multicentered clinical trial. In: Second European Congress of Viscero Synthesis, Luxembourg, 10–12 September 1992.

68

Laparoscopic Repair of Recurrent Groin Hernias

EDWARD L FELIX, CONSTANTINE A MICHAS AND ROBERT L MCKNIGHT Jr

Some 50 000 recurrent hernias are repaired each year in the USA[1]. Up to one-third of these repair fail[2]. The surgical techniques used vary widely but the majority are fixed using an anterior approach. The reviews of Nyhus[3] and Stoppa[4] suggest that a mesh-buttressed posterior approach may reduce recurrence to less than 3%. When Schapp, however, altered their technique by using only small pieces of mesh or no mesh at all, his recurrence rate reached 33%[5]. It therefore appears that the extent of dissection and the size of mesh are crucial. In an effort to reduce the morbidity and recovery time seen with the traditional posterior approach, but still achieve its low recurrence rate, we extended the original principles of a total mesh-buttressed repair to a laparoscopic approach. This approach was recently shown to be technically reliable for the repair of primary hernias. The recovery time was shorter and the postoperative discomfort less[6]. This chapter reviews our experience with the laparoscopic repair of recurrent groin hernias performed over an 18-month period in a community outpatient setting.

Operative technique

From November 1991 to May 1993, 54 recurrent groin hernias were repaired in 50 patients: 48 were men and two were women. Patients' ages ranged from 12 to 86 years, with a mean of 55 years. Eleven patients underwent simultaneous bilateral repairs, seven of which were for new contralateral hernias. Twenty-seven patients had a history of bilateral repairs either staggered or simultaneous, and 13 had new hernias on the contralateral side and were given the option of a simultaneous bilateral laparoscopic repair.

Patients received 1 g of cephazolin (cefazolin) intravenously prior to general tracheal anaesthesia. After induction of anaesthesia the patient was placed in the Trendelenburg position and insufflated with either a Verres needle or the Hassan technique. A 10/11 mm disposable trocar was placed in the umbilicus, and under direct vision a similar trocar was positioned lateral to the rectus muscle on each side at approximately the level of the initial puncture. A high-flow CO_2 insufflator maintained the intra-abdominal pressure at 15 mmHg until closure of the peritoneum, at which time it was reduced to 8–10 mmHg.

The hernia was identified and the contents were reduced if necessary. The peritoneum was incised from lateral to medial and the preperitoneal space opened. Both the medial and lateral floor were exposed. The hernia sac was dissected out of the recurrent defect using blunt and scissors dissection with unipolar cautery as needed. Any persistent lipoma of the cord was removed. An oval mesh with a slit for the cord structures was cut from a 10 × 6 cm (4 × 2½ inch) polypropylene sheet. The wings of the slit were brought around the cord medially and stapled to Cooper's ligament. The upper portion of the mesh was stapled to the transversalis fascia and the lower part to the iliopubic tract. A larger piece of mesh cut from a 15 × 15 cm (6 × 6 inch) polypropylene sheet was placed over the first piece to repair the direct floor and secure the area over the slit. It was stapled in place with a multifire hernia stapler. The peritoneum was closed with a running Gore-Tex suture or staples. The fascial incisions were closed and the adhesive skin closures applied to the skin. Patients were discharged from the short-stay area and were told to resume normal activity as tolerated.

Results

Laparoscopic hernia repair was completed in the 50 patients explored. Two female and 48 male patients underwent repair. Forty-six recurrent hernias were unilateral and four bilateral. In only ten patients was the contralateral side normal. Twenty-seven had a previous repair on the opposite side and 13 had a new contralateral hernia, seven of which were repaired. The recurrent hernias were composed of 25 direct, 19 indirect, ten pantaloon, and two with a femoral component. In 39 patients it was their first recurrence, in ten their second, in four their third and in one his fourth. Male patients were repaired using a double-buttress technique and the two female patients were repaired using only a single sheet of mesh. The repairs were done on an outpatient basis and the patients discharged home from the recovery room.

Examination of the patients took place at one week, three months, six months, and every six months thereafter. Follow up ranged from one to 18 months, with a mean of eight months. To date no recurrences have been found and none of the patients in this small group has been lost to follow up.

The most common complication was seroma formation which occurred in 10% of the patients. These resolved spontaneously in most patients and were aspirated successfully in the others. One small bowel injury resulted from lysis of adhesions in a patient with a history and a previous ruptured appendix. This was repaired through the lateral port site. The patient has done well and shows no evidence of infection or recurrence over one year after his operation. Other complications included urinary retention in one patient and a lateral cutaneous neuralgia in one patient who was undergoing his fourth repair for an incarcerated hernia. The pain and paraesthesia lasted almost six months, but then resolved completely. Several patients have had transient scrotal discomfort with hyperaesthesia following surgery, but all resolved spontaneously.

Conclusions

The anterior floor repair of Bassini[7] was introduced a little over one hundred years ago and revolutionized inguinal herniorrhaphy. Recurrence rates were reduced to 10%, where they remain today except in a few specialist centres. Failure of primary hernia repairs appears to be caused by multiple factors. About 40–59% of all recurrences are indirect and, of these, 24% are due to missed hernias[8,9]. Technical errors such as not dissecting or finding the sac, leaving too long a peritoneal stump and incorrect closure of the hernial orifice lead to early indirect failures[10,11]. From 30 to 53% of recurrences are direct[8,12]. Most of these are due to repairs under tension which result in holes, usually near the pubic tubercle[13,14]. Failure to identify and repair co-existing floor defects also causes early direct recurrences. Femoral hernias represent about 4% of recurrences and are due to missed hernias or are caused by upward traction on the iliopubic tract[8,12]. In addition, studies have shown that intrinsic fascial weakness due to abnormal collagen may play some role in influencing the fate of the hernia repair[15]. Of the patients we saw for a recurrent hernia 80% had bilateral disease, either previously repaired or new, suggesting that an intrinsic floor defect may be partially responsible for the failure of the previous repair.

Once a hernia repair has failed, the results of further efforts to correct the problem are even worse than with the primary repair. Recurrence rates for repair of previously repaired groin hernias have been reported to be as high as 39%[16]. There have been reports of improved results with the use of mesh-buttressed repairs and a posterior approach[3,17,18]. When one analyses the causes of recurrence (missed hernias, tension-disruption, intrinsic collagen weakness, and the late development of a new defect), improved results seem logical. The posterior or preperitoneal approach avoids previous scar and dissects the entire inguinal floor. It clearly identifies the hernia and any other potential sites of failure. This technique should eliminate missed hernias; in Stoppa's report, his only failures were technical and occurred within one year after surgery[4]. Open posterior repairs, however, have a long and uncomfortable recovery – up to six weeks.

Laparoscopic preperitoneal hernioplasty, when first developed to reduce this recovery period, failed to heed the lessons taught by the open preperitoneal approach. Early investigators used small pieces of mesh or none at all and failed to expose the entire floor[19]. They consequently had a high early recurrence rate. More recent studies, which have used a larger mesh buttress, dissected the entire floor to avoid missing subtle defects and stabilized the mesh with staples, have had very low early recurrence rates[6,20].

The present study applied these principles to a laparoscopic repair of recurrent hernias. A double-buttressed repair, as described in this chapter, was used to ensure adequate closure of the internal ring and complete coverage of the entire floor. As in other studies using the laparoscopic approach to the inguinal hernia repair[6,21], recovery time and postoperative pain were reduced. Early recurrences in the present study were not seen on close follow up. Recurrence rates at one year in several studies of open hernia repairs represented from 25 to 50% of their long-term rate and ranged from 4 to 11%[4,5,12,22]. Although the mean follow up of our study was obviously short – eight months – the lack of any early recurrence appears to make it meaningful. It is almost certain that the words of Stoppa ('A hundred years after the famous Bassini it is not possible these days to ignore the extraordinary possibilities offered by prostheses in groin hernia surgery'[23]) will be applied to the laparoscopic approach of inguinal hernioplasty for the repair of recurrent hernias.

References

1. Nyhus L. Recurrent groin hernia. *World J Surg* 1989; **13**: 541–4.
2. Glassow F. Inguinal hernia repair: a comparison of the Shouldice and Cooper ligament repair of the posterior inguinal wall. *Am J Surg* 1976; **131**: 306–3.
3. Nyhus LM, Pollak R, Rombeck CT, Donahue P. The preperitoneal approach and prosthetic buttress repair for recurrent hernia. *Ann Surg* 1988; **208**: 733–7.
4. Stoppa R. The treatment of complicated groin and incisional hernias. *World Surg* 1989; **13**: 545–54.
5. Schapp HM, van de Pavoordt HD, Bast TJ. The preperitoneal approach in the repair of recurrent inguinal hernias. *Surg Gyn Obs* 1992; **174**: 460–4.
6. Felix E, Michas C. The double-buttress laparoscopic herniorrhaphy. *J Laparoendosc Surg* 1993; **1**: 1–8.
7. Bassini E. Nuovo metodo sulla cura radicale dell' ernia inguinale. *Arch Soc Ital Chir* 1887; **4**: 380.
8. Postlethwait RW. Causes of recurrence after inguinal herniorrhaphy. *Surgery* 1971; **69**: 772–5.
9. Shulman AG, Amid PK, Lichtenstein IL. The plug repair of 1402 recurrent inguinal hernias: a 20 year experience. *Arch Surg* 1990; **125**: 265–7.
10. Glassow F. Recurrent inguinal and femoral hernia. *BMJ* 1970; **1**: 215–19.
11. Ryan EA. Recurrent hernias: an analysis of 369 consecutive cases of recurrent inguinal and femoral hernias. *Surg Gynecol Obstet* 1953; **96**: 343–54.
12. Marsden AJ. Recurrent inguinal hernia: a personal study. *Br J Surg* 1988; **75**: 263–6.
13. Postlethwait RW. Recurrent inguinal hernia. *Ann Surg* 1985; **207**: 277–82.
14. Shulman AG, Amid PK, Lichtenstein I. Plug repair of recurrent inguinal hernias. *Contemp Surg* 1992; **40**: 30–3.

15. Shulman AG, Amid PK, Lichtenstein I. The safety of mesh repair for primary inguinal hernias: results of 3019 operations from five diverse surgical sources. *Am Surg* 1992; **58**: 255–7.

16. Clear J. Ten year statistical study of inguinal hernia. *Arch Surg* 1976; **46**: 70–5.

17. Stoppa RE, Rives JL, Warlaumont CR, *et al.* The use of Dacron in the repair of hernias of the groin. *Surg Clin North Am* 1984; **64**: 269–85.

18. Rignault DP. Preperitoneal prosthetic inguinal herniorrhaphy through a Pfannenstiel approach. *Surg Gynecol Obstet* 1986; **163**: 465–8.

19. Schultz, L, Graber J, Pietrafitta J, Hickok P. Laser laparoscopic herniorrhaphy: a clinical trial. Preliminary results. *J Laparoendosc Surg* 1990; **1**: 41–5.

20. Ferzli GI, Massaad A, Albert P. Extraperitoneal endoscopic inguinal hernia repair. *J Laparoendosc Surg* 1992; **2**: 281–6.

21. Voeller GR, Mangiante EC, Britt LG. Preliminary evaluation of laparoscopic herniorrhaphy. *Surg Laparosc Endosc* 1993; **3**: 100–5.

22. Read R. Recurrence after preperitoneal herniorrhaphy in the adult. *Arch Surg* 1975; **110**: 666–71.

23. Stoppa RE, Walaumont CR, Verhaeghe PJ, Romero ER, M'Balla-N'-Di CJ. Prosthetic repair in the treatment of groin hernias. *Int Surg* 1986; **71**: 154–8.

69

The Laparoscopic Preperitoneal Prosthetic Repair of Recurrent Inguinal Hernia

ARNOLD S SEID

Recurrent inguinal hernias continues to be a surgical challenge with significant morbidity and an unacceptable incidence of failure, resulting in repeat recurrences. Series published in the last few years report re-recurrence rates of 23% and 33%[1,2]. However, series limited to preperitoneal prosthetic repairs reported significantly better results[3–5].

Since December 1990, we have repaired recurrent inguinal hernias laparoscopically, using a preperitoneal prosthetic mesh repair. Our early results suggest that this approach provides excellent anatomical exposure, minimal morbidity and a low re-recurrence rate.

Materials and methods

Between December 1990 and May 1993 we treated 33 recurrent inguinal hernias. A total of 25 patients had had a single previous repair, five patients had had two previous recurrences and three had had three previous repairs. In all, 30 patients had had conventional repairs previously; three initially had laparoscopic herniorrhaphy.

All the operations were performed under general anaesthesia with the groin approached laparoscopically. Complete groin dissections revealed that 24 were direct hernias (73%), four were indirect hernias (12%), three were femoral hernias (9%) and two combined direct and femoral hernias with cord lipoma. All the repairs were completed with polypropylene mesh prosthetic.

Operative technique

A 10-mm laparoscope is inserted into the peritoneal cavity through a subumbilical incision. Two operating trocars (5 mm and 11 mm) are inserted under direct vision at the lateral border of the rectus muscle at the level of the umbilicus. The peritoneum is then opened from the medial umbilical ligament to a point 3 cm lateral to the internal inguinal ring. Flaps are developed superiorly and inferiorly and the entire groin anatomy is evaluated. An indirect or femoral sac is dissected out and included in the peritoneal flap.

No attempt is made to approximate the hernial defect with endogenous tissue. The entire groin floor is reinforced with a polypropylene rectangle 10 × 7 cm. The mesh is affixed to the anterior abdominal wall with staples – medially to the symphysis, inferiorly to Cooper's ligament and superiorly to the aponeurotic arch. Staples must avoid the area inferior to the iliopubic tract, from the vas deferens to the anterior superior iliac spine, thereby preventing injury to the vas deferens, external iliac vessels, spermatic vessels and femoral branch, femoral nerve, femoral branch of the genitofemoral nerve and lateral femoral cutaneous nerve. The peritoneum is then closed with the same staples to isolate the mesh from intraperitoneal structures.

In two patients, the laparoscopic approach was converted to a conventional repair. One patient had had a previous conventional herniorrhaphy, but in the interim period had developed a colovesical fistula which had required a sigmoid colon resection with a Hartmann's procedure and subsequent reanastomosis. There were dense pelvic adhesions which prevented easy access to the groin and thus the procedure had to be converted to a conventional approach. The other patient had originally undergone laparoscopic repair and had a direct recurrence just lateral to the symphisis pubis. There was significant fibrosis associated with the previous mesh repair which prevented a complete dissection of the groin. Therefore, the operation had to be converted to a conventional repair.

Results

Follow-up was from 1 to 28 months. All the patients were examined postoperatively by the author. There was one asymptomatic recurrence, observed after nine months. There was no infections, nerve injuries or testicular complications.

The sole recurrence was discovered in follow-up examination. Because it is small and asymptomatic, the patient has chosen to defer repair until symptoms or a noticeable bulge appear.

Conclusions

The disappointingly high incidence of re-recurrence after repair of recurrent inguinal hernia seems to have multiple causes. Technical error, missed hernia and collangenolysis all contribute to the poor results[6,7]. Additionally, the anterior approach to recurrent hernia demands dissection through distorted anatomy and scarred tissue, resulting in significant morbidity from nerve injury and testicular atrophy. The preperitoneal prosthetic repair originally described by Nyhus theoretically offers advantages over the conventional approach. The preperitoneal prosthetic repair is performed through undisturbed tissue and offers the opportunity to observe the entire groin with undistorted anatomy. Avoiding the scarred tissue encountered in the anterior approach results in marked reduction in testicular injury. In the anterior approach to recurrent hernia repair, Ijzermans reported a 4% rate of testicular atrophy[1]. Fong and Wantz reported a 2.25% rate of ischaemic orchitis when the anterior approach was employed, and only a 0.4% rate when the preperitoneal approach was used[3]. The use of prosthetic mesh reinforces the entire groin, decreases tension and pain, and seems to prevent future recurrence due to the collagenolysis of the groin tissues.

The lowest rates of re-recurrence in the literature are in the series that employ the preperitoneal prosthetic repair: Fong reports 5.3%, Nyhus reports 1.7% and Mozingo reports 3%[3,5,4].

The laparoscopic approach promises to be a further evolution in herniorrhaphy technique. Through the laparoscope, the classic Nyhus repair can be performed with the scope affording magnification and high resolution, resulting in excellent visualization of the groin area. The only technical difference between the two techniques is using staples instead of sutures to affix the mesh.

Assuming that the preperitoneal prosthetic repair is the optimal method for repairing a recurrent inguinal hernia, the question of whether to employ the conventional or laparoscopic approach remains. The conventional method can be performed with local anaesthesia whereas the laparoscopic technique demands general anaesthesia. The conventional operation has caused hernias at the incision site. The laparoscopic technique potentially can result in bowel and vascular injuries during the peritoneal portion of the procedure. In addition, future problems with trocar site hernia and intraperitoneal adhesions remain to be evaluated. Contraindications to the laparoscopic approach include extensive previous pelvic surgery and prior laparoscopic hernia repair.

Summary

The laparoscopic preperitoneal prosthetic approach to the repair of recurrent groin hernias permits excellent anatomical visualization, is well tolerated with minimal morbidity and has minimal complications. Early results of a 3% recurrence rate are encouraging and suggest that this approach may prove to be excellent for the repair of recurrent inguinal hernia.

References

1. Ijzermans J, De Wilt H, Hop WCJ, Jeekel H. Recurrent inguinal hernia treated by classic hernioplasty. *Arch Surg* 1991; **126**: 1097–100.

2. Schaap HM, van de Pavoordt HDWM, Bast TJ. The preperitoneal approach in the repair of recurrent inguinal hernias. *Surg Gynecol Obstet* 1992; **174**: 460–4.

3. Fong Y, Wantz G. Prevention of ischemic orchitis during inguinal hernioplasty. *Surg Gynecol Obstet* 1992; **174**: 399–402.

4. Mozingo D, Walters M, Otchy D, Rosenthal D. Preperitoneal synthetic mesh repair of recurrent inguinal hernias. *Surg Gynecol Obstet* 1992; **174**: 33–5.

5. Nyhus L, Pollak R, Bombeck C, Donahue P. The preperitoneal approach and prosthetic buttress repair for recurrent hernia: the evolution of a technique. *Ann Surg* 1988; **208**: 733–7.

6. Peacock EE, Madden JW. Studies on the biology and treatment of recurrent inguinal hernia. II: Morphological changes. *Ann Surg* 1974; **179**: 567–71.

7. Read RC. Bilaterality and the prosthetic repair of large recurrent inguinal hernias. *Am J Surg* 1979; **138**: 788–92.

70

Laparoscopic Inguinal Hernia Repair: Total Extraperitoneal Laparoscopic Hernia Repair with Prosthetic Replacement

DANIEL CASTRO, MAURICE E ARREGUI, CIHAT TETIK AND ROBERT F NAGAN

In the United States, repair of inguinal hernia constitutes the second most common procedure performed by the general surgeon. The recurrence rate is related to the repair and type of hernia. This constitutes a major economic expense, including not only the cost of the procedure but the loss of productivity, as well as significant pain and discomfort to the patient undergoing re-operation.

The intent with these new techniques is to reduce the pain, speed the convalescence, and the recurrence rate. At St Vincent Hospital, from October 1990 to April 1993, we have performed 202

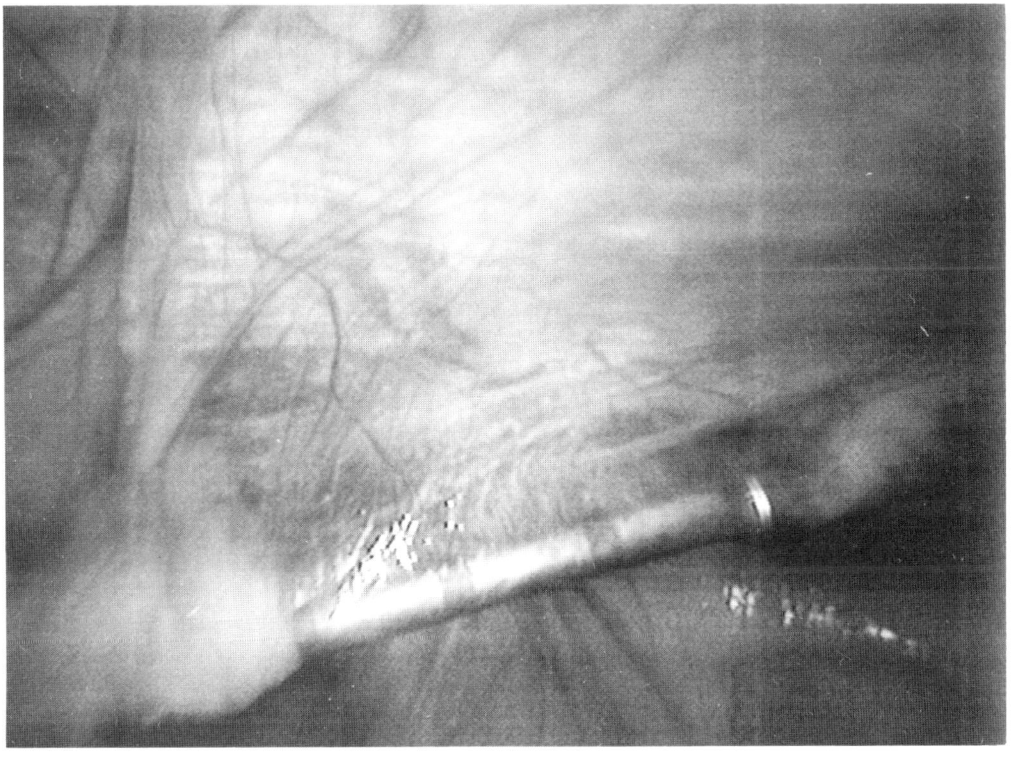

Figure 70.1: Transperitoneal view of dissection with a blunt forceps. The preperitoneal space on the right side is entered. (From Arregui ME *et al.* Laparoscopic inguinal hernia repair with preperitoneal prosthetic replacement, Fig. 15, In *Prostheses and abdominal wall surgery*, RG Landes Co, 1994, in press, with permission.)

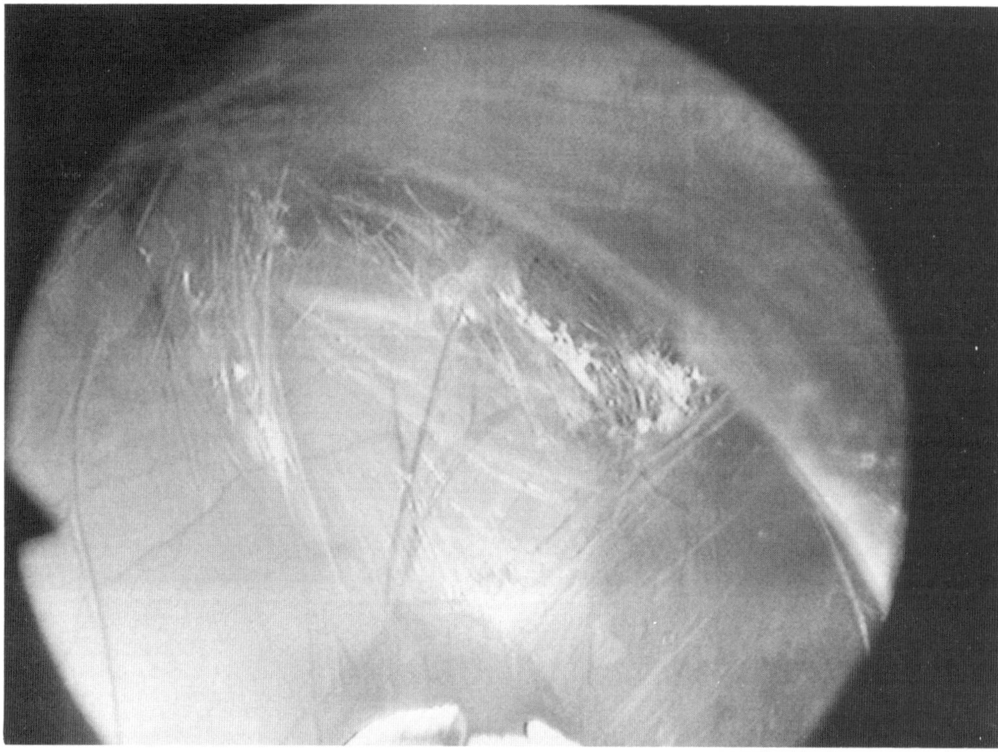

Figure 70.2: Dissection is carried out using a blunt forceps. Note the blood supply of the preperitoneal fascia. This is separate to that of the anterior abdominal wall including the transversalis fascia.

laparoscopic hernia repairs on 156 patients. The ages ranged from 12 to 83 years old. There were 113 indirect, 68 direct, 34 bilateral, 31 recurrent, 12 femoral, four obturator hernias, and five mixed. One hundred and seven hernias were repaired using the transabdominal preperitoneal approach, 90 were repaired with the extraperitoneal approach and five were repaired with simple closure of the orifice of the congenital indirect hernia. The vast majority were released the same day of surgery. To date, we had two recurrences (2/202—1%). One recurrence with transabdominal preperitoneal and one with total extraperitoneal mesh technique. We have had three intraoperative complications. One related to general anaesthesia, the second was loss of a needle in the anterior abdominal wall and the third was that the tip of the hernia stapling device broke. There were 22 (15%) minor postoperative complications. Patients were allowed to return to full activity without restriction within one week.

Technique of total extraperitoneal hernia repair

Upon induction of general endotracheal anaesthesia, the patient is given one gram of cephomandole or other second generation cephalosporine (there are no clinical data to support the need to use prophylactic antibiotics and this may not be necessary). A Foley catheter is inserted to maintain an empty bladder. The abdomen is not shaved. After the abdomen is prepped and draped, a 1 cm incision is made in a longitudinal crease in the lower part of the umbilicus for insertion of a Verres needle. Insufflation with CO_2 is created to a pressure of 15 mmHg. An 11 mm reusable trocar is inserted and inspection of the peritoneal cavity is carried out followed by an inspection of both inguinal areas (Figure 70.1). If a unilateral hernia is encountered, dissection is only on one side.

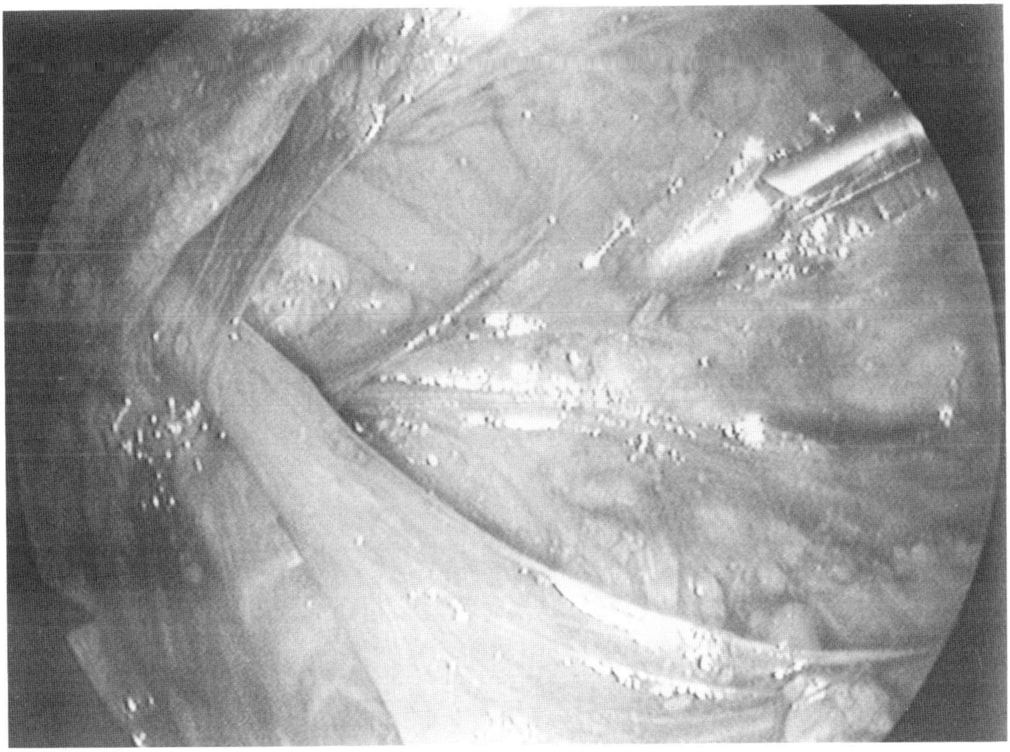

Figure 70.3: Exposure of the cord structures and enveloping preperitoneal fascia which will form the internal spermatic fascia. The internal ring is formed by the transversalis sling. The lateral iliopubic tract is exposed. This is the right inguinal area.

Bilateral hernia will require exposure of both sides. A 45° angle view laparoscope is used. The procedure is performed with the patient in Trendelenburg position with the side of the hernia tilted upward. The surgeon stands on the side opposite the hernia. Using a 5 mm trocar inserted lateral to the rectus sheath and well above the level of the anterior superior iliac spine, the space between the peritoneum and transversalis fascia is carefully entered. Blunt dissection is then carried out medially and inferiorly being careful to stay deep to the epigastric vessels and posterior lamina of the transversalis fascia to avoid tearing blood vessels and creating a blood field (Figure 70.2). In this moment, the CO_2 insufflator with the same pressure is switched to other trocar. This manoeuvre helps to dissect this space. If bilateral hernias are being repaired, a trocar is inserted into the preperitoneal space in a similar fashion on the contralateral side. At this point, the 45° view scope is removed and operating laparoscope with a 5 mm central channel is substituted. Both laparoscope and trocar are slowly pulled back into the umbilicus until the posterior rectus sheath is seen. Carefully the plane between the posterior rectus sheath and the preperitoneal fascia containing the umbilical ligaments is entered. If an unilateral hernia is being repaired, a 5 mm trocar is inserted in the middle at one third between the pubis and umbilicus. Blunt dissection is carried out until the symphysis pubis and Cooper's ligament are identified. If a direct hernia is encountered, it is reduced fairly easily. After the peritoneum and the preperitoneal tissues have been reduced, it is grasped and inverted into the preperitoneal space. With suture or clip, it is anchored onto Cooper's ligament. The inversion of the sac eliminates the space in the inguinal area which will accumulate blood or serous fluid which could result in a haematoma bulging outward.

This could be perceived by the patient as a recurrence. An indirect hernia, especially if large, is somewhat more difficult to manage. A 45° view laparoscope is then reintroduced for the remainder

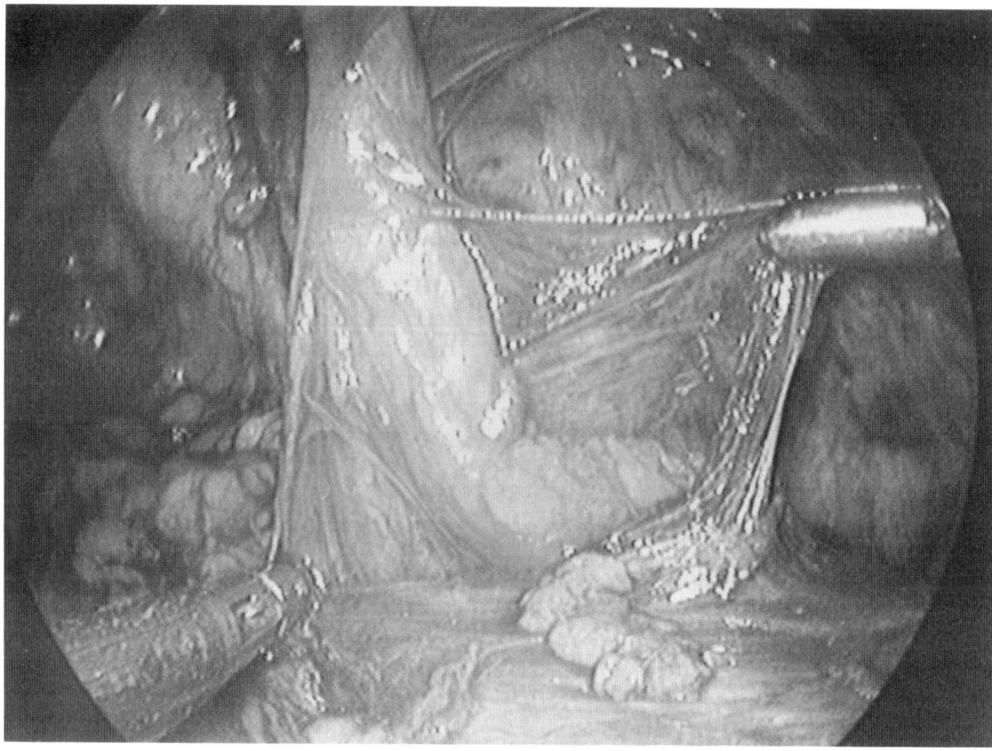

Figure 70.4: Same patient as in Figure 69.3. The preperitoneal fascia has been opened to expose the cord structures. (From Arregui ME *et al.* Laparoscopic inguinal hernia repair with preperitoneal prosthetic replacement, Fig 19, In *Prostheses and abdominal wall surgery*, RG Landes Co, 1994, in press, with permission.)

of the procedure. After separating the preperitoneal fascia surrounding the hernia sac and cord structures, the hernia sac is carefully dissected free from the blood supply and cord to the testicle (Figure 70.3 and 70.4). If it is a long sac, a zero chromic suture is placed around and extracorporeal knot created for high ligation. Distally the sac is transected using a scissors with monopolar coagulation. The distal sac is left in place. The peritoneum is then dissected laterally and proximally to allow placement of a large mesh 10 by 15 cm which has been soaking in 500 ml of normal saline containing 500 mg of cephalothin, to cover the myopectineal orifice of Fruchaud. Complete medial dissection requires good exposure of Hesselbach's triangle and the transversus abdominis aponeurotic arch. Dissection is carried lateral to the internal ring. The lateral iliopubic tract is exposed. Care must be taken not to injure the genitofemoral and lateral femoral cutaneous nerves which are located inferior to the lateral iliopubic tract. The mesh is introduced by rolling it, grabbing one end with grasping forceps, and stuffing it through the 11 mm trocar (Figure 70.5). The laparoscope is then reintroduced, and the mesh is unrolled and positioned. The mesh is fixed with sutures or staples. If sutures are used, a stitch is placed on Cooper's ligament, transversus abdominis aponeurotic arch, and lateral to the internal ring. This suture should be a non-absorbable material. No sutures or staples are placed between the cord structures and the lateral aspect of the iliopubic tract. Care is taken to overlap the hernia defect by at least 3–4 cm on all sides and potential place for hernia formation. Upon completion, the laparoscope is returned to the peritoneal cavity and the CO_2 is evacuated from the preperitoneal space and 20 cc of marcaine 0.5 is infunded. The mesh is then inspected to see that it is resting flat without curling of its edges. Inspection is also carried out to be certain that there are no tears in the peritoneum which could allow adhesions or internal herniation.

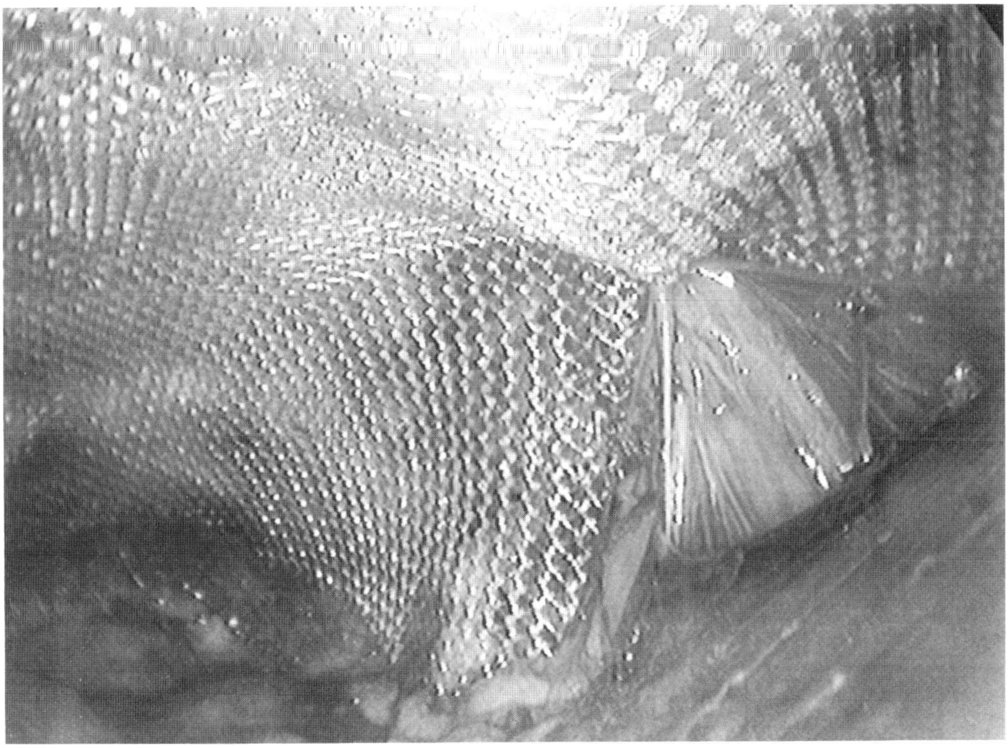

Figure 70.5: In this case, a slit has been made in the mesh to wrap it around the cord structures. (From Arregui ME *et al.* Laparoscopic inguinal hernia repair with preperitoneal prosthetic replacement, Fig 23, In *Prostheses and abdominal wall surgery*, RG Landes Co, 1994, in press, with permission.)

Any tears should be repaired. After removal of the trocars, all fascial defects 10 mm or larger are closed with 2-0 vicryl suture. Marcaine 0.5 is injecting in the aponeurosis. The incisions are closed with 3-0 subcutaneous vicryl suture. Collodion is then applied to the wounds. No bandages or bandaids are used. The patient is transferred to the recovery room for one hour, and then to the holding area for one or two hours before going home.

Conclusion

Access to the extraperitoneal space requires experience and good knowledge of the anatomy. A superficial understanding of this area will lead to confusion, bleeding, and potential injury. Total extraperitoneal repair is the choice approach for bilateral or direct hernias. The procedure is safe and the recurrence rate is low. Total extraperitoneal mesh technique eliminates the peritoneal defect and avoids the potential for small bowel obstruction.

71

Laparoscopic Herniorrhaphy: a Case for the Extraperitoneal Approach

GEORGE S FERZLI AND FRANCIS A DYSARZ

Man has been affected by inguinal hernia for thousands of years. Successful methods of surgical correction have existed since the late ninth century[1]. The recent widespread application of minimally invasive surgery has led to the development of ways enabling hernia repair to be done laparoscopically.

Multiple techniques of laparoscopic herniorrhaphy have been described since 1990[2,3]. The transabdominal preperitoneal repair (TAPP) and the extraperitoneal endoscopic herniorrhaphy (EEPH) are two such techniques[4,5]. Both attempt to copy the conventional preperitoneal repair with prosthetic mesh described by Nyhus, Stoppa and Rignault[6–8]. EEPH avoids the potential complications inherent in the TAPP method. The purpose of this chapter is to analyse the advantages of EEPH and to report the clinical experience with EEPH using CO_2 insufflation and, more recently, without CO_2 insufflation.

Transabdominal preperitoneal repair

The TAPP repair remains less technically demanding and has therefore become more popular than the EEPH repair. Multiple complications have been reported as resulting from the TAPP method. These include bowel obstruction, orchitis, neuralgias, haematoma formation, hydrocele formation and bladder injuries[9,10].

Creating the pneumoperitoneum for transabdominal hernia repair techniques may cause hypothermia, hypercarbia, venous stasis and cardiopulmonary haemodynamic changes intraoperatively[11]. Abdominal distension and diaphragmatic shoulder pain may be seen postoperatively. The Verres needle puncture and initial umbilical trocar placement are done blindly, and have the potential for injury to blood vessels or bowel. Furthermore, accessory trocar placement can injure the epigastric vessels[12]. Significant dissection is frequently needed in the TAPP method to gain exposure to the operative area in patients with prior abdominal surgery. Sigmoid colon fixation by adhesions may be present, which would necessitate lysis. All of the aforementioned problems are avoided by EEPH because it does not involve peritoneal violation[5,13,14].

The division of the peritoneum required by the TAPP approach is frequently done with electrocautery to obtain haemostasis. Electrocautery has the potential to injure the lateral femoral cutaneous nerve, the genital branch of the genitofemoral nerve and the spermatic cords (Figure 71.1). The spermatic cords are also more likely to be injured when they become obscured following the invagination of an indirect hernia sac, prior to its division (Figure 71.1). Also, the invagination may cause kinking of the cord structures, resulting in a higher incidence of spermatic cord injury and orchitis.

Reducing bowel contents present in an indirect hernial sac may lead to injury if adhesions are present. Medial dissection for a large direct hernia may result in bladder injury (Figure 71.1). EEPH

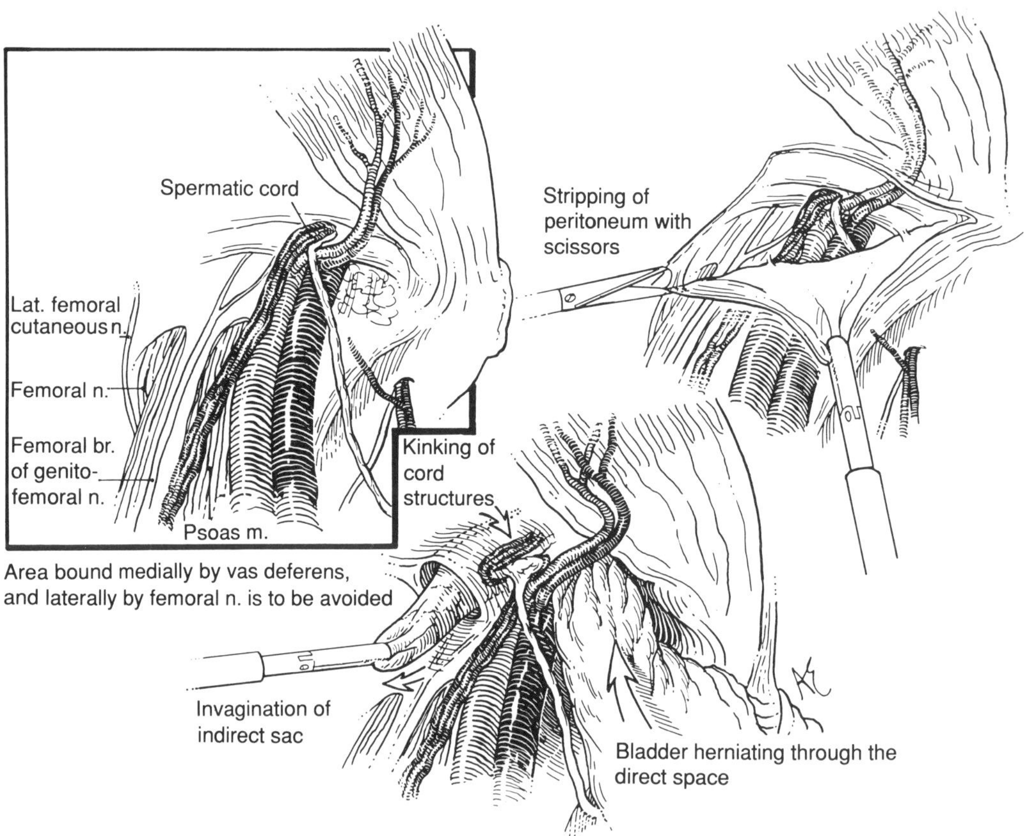

Figure 71.1: The trapezoidal area where complications are likely to arise, bounded medially by the vas deferens and laterally by the femoral nerve. Stripping of peritoneum. Bladder herniating through the direct space. Kinking of the cord structures. Invagination of indirect sac.

avoids peritoneal stripping, allows an approach to direct and indirect hernias from above the bladder, as in conventional surgery.

The TAPP approach subjects neurovascular structures in the trapezoidal area to injury when stapling the polypropylene mesh in place (Figure 71.1). It requires closing the peritoneum over mesh, adding to the number of staples required, increasing the likelihood of injury to the neurovascular structures. Also this closure may leave openings in the peritoneum that can allow herniation and entrapment of small bowel, as well as potential adhesion formation. The ideal closure would involve mesh placed anteriorly without any staples in the trapezoidal area and continuous suture closure of the peritoneum.

Extraperitoneal endoscopic herniorrhaphy

Extraperitoneal endoscopic herniorrhaphy avoids the previously mentioned laparoscopic hazards. In EEPH, the endoscopic stapler remains parallel to the psoas muscle, decreasing the risk of entering the trapezoidal area and eliminating the risk of future herniation through the peritoneum.

A total of 100 patients underwent EEPH using CO_2 insufflation via the previously described technique[5]. The patients ranged in age from 18 to 78 (mean 66.8) years of age. Nineteen patients had had prior abdominal surgery; seven patients had had a contralateral hernia repaired previously through an anterior approach. A total of 62 direct, 49 indirect, nine pantaloon, two femoral, six recurrent and 22 bilateral hernias were repaired in these 100 patients. The recurrences followed three modified Bassini repairs, one Lichtenstein, one Shouldice and one laparoscopic plug and patch repair.

Six patients underwent concomitant extraperitoneal endoscopic lymph node dissections (EEPLND) for the staging of prostatic carcinoma, and two other patients had concomitant left varicocelectomy. Mean operative time was 73 minutes, ranging from 30 to 165 minutes. All repairs were done with polypropylene mesh measuring at least 10 × 12 cm. Bilateral repairs were done with one large sheet of mesh in three patients, and all others received two separate pieces of mesh overlapping in the midline.

Five operations were converted: two to an open inguinal repair and three to a laparoscopic transabdominal preperitoneal repair. All conversions were secondary to disruption of the peritoneum. However, as experience was gained, disruption no longer required a conversion.

The six patients who underwent EEPLND were admitted to the hospital for up to 72 hours. The other 84 patients were all operated on on a day-surgery basis, but 14 were held for 24 hours. Overall average hospital stay was eight hours. Postoperative analgesic requirements varied from none to 12 tablets of Percocet (oxycodone) or Tylenol (paracetamol) with codeine. All patients returned to normal activity four to six days postoperatively. To date, there have been no recurrences.

Postoperative follow up ranges from six to 20 months, with a mean of 12 months. Seven patients who had contralateral hernias repaired previously via the standard, open method, were far more satisfied over all with the endoscopic repair.

Results

There were no deaths in the series. Minor complications were seen in six patients and included urinary retention in two patients, groin haematoma in two patients (one of whom had also undergone a simultaneous EEPLND), one trocar site infection, and one left lateral femoral cutaneous nerve neuralgia, seen in a patient converted to a laparoscopic transabdominal approach.

It is possible to perform the EEPH under epidural, rather than general anaesthesia, when patients are considered high surgical risks. However, leakage of CO_2 into the abdominal cavity would occur in the event of a peritoneal disruption during dissection of the extraperitoneal space. This would necessitate an intraoperative conversion of the procedure to general anaesthesia. A method has been devised to perform the EEPH without CO_2 insufflation, lifting the anterior abdominal wall rather than inflating it, thereby allowing epidural anaesthesia to be used exclusively (Figure 71.2).

Gas-free EEPH

Type III endoscopic extraperitoneal herniorrhaphies were performed recently in five patients. The repairs were entirely gas free in three patients. In order to explore the differences between CO_2 and non-CO_2 insufflated procedures, endoscopic herniorrhaphies in the other two patients were performed with CO_2 insufflation added midway throughout the procedure.

Several differences exist for non-CO_2 insufflated extraperitoneal inguinal herniorrhaphies. Diffuse, pinpoint peritoneal bleeding can occur, making the field more bloody. Dissection of large indirect hernia sacs is easier, as opening them will not risk leakage of CO_2 into the peritoneal cavity. Recognition of large direct defects requires more experience because intracavity pressure is not increased as it would be if CO_2 were used. Defects do not bulge out, thereby making them more difficult to identify.

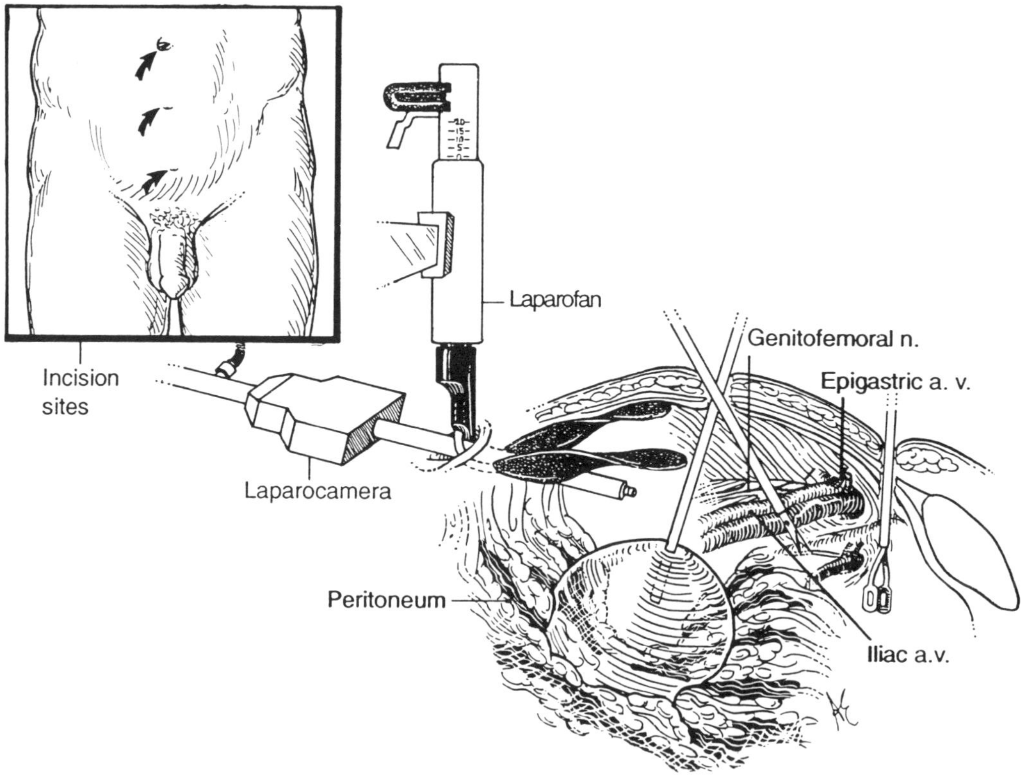

Figure 71.2: Incision placement sites. Laparolift and Laparofan in place, the camera in the extraperitoneal space, balloon retraction of the peritoneum, and instruments used without trocars.

With CO_2 insufflated midway to examine the differences, the operative field becomes dry; again, direct defects become more easily recognizable at a pressure of 8 mmHg. Trocars are not required, yet standard laparoscopic instruments may be used. Certain standard surgical instruments (DeBakey forceps, Hemoclips, etc.) may be used. But, exposure obtained without CO_2 insufflation is not as broad as that obtained with it.

Since April 1993, this approach has been used on five patients. All five tolerated the procedure well, regardless of whether or not CO_2 was added midway throughout the case. No known additional morbidities or mortalities have resulted as yet in these patients, compared to patients whose extraperitoneal herniorrhaphies were done entirely with CO_2 insufflation.

Conclusions

The non-insufflated extraperitoneal repair appears to be a viable alternative. The ability to do the EEPH without CO_2 insufflation alleviates problems for patients unable to tolerate general anaesthesia, while maintaining the benefits of minimally invasive surgery. The method eliminates the need for standard trocars, allows some standard surgical instruments to be used in a laparoscopic situation, and can be done entirely under epidural anaesthesia. However, more laparoscopic skill on the part of the surgeon will be required to accomplish the repair well because of the diminished exposure available.

The technique of CO_2-insufflated endoscopic extraperitoneal herniorrhaphy with the placement of a polypropylene mesh appears to have excellent results, with and without CO_2 insufflation. In the series of 100 patients with 122 hernias, no recurrences after repair have yet been seen, EEPH appears to have the efficacy of the standard, open herniorrhaphy with reduced convalescence time, and less postoperative pain due to the nature of minimally invasive surgery.

References

1. Bassini E. Sulla cura radicale de hernia inguinale. *Arch Soc Ital Chir* 1887; **4**: 380.
2. Ger R, Monroe K, Duvivier R, Mishrick A. Management of indirect inguinal hernias by laparoscopic closure of the neck of the sac. *Am J Surg* 1990; **159**: 370.
3. Schultz L, Graber J, Pietrafitta J, Hickok D. Laser laparoscopic herniorrhaphy: A clinical trial. Preliminary results. *J Laparoendosc Surg* 1990; **1**: 41–5.
4. Arregui ME, Davis C, Osman Y, Nagan RF. Laparoscopic mesh repair of indirect inguinal hernia using a preperitoneal approach: a preliminary report. *Surg Laparosc Endosc* 1992; **2**: 53–8.
5. Ferzli GS, Massaad A, Albert P. Extraperitoneal endoscopic hernia repair. *J Laparoendosc Surg* 1992; **2**: 281–6.
6. Nyhus LM, Pollack R, Rombeck CT, Donohue P. The preperitoneal approach and prosthetic buttress repair for recurrent hernia. *Ann Surg* 1988; **208**: 733–7.
7. Stoppa RE, Warlaumont CR. The preperitoneal approach and prosthetic repair of groin hernia. In: Nyhus LM, Condon RE, eds. *Hernia*, 3rd ed. Philadelphia: JB Lippincott, 1989: 199–225.
8. Rignault D. Preperitoneal prosthetic inguinal hernioplasty through a Pfannenstiel approach. *Surg Gynecol Obstet* 1986; **163**: 465.
9. MacFadyen B, Arregui M, Corbitt J, *et al.* Complications of laparoscopic hernia. *Surg Endosc* 1993; **7**: 155.
10. Fitzgibbons Jr F, Annibali R, Litke B, Filipi C, Salerno G, Cornet D. Multicentered clinical trial on laparoscopic inguinal hernia repair: preliminary results. *Surg Endosc* 1993; **7**: 115.
11. Beebe DS, McNevin MP, Crain JM, *et al.* Evidence of venous stasis after abdominal insufflation for laparoscopic cholecystectomy. *Surg Gynecol Obstet* 1993; **175**: 443–7.
12. Felix E, Michas C. Double buttress laparoscopic herniorrhaphy. *J Laparoendosc Surg* 1993; **3**: 1.
13. Ferzli GS, Massaad A, Albert P, Worth M. Endoscopic extraperitoneal herniorrhaphy vs conventional hernia repair. *Curr Surg* 1993; **50**: 291–4.
14. McKernan JB, Laws HL. Laparoscopic repair of inguinal hernias using a totally extraperitoneal prosthetic approach. *Surg Endosc* 1993; **7**: 26–8.

72

Laparoscopic Inguinal Hernia Repair Without Fixation of the Prosthesis

CORNELIS J VAN STEENSEL AND WIBO F WEIDEMA

In the Reinier de Graaf hospital in Delft, The Netherlands, repair of inguinal hernia has been performed by laparoscopic technique since August 1991. The operation can be looked upon as comprising two aspects: the approach and the repair. The basic principle of the repair of the abdominal wall is based on the Stoppa technique in which the mesh prosthesis is anchored by intra-abdominal pressure. Therefore, we do not use any sutures or staples for fixation of the prosthesis.

There are two laparoscopic approaches in this series: the transabdominal preperitoneal procedure and the laparoscopic extraperitoneal route.

Technique

Transabdominal preperitoneal procedure (TAPP)

Three trocars are introduced: one under the umbilicus for the optical system and two working channels at each side of the umbilicus in the semilunar line. The hernial sac is grasped and inverted. Then the peritoneum is opened and the sac is freed from its adhesions. The surrounding peritoneum is mobilized to make room for the mesh. The polypropylene mesh prosthesis is introduced into the abdomen with the help of a trocar reduction sleeve. It is placed preperitoneally, covering the defect. The prosthesis is held in place by the intra-abdominal pressure, and no sutures or staples are used. To prevent the formation of adhesions to the bowel and the formation of fistula, the peritoneum must be closed. This is accomplished by suturing the peritoneum with a running polydioax-anone (PDS) suture.

Laparoscopic extraperitoneal method (LEP)

After developing the preperitoneal space, a pneumopreperitoneum is developed and three trocars are placed: one under the umbilicus for the optical system, one halfway between the umbilicus and the symphysis pubis, and the third at the lateral side of the umbilicus in the semilunar line.

At present we use the peritoneal dissection balloon to create the preperitoneal space. The placement of the mesh is accomplished just as in the TAPP. Closure of the peritoneum is not necessary.

Results

Between August 1991 and May 1993, 251 hernias were repaired in 213 patients. In this group there were only three women (1.2%); the mean age was 56 years (range, 24–82 years).

Both direct and indirect hernias were operated on; even large defects (Nyhus IIIB) were repaired (11%). In only two patients was a femoral hernia repaired. Recurrent hernia accounted for 25% of the operations in this study. The recurrences resulting from primary repairs with an anterior approach were quite easy to repair; similarly, recurrences from preperitoneally placed Marlex, including our own laparoscopic recurrences, caused no problems when a laparoscopic repair was performed.

In the first period the plug and patch method as described by Schultz was used. Recurrences occurred predominantly in this period when small size prosthesis were used (4 out of 34). The recurrence rate was the reason why the prosthesis in the second group was enlarged to a size of 10 × 15 cm. Because the plugs were palpable in a considerable number of patients, the plugs were left out in the last group. So finally only a 10 × 15 cm prosthesis was used, in which fixation of the prosthesis was accomplished by intra-abdominal pressure alone. With the larger prosthesis this recurrence rate dropped from 12% to 1.9%.

Both working and retired patients are returning to normal daily life within 14 days (mean, four days).

Complications

The peroperative complications rate was 3.6%. Bleeding led to conversion and anterior repair after haemostasis. In three patients a bladder perforation occurred. One, a perforated diverticulum was resected after conversion and an anterior repair was done. One perforation was noticed after operation and conservative treatment with bladder decompression appeared to be successful. In the third patient the bladder perforation was noticed during operation and the bladder was sutured laparoscopically. On one patient a spermatic duct lesion occurred and once a lost needle could not be retrieved.

Five procedures were converted to an anterior approach: three massive haemorhages, one bladder perforation and one because of malfunctioning of the optical system.

The postoperative course in these patients was uneventful. Minor wound haematomas and infections were seen in some patients but resolved spontaneously within three weeks. No nerve damage or graft infection was encountered.

Conclusion

The laparoscopic method is a safe technique for the repair of an inguinal hernia. The return to normal daily life – in the majority of the patients within a week – can be viewed as an indication of the very low morbidity.

Although the follow-up period is short as yet, the recurrence rate supports the fact that intra-abdominal pressure alone is sufficient to prevent dislocation of the mesh prosthesis.

Further Reading

Stoppa RE, Warlaumont CR. The preperitoneal approach and prosthetic repair of groin hernia. In: Nyhus LM, Condon RE, eds. *Hernia*. Philadelphia: JB Lippincott, 1989; 199–255.

Steensel CJ van, Weidema WF, Gerritson van der Hoop A. Laparoscopic inguinal hernia repair I: one-year follow-up of 34 laparoscopic plug and patch repairs for inguinal henia. *Surg Laparosc Endosc* 1993, in press.

Steensel CJ van, Weidema WF, Gerritsen van der Hoop A. Laparoscopic inguinal hernia repair II: development of the laparoscopic transabdominal preperitoneal procedure based on the preliminary results of 77 inguinal hernia repairs. *Surg Laparosc Endosc* 1993, in press

73

Inguinal Herniorrhaphy using Intraperitoneal Placement of an Expanded Polytetrafluoroethylene Patch

KARL A LEBLANC, ALBERT T SPAW AND WILLIAM V BOOTH

The repair of inguinal hernias using a laparoscopic approach remains a controversial subject. This chapter does not attempt to resolve these issue, which will doubtless be answered over time, when enough long-term data are available to determine definitively the efficacy not only of each technique but also of the entire arena of laparoscopic inguinal hernia repair. Instead, we focus on the intraperitoneal placement of an expanded polytetrafluoroethylene (ePTFE) patch (Gore-Tex Soft Tissue Patch) to repair these hernias.

We first began to experiment with this repair in 1990. At that time, because of our unfamiliarity with the laparoscopic view of the inguinal anatomy, we limited our use of the technique. Since that time, we have developed a fairly standardized technique that we have been able to apply to a growing series of patients. Although there are minor variations in technique among the authors, the general approach and results are the same.

Technique

General anaesthesia is administered via tracheal intubation. The urinary bladder is decompressed with an indwelling catheter. The scrotum is frequently prepared and draped into the operative field. A monitor is placed at the foot of the table. The surgeon stands on the side contralateral to the hernia and the assistant surgeon (if used) stands on the side ipsilateral to the hernia.

With the patient in the Trendelenburg position, a midline incision is made at the umbilicus, through which a 10-mm trocar is inserted, and the abdomen is insufflated with CO_2. At this point, the surgeon should examine the abdominal cavity and the inguinal region to identify any unsuspected pathology or the presence of an unsuspected bilateral hernia, and to determine the type and extent of the hernia present. Two or three additional incisions are made (depending on the location of the defect and the surgeon's preference) laterally, through which 5- or 10-mm trocars are inserted (the size of the trocar also depends on the surgeon's preference). Either a 0° or a 30° laparoscope can be used. The laparoscope can be placed through the internal spermatic ring directly into the hernia sac, through the inguinal canal and into the distal extent of the sac.

The surgeon defines the location of the 'triangle of doom' between the vas deferens and the spermatic vessels. The peritoneum is dissected off anteromedial to the vas deferens, exposing Cooper's ligament and the medial portion of the iliopubic tract. If a lipoma of the spermatic cord is present, it is dissected. However, the hernia sac, if present, is not ligated.

A 7.5 × 10 or 8 × 12 cm ePTFE patch is then rolled, inserted through the trocar, unrolled and placed over the defect, along the entire length of the inguinal floor. A laparoscopic stapler is inserted

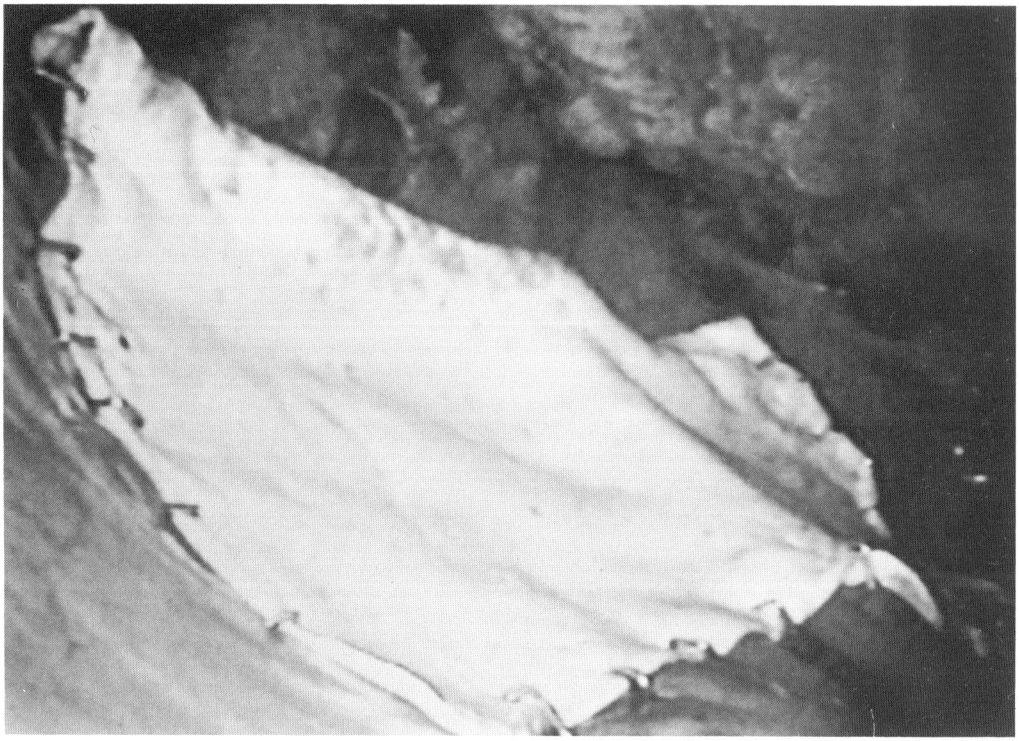

Figure 73.1: A completed right inguinal herniorrhaphy.

and the patch is stapled in place, taking care to affix the patch starting from Cooper's ligament medially to the iliopubic tract lateral to the internal spermatic ring. Because of the potential space overlying the triangle of doom, we frequently affix the peritoneum to the patch using about three staples.

The patch is initially stapled along this inferior edge and then flipped upward onto the anterior abdominal wall. The anterior edge of the prosthesis is stapled to the transversalis fascia overlying the rectus sheath medially and transversalis fascia superiorly and laterally. Staples must never be placed in the area of the triangle of doom. Care must also be taken to prevent injury to the inferior epigastric vessels. Figure 73.1 shows a completed repair.

The CO_2 is allowed to escape the abdominal cavity with the trocars in place to prevent the abdominal contents from being pushed into the fascial defects made by the trocar holes. This could predispose these sites to the creation of a new hernia defect almost immediately. Removal of the lateral trocars must be performed under direct visualization to identify any injured vessels within the abdominal wall.

Results

After learning the technique, the average time in surgery is 30 minutes. All procedures are performed on an outpatient basis and patients are often discharged from the hospital within two hours postoperatively.

Between September 1991 and May 1993, we used this technique to repair 264 inguinal hernias. Average patient age was 49.54 years (range 18–86 years). There were 123 direct and 141 hernias, including ten sliding and four incarcerated hernias. Fifty-five of the defects were recurrent; the remainder were primary.

Patients took an average of 6.55 tablets for postoperative pain (usually hydrocodone 7.5 mg and returned to work in an average of 6.05 days.

Average follow-up time is nine months (longest: 20 months). Follow up is conducted by physical examination one and three weeks and three, six, nine and 12 months postoperatively, followed by yearly examinations thereafter.

Four patients have presented with recurrences. Three were early in the series and probably resulted from improper positioning of the patch and inadequate fixation to Cooper's ligament. One recurrence was repaired using an open technique and the reason for the recurrence is unknown.

One patient bled from a lateral trocar site, probably as a result of injury to the inferior epigastric vein. Two patients experienced transient genitofemoral neuralgia that resolved within a few days.

Lessons learned

Although the field of laparoscopic repair of inguinal hernias is still young and many questions remain unanswered, the technique presented here seems promising. It is fairly easy to learn and, once learned, quick to perform, with an average time in surgery of 30 minutes. Anyone who can tolerate general anaesthesia is a candidate for the procedure, but it is especially well suited for patients with recurrent and bilateral hernias. Anecdotally, patients with recurrent hernias verify markedly reduced postoperative pain and quicker return to normal activity levels.

Early in the series, we did not routinely dissect lipomas of the cord. However, we found that leaving the lipoma *in situ* often created an inguinal bulge that patients could confuse with a recurrence, so we now routinely dissect any lipomas.

The choice of prosthetic is an extremely important consideration with this technique. We use only the ePTFE patch because it is strongly and extremely inert, exhibiting very good tissue ingrowth with little or no fibrotic response. If another material is used, such as a polypropylene mesh, the peritoneum must be closed over the mesh to prevent the risk of injury to the viscera from the adhesions that will form. However, closing the peritoneum is time-consuming and negates the inherent simplicity of the technique. Also, some surgeons have been hesitant about using the ePTFE patch because it is opaque, obscuring the anatomy lying beneath it. We have found that stapling the inferior edge of the patch first and then flipping the patch upward, combined with a thorough knowledge of the inguinal anatomy from the laparoscopic perspective, allows the surgeon to position and affix the patch with confidence, obviating any need for a transparent prosthesis.

We feel that the technique definitely reduces postoperative morbidity and significantly speeds recovery time to full activity. Although many surgeons report that their patients return to work within a week or less using an open, tension-free technique, the average return to full activity for our patients repaired with an open, tension-free repair was 45 days.

Although we are encouraged by our early results, we will continue to monitor our patients closely to determine long-term recurrence and complication rates. This will be the true measure of the success of the technique.

74

Gore-Tex Peritoneal Onlay Laparoscopic Hernioplasty

FREDERICK K TOY

The Gore-Tex peritoneal onlay laparoscopic inguinal hernioplasty has been performed on 170 patients (male, female) with a total of 212 hernioplasties over the past 32 months, from February 1991 to August 1993. The age range was 17–89 years, with an average of 60.3 years. Forty-two of the patients had bilateral hernias repaired; 147 direct hernias; 52 indirect hernias; 10 pantaloon hernias; and seven femoral hernias. Thirty two of the repairs were for recurrent hernias.

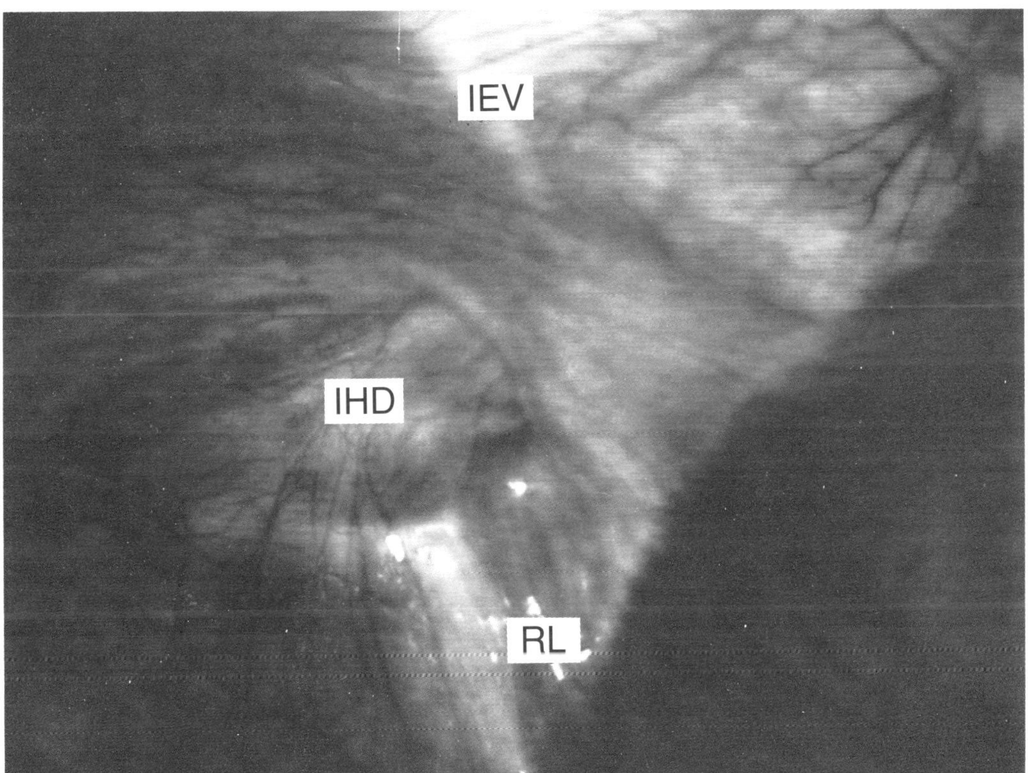

Figure 74.1: Indirect inguinal hernia in a female. IEV, inferior epigastric vessels; IHD, indirect hernia defect; RL, round ligament.

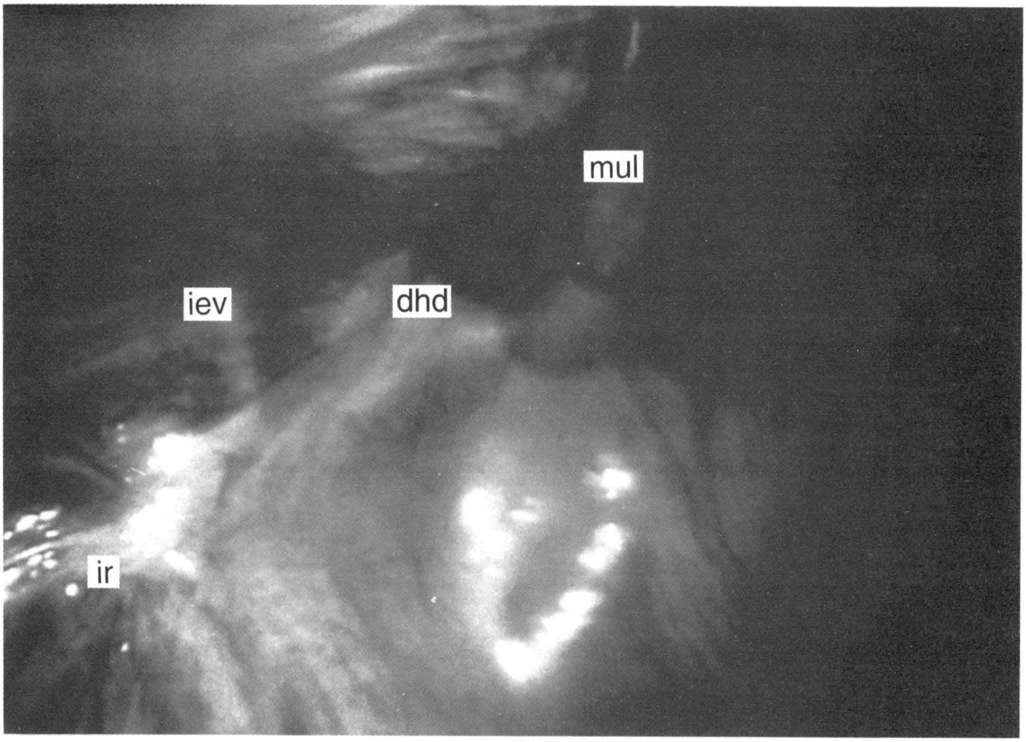

Figure 74.2: Direct hernia. dhd, direct hernia defect, iev, inferior epigastric vessels; ir, internal ring; mul, medial umbilical ligament.

Operative procedure

The procedure is performed under general anaesthesia. The patients is given antibiotic prophylaxis, and the bladder is decompressed with a Foley catheter; the stomach is decompressed with a nasogastric tube. The patient is supine in the Trendelenburg position. A skin incision is made at the superior edge of the umbilicus, and a Veress needle is used to insufflate CO_2 for the visualization of the peritoneal cavity.

An 11 mm trocar is inserted into the peritoneal cavity via the umbilical incision, through which a 0° laparoscope is introduced. The abdominal cavity is then explored and the hernia defects are confirmed (Figures 74.1 and 74.2). Two additional 11 mm trocars are inserted under direct vision. These are placed at the level of the umbilicus along the anterior axillary lines (Figure 74.3).

The contents of the sac, if present, are reduced into the peritoneal cavity. This is usually quite easy; however, it can be the most difficult part of the procedure, especially on large, direct hernias. These may be sliding hernias and have colon (usually sigmoid on the left and caecum on the right) making up the inferior portion of the sac (Figure 74.4) and/or bladder making up the medial portion of the sac. The bowel or bladder fat is grasped with an atraumatic babcock and retracted cephalad. The peritoneal reflection between bowel and hernia sac is easily identified and incised with endoscopic shears, delivering the bowel back into the peritoneal cavity.

The demarcation between the bladder and the hernia sac is not so obvious. For this reason, on large, direct hernia defects, dissection is started on the anterior abdominal wall component of the medial umbilical ligament and carried inferiorly, incising only the peritoneum and teasing bluntly all bladder and perivesical fat from the medial portion of the hernia sac. This safely reduces

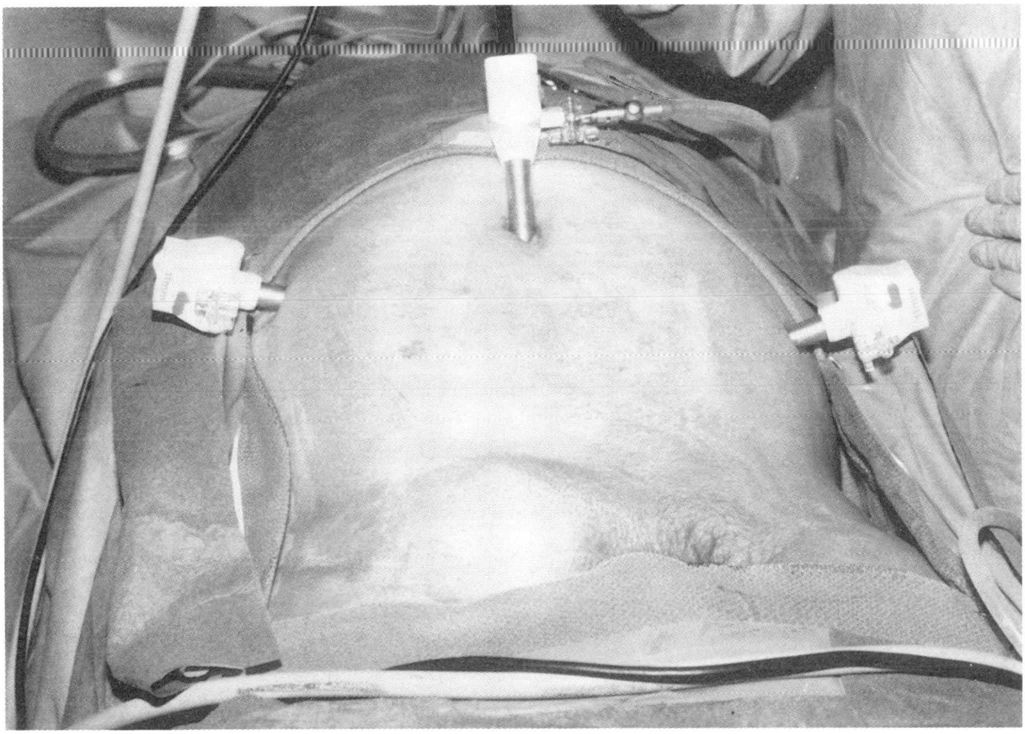

Figure 74.3: Trocar placement. Note the right inguinal hernia bulge with insufflation.

the bladder into the peritoneal cavity and clears the medial edge of the hernia defect for patch fixation.

The sac is left *in situ* with no ligation of the internal ring. The medial umbilical ligament is incised laterally and reflected medially with endoscopic scissors. This exposes the pubic tubercle and Cooper's ligament (Figure 74.5). The dissection is carried laterally along Cooper's ligament up to the vas deferens, which courses over the external iliac vein at this level. Any redundant, floppy, medial umbilical ligament is stapled medially to the anterior abdominal wall to prevent its obstructing one's view.

The repair

An e-PTFE soft tissue patch, 1 mm thick (W.L. Gore & Associates Inc., Flagstaff, Arizona), is cut to 8 × 12 cm in size and tailored inferiorly to conform with the oblique Cooper's ligament and iliopubic tract. The edge to be stapled to Cooper's ligament is highlighted with a marker for easy orientation. The patch is then attached to a two-pronged Nanticoke Endo-patch spreader (Nanticoke Surgical Instruments, Seaford, Delaware) (Figure 74.6) with 2-0 Ethibond sutures. The medial (pubic tubercle) corner of the patch is attached to the short prong (Figure 74.7). This greatly facilitates the introduction of the patch into the peritoneal cavity and the spreading and positioning of the inferomedial edge of the patch over the pubic tubercle and Cooper's ligament.

The Endo-patch spreader is inserted through the contralateral 11 mm trocar. Through the ipsilateral 11 mm trocar, the Endopath EMS hernia stapler (Ethicon Inc., Cincinnati, Ohio) (Figure 74.8) is inserted, and several staples are placed, securing the Gore-Tex patch to the pubic tubercle and Cooper's ligament up to the external iliac vein (Figure 74.9).

The sutures attaching the patch to the spreader are then cut, and the Endo-patch spreader is removed. The inferior lateral corner is grasped and positioned over the iliopubic tract and fixed

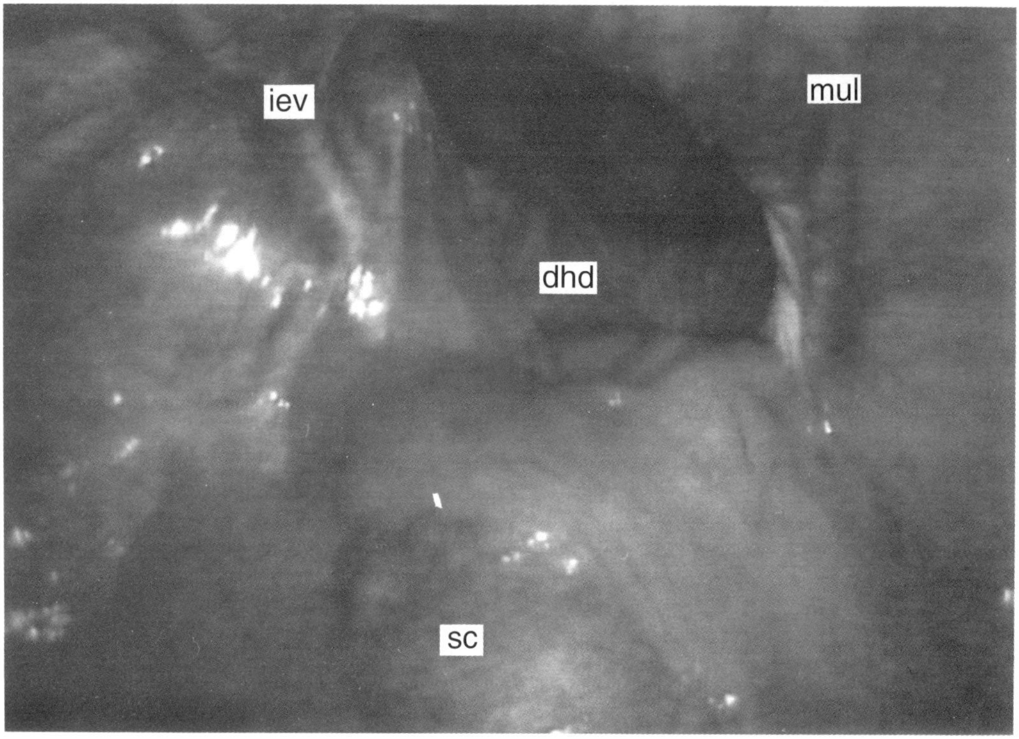

Figure 74.4: Direct sliding hernia with sigmoid colon. dhd, direct hernia defect; iev, inferior epigastric vessels; mul, medial umbilical ligament; sc, sigmoid colon.

with staples. The iliopubic tract is easy to identify without any dissection. The iliopubic tract lies parallel and deep to the inguinal ligament (Poupart's ligament). Anterior abdominal wall countertraction is applied just above the inguinal ligament; this countertraction can be seen laparoscopically and palpated with the stapler head. The stapler head is then rolled inferiorly, just below the operator's palpable fingers. This is the iliopubic tract from the laparoscopic perspective.

It is paramount not to staple inferior to the iliopubic tract, so as to prevent injury to the femoral, genitofemoral and/or lateral femoral cutaneous nerves (Figure 74.10). At this point, the patch is grasped at its superior edge via the ipsilateral trocar and folded up over the hernia defect. The EMS stapler is introduced via the contralateral trocar, and the patch is stapled anteriorly to the transversalis fascia and laterally to the endoabdominal fascia. Good fascial fixation of the staples anteriorly and laterally is facilitated by anterior abdominal wall countertraction (Figure 74.11) This provides secure and reliable fixation of the patch to the fascial structures, covering the indirect, direct and femoral hernia spaces (Figure 74.12).

The area of repair is then irrigated and the security of the patch verified. The pneumoperitoneum is released, and the trocars are removed. The skin is closed with 4-0 Vicryl, subcuticular sutures. The patient is discharged home when fully recovered which is usually about four hours post-operatively.

Results

There were a total of five different complications. One major complication was a bladder injury that required an open repair of the bladder and then an open, conventional hernioplasty. The other more

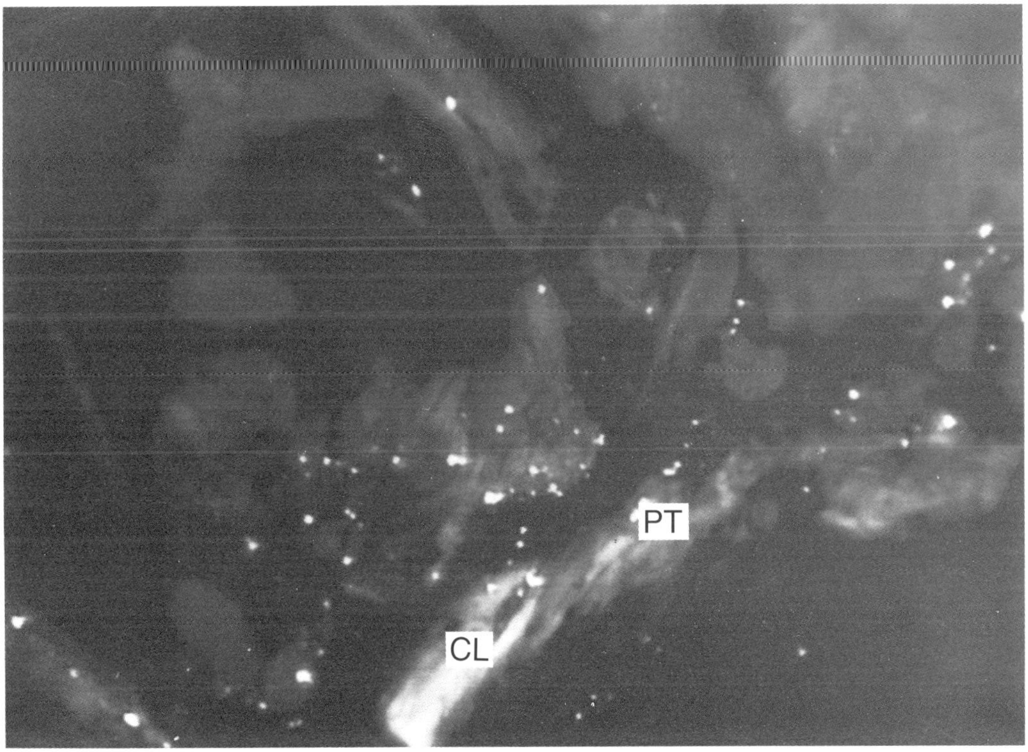

Figure 74.5: Direct hernia defect with pubic tubercle (PT) and Cooper's ligament (CL) exposed.

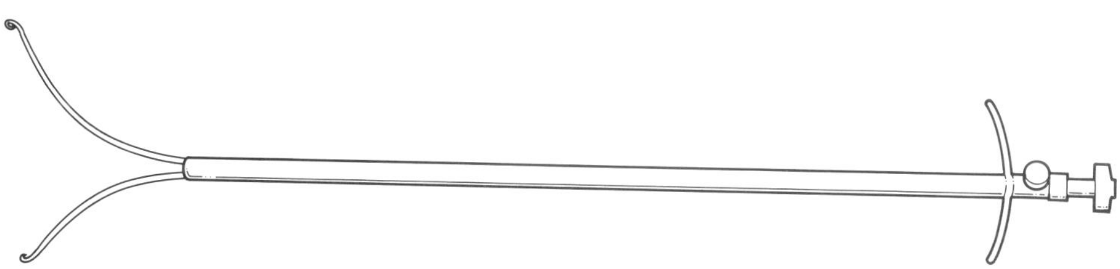

Figure 74.6: Nanticoke two-pronged Endo-patch spreader (Nanticoke Surgical Instruments, Seaford, Delaware).

minor, complications were urinary retention, pubic osteitis, anterior thigh pain and abdominal wall haematoma, all of which resolved spontaneously by the third postoperative week. Postoperative pain and discomfort were minimal. Normal, unrestricted activity, including heavy manual labour, was resumed at an average of 5.3 days postoperatively. With the maximum follow up now of 32 months, five recurrences (2.7%) have been noted; they were in patients early in the evolution of the procedure. These recurrences have resulted in several modifications in the procedure. There have been no recurrences in the past 23 months.

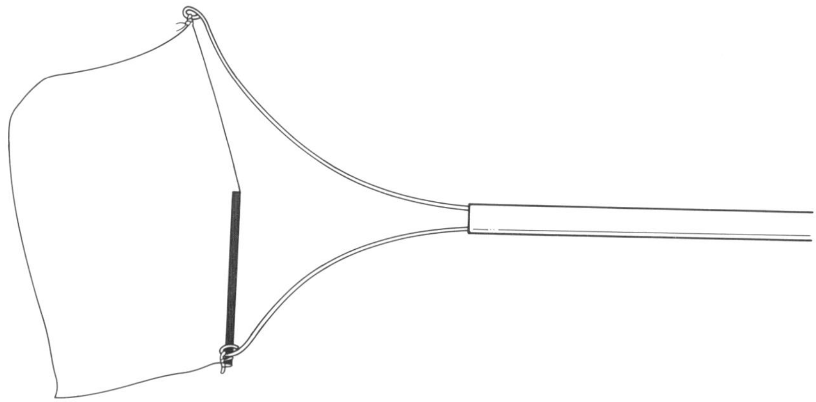

Figure 74.7: An 8 × 12 cm Gore-Tex soft tissue patch attached to the Nanticoke Endo-patch spreader. Note that the medial corner is attached to the shorter prong.

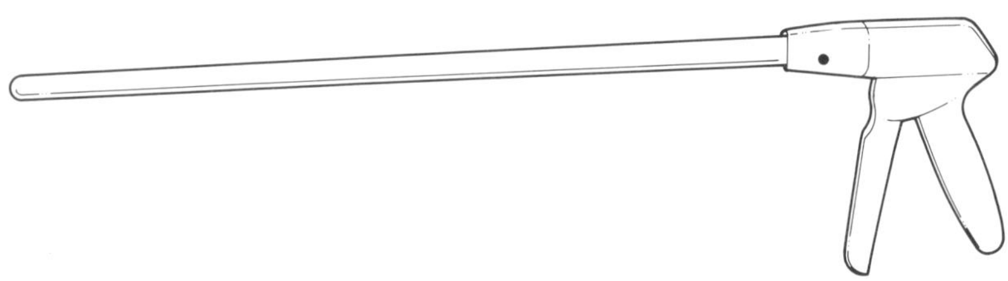

Figure 74.8: Endopach EMS hernia stapler (Ethicon Inc, Cincinnati, Ohio).

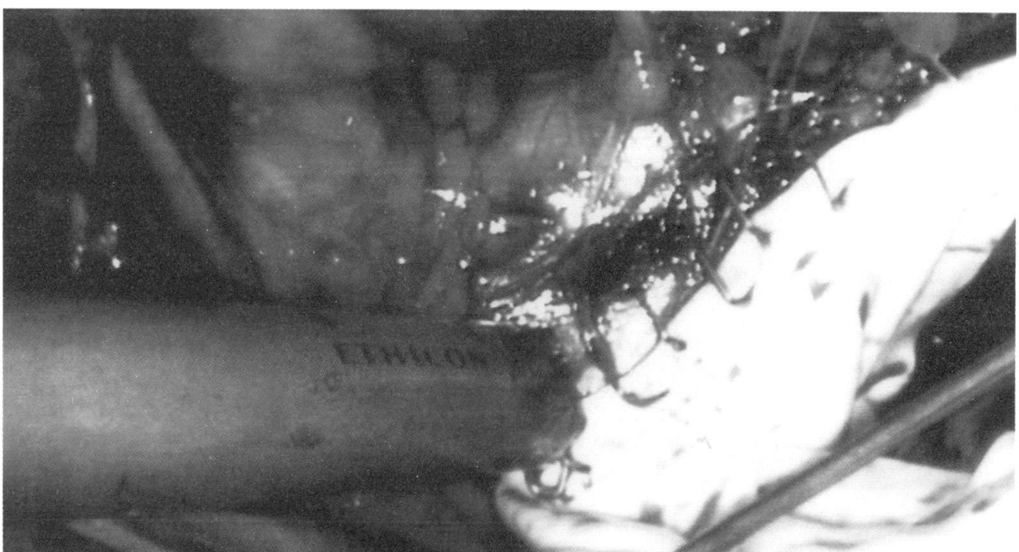

Figure 74.9: Stapling the Gore-Tex soft tissue patch to the pubic tubercle and Cooper's ligament.

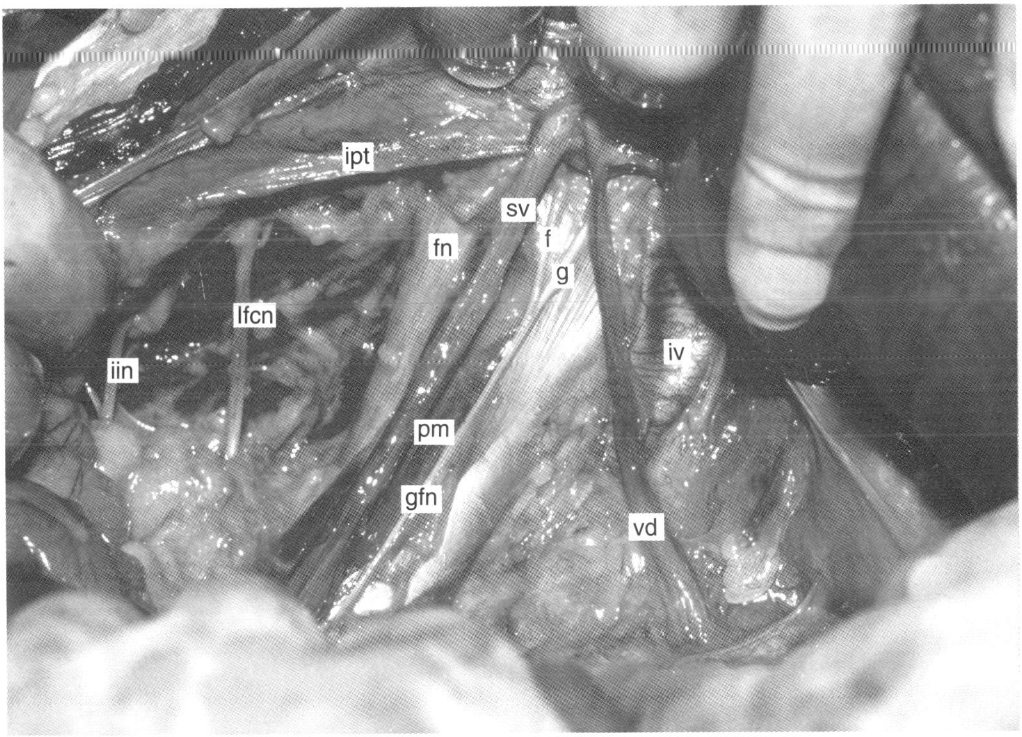

Figure 74.10: Nerve anatomy. f, femoral branch of the genitofemoral nerve; fn, femoral nerve, g, genital branch of the genitofemoral nerve; gfn, genitofemoral nerve; iin, ilioinguinal hernia; ipt, iliopubic tract; iv, iliac vessels; lfcn, lateral femoral cutaneous nerve; pm, psoas muscle; sv, spermatic vessels; vd, vas deferens.

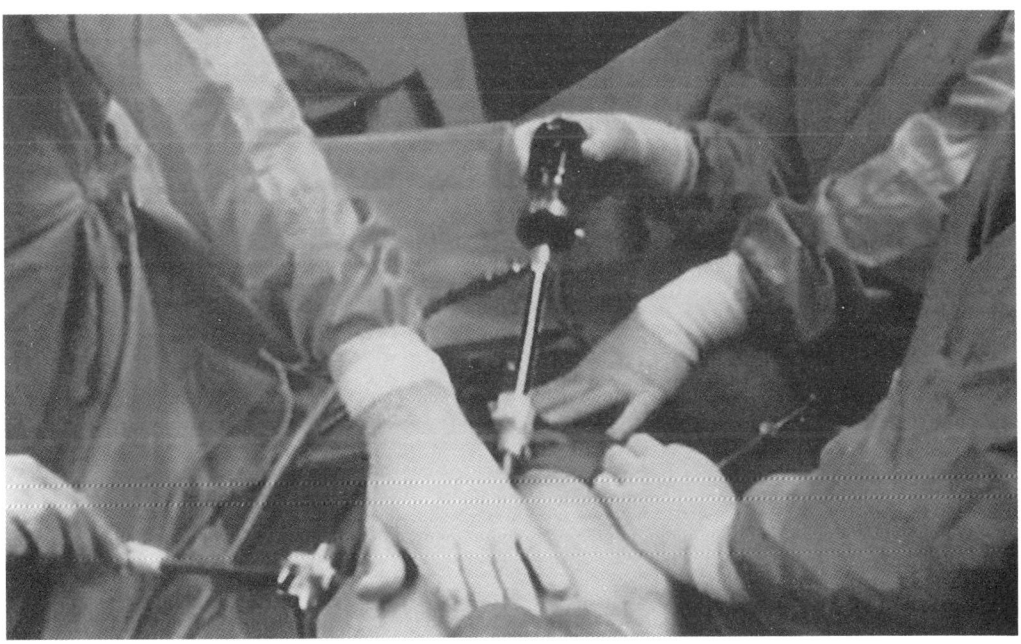

Figure 74.11: Applying countertraction on the anterior abdominal wall for good staple fixation.

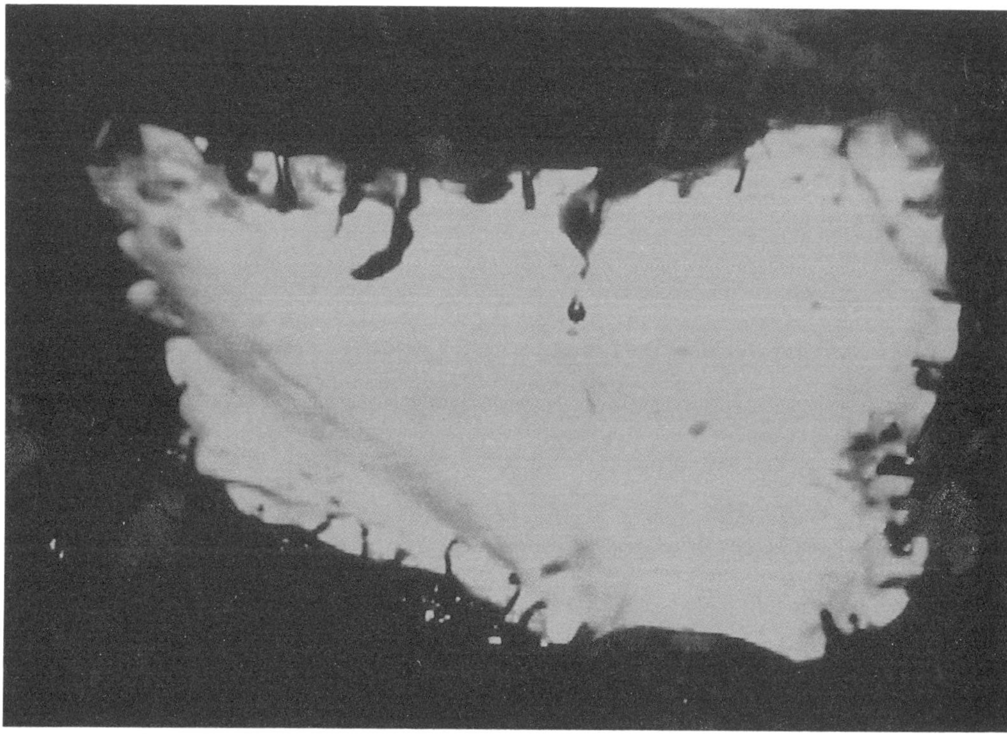

Figure 74.12: Completed repair of right inguinal hernia.

75

Paediatric Laparoscopic Herniorrhaphy (Ultra-high Ligation)

LUIS I CAMPOS

The laparoscopic approach was carried out using 5 mm ports, the umbilicus for the camera and two accessory ports for a dissector and micro-scissors. The high ligation of a standard paediatric herniorrhaphy, done previously by another surgeon, was found to be noticeable as a small sinus intra-abdominally. This patient had been referred for an undescended testicle, which was found intra-abdominally with an associated hernia. Because the laparoscopic approach is higher and leaves no residual sinus, the term 'ultra-high ligation' was adopted for this procedure. The ligation was carried out using endoscopic loops pre-made with absorbable suture material. One 8-year-old boy had an iatrogenic vasectomy that required an immediate conversion to an open procedure with repair of the transected vas with one-layer vasovasotomy.

Laparoscopy in children has been done for the last 30 years, to aid diagnosis in difficult clinical situations or for the evaluation of jaundice[1]. Paediatric surgeons have used pneumoperitoneum to insufflate and diagnose inguinal hernias. The Goldstein test is the insufflation of air through the hernia sac at the time of repair of a symptomatic inguinal hernia. Goldstein had vast experience with his procedure requiring between 200 and 2000 ml of insufflation. The number of patients exceeded 5000[2]. The duration of pneumoperitoneum was relatively short, never exceeding 2–4 minutes.

The safest gas to insufflate the abdomen for a procedure lasting several minutes is carbon dioxide. Unfortunately, CO_2 presents several problems in children. On of these its potential for hypothermia. The gas gets colder as it is released from its liquid pressurized form. Operating rooms keep these pressurized tanks at a temperature of 15.5–21 °C (60°–70 °F). The release (flow rate) to normal atmospheric pressures changes the pressurized liquid to its gas form; once in gas form, the temperature of the gas is the same as the environment. Another disadvantage of using CO_2 is hypercarbia. Hypercarbia (or excess carbon dioxide in the circulation) is typically seen in patients who have no pulmonary compensation (anaesthetized and breathing spontaneously); thus it is imperative that airway control be provided by a tracheal tube in order to hyperventilate the patient if a dangerous accumulation of CO_2 is detected. The prolonged increase of intra-abdominal pressure (if it is not controlled) may give rise to bradyarrhythmias, with potentially lethal consequences. Animal experimentation by Booker[3] in the 1940s demonstrated that catastrophic events (lethal doses of CO_2) occurred faster in smaller dogs than in larger ones.

With these considerations in mind, laparoscopic surgery in children is possible but requires tracheal anaesthesia, CO_2 monitoring, environmental temperature control, patient temperature monitoring and paediatric-size laparoscopic instruments. The results of the author's initial experience is presented in this chapter, with the performance of ultra-high ligation performed through the laparoscope for the treatment of symptomatic inguinal hernias in children aged 2 years or over.

Operative procedure

There were 12 patients (five girls and seven boys) in this series. Their ages ranged from two to 14 years (average age, 7 years). The first case performed has been followed for nine months, with most of the cases followed at least 6 months; the shortest follow up has been two months. The patients' weight ranged between 12 and 50 kg (average, 27 kg). The patients' weights and ages were plotted against the charts published by the National Health Center for Statistics to obtain the corresponding percentile group. They ranged between the 10th percentile to the 95th percentile with an average of 50. One of the five girls had bilateral inguinal hernias, one had a right inguinal hernia (Figures75.1 and 75.2) and two had left inguinal hernias. Of the seven boys, three had bilateral inguinal hernias and four had right inguinal hernias. There was a total of 16 hernias.

The parents and paediatricians were informed about the procedure, and the consent form specified the use of laparoscopic surgery for inguinal hernia repair. The operating room setting included a video monitor at the foot of the table. A Verres needle (disposable type) was used in all cases, to create a pneumoperitoneum. The intra-abdominal pressure was maintained between 6 and 10 mmHg depending on the size and age of the patient: the smaller the individual, the lower the pressure. The initial amount of CO_2 necessary to obtain a pneumoperitoneum was directly proportional to the size of the abdomen. The flow rate was never increased beyond 3 l/minute. All the patients had a tracheal tube, CO_2 monitoring, core temperature monitoring and an anaesthesiologist with experience in paediatric surgery.

One 2–0 chromic laparoscopic endoligature was used to tie the inverted sac. In girls an attempt was made to include the round ligament. Boys required dissection of the sac in order to prevent the inadvertent ligature of testicular artery and/or the vas deferens.

Insufflation of the pneumoperitoneum was carried out by calculating the initial volume of CO_2 necessary, according to the formula:

$$\text{Initial volume} = 200\ \text{ml} + (\text{age in years} \times 100)$$

This formula was developed based on the experience accumulated with the published data on the Goldstein test. The insufflator had no gas-heating capabilities. In the last four cases an insufflator with automatic gas heating was used.

Results

No complications were found in 11 patients. One patient (14 years old) had an iatrogenic transection of the right vas deferens; this was recognized, the operation converted to an incisional procedure and a one-layer vasovasotomy using 7–0 Vicryl performed. The technique used consisted of an end-to-end (spatulate) anastomosis, patency being confirmed by injecting methylene blue into the lumen and observing that there was no extravasation of the dye. This patient was followed up in conjunction with a urologist.

One patient had previously undergone left inguinal herniorrhaphy (high ligation) by another surgeon. He was found to have a right inguinal hernia with an undescended testicle, and a first-stage orchiopexy was performed with laparoscopic ultra-high ligation. This patient required a subsequent orchiopexy at another date by a urologist.

The core temperature, monitored by an oesophageal probe, reflected a slight change (hypothermia). This change occurred in spite of the precaution of avoiding both high-flow insufflation (flow used ranged between 2 and 3 l/minute) and large amounts of CO_2, known to cause this complication. The use of a heated insufflator improved the temperature and in one patient corrected the temperature during the procedure. This observation will require a larger number of cases to determine its clinical significance.

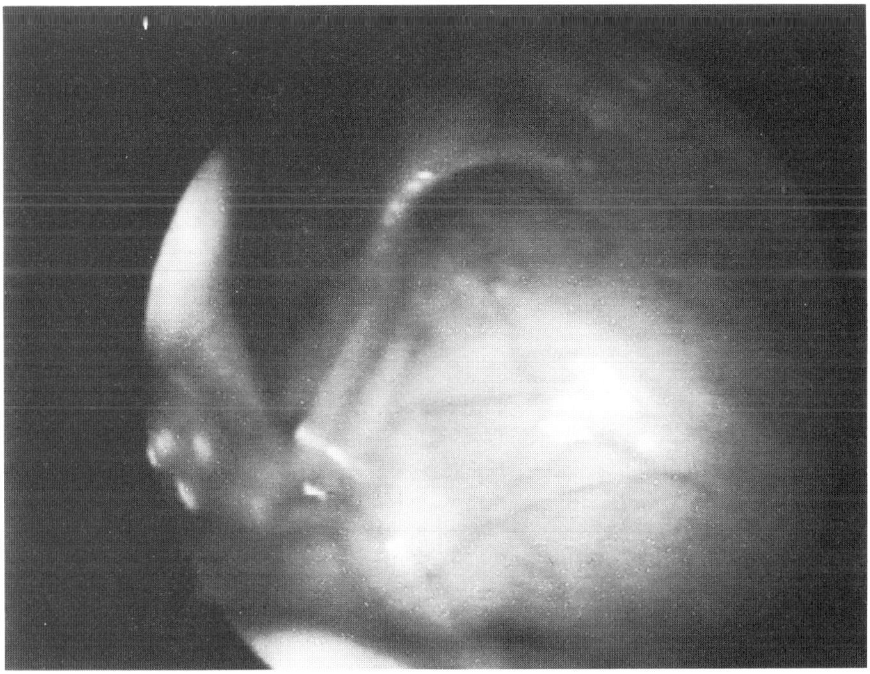

Figure 75.1: The photograph demonstrates a right inguinal hernia in a 2-year-old female with a unilateral symptomatic inguinal hernia.

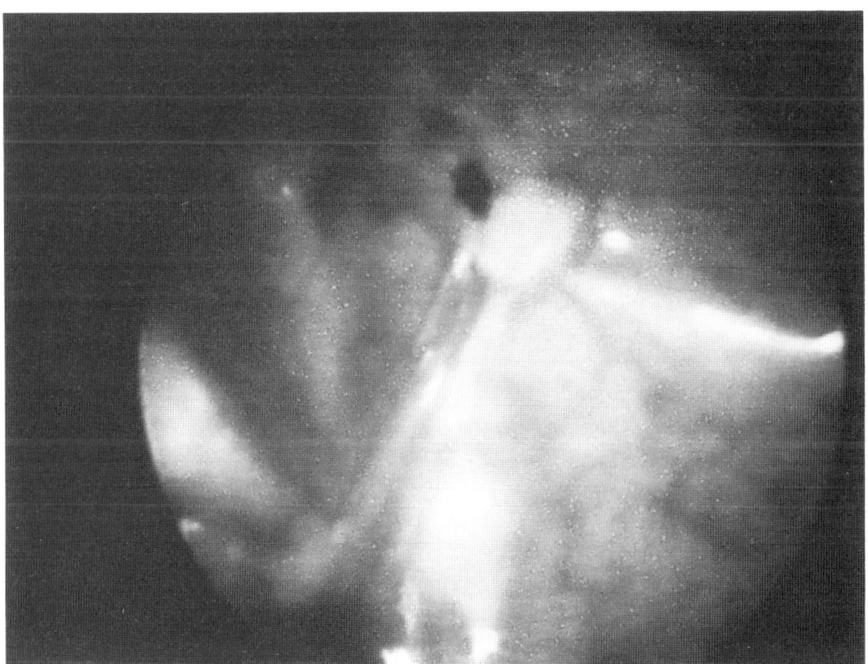

Figure 75.2: The patient in Figure 75.1 after her hernia was inverted and ligated with a 2–0 chromic catgut endoligature.

The operative time ranged between 17 and 70 minutes, this wide range is because of the patient requiring 70 minutes who was the one requiring the repair of the complication. The average operative time was 33 minutes.

The results are summarized in Table 75.1.

Table 75.1: Summary of the results in the 12 children in the series

Patient	*Age* (years)	*Weight* (kg)	*Percentile*	*Complication*	*Temp. change*	*Sex*	*Side*	*CO_2*	*OR time* (min)
1	10	28	25	Nil	−2 °C	M	Rt	Standard	39
2	3	12	10	Nil	−1 °C	M	Rt	Standard	40
3	6	27	95	Nil	−2 °C	F	B	Standard	20
4	4	15	25	Nil	−1 °C	M	Rt	Standard	35
5	8	25	50	Nil	−2 °C	F	Lt	Standard	19
6	7	23	23	Nil	−2 °C	M	Rt	Standard	42
7	11	29	10	Nil	−1 °C	F	Rt	Standard	20
8	2	13	75	Nil	−1 °C	M	B	Standard	45
9	5	19	50	Nil	No change	M	B	Heated	35
10	14	50	50	Vas injury	No change	M	B	Heated	70
11	4	16	50	Nil	−1 °C	F	Lt	Heated	17
12	6	18	25	Nil	No change	F	Lt	Heated	19
Average	7 years	27 kg	40%	–	–	–	–	–	33

B = bilateral

The patients' tolerance and their parents' acceptance was excellent because of the immense popularity of laparoscopic surgery for adults these days. There was no difference in the response of the patients to anaesthesia, and the hospital stay was the same as if the repair had been done with a standard transverse incision. The initial six patients have had a follow up of six months with no recurrences, and the initial scepticism of the paediatricians has diminished in view of the added diagnostic properties of the new procedure.

The author feels that diagnostic laparoscopy (umbilical visualization as compared to contralateral hernioscopy), with or without ultra-high ligation, is possible and is the procedure of choice in females with bilateral inguinal hernias. On the other hand, laparoscopic ultra-high ligation, a tedious and time-consuming procedure in males, is possible in skilful hands, but is not appropriate because a similar result can be obtained through an incision, and with less risk. Laparoscopic hernia management should be limited to surgeons who understand and can repair its complications and prevent its risks.

Conclusions

Laparoscopic hernia repair should be performed by surgeons with advanced training in paediatric laparoscopy. This group of patients illustrates the potential complications when trying to dissect a hernia sac in a boy. Because the anatomical structures are less likely to be injured in a girl, the procedure is safer in females. Ultra-high ligation gives the patient a more anatomical repair with a higher diagnostic value. The Goldstein test (pneumoperitoneum through the hernia sac) was not performed because of the greater value of umbilical laparoscopic visualization[4]. Since laparoscopy was added to the diagnostic tools, the paediatricians' referrals and acceptance has increased even when there was an initial reluctance to implement a new procedure. The surgical metabolism of children, especially their poor thermoregulation, is a major concern when using CO_2 insufflation. Carbon dioxide kept in liquid form in pressurized tanks is released to the environment through regulating valves; the higher the flow, the colder the gas released. The gas rapidly equilibrates its temperature to the environment. Room temperature should be kept higher than normal or a thermal blanket used.

Parents' acceptance was excellent owing to the popularity of laparoscopy for cholecystectomy and other common surgical procedures. They had been informed of the potential for complications and the risks involved in the procedure. The use of a Verres needle in children requires the same precautions as with adults. Although no complications were found with this blind approach, it should be kept in mind that careless insertion in a thin abdomen may perforate a viscus[5]. The author believes that there is a definite role for laparoscopy in paediatric hernia surgery because it will eliminate unnecessary contralateral explorations, will result in earlier diagnosis of undescended intra-abdominal testicles, and will help in the diagnosis of adnexal pathology in females[6].

Acknowledgements

The author thanks the Pediatric Department at Sacred Heart Hospital in Allentown PA, Wanda Morgan for her review of the original manuscript, Dennis Richard from Snowden Pencer for his assistance with the heated insufflator, Jill Dooling from US Surgical Corporation for her help in the course 'Advanced Pediatric Laparoscopy and Thoracoscopy', and also the office staff, wife Rosalia and four children Luis, Jose, Carlos and Nicolas for their patience and support.

References

1. Gans S, Berci G. Peritoneoscopy in infants and children. *J Pediatr Surg* 1973; **8**: 418–21.
2. Powel W. Intraoperative diagnostic pneumoperitoneum in pediatric patients with unilateral inguinal hernias: the Goldstein test. *J Pediatr Surg* 1985; **20**: 399–405.
3. Booker WM, French DM, Molano P. Further studies on the acute effects of intra-abdominal pressure. *Am J Physiol* 1947; **149**: 292.
4. Lobe T. Response in 'Letter to the Editor'. *J Laparoendosc Surg* 1993; **3**: 361.
5. Orsa K, Fisher J. Aorta laceration: a rare complication of laparoscopy. *J Laparoendosc Surg* 1992; **25**: 235–7.
6. Shalev E, Mann S, Romano S, Rahav D. Laparoscopic detorsion of adnexa in childhood: a case report. *J Pediatr Surg* 1991; **26**: 1193–4.

76

Laparoscopic Hernioplasty using a Regular or a Self-expanding Prosthesis: Follow Up

JACQUES M HIMPENS, GUY B CADIERE AND JEAN A BRUYNS

Most of the techniques of laparoscopic hernioplasty involve the placement of a mesh in synthetic material[1–3]. In our search for the ideal laparoscopic mesh insertion, we had the experience of open procedures guide us which is in accordance with a general policy in laparoscopy[4].

There are several technique of 'open' herniorrhaphy involving the placement of a mesh. One of the most popular, with excellent results, is Lichtenstein's[5]. Because it consists of suturing a mesh *superficial to* the transversalis fascia, however, it is not suitable for the laparoscopic approach, which involves dissection of the *deep* side of this fascia. We therefore focus on the 'open' hernioplasty procedures in which the prosthesis is placed in a preperitoneal position.

Two different techniques can be mentioned. One is Rives'[6], in which a mesh is placed behind the transversalis fascia, via an inguinal approach. The mesh is then tacked to the edges of the so-called 'myopectineal defect' by several stitches. The other technique is Stoppa's[7]. Here, a prosthesis is placed between the inguinal wall and the peritoneum, but either is not fixed at all, or, more recently, is fixed in one or two places to prevent migration. The approach can be midline preperitoneal (Stoppa), suprainguinal (Nyhus[8]) or Pfannenstiel (Rignault[9]). In this technique, immobilization of the prosthesis is obtained by intra-abdominal pressure.

Materials and methods

In this series, 100 consecutive patients with 148 inguinal hernias were treated laparoscopically in our department. They were randomly assigned to undergo either the 'Rives' or the 'Stoppa' technique. After reduction of the hernia sac, incision of the peritoneum and dissection of the transversalis fascia and the spermatic cord, a prosthesis was inserted. Depending on the type of mesh handed to the surgeon at that point, a technique was chosen.

Rives' technique

A 15 × 10 cm polypropylene prosthesis was stapled to the inguinal floor and to Cooper's ligament by several staples rather than by stitches, which are tedious to place laparoscopically. Care was taken not to insert any staples distal to Poupart's ligament so as to prevent injury to the nerves in that area. Thus, in this technique, one relies on the staples to maintain the prosthesis in the correct position.

Stoppa's technique

A large piece of soft mesh (polyester) was introduced between the inguinal floor and the peritoneum without tacking it down. Because doubt remains about the prosthetic sheet maintaining its correct position during closure of the peritoneum and after deflation of the pneumoperitoneum, the mesh is contained by a frame of superelastic metal material (Nitinol; Cook Europe Inc., Bjaeverskov,

Denmark). This frame remains attached to the mesh. The metal skeleton facilitates the placement of the prosthesis and prevents its folding at the conclusion of the procedure[10]. Because Nitinol is radio-opaque, correct placement of the mesh can be verified postoperatively at any time.

As displacement occurred in the first few patients treated, a one-point fixation was carried out with effect from patient number 10.

In order to perform a prospective randomized study, both types of mesh were stored in similar packages. The patients thus underwent identical procedures up to the point of insertion of the prosthesis. Only at that time was the package opened and the type of prosthesis revealed. Patients with bilateral hernias could therefore receive one 'regular' and one 'reinforced' prosthesis.

This study reports the findings with a follow up of six months, minimum: recurrence after hernioplasty with mesh recurs before six months (Stoppa, personal communication, May 1993).

Results

Between 1 November 1991 and 18 September 1992, 148 hernias were treated (in 100 patients). Seventy-eight hernias were repaired with a 'regular' prosthesis (group A) and 70 with a 'reinforced' prosthesis (group B). Details of the two groups are listed in Table 76.1.

One reoperation had to be performed in group B, because of early obstruction (day 6). A loop of small bowel had to be released by laparotomy after incarceration in a gap in the peritoneal closure. There were no testicular or neural problems in this group. Two reoperations were performed for reasons other than recurrence before three months in group A. In both cases, nerve entrapment (one ilioinguinal, one cutaneous femoris lateralis) was treated by removing the staple, with good results in only one. Persistent neuralgia of the ilioinguinalis nerve in the other one had to be treated by alcoholization. There was one case of orchitis after an inguinoscrotal hernia repair in this group.

Two severe late postoperative complications occurred in group A. Both patients presented with small bowel obstruction due to adhesions to the repair area (one after four months and one after six months). In both cases, the Prolene prosthesis was clearly visible, despite adequate closure of the peritoneum. After unsuccessful laparoscopic adhesiolysis, laparotomy and finally small bowel resection had to be performed. Resection was unavoidable owing to over dense inflammatory adhesions. There were no infections in any of the cases under investigation.

Recurrences occurred in both groups. Early recurrence occurred only in the patients in whom no fixation of the mesh had been carried out (two recurrences out of ten in group B). Treatment consisted of laparoscopic repair with a new mesh in one and of open repair in the other. Late recurrence occurred in one patient each in groups A and B. At re-laparoscopy the prosthesis appeared to have been placed too medially in both, and had resulted in a lateral recurrence.

Table 76.1: Comparison of operations using 'regular' prosthesis (group A) and a 'reinforced' prosthesis (group B)

	Group A (n = 78)	*Group B* (n = 70)
Distribution of hernias:		
Indirect	37 (2 recurrent)	34 (3 recurrent)
Direct	32 (11 recurrent)	28 (5 recurrent)
Combined direct/indirect	3	1
Femoral	2	2
Lost to follow up	4	5
Mean operating time per hernia	63 min (45–120 min)	39 (15–72 min)
Perioperative complications	1*	nil
Mean hospitalization time per hernia	36 hours (8–72 hours)	34 hours (8–140 hours)
Follow-up period	11 months (6–16 months)	10 months (6–16 months)

* Staple injury of epigastric artery, treated by clipping

Conclusions

Laparoscopic inguinal hernioplasty has revealed an array of complications. Nerve entrapment is not something new in hernia surgery[11]. Because the dissection is more limited than with the conventional approach, nerve damage is likely to occur during stapling. It is possible to remove those staples at a repeat laparoscopy, as was done in our series. It is remarkable, however, that the neural pain in the two patients mentioned was very debilitating, probably more so than with the conventional technique. Reoperation at that point is therefore almost unavoidable.

An even more serious complication is postoperative obstruction. Whereas the early obstruction in group B was clearly due to a technical shortcoming, the two late obstructions in group A occurred because of adhesions over the entire surface of the prosthesis, possibly because of dehiscence of the peritoneal suture line. The adhesions with the polypropylene mesh were so intense, that they could not be dissected free, either laparoscopically or by open surgery. The bowel resection that was necessary raises serious doubts as to the acceptability of the transperitoneal laparoscopic approach with staples closure of the peritoneum.

We think that this severe complication could be avoided in two different ways. First, suturing rather than stapling of the peritoneum gives a much more satisfactory result. It is unlikely that the successful extracorporeal tie of a purse-string suture will be undone postoperatively. The bites taken by a needle are bigger and therefore more secure than a staple in an often torn peritoneum[12]. Second, the preperitoneal approach most certainly will avoid this severe drawback. The technical difficulty so far precluded its widespread application. Increasing laparoscopic experience and encouraging reports from different sources[13] prompted us and others to use this approach in our most recent cases. The addition of the self-expanding Nitinol mechanism offers a remarkable improvement in the positioning of the prosthesis in the restricted preperitoneal space. Curling of the mesh, which in our hands is a real problem[14] in this approach, is virtually impossible with the Nitinol support.

This study seems to indicate that the transperitoneal laparoscopic placement of a stapled preperitoneal prosthesis carries a considerable long-term morbidity. This morbidity can be prevented by reducing the number of staples, which is made possible by reinforcing the prosthesis and stapling it in only one spot. Problems of long-term adhesion formation can perhaps be prevented by using a softer mesh[15], by the meticulous suture closure of the peritoneum and, ideally, by a strictly preperitoneal approach.

More and more long-term clinical studies will give us the answers to the questions about which approach to use[4] and which prosthesis to choose.

References

1. Arregui ME, Davis CJ, Yucel O, Nagan R. Laparoscopic mesh repair of inguinal hernia using a preperitoneal approach. *Surg Laparosc Endosc* 1992; **2**: 53–8.
2. Hawasli A. Laparoscopic inguinal herniorrhaphy: the mushroom repair. *Surg Laparosc Endosc* 1992; **2**: 111–16.
3. Seid A, Deutsch H, Jacobson A. Laparoscopic herniorrhaphy. *Surg Laparosc Endosc* 1992;**2**: 59–60.
4. Colver RM. Laparoscopy: basic technique, instrumentation and complications. *Surg Laparosc Endosc* 1992; **2**: 35–40.
5. Lichtenstein IL, Shulman AJ, Amid PK, *et al.* The tension-free hernioplasty. *Am J Surg* 1989; **117**: 188–93.
6. Rives J, Lardennois B, Flament JB, Convers G. La Pièce en tulle de dacron, traitement de choix des hernies de l'aine de l'adulte. A propos de 183 cas. *Chirurgie* 1973; **99**: 564–75.
7. Stoppa RE, Rives JL, Warlaumont CR. The use of Dacron in the repair of hernia of the groin. *Surg Clin north Am* 1984; **64**: 269–85.

8. Nyhus LM, Pollak R, Bombeck TC, Donahue PE. The preperitoneal approach and prosthetic buttress repair for recurrent hernia. *Ann Surg* 1988; **208**: 733–7.

9. Rignault DP. Properitoneal prosthetic inguinal hernioplasty through a Pfannenstiel approach. *Surg Gynecol Obstet* 1984; **158**: 181–9.

10. Himpens JM. Laparoscopic hernioplasty using a self-expandable (umbrella-like) prosthetic patch. *Surg Laparosc Endosc* 1992; **2**: 312–16.

11. Madden JL. Indirect inguinal hernia – anatomic method of repair. In: Maddan JL, ed. *Atlas of Technics in Surgery*, vol 1. New York: Appleton-Century-Crofts, 1958; 68.

12. Toy FK, Smoot RT. Toy–Smoot laparoscopic hernioplasty. *Surg Laparosc Endosc* 1991; **1**: 151–5.

13. McKernan JB, Laws HL. Laparoscopic repair of inguinal hernias using a totally extraperitoneal prosthetic approach. *Surg Endosc* 1993; **7**: 26–8.

14. Burkel WE, Kahn RM. Biocompatibility of prosthetic grafts. In: Stanley JC, ed. *Biologic and Synthetic Vascular prostheses*. New York: Grune and Stratton, 1982: 221–7.

15. Alexander JM, Dupin PM, Levard M, Billevaud T. Cure des hernies de l'aine par prothèse de mersilene 'non fendue'. Intérêt de la pariétalisation du cordon et de la ligature des vaisseaux épigastriques. *Pressé Méd* 1984; **13**: 161–3.

77

Techniques and Safety Issues With Gasless Laparoscopy

W STEVE EUBANKS, LUCIAN NEWMAN Jr III AND GEORGE W LUCAS

Laparoscopic herniorrhaphy is currently a topic of much controversy and debate. Minimally invasive techniques are being used by many surgeons across the USA and around the world for the treatment of groin hernias. The debate over the proper utilization of laparoscopy in the treatment of hernia defects centres around several issues. One of these concerns is related to the need for general anaesthesia during the performance of laparoscopic procedures. Many surgeons feel that the repair of the groin hernia is a procedure that should routinely be done with local or regional anaesthesia. Another area of criticism of laparoscopic hernia repair relates to the complications inherent to laparoscopy. Documented complications of laparoscopy include diminished cardiac output[1–7], pulmonary changes including increased peak respiratory pressures[1,7–12] and injuries related to trocar insertion[11,13,14].

This study using gasless laparoscopy addresses some of the criticisms of laparoscopic hernia repair. The gasless approach eliminates the need for pneumoperitoneum and therefore eliminates the cardiovascular and pulmonary complications which may be encountered during the use of pneumoperitoneum. The elimination of the pneumoperitoneum also relieves the surgeon of the necessity of performing this procedure under general anaesthesia.

The study

Under Institutional Review Board (IRB) approval, the study of gasless laparoscopic techniques was undertaken at Georgia Baptist Medical Center in January 1993. Patients undergoing laparoscopic herniorrhaphy by the authors were offered the opportunity to enroll in this study. Each patient was given a detailed explanation of the risks and benefits associated with this procedure, and an IRB approved consent form was signed by all patients choosing to enter. The procedures were performed under general anaesthesia (except for one) utilizing the Laparolift™ and Laparofan™ devices by Origin Medsystems (Menlo Park, California). This mechanical abdominal wall retracting device was developed specifically for use with laparoscopic surgery. The device consists of a hydraulic arm, which may be mounted to the side of the operating table (Figure 77.1), and contains a telescoping arm that extends over the patient's abdomen. The Laparofan is the device that may be inserted through an umbilical incision, the fan blades spread and then connected to the Laparolift arm (Figure 77.2). The hydraulic arm is then used to elevate the abdominal wall to provide a space within the peritoneal cavity for the performance of laparoscopic operations.

The study was designed to evaluate the feasibility of performance of laparoscopic herniorrhaphy using the Laparolift and Laparofan. Complications related to the use of the gasless technique and to the performance of laparoscopic herniorrhaphy were assessed in each patient.

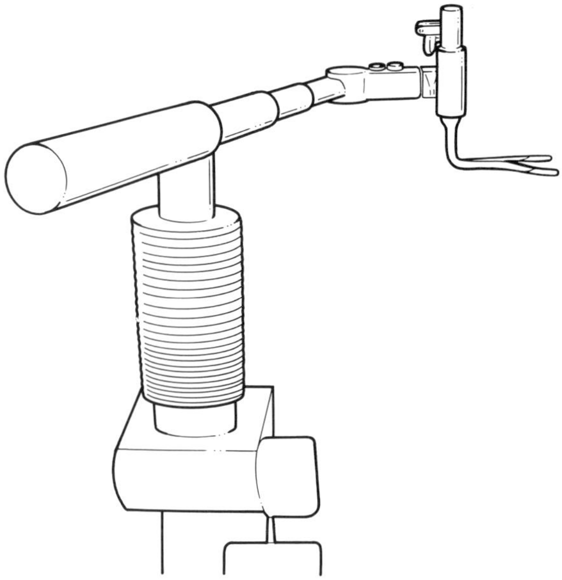

Figure 77.1: The Laparolift device (courtesy of Origin Medsystems).

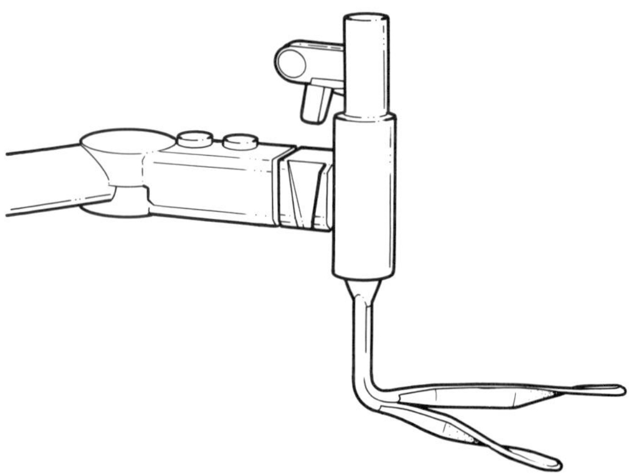

Figure 77.2: The Laparofan device (courtesy of Origin Medsystems).

Operative technique

All patients in this study underwent a transabdominal preperitoneal (TAPP) laparoscopic hernia repair[15]. This repair is performed by grasping the medial umbilical ligament from the contralateral side and retracting it in a medial direction. The endoshears are used to create a peritoneal flap. The peritoneal flap is then bluntly swept from the anterior abdominal wall. The properitoneal fat is bluntly dissected off the abdominal wall structures to which the mesh will be secured. These structures include Cooper's ligament, the iliopubic tract and the transversus abdominis aponeurotic arch. Also identified are the epigastric vessels and the region containing the spermatic cord, vas deferens and iliac vessels.

A 7.5 × 12.5 cm (3 × 5 inch) piece of Surgi-Pro (US Surgical, Norwalk, Connecticut) mesh is then inserted into the abdominal cavity and secured to Cooper's ligament, the iliopubic tract and the transversus abdominis aponeurotic arch using a hernia stapler. The lateral attachments of the mesh are the superior edge of the iliopubic tract and the lateral extension of the transversus abdominis aponeurotic arch. Stapling is not performed below the iliopubic tract lateral to the internal inguinal ring, to prevent injury to the lateral femoral cutaneous nerve[16]. The mesh is covered with the already dissected peritoneal flap and the flap is approximated to the cut edge of peritoneum using the hernia stapler.

The laparoscopic instruments are removed from the abdominal cavity and the lateral trocars are removed from the abdominal wall. The removal of these trocars is performed under direct vision of the camera. All port sites greater than 5 mm are closed at the fascia level in order to prevent an abdominal wall hernia, a Richter's hernia or the entrapment of omentum in the cannula site which might lead to subsequent small bowel obstruction.

Several techniques for closing these lateral port sites have been used by these authors. Initially, we and others used a simple suture closure of the anterior fascia. This technique allowed an opening in the peritoneum, posterior fascia and muscle to remain, and repeat laparoscopy on several patients who had undergone other procedures revealed entrapped omentum in these wounds. Subsequently, a second technique was employed which involved placing a Keith needle inside the skin wound but through all other layers of the anterior abdominal wall, grasping the needle inside the abdominal cavity and passing the needle back through the abdominal wall structures on the other side of the defect. The suture could then be tied within the skin wound, leaving the knot buried. This technique was somewhat slow and cumbersome and therefore a third technique was developed.

The current practice of the authors is to close the port site using a Grice needle (Ideas for Medicine, Clearwater, Florida) which facilitates suture closure of the abdominal wall wound. The closure of cannula sites is greatly facilitated by the gasless technique because the peritoneal space is maintained and there is no problem of ongoing loss of pneumoperitoneum. Two instruments or the laparoscope and an instrument may be placed through the umbilical wound simultaneously, thereby facilitating wound closure. This closure is performed under direct vision and thereby diminishes the possibility of bowel entrapment in suture closure. Finally, the umbilical trocar and Laparofan are removed and the umbilical wound is closed with the previously placed fascial sutures. All skin wounds are closed with subcuticular sutures.

Results

Between 1 January 1993 and 15 May 1993, 40 patients were operated on using gasless laparoscopy. These procedures included laparoscopic herniorrhaphy, laparoscopic cholecystectomy, laparoscopic tubal ligation and laparoscopic laser ablation of endometriosis. In all, 75% of the attempted gasless laparoscopic procedures were completed successfully. The remaining 25% of these procedures were converted to pneumoperitoneum in which all were successfully completed with laparoscopic techniques.

The primary reason for conversion to pneumoperitoneum from gasless laparoscopy was difficulty with visualization secondary to intestinal distension and problems with bowel retraction. The second most common reason for conversion to pneumoperitoneum was an endomorphic body habitus, leading to difficulty with retraction of the lower abdominal wall.

A total of 18 patients underwent attempted gasless laparoscopic hernia repair: 13 (72%) were completed successfully; five procedures were converted to pneumoperitoneum cases because visualization was less than optimal.

During the same period, 16 patients underwent attempted gasless laparoscopy for gynaecological procedures. Of these, 14 (87.5%) were successfully completed using the Laparolift.

Six patients underwent laparoscopic cholecystectomy using the Laparolift for abdominal wall retraction. Three of them (50%) required conversion to pneumoperitoneum because of inadequate exposure of the right upper quadrant. The remaining three patients received a laparoscopic cholecystectomy employing gasless techniques.

The operative time for gasless laparoscopic procedures was identical to those in which pneumoperitoneum was used. There were no complications in any of these 40 cases related to the use of a gasless technique. One patient in this series sustained a severe complication of a Richter's hernia at the site of a 12 mm lateral cannula. The surgeon in this case varied from the normal practice of closing the lateral port sites and the patient subsequently presented on the third postoperative day with signs and symptoms of a small bowel obstruction. The patient underwent an exploratory laparotomy and was found to have a Richter's hernia at the lateral port site with non-viable bowel entrapped in the defect. This finding necessitated a small bowel resection with a primary anastomosis.

The final patient entered in this study of laparoscopic hernia repair underwent a successful laparoscopic herniorrhaphy under epidural anaesthesia. The procedure was performed uneventfully and the patient tolerated all aspects of the operation and convalescence without problems.

Conclusions

Laparoscopic procedures without pneumoperitoneum have been shown to be technically feasible. A device such as the Laparolift and Laparofan greatly facilitates the ability of the surgeon to perform gasless laparoscopy. The devices previously proposed by Japanese investigators[17,18] have received little support in the USA. The gasless approach to laparoscopy provides adequate exposure in the majority of the patients but is currently not optimal in all patients. The exposure provided by the abdominal wall retraction device generally approaches but does not equal that encountered with pneumoperitoneum. There is less 'ballooning' of the hernia defect when gasless techniques are used. The lack of distension of the hernia sac makes identification of the borders of the hernia and the surrounding structures slightly more difficult. These problems may make gasless laparoscopic hernia repair quite difficult for the novice laparoscopic herniotomist.

Summary

The gasless approach to laparoscopic hernia repair is technically feasible and warrants further investigation. The development of new technology in this field with modifications of existing devices is likely to provide increased visualization and to facilitate the use of the gasless approach. The gasless approach to laparoscopy eliminates the potential for complications directly attributable to pneumoperitoneum. These techniques provide an alternative to current laparoscopic hernia repair procedures in patients who are unable to withstand general anaesthesia, in patients who refuse general anaesthesia and for surgeons who feel that general anaesthesia is inappropriate for the repair of hernia defects. The gasless approach also provides a markedly improved means of closing lateral port sites. The subject of cannula site closure is likely to become an increasingly important topic, as a larger number of complications related to the lack of closure of port sites is reported in the literature.

The authors recommend that further investigation of gasless laparoscopic techniques be performed by experienced laparoscopic herniotomists. All investigators should proceed with these studies under IRB (or similar) approval. A low threshold for conversion to pneumoperitoneum is advised in the event that optimal visualization is not provided.

References

1. Hashimoto S, Munakata Y, Hashikusa Y, *et al.* Cardiovascular and respiratory effects of intraperitoneal insufflation with carbon dioxide at laparoscopic cholecystectomy. [Abstract] *Surg Laparosc Endosc* 1992; **2**: 174.
2. Ivankovich AD, Albrecht RF, Zahed B, *et al.* Cardiovascular collapse during gynecological laparoscopy. *Ill Med J* 194; **145**: 58–61, 77
3. Kelman GR, Swapp GH, Smith I, *et al.* Cardiac output and arterial blood gas tension during laparoscopy. *Br J Anaesth* 1972; **44**: 1155–62.
4. Liu SY, Leighton T, David I, *et al.* Prospective analysis of cardiopulmonary responses to laparoscopic cholecystectomy. *J Laparoendsoc Surg* 1991; **1**: 241–6.
5. Morison DH, Riggs JRA. Cardiovascular collapse in laparoscopy. *Can Med Assoc J* 1974; **11**: 433–7.
6. Motew M, Ivankovich AD, Bieniarz J, *et al.* Cardiovascular effects and acid–base and blood gas changes during laparoscopy. *Am J Gynecol* 1973; **115**: 1002–12.
7. Wittgen CH, Andros CH, Fitzgerald SD, *et al.* Analysis of hemodynamic and ventilatory effects of laparoscopic cholecystectomy. *Arch Surg* 1991; **126**: 997–1001.
8. Barnett RB, Clement GS, Prizin GS, *et al.* Pulmonary changes after laparoscopic cholecystectomy. *Surg Laparosc Endosc* 1992; **2**: 125–7.
9. Holzman H, Sharp K, Richards W. Hypercarbia during carbon dioxide gas insufflation for therapeutic laparoscopy: a note of caution. *Surg Laparosc Endosc* 1992; **2**: 11–14.
10. Newman L, Luke JP, Ruben DM, Eubanks S. Laparoscopic herniorrhaphy without pneumoperitoneum. *Surg Laparosc* 1993; **3**: 213–15.
11. Baadsgaard SE, Bille S, Egeblad K. Major vascular injury during gynecologic laparoscopy. Report of a case and reviews of published cases. *Acta Obstet Gynecol Scand* 1989; **68**: 283–5.
12. Root B, Levy M, Pollack S. Gas embolism death after laparoscopy delayed by trapping in the portal circulation. *Anesth Analg* 1978; **7**: 232–7.
13. Mintz M. Risks and prophylaxis in laparoscopy: a survey of 100,000 cases. *J Reprod Med* 1977; **18**: 269–72.
14. Vilardell F, Seres I, Marti-Vicente A. Complications of peritoneoscopy: a survey of 1,455 examinations. *Gastrointest Edosc* 1968; **14**: 178–80.
15. Newman L, Eubanks WS, Mason E, Duncan T. Is laparoscopic herniorrhaphy an effective alternative to open hernia repair? *J Laparoendosc Surg* 1993; **3**: 121–8.
16. Eubanks S, Newman L, Goehring L, *et al.* Meralgia paresthetica: a complication of laparoscopic herniorrhaphy. *Surg Laparosc Endosc* 1993; **3**: 381–5.
17. Kitano S, Tomikawa M, Iso Y, *et al.* A safe and simple method to maintain a clear field of vision during laparoscopic cholecystectomy. *Surg Endosc* 1991; **6**: 197–8.
18. Nagai H, Inaba T, Kemia S, *et al.* A new method of laparoscopic cholecystectomy. An abdominal mass lifting technique without pneumoperitoneum. [Abstract] *Surg Laparosc Endosc* 1991; **1**: 126.

Poulin EC, Mamazza J, Breton G, *et al.* Evaluation of pulmonary function in laparoscopic cholecystectomy. *Surg Laparosc Endosc* 1992; **2**: 292–3.

78

Advances in Extraperitoneal Dissection and Hernia Repair

MACIEJ J KIETURAKIS

Today, a common inguinal hernia rarely contributes to mortality among the members of industrialized countries. Routine physical examinations and patient awareness will almost always lead to prompt diagnosis and treatment of inguinal hernia. The infection rate in elective hernia operations is about 1%, haematomas less than 10%, recurrence rate of 1–10% for indirect and up to 28% for direct hernia repair[1]. Neuropathies involving ilioinguinal and genitofemoral nerves are not that uncommon (and mild forms are probably much more frequent than generally reported in the medical literature). There are a number of commonly accepted herniorrhaphies used by surgeons with highly variable degrees of success. Usually the excellent operative results obtained by the original authors cannot be reproduced by other surgeons[2]. Discrepancies over the reported results of a particular technique imply that the definition of successful hernia repair remains controversial. The continuing proliferation of different techniques, and frequent arguments in the medical literature over the optimal approach, indicates that no one technique is vastly superior to any other.

There is one common disadvantage to all these traditional open techniques: three to six or more weeks of postoperative recovery time is required before patients are allowed to return to regular physical activity. Open techniques that incorporate mesh into the repair of the hernia defect may decrease the recurrence rate and postoperative discomfort, but still carry the same disadvantages of a prolonged total recovery period. Enthusiasts of newer anterior approaches (eg Lichtenstein repair) contend that patients may return to work days after the procedure. This apparent advantage is tempered by the fact that every 10 cm skin and adipose tissue incision (not mentioning fascias and ligaments) still needs about three weeks of healing to achieve just 15% of normal tissue strength, which may be considered relatively secure adhesion[3].

It seems that the most natural way to shorten the healing period and accelerate recovery is to reduce the size of the incision and to avoid the temptation to rearrange the anatomy surrounding the hernia defect. This alternative may be provided by laparoscopic techniques. Such procedures usually leave three very small wounds, each up to 10 mm in diameter. The healing of such small incisions or 'puncture' wounds is not impaired by mechanical disruptive forces created by the patient's musculature during strenuous physical activity. Also, the mesh patch may be spread at the inner surface of the inguinal floor, creating a mechanically appealing arrangement. The intra-abdominal forces generated during physical activity will press the mesh patch against the surface of the abdominal wall neighbouring the hernia defect, minimizing the chance of recurrent herniation during the mesh 'healing in' period.

Over the last few years a number of laparoscopic techniques have been added to the armamentarium of inguinal herniorrhaphies[4]. Intraperitoneal onlay mesh repair (IPOM) and transabdominal preperitoneal repair (TAPP) both utilize the principles of conventional laparoscopy. Trauma to the abdominal wall is minimal, the mechanics of the repair are appealing, postoperative pain presents a fraction of that observed after any anterior repair, and recovery takes just several days. Unfortunately, both repairs violate the integrity of the peritoneal cavity. The IPOM technique introduces the mesh patch intraperitoneally, which remains in contact with intra-abdominal viscera. The TAPP technique leaves a peritoneal suture line which has the potential to form adhesions and other related complications. There is a risk of suture line dehiscence[5] which results in inadvertent exposure of the mesh patch inside the peritoneal cavity.

Totally extraperitoneal hernia repair (laparoscopic extraperitoneal; LEP) with the use of the laparoscope (popularized in the USA by Barry McKernan) constitutes another route[6]. The currently accepted technique involves insertion of the trocar through an infraumbilical incision posterior to the rectus muscle. An operative laparoscope is then introduced and further dissection is accomplished with the use of a blunt cannula. Next, the accessory trocars are introduced and the pertinent anatomy is identified with the help of standard laparoscopic instrumentation. The sac is isolated from surrounding structures, inverted or ligated and then the inguinal floor is covered with a mesh prosthesis. Staples are usually employed to secure the mesh position, anchoring it to Cooper's ligament, the transversus abdominis arch and fascia.

The extraperitoneal technique has several advantages over the transabdominal approaches. Most importantly, it does not violate the integrity of the peritoneal cavity, decreasing the likelihood of adhesion formation and related complications. The pneumoextraperitoneum is limited to the infraumbilical region, allowing spinal or epidural block to be used as anaesthetic alternatives. This procedure also avoids complications that may occur during routine laparoscopy due to increased intra-abdominal insufflation pressures.

The major disadvantage of laparoscopic extraperitoneal inguinal hernia repair is a somewhat cumbersome and time-consuming surgical dissection in the extraperitoneum, which strongly limits the attractiveness of this procedure[4,7]. A number of arguments have been presented in the surgical literature to increase the popularity of the current laparoscopic extraperitoneal hernia repair[6–8]. The technique presented here continues to improve upon the current approach and may provide a more compelling argument for surgeons to embrace the laparoscopic extraperitoneal herniorrhaphy procedure.

Principle

The main focus of this study was to evaluate a balloon dissecting instrument, which was designed to facilitate extraperitoneal dissection and reduce the operating time of laparoscopic inguinal herniorrhaphy.

Materials

The balloon dissector (General Surgical Innovations Inc., Portola Valley, CA) is a device designed to facilitate dissection for laparoscopic extraperitoneal procedures (Figure 78.1). It dissects a predetermined-shaped cavity so that accessory trocars can be introduced safely and the hernia repair can be completed promptly. The balloon dissector also incorporates the primary 10/11 mm trocar through which the 10 mm, 30° laparoscope is placed. The polypropylene mesh patch (Prolene, Ethicon Inc., Somerville, NJ) is a loosely woven filament network which is supple and adheres well to soft tissues. It allows for rapid cellular ingrowth and stimulates a strong fibroblastic reaction in tissue. To secure the mesh patch in place, the hernia stapler (EMS stapler, Ethicon Inc.) is used. It produces strong box-shaped staples with adequate depth of tissue penetration. Secondary trocars (10/11 mm, stylet tip, Ethicon Inc.) penetrate the abdominal wall relatively easily. Their diameter will accommodate the size of the hernia stapler and the rolled mesh patch, and will allow for removal of large hernia sacs or cord lipomas. A standard CO_2 insufflator is set to 8 mmHg of insufflation pressure and 'high flow' mode after initial balloon dissection has been accomplished.

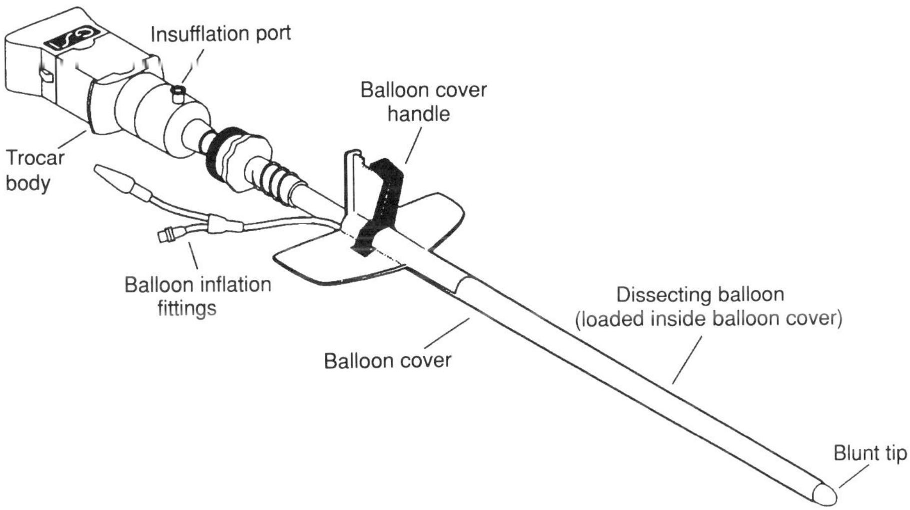

Figure 78.1: Extraperitoneal balloon dissector (General Surgical Innovations Inc., Portola Valley, CA).

Methods

Preparation

The skin is shaved from the periumbilical area to the mons pubis. The preparation is done with iodine soap and solution. On larger hernias the perineum is prepared as well because manipulation of the scrotum may be necessary to reduce the hernia contents. Patients are voided on call to the operating room so that they are not catheterized later. It appears that some distension of the urinary bladder does not compromise the exposure of the inguinal floor. Besides, no sharp instruments (Verres needle or umbilical trocar) are introduced into the abdominal cavity, which obviates the risk of bladder perforation. Anti-embolic prophylaxis (sequential compression boots and medication) are not routinely used because the procedure is performed under low insufflation pressures and limited pneumoextraperitoneum. A single dose of intravenous antibiotic solution is given preoperatively.

Anaesthesia

In all cases but one, a general anaesthesia with tracheal intubation was used. One patient with a large bilateral inguinal hernia was operated on in epidural block; the operation was uneventful.

Laparoscopy equipment

We usually use two video monitors for bilateral hernias. They are positioned at the patient's feet, each one within the surgeon's (or assistant's) view, with the hernia site in between. For unilateral hernias the video monitor is positioned on the hernia side. The 10 mm, 30° laparoscope is used. The 30° wide-angle scope is often very useful, particularly during mesh placement.

Technique

The patient is placed on the operating table in the supine position. A small infraumbilical (1 cm) incision is made and blunt dissection is used to visualize the fascia. The most consistent approach to enter the correct anatomical layer is to make the incision in the fascia somewhat lateral to the midline, directly over the medial border of the rectus muscle belly on the side of the hernia. This technique distances the dissector insertion site slightly from the area where the abdominal layers are fused. The rectus muscle is then retracted laterally, which exposes the posterior rectus sheath. The balloon dissector is introduced into the incision (Figure 78.2).

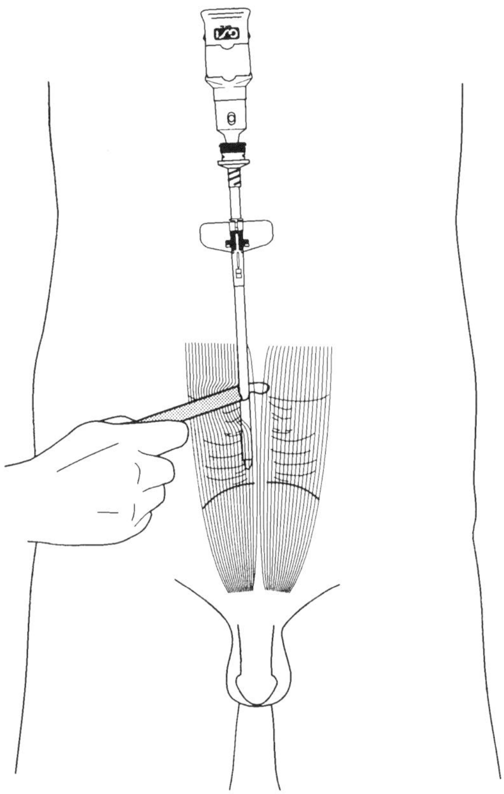

Figure 78.2: Insertion of the balloon dissector.

The dissector is advanced bluntly in between the rectus muscle and the posterior rectus sheath along the midline toward and eventually below the symphysis pubis (Figure 78.3a). The dissector probe meets minimal tissue resistance. By removing the external sheath of the dissector probe, the balloon is deposited into the desired space. Instillation of the recommended volume of saline solution (typically 500 ml) allows the balloon to inflate within the extraperitoneal region (Figure 78.3b). After dissection is completed, the balloon is deflated and removed. Next, the primary 10/11 mm trocar, which constitutes the handle of the device, is advanced over the guide rod which maintains unobstructed entry into the newly created extraperitoneal space (Figure 78.3c). The guide rod is removed and the CO_2 line is connected to the primary trocar to insufflate the extraperitoneal space (Figure 78.3d).

The laparoscope is introduced. Two additional trocars are inserted; one midline suprapubic and another one in between the two previous trocars. If the surgeon chooses to arrange the accessory trocars in this manner, there is only a short distance between the suprapubic trocar insertion site and the area of surgical dissection. However, this arrangement allows comfortable access to bilateral hernias, minimizes the risk of injury to the epigastric vessels and is cosmetically superior. Standard surgical dissection is then used to complete visualization of all the anatomical landmarks and structures necessary to achieve safe and secure repair of the hernia defect. The lateral segment of Cooper's ligament is visualized; care is taken not to injure the small, crossing pubic branch of the obturator artery.

Direct hernia defects are then reduced. The dissection of the internal ring is started laterally, down to the surface of the transversus abdominis fascia. The 'funnel' of the indirect sac is then identified and separated from the spermatic vessels and duct. The sac is stabilized with graspers. The spermatic duct and vessels are displaced by manipulating the attenuated transversalis fascia, which minimizes the possibility of injury to these structures. Smaller sacs are inverted, larger sacs are ligated at the neck and divided. The distal sac is allowed to retract into the inguinal canal. A

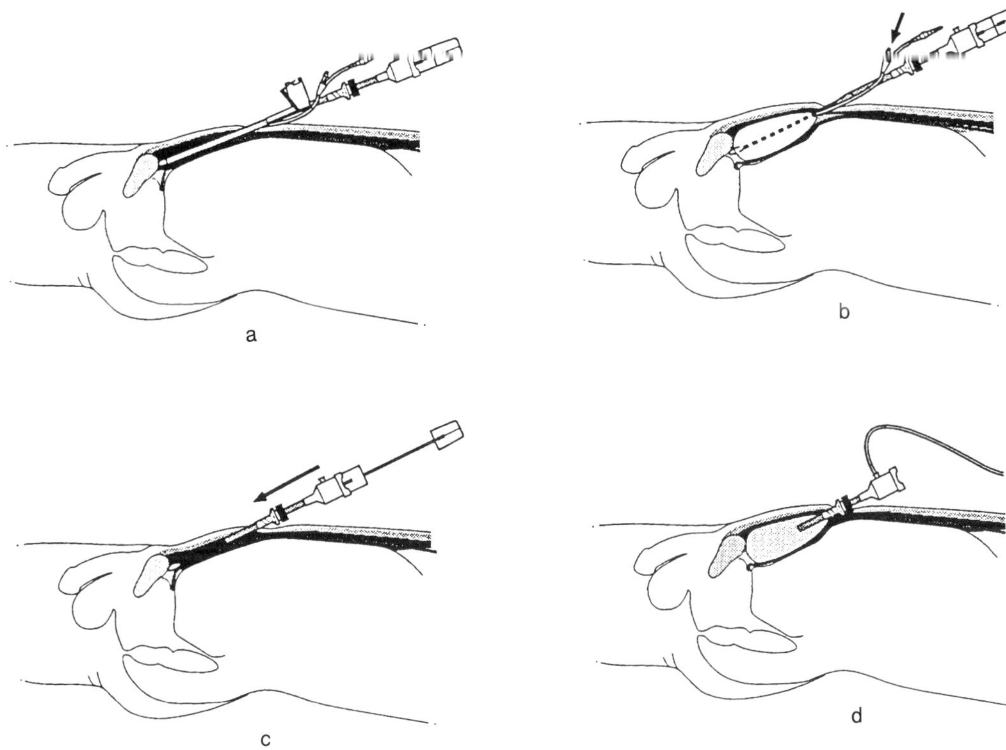

Figure 78.3: (a) The balloon dissector (rigid before balloon is exposed) is inserted in between the rectus muscle and transversalis fascia, and is advanced to the level of the symphysis pubis. (b) The dissecting balloon is exposed and inflated (using physiological saline) within the extraperitoneal region. The balloon is attached to guide rod during inflation. (c) The dissecting balloon is removed. The integral trocar is advanced over the guide rod into the dissected extraperitoneal space. (d) The guide rod is removed and the extraperitoneal space insufflated.

7.5 × 12.5 cm sheet of Prolene mesh patch is introduced into the extraperitoneal space and then secured with staples to Cooper's ligament, the transversus abdominis aponeurosis arch and muscle and the rectus muscle. It is very important not to anchor any staples over, lateral to and posterior to the iliac vessels or anywhere that the surgeon's hand placed over the abdomen cannot meet the head of the hernia stapler. Inadvertent staple placement in this region may result in femoral, genitofemoral or lateral cutaneous femoris neuropathy. Next 100 ml of 0.15% bupivacaine (Marcaine) solution is injected into the extraperitoneal space and the CO_2 is released. The inner surface of the suprapubic incision is covered automatically by the mesh used for the repair. The infraumbilical incision is secured anatomically by the intact posterior rectus sheath. These incisions are approximated only at skin level. The middle incision may not be protected by the posterior rectus sheath owing to an inconsistent level of the arcuate line; therefore a single Vicryl 0 stitch is used to close the fascia.

Mechanics of balloon dissection

The balloon used for dissection is made of relatively non-elastomeric material, an important feature for predictable and consistent dissection. The balloon is distended with saline solution to a predetermined volume. At this stage, the balloon assumes its final shape, which has been calculated

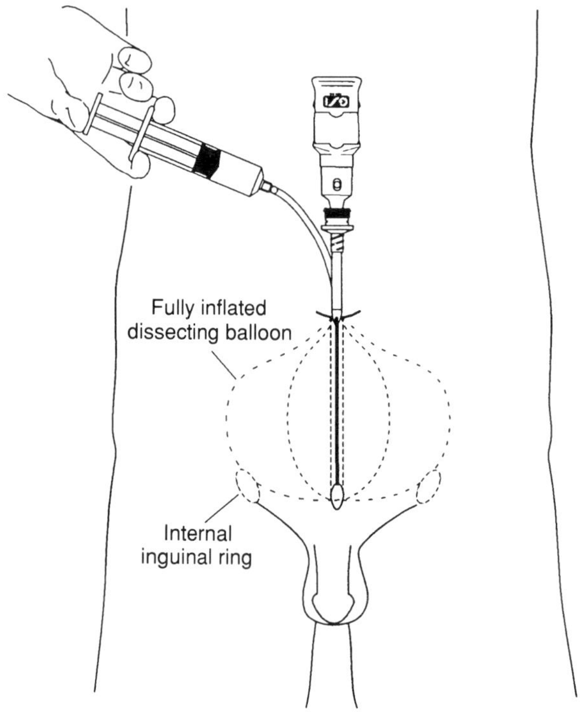

Figure 78.4: Outline of the inflated dissecting balloon within the extraperitoneal region.

to provide a comfortable working space to accommodate the repair procedure without extraneous dissection (Figure 78.4). Because the balloon is attached to a central rod, it has little tendency to migrate from the desired location during the inflation process. The non-compressible character of saline used for balloon inflation gives the operating surgeon precise knowledge of the dissected volume.

Accidental leakage or rupture of the balloon is of no consequence because the saline volume delivered to the balloon is equal to the volume of the dissected space. The use of air or CO_2 is not recommended for inflation because, by its compressible nature, the volume of a gas infused does not correspond to the size of the dissected cavity and the surgeon cannot control the size of cavity that will be produced. More importantly, if gas is used as the medium for balloon expansion, the inadvertent rupture of the balloon would result in a sudden egress of compressed gas which could lead to vascular gas emboli. Considering the pressure difference between the lumen of a dissecting balloon (up to as much as 300 mmHg) and the venous pressure (0–5 mmHg) the potential danger of this complication cannot be neglected[9].

During inflation, a non-elastomeric balloon fills out to a predefined shape and volume, and bluntly propagates tissue dissection along the natural cleavage plane (between the rectus muscle and the transversalis fascia). Conversely, use of an elastomeric material (eg latex) for this dissection application will allow the balloon membrane to follow a (potentially undesirable) path of minimal resistance and continues to do so as long as inflation continues. This concept has been previously documented in other anatomical locations by Fogarty *et al.*[10]. Our initial use of an elastomeric material for extraperitoneal dissection was abandoned early in the series. We found that an elastomeric membrane could inflate uncontrollably in the direction of least resistance, resulting in balloon migration and the creation of a space in an undesired location.

The balloon dissector (GSI, Portola Valley, CA) facilitates dissection for laparoscopic extraperitoneal procedures (*see* Figure 78.2). It incorporates a trocar, guide rod, dissecting blunt probe and a balloon system. The probe resembles and behaves like a Hegar-type dilator. The probe is introduced via the infraumbilical incision directly posterior to the rectus muscle and is advanced to the symphysis pubis. During inflation, the non-elastomeric balloon unrolls sideways and exerts a perpendicular

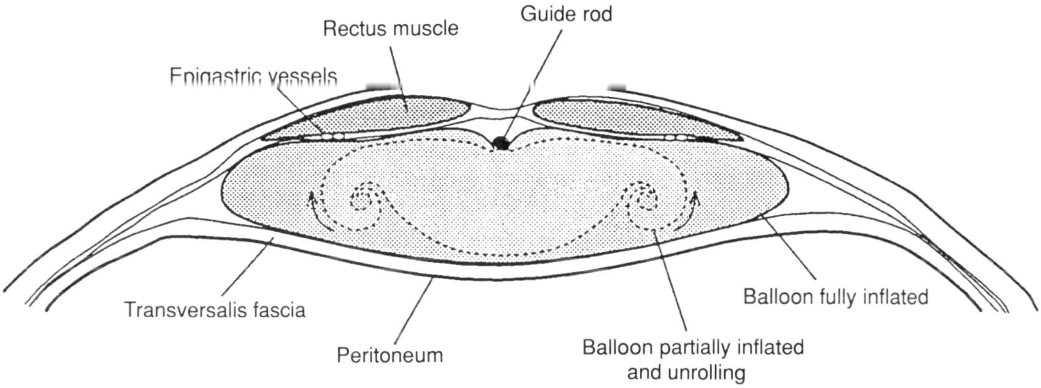

Figure 78.5: Cross-sectional view of the dissecting balloon partially and fully inflated within the extraperitoneal region.

force along the sagittal axis on the rectus muscle anteriorly, and peritoneum with transversalis fascia posteriorly. At the same time the balloon moves along the coronal plane, propagating a blunt tissue cleavage line in between the rectus muscle and transversalis fascia (Figure 78.5). The balloon in its compact phase is packed in such a way that, during the deployment phase, the wall of the balloon facing the rectus muscle and epigastric vessels will not slide against those structures but will simply roll over them. This minimizes the potential injury to the epigastric vessels. The non-elastomeric character of the balloon creates a very predictable size and shape of the extraperitoneal working space. The balloon's intraluminal pressure during the insufflation phase typically ranges from 50 to 100 mmHg. The final distension pressure is between 100 and 140 mmHg. The dissection process takes about 45 seconds and creates a practically bloodless working space large enough to accommodate standard laparoscopic instruments and mesh patches.

Results

A series of 60 patients with 80 hernias were studied. Most of the patients selected to the initial group had bilateral hernias because anticipated decreased morbidity resulting from laparoscopic repair would provide maximal benefits compared to a bilateral open procedure. A summary of the clinical series appears in Table 78.1.

There were no infections observed in any of the incisions. One patient early in this series with bilateral hernias developed an immediate right-sided recurrence, which was most likely due to shallow staple placement. The patient was treated with a standard Bassini procedure about three weeks after the initial operation. Two patients developed neuropathies within the region of the lateral cutaneous femoris nerves. One of them subsided spontaneously after two and a half weeks, the other one after ten days. Interestingly, both were women. One recent patient developed a neuropathy of one of the cutaneous nerves originating from the T11 or T12 intercostal nerves, which is subsiding at three weeks after the procedure. Two peritoneal tears occurred early in the series, which were related to the learning curve regarding establishing the optimal anatomical dissection plane. One patient was converted to a Stoppa operation and the other was repaired extraperitoneally after reapproximation of the peritoneum. One giant scrotal hernia was converted to an open procedure after it was determined that the benefits associated with the laparoscopic approach would be outweighed by the longer operating time.

Typical postoperative pain presented in the form of diffuse discomfort in the lower abdomen, which was very well tolerated with minimum doses of oral analgesics. Some patients did not take any pain medication at all. A small group took medication for up to one week. Two patients with neuropathies continued with pain medication throughout the duration of symptoms. Almost all

Table 78.1: A summary of the series

Number of patients	60 (54 men, 6 women)
Patients age	23–84 years (mean, 50)
Follow up	Up to 21 months (mean, 5.6)
Total number of hernias	80 (40 unilateral, 20 bilateral)
Type of hernia:	
Indirect	49
Direct	27
Scrotal	2
Sliding	1
Spigelian	1
Complications:	
Recurrence	1
Haematoma	2
Transient neuropathy	3
Urinary retention	1
Peritoneal tear	2
Infection	0
Orchitis	0

patients returned to work within several days, which was usually related to the amount of interest they had in resuming work.

Conclusions

Both the extraperitoneal (LEP) and transabdominal preperitoneal (TAPP) mesh patch repair have been performed in many medical centres and by a number of individual surgeons. Currently available results show an early recurrence rate of less than 1%, which compares favourably to open anterior or preperitoneal techniques. Long-term results will be forthcoming as follow-up time increases. Because the mechanics of preperitoneal laparoscopic mesh patch repair are virtually identical to open preperitoneal repair performed by Stoppa[11], Rignault[12] and Nyhus[13], one could expect the overall recurrence rate to be within the range of 1–2%. Initial findings in this series parallel those above.

Our experience with 80 herniorrhaphies has confirmed the initial assumptions. Balloon dissection is safe. The non-elastomeric character of the balloon and the guide rod minimize undesired migration of the balloon during the dissection process. The separation of the extraperitoneal space is so anatomical that in this series there were no cases of bleeding related to balloon dissection. Balloon dissection is very reliable. It has consistently produced a well-defined, predictable size and shape working space in approximately one minute of dissection time. Additionally, dissection does not require specialized skills and the hernia repair may be carried out in a standardized fashion using familiar laparoscopic instruments. Extraperitoneal hernia repair provides the advantages of laparoscopy and time-tested open preperitoneal procedures. Extraperitoneal balloon dissection minimizes the time required to create an extraperitoneal working space. The balloon dissector, because of its safety and simplicity, may help bring extraperitoneal hernia repair to the circle of procedures widely accepted by the surgical community.

References

1. Lange Medical Publications. *Current Surgical Diagnosis and Treatment*. Los Altos, CA: Lange Medical Publications, 1988.

2. Wantz GE. Complications of inguinal hernia repair. *Surg Clin North Am* 1984; **64**: 287–98.

3. Levenson SM, Geever EF, Crowley LV, Oates JF, Berard CW, Rosen H. The healing of rat skin wounds. *Ann Surg* 1965; **161**: 293.

4. Filipi CJ, Fitzgibbons RJ, Salerno GM, Hart RO. Laparoscopic herniorrhaphy. *Surg Clin North Am* 1992; **72**: 1109–24.

5. Wissing J, van Vroonhoven ThJMV, Schattenkerk ME, Veen HF, Ponsen RJG, Jeekel J. Fascia closure after midline laparotomy: results of a randomized trial. *B J Surg* 1987; **74**: 738–41.

6. McKernan JB: Laparoscopic preperitoneal prosthetic repair of inguinal hernias. *Surg Rounds* 1992; **15**: 597–610.

7. Dion Y-M, Morin J. Laparoscopic inguinal herniorrhaphy. *Can J Surg* 1992; **35**: 209–12.

8. Ferzli G, Massaad A, Albert P, Worth M. Endoscopic extraperitoneal herniorrhaphy vs conventional hernia repair: a comparative study. *Curr Surg* 1993; **50**: 291–4.

9. Greville AC, Clements EAF, Erwin DC, McMillan DL, Wellwood JMcK. Pulmonary air embolism during laparoscopic laser cholecystectomy. *Anaesthesia* 1991; **46**: 113–14.

10. Fogarty TJ, Chin A, Shoor PM, Blair GL, Zimmerman JJ. Adjunctive intraoperative arterial dilation. *Arch Surg* 1981; **116**: 1391–8.

11. Stoppa RE, Rives JL, Warlaumont CR, Palot JP, Verhaeghe PJ, Delattre JF. The use of Dacron in the repair of hernias of the groin. *Surg Clin North Am* 1984; **64**: 269–85.

12. Rignault DP. Properitoneal prosthetic inguinal hernioplasty through a Pfannensteil approach. *Surg Gynecol Obstet* 1986; **163**: 465–8.

13. Nyhus LM, Pollak R, Brombeck CT, *et al.* The preperitoneal approach and prosthetic buttress repair for recurrent hernia. *Ann Surg* 1988; **208**: 733–7.

79

Learning Laparoscopic Hernia Repair: Pitfalls and Complications among 178 Repairs

ALBERIC GTW FIENNES AND ROBERT S TAYLOR

Laparoscopic inguinal hernia repair has been reported since about 1990 and we have undertaken the procedure since May 1991 (RST) and December 1991 (AGF). Over this period our personal development of the procedure has been an abbreviated recapitulation of the evolution reflected throughout this volume (Tables 79.1 and 79.2).

Patients and techniques

A first few plug repairs yielded the same poor results as in other hands, and we moved to transperitoneal placement of a modest sized (4.5 × 7.5 cm) expanded PTFE patch sutured to Cooper's ligament and to the muscle around the defect by continuous 3/0 monofilament polypropylene, the ends of which were secured by haemostatic clips. The overlying peritoneum was reflected medially, as the cover of a book, and subsequently closed over the patch by the same suture technique.

With increasing awareness of the work of Stoppa[1] and of others advocating wide overlap with the tissues around the defect, we progressed to the largest PTFE patch available to us (6 × 11 cm). At about this time we had access to prototype staplers, which were used in a few cases to fix the patch.

In September 1991 one of us (AGF) learned of the pioneering work of Dulucq[2], who had developed the totally extraperitoneal approach, and we were privileged to learn the technique from him in February 1992.

Table 79.1: Evolution of technique over time

Suture mesh plug (6 only, 1 of the 6 recurred)
Sutured transperitoneal patch (PTFE, 4.5 × 7.5 cm)
Dulucq extraperitoneal repair (Prolene mesh)
Modified Dulucq procedure
Selective trans-/extraperitoneal preperitoneal patch

Table 79.2: Evolution of patch fixation over time

Continuous 2/0 Prolene suture
Interrupted Vicryl sutures:
many
two
No fixation: large patch
Stapling: various types
Selective fixation

Dulucq originally advocated fixation of a moderate sized polypropylene patch by means of two interrupted braided sutures, placed one on the ligament of Cooper and one on the psoas lateral to the testicular vessels. We duly used his technique with our existing PTFE patch (6 × 11 cm). However, these patches became difficult to obtain, concerns arose as to the adequacy of their size and light reflection in the confined space was a problem. The availability of a 7.5 × 12.5 cm braided polypropylene patch (US Surgical), and subsequently of larger sheets of the same material, led us to enlarge the patch (aiming for 11 × 15 cm) in accordance with the theory of Stoppa. We have previously[3] argued that adequate patch size obviates patch fixation by this approach, but more recently we have adopted a selective approach to patch size and fixation. Furthermore, a Dulucq approach is not suitable for every hernia, just as not every patient or hernia is suitable for laparoscopic surgery.

At the time of writing we have completed over 250 hernia repairs, but the present review relates to the initial 178 repairs prior to April 1993 and the techniques discussed relate to this initial cohort (see Tables 79.1 and 79.2). The follow up is short (1–23 months) and we concentrate here on perioperative complications. We have tried to learn from the complications and pitfalls to be presented and our current protocol is presented toward the end of this chapter.

Results

Amid 178 hernia repairs, a total of 19 complications were identified perioperatively (ie within 28 days of surgery), a crude complication rate of 11%. These may be subdivided into complications of prosthesis fixation, complications of catheterization, complications of dissection and complications of insufflation (Table 79.3).

Complications of prosthesis fixation

Staples

Three patients (1.7%) developed genitofemoral or ilioinguinal neuralgia. In all of these patients the patch had been stapled to the psoas muscle. All resolved spontaneously.

One patient returned to hospital within two weeks of surgery with a small bowel volvulus, within which a loose staple was found at laparotomy. The hernia repair was noted to be intact.

Recurrence

The single largest group of complications were recurrences within one month of repair (six patients, 3.4%). The time of occurrence is given in Table 79.4. The first recurrence in a plug repair at two weeks prompted the abandonment of this technique, in accordance with world-wide

Table 79.3: Complications (19)

Patch fixation	10
Catheterization	4
Extensive dissection	4
Hypercarbia	1

Table 79.4: Recurrences: 6 in 178 repairs (3.4%)

Among six plug repairs	1
Noted at two weeks	2
Verified superolateral displacement:	
noted immediately	2
noted at three weeks	2

experience. Of the remaining five recurrences, four were shown by laparoscopic transperitoneal inspection to have passed inferomedially under the patch. There was no preponderance of fixed or unfixed patches among the recurrences.

Complications of bladder catheterization

Three patients (1.7%) went into retention of urine, two subsequently requiring prostatic resection. An additional patient developed urinary infection with fever and rigors 24 hours after discharge following hernia surgery. Investigation revealed a high residual urine volume, and prostatic resection was undertaken.

Complications of sac dissection

Four patients (2.2%) developed scrotal haematomas. All had had long indirect sacs laboriously dissected out and inverted into the peritoneum. All had also had subcutaneous heparin as thromboprophylaxis and rectal diclofenac as analgesia.

Complications of insufflation

One patient, a 74-year-old man, became significantly hypercarbic, developed respiratory depression and suffered a myocardial infarction. There was no prior history of significant exercise intolerance. The end-tidal CO_2 concentrations were, however, normal throughout surgery.

Discussion

The initial world literature on laparoscopic inguinal hernia repair presents a picture of a simple, painless and complication-free treatment for a ubiquitous disorder. We believe that the benefits to patients of successful laparoscopic hernia surgery are self-evident (we are currently undertaking a randomized prospective trial controlled against the Lichtenstein repair). However, boundless optimism does not serve that aim of *successful* surgery: it is not educational . The techniques are not easy to learn, and only facing the complications critically, considering their significance and modifying our approach will lead to a reliable set of definitive techniques.

Understanding our complications

Staples

Genitofemoral neuralgia following injury of the nerve in the inguinal canal occurs as a recognized complication of open hernia repair, but in the laparoscopic procedure the injury is a different one: the operator cannot see what lies beneath the patch at the moment of stapling. Staples applied to the inferolateral corner of the patch may impinge on the nerves as they cross the belly of the psoas major muscle.

Staples are easily lost within the peritoneal cavity, but the mechanism by which a volvulus can form around a loose staple is far from clear, save that fibroblasts are easily able to adhere to titanium[4]. Health-economic pressures militate strongly against the use of staplers, some of which are certainly convenient, but it is for the above clinical reasons that we have discontinued their use in all but exceptional cases.

Fixed or unfixed patch?

We have argued elsewhere[3] that the practice of circumferential patch fixation is contrary to Stoppa's postulate of a tension-free repair, because the fixation points act as stress risers. According to Stoppa, the 'Pascal forces' pressing the patch against the intact abdominal wall surrounding the defect always suffice to resist pulsion forces pushing the patch through the defect (Figure 79.1). If sufficient overlap is obtained all around the defect, Stoppa's own experience with open mesh repair is repeatable

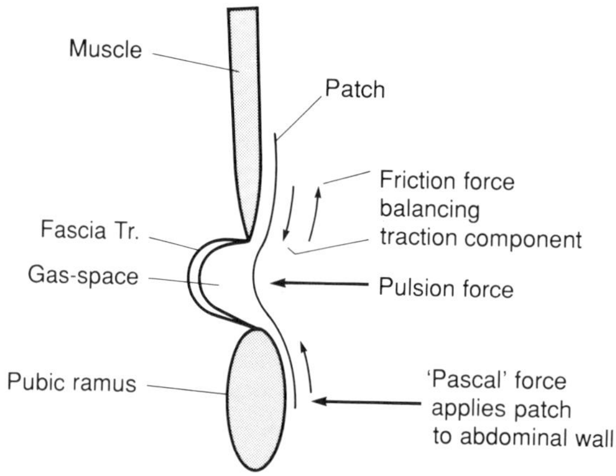

Figure 79.1: Forces in equilibrium on unfixed patch across direct defect.

laparoscopically by the extraperitoneal approach, obviating the time, cost and hazards of suturing or stapling. However, there is no means to know what is *sufficient* overlap. The coefficient of friction between patch and abdominal wall is least inferomedially, where the patch lies against relatively smooth periosteum and fat and is not firmly sandwiched on desufflation as it is around the other three sides. This accords with the majority of our observations on the pathway of recurrence: as long as the patch remains where it was placed, the Stoppa theory will hold good, but there is a tendency for the lower edge of the patch to lift up like a flange on desufflation. Pulsion of the patch through the defect in the immediate postoperative phase will withdraw the inferomedial corner from the cave of Retzius and lead to breakdown of the Pascal forces in this region. Although we have no data to incriminate non-fixation as a specific cause of early recurrence, we now leave the patch unfixed only in indirect hernias with narrow deep rings. In all other hernias, one or two interrupted sutures secure the patch to Cooper's ligament, thus preventing patch *migration* that might result in loss of Pascal forces. The stress transfer from abdominal wall to patch periphery remains continuous. We remain sceptical of the need for any additional fixation. In all hernias with wide defects we now cut a patch according to Figure 79.2, providing a long inferomedial tongue which reaches down behind the pubic ramus, enhancing the frictional forces in this area.

The early recurrences we have seen after laparoscopic repair are thus technical errors rather than the fate of the repair over time. There has been no recurrence beyond the first month after operation. A single additional patient presented at six months with a recurrence after totally extraperitoneal unsutured patch repair of a direct inguinal hernia. This was one of the first procedures performed by one of us (AGF), and at repeat (laparoscopic) operation there was a primary indirect hernia passing lateral to the patch. At initial operation the direct sac had been dealt with and the vasovascular triangle at the root of the cord left undisturbed. A coexisting indirect hernia was thus missed, and the patient had noticed symptoms within a month of the first surgery.

Suture fixation

A large patch is not easy to manoeuvre within the confined space of the extraperitoneal pouch. By placing a double-ended Prolene suture in Cooper's ligament and passing both needles through the patch before the latter is introduced, an external knot can be used to locate and orientate the patch correctly from the outset.

Other aspects of recurrence

Large direct hernias leave a gas-filled space outside the patch after desufflation and this actual space may provide a route for early displacement of the patch. We therefore advocate using a single interrupted suture to invert the transversalis fascia 'pseudosac' and apply it to the deep aspect of the abdominal wall muscle above the defect.

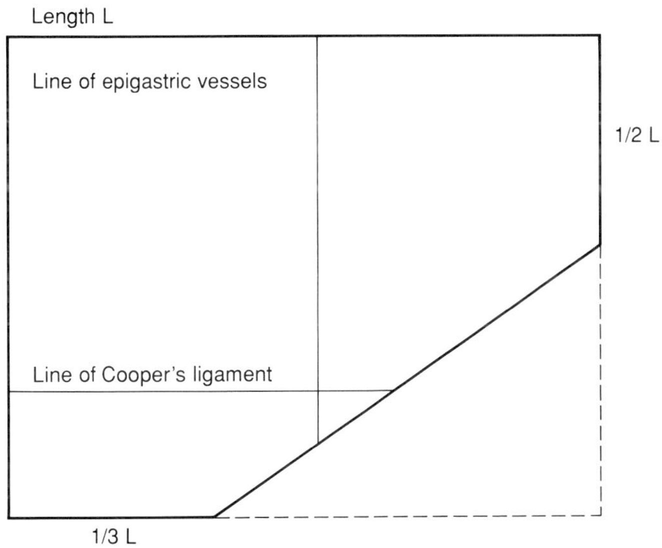

Figure 79.2: Standard patch dimensions. L = length of inguinal ligament. H = L minus 2 cm.

Violent coughing by the patient on reversal of neuromuscular blockade is a psychological burden to the surgeon and may contribute to immediate recurrence. It would be of interest to know if this problem is less common in centres where patients are ventilated mechanically until the blockade wears off.

The bladder

Surgeons catheterize patients for laparoscopic surgery in the belief that the bladder is at risk or will be an obstacle. In fact, the bladder injuries reported by other authors occurred in patients who were catheterized, and a partially filled bladder has not proved a hindrance in our hands.

Accordingly we do not now catheterize patients routinely, but have them void to the best of their ability at the time of premedication.

Dissecting the sac

Dulucq demonstrates dissection and inversion into the peritoneal cavity of every indirect sac. That we are unable to emulate this feat may be a matter of personal technical ability, but, because of the haematomas we have seen, we no longer advocate this manoeuvre for the long or difficult sac. Heparin prophylaxis is difficult to abandon, but we are considering whether the antiplatelet activity of diclofenac could provide adequate prophylaxis. The two agents together constitute a bleeding hazard. If heparin remains an indispensable practice, alternative non-opiate analgesia needs to be investigated.

We routinely ligate and divide long sacs by the extraperitoneal route or circumcise the sac by the transperitoneal route. This policy builds on the experience in open hernia surgery that the distal sac is not a source of problems if left within the cord, but that ambitious dissection may be.

Insufflation

Patients with so severe a gas-transfer defect that the end-tidal CO_2 is not in equilibrium with the pulmonary capillary CO_2 have marked impairment of exercise tolerance, so our patient's complication is not easily explained. However, it is presented here as an important caution. In particular, note that an extraperitoneal approach was employed. The totally extraperitoneal approach dramatically reduces the inflation pressure required for ventilation, but does not reliably reduce CO_2 absorption.

We do not now offer laparoscopic hernia surgery to patients with severely reduced exercise tolerance or with known reduced myocardial reserve.

Learning aspects

The Dulucq approach

Laparoscopic hernia repair is technically taxing and the Dulucq technique is generally regarded as particularly difficult. Blind suprapubic puncture and insufflation is a psychological hurdle to overcome, but there are no reported complications if the puncture is kept suprapubic: The Verres needle is then within the fat in the cave of Retzius. By contrast, passing the cannula subcutaneously to enter the correct plane behind the recti can be learned only by experience. The certainty of orientation and the anatomical access afforded by mastery of this technique fully justify the apprenticeship. Lastly, it is important to appreciate the potential for inadvertent peritoneal puncture when introducing the lateral cannula: the peritoneum is adherent to the abdominal wall at the lateral margin of the rectus muscle and a double layer of peritoneum is easily impaled on the trocar.

Suturing

Laparoscopic hernia surgery is an elysian field for stapling, because of the administrative and physiological pressures for rapid operation. We believe that an irreversible tide is flowing against this expensive technology, the complications of which we have experienced. Laparoscopic hernia repair must grow beyond stapling, and we believe that our evaluation of patch fixation contributes to such a development.

Learning to suture is essential for progress in laparoscopic hernia surgery. The simple box simulator is a poor tool in this learning process. Only by consistently employing suture techniques during clinical surgery can the necessary dexterity be acquired in the real world.

Whilst there are arguments for internal knots, the externally tied self-locking slip-knot on a Prolene suture seems a quick, safe, solid technique for hernia repair.

Conclusion: current protocol and future perspectives

We inform all our patients that the long-term results of laparoscopic hernia surgery are unknown. Preoperative preparation does not include catheterization. Our approach of choice is extraperitoneal. Patients with huge inguinoscrotal hernias and previous scars affecting the muscle coat of the abdomen are treated by the transperitoneal approach (unless the scars are very old indeed). Patients with recurrent hernias and extensive scarring are treated the same way. Large direct defects receive a suture to invert the transversalis pseudosac. All extraperitoneal patches are polypropylene mesh and we employ a giant patch in all but small indirect hernias. All patches are fixed to Cooper's ligament by Prolene suture. Non-fixation or additional fixation has to be argued case by case. Where an intraperitoneal patch is needed, expanded PTFE is used. Patients with significant cardiopulmonary impairment have open hernia surgery.

Three major developments are needed to promote laparoscopic inguinal hernia repair:

- more rapid extraperitoneal dissection, for which the Kieturakis balloon dissector offers good prospects

- cheaper, more rapid patch fixation, for which the ideal technology is awaited
- laparoscopic hernia surgery must be possible as day care. We are currently studying the role of an outreach nurse as facilitator of this advance.

References

1. Stoppa R, Rives JL, Warlaumont CR *et al.* The use of Dacron in the repair of hernias of the groin. *Surg Clin North Am* 1984; **64**: 269–85.
2. Dulucq J-L. The treatment of inguinal hernias by implantation of mesh through retroperitoneoscopy. *Postgrad Gen Surg* 1992; **4**: 173–4.
3. Taylor RST, Fiennes AGTW. A tension free modification of the Dulucq preperitoneal laparoscopic hernioplasty. *Minimally Invasive Ther* 1992; **1**, suppl 1: 100.
4. Steinemann SG, Mäusli PA. Titanium alloys for surgical implants. Biocompatibility from physico-chemical principles. At: *Sixth World Congress on Titanium*, Cannes. 1988.

80

Safe Areas for Mesh Stapling in Laparoscopic Hernia Repair

H VAN MAMEREN AND PMNYH GO

In laparoscopic hernia repair the parietal peritoneum surrounding the internal inguinal ring is released. Then a prosthetic mesh is usually placed at the inner side of the abdominal wall to cover the hernia defect. To prevent displacement, the mesh is fixed to the abdominal wall with staples. Both peritoneum dissection and inappropriate stapling may result in vascular lesions and nerve injury, causing haematomas, pain and numbness after the operation. Fitzgibbons *et al.*[1] reported the occurrence of local haematomas in 7.5% of patients, pain or numbness in the ventrolateral region of the upper leg in 3.9% and groin pain in 12.9% after laparoscopic hernia repair. Long-term complications (4.2%) are related to nerve injury, usually resulting in groin pain. MacFadyen[2,3] observed vascular lesions resulting in scrotal, inguinal canal, anterior abdominal wall and preperitoneal haematomas. Impaired sensibility and pain are suggested to be related to cutaneous nerve injury[3].

The occurrence of these complications may be reduced by a better understanding of the topographical anatomy of this region[4]. Therefore, we performed dissections on human cadavers to demonstrate the topography of vessels and nerves which can easily be injured by release of the peritoneum or by blind stapling.

Operative procedure

The preperitoneal tissue in the inner inguinal region has been studied in six preserved human male cadavers. They are sawn transversely with a bandsaw at the level of the umbilicus in deep frozen state. After thawing, the remaining parts of the intestines, together with their mesenteries up to the peritoneal reflexion of Douglas, are removed. This gives optimum insight into the region of interest (a view comparable to the one during laparoscopic hernia repair). Besides, the entire abdominal wall caudal to the umbilicus is intact.

The parietal peritoneum is incised transversely cranial to the iliopubic tract from the medial umbilical ligament up to the inner side of the anterior superior iliac spine. The peritoneum is released from the preperitoneal adipose tissue in cranial and in caudal direction. Consequently, blood vessels, nerves and ductus deferens are dissected. This is carried out in the adipose tissue overlying the medial part of the superior pubic arch, the external iliac vessels and the iliopsoas muscle up to their passage below the iliopubic tract and in the region of the inferior epigastric vessels (Figure 80.1).

Results

The testicular vessels entering the deep inguinal ring can be distinguished in the medial part of the operating field of transabdominal laparoscopic hernia repair, superficial to the external iliac vessels. Near this ring, the genital branch of the genitofemoral nerve and the ductus deferens join into the

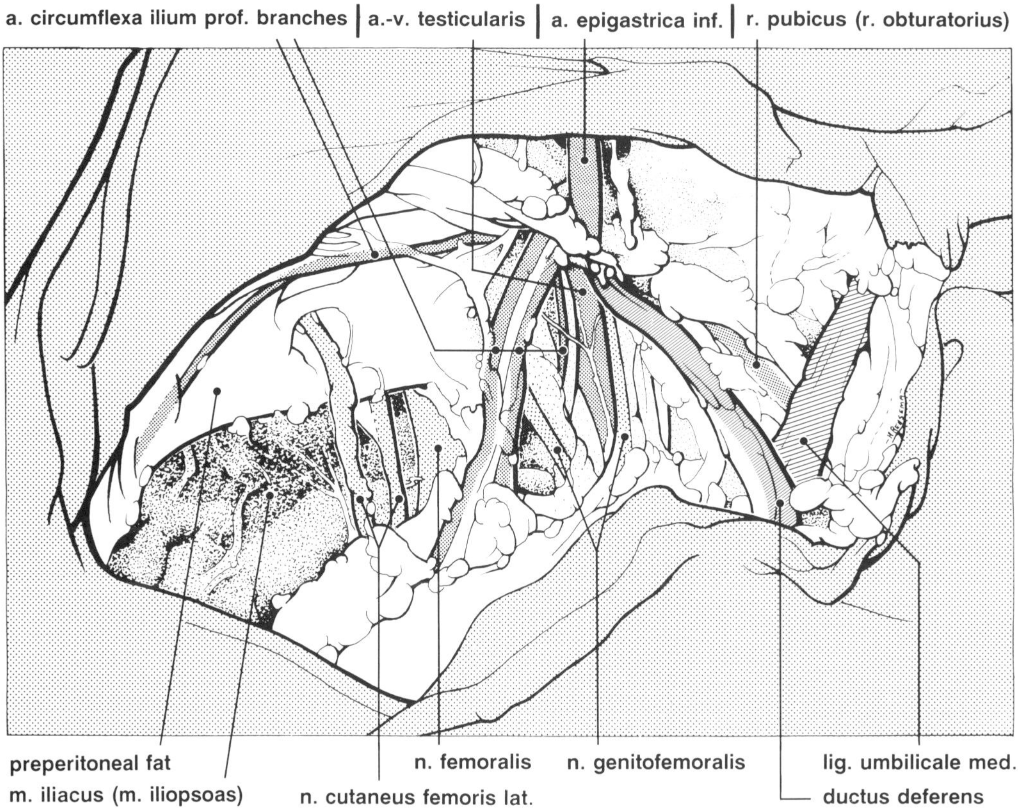

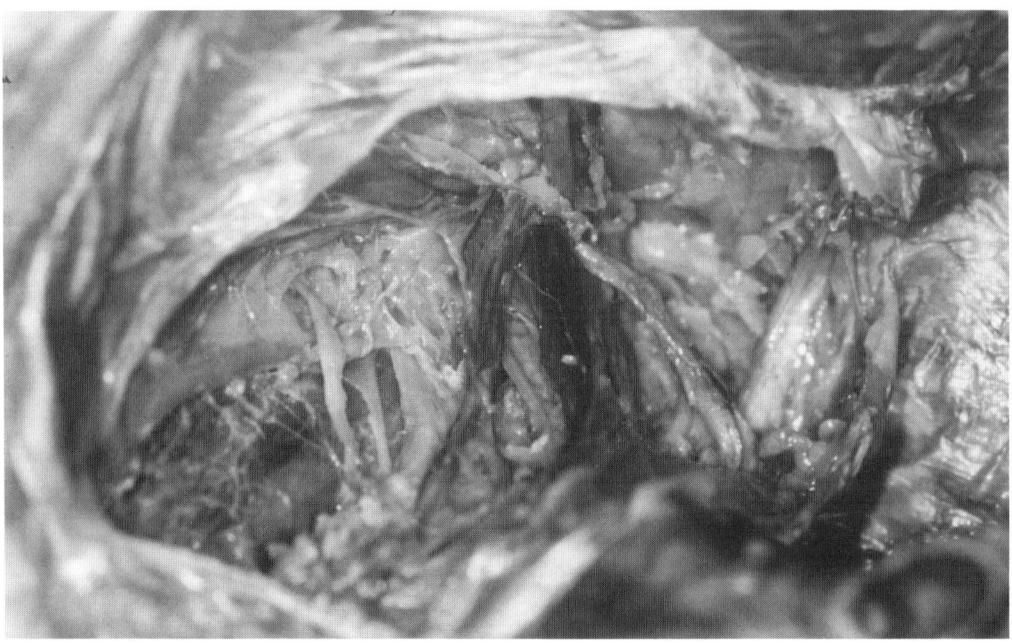

Figure 80.1: The dissected region in the area of the inner inguinal ring. Preperitoneal adipose tissue has been removed. Structures that can be injured easily are given in the schematic drawing.

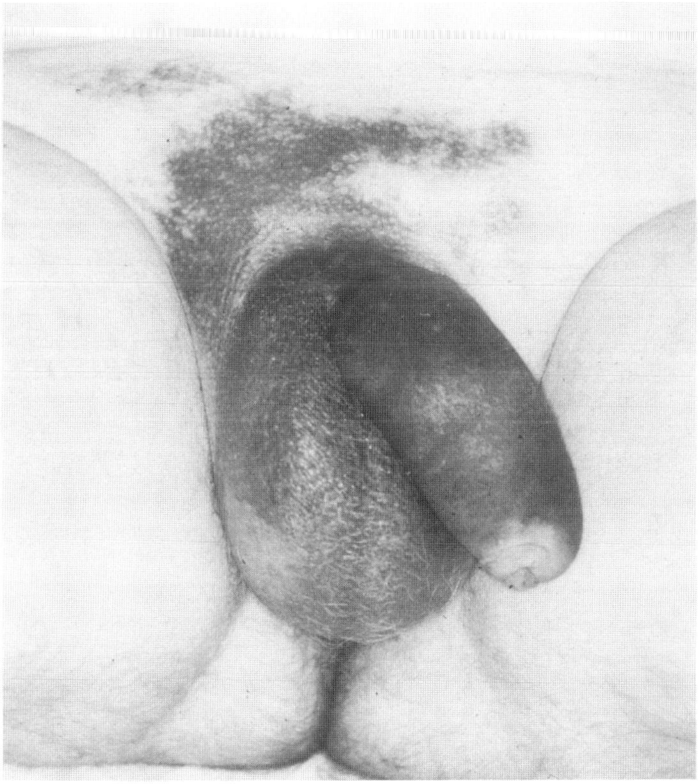

Figure 80.2: A patient showing haematomas in the scrotal region after laparoscopic hernia repair.

spermatic cord. Usually, the testicular vessels and the ductus deferens (landmarks during laparoscopic hernia repair) are already visible through the intact peritoneum. This also holds true for the peritoneal folds over the obliterated umbilical artery (medial umbilical fold) and over the epigastric vessels (lateral umbilical fold). Deep in the adipose tissue, overlying the inner side of the superior pubic arch, a branch of the epigastric artery is found. It runs to the obturator foramen. It is classically called the pubic or obturator branch.

In the lateral region of the operating field, bordered by the iliopubic tract and external iliac artery and superficial to the iliopsoas muscle, many blood vessel branches of the deep circumflex iliac artery are found. The lateral femoral cutaneous nerve and one or more femoral branches of the genitofemoral nerve lie in the adipose tissue of this region. Laterally, the ilioinguinal nerve penetrates into the abdominal wall muscles. The femoral nerve is situated at the medioventral side of the iliopsoas muscle. This large nerve lies deep in the centre of the operating field. Figure 75.1 shows the topographic relations of the structures mentioned.

Discussion

Inadvertent lesions of nerves and blood vessels during laparoscopic dissection may result in patient discomfort. Due to the superficial course, as seen from the intra-abdominal side, the genitofemoral, the lateral femoral cutaneous and the ilioinguinal nerve are easily severed by stapling. This results in impaired sensibility, including pain, paraesthesia and loss of sensibility in specific areas.

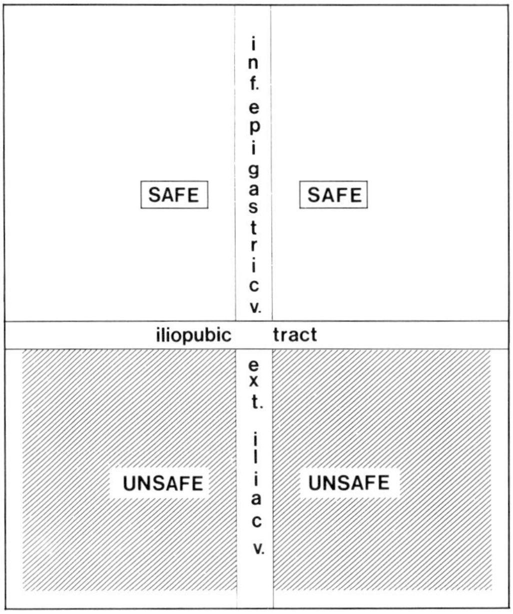

Figure 80.3: Schematic drawing of the inner inguinal region showing 'safe' and 'unsafe' quadrants for mesh stapling.

- Lesion of the genitofemoral nerve leads to impaired sensibility in the scrotal area.
- Lesion of the lateral femoral cutaneous nerve results in discomfort in the ventrolateral side of the proximal upper leg.
- Lesion of the ilioinguinal nerve affects the ventromedial side of the proximal upper leg.

Blood vessel lesions result in haematoma. Lesions of the branches of the epigastric vessels or of their pubic (obturator) branch leads to scrotal haematoma or their surrounding (Figure 80.2). The deep circumflex iliac vessels and their branches run superficially behind the iliopubic tract. Injury of these vessels may result in an anterior abdominal haematoma.

The inguinal area as seen from the intra-abdominal side can be divided into quadrants (Figure 80.3): two above and two below the iliopubic tract. The area above the iliopubic tract is divided in a lateral and a medial quadrant by the epigastric vessels and the area below the iliopubic tract is divided by the external iliac vessels. Most vessels and nerves that can be injured easily run below the iliopubic tract. Therefore, the use of stapling for mesh fixation should be avoided in the lower two quadrants. If staple fixation is necessary, this should be done lateral and medial to the epigastric vessels.

If the hernia defect is not too large and a considerable surface area can be covered by a prosthetic mesh, the use of staplers may be superfluous. It may be supposed that the interstices in the mesh allow for tissue ingrowth and incorporation into the inguinal floor, as has been investigated in anterior inguinal hernia repair[5]. Using a transabdominal laparoscopic hernia repair without fixation of the prosthetic mesh, Van Steensel *et al.*[6] reported a recurrence rate of 1.9% in 254 laparoscopic hernia repairs. No nerve injuries and six haematomas were observed.

Avoidance of stapling reduces nerve and vessel injuries. In addition, the cost of the laparoscopic hernia repair can be reduced by omitting the use of stapling devices.

Acknowledgements

We thank Prof. Dr J Drukker for this helpful comments on the manuscript and Mr H Rensema for the preparation of the Figures.

References

1. Fitzgibbons R, Annibali R, Litke B, Filipi C, Salerno G, Cornet D. A multicentered clinical trial on laparoscopic inguinal hernia repair: preliminary results. *SAGES Symposium*, 1993: S07 (abstract).

2. MacFadyen B. Complications of laparoscopic herniorrhaphy. *SAGES Symposium* 1992; **5**: 9–10 (abstract).

3. MacFadyen Jr BV, Arregui ME, Corbitt JD, *et al.* Complications of laparoscopic herniorrhaphy. *Surg Endosc* 1993; **7**: 155–8.

4. Kraus MA. Laparoscopic identification of preperitoneal nerve anatomy in the inguinal area. *SAGES Symposium* 1993; S02 (abstract).

5. Lichtenstein IL, Shulman AG, Amik PK, *et al.* The tension free hernioplasty. *Am J Surg* 1989; **157**: 188–92.

6. Van Steensel CJ, Weidema WF. Laparoscopic inguinal hernia repair without fixation of the prosthesis. Symposium: *Hernia '93: Advances or Controversies 1993* (abstract).

81

Complications of Laparoscopic Inguinal Hernia Repair

ROBERT W SEWELL AND ROBERT L WADDELL

Laparoscopic techniques have been used to perform inguinal hernia repairs for the last several years and, like all surgical procedures, these operations carry with them some risk of complications. Most of these complications can be avoided if the surgeon has a clear understanding of the anatomy, employs careful laparoscopic techniques and adheres to fundamental surgical principles. These basics of operative surgery are particularly important in laparoscopic procedures because tactile feedback and three-dimensional vision are virtually eliminated.

Complications associated with laparoscopic hernia repair can be separated into two major categories: those that are common to all laparoscopic procedures, and those that are specific to the hernia repair procedure. Also, since there are at least three different laparoscopic techniques currently being employed, each technique may have specific complications that are more likely. The following series of complications is by no means a complete summary of this topic, but rather is a collection of specific complications encountered by the authors.

The incidence of complications in our series of laparoscopic hernia repairs has decreased perceptibly as each surgeon has become thoroughly familiar with the inguinal anatomy from the laparoscopic viewpoint. This region looks quite different from inside the abdominal cavity than it does through the conventional anterior approach. For this reason, laparoscopic inguinal hernia repair is technically more difficult to master than laparoscopic cholecystectomy, and should be approached cautiously.

Trocar injury to the inferior epigastric vessels

During the introduction and manipulation of laparoscopic instruments the vessels of the abdominal wall may be injured, with the epigastric vessels at particular risk. Accordingly, each cannula should be viewed laparoscopically as it is placed, and if significant bleeding is identified it should be controlled immediately. This particular complication was managed in one case by placing percutaneous 'U' stitches of no. 2 nylon, both above and below the site of injury. There sutures were tied externally and left in place for 24 hours. The hernia repair then proceeded uneventfully.

Trocar site hernia

A somewhat delayed complication of laparoscopic procedures may be the occurrence of a hernia in one of the trocar sites. Such hernias may involve bowel or omentum and probably occur immediately upon removal of the cannula. Even when trocars are inserted obliquely through the abdominal wall, penetrating each successive fascial layer at a slightly different point, a hernia may develop. One such complication occurred in our series. The patient presented three days after his hernia repair with signs and symptoms of a small bowel obstruction, along with a small mass in the region of the right flank trocar site. Laparoscopic exploration was performed and a loop of small bowel was incarcerated within the fascial defect where the trocar had been placed. The fascial defect was enlarged, allowing the bowel to be reduced back into the abdomen while being observed laparoscopically. This segment of the bowel was found to be necrotic and required segmental resection with primary anastomosis. The resection was performed extracorporeally through an expanded umbilical incision.

One factor in the development of trocar site hernias may be the common practice of applying significant extrinsic compression on the abdominal wall in an effort to force carbon dioxide gas out during cannula removal. This practice may actually force bowel or omentum into the end of the cannula, which is then literally dragged out through the fascial opening. The same situation may result when muscular relaxation is inadequate at the end of the procedure, causing the patient to start 'pushing' when the cannulas are being removed. For these reasons it is recommended that all trocars be removed under continuous laparoscopic visualization, and that abdominal wall relaxation be maintained until all fascial incisions have been sutured closed.

Nerve injuries

Nerve injuries are among the more common complications of any type of inguinal hernia repair. In conventional hernia repairs, such injuries typically occur either due to incomplete dissection of the region or because the normal anatomy is obscured by large or recurrent hernias[1]. Nerve injuries may also occur during laparoscopic hernia repairs but the means of injury is somewhat different. The nerves most likely to be injured include the ilioinguinal, genitofemoral and femoral. There have been no femoral nerve injuries in our series, but we have had patients experience transient neuritis of the genitofemoral and ilioinguinal nerves. We presumed that these injuries were due to one of the following mechanisms.

Ilioinguinal nerve injury

The ilioinguinal nerve is not visible during the preperitoneal dissection of the inguinal floor, as it lies superficial to the transversus abdominis and internal oblique layers. However, it is possible to injure this nerve by the indiscriminate use of electrocautery for dissection around the internal inguinal ring. During staple fixation of the mesh prosthesis it is possible for the abdominal wall to be compressed sufficiently to bring this nerve within reach of a staple as it is being applied. This type of nerve entrapment has not been seen thus far in our experience, but other surgeons have indicated that reoperation for staple removal has been required to resolve this problem.

Genitofemoral nerve

The genital branch of the genitofemoral nerve accompanies the cord structures down the inguinal canal. This nerve is usually somewhat difficult to see and may easily be injured during excessive dissection around the internal inguinal ring. This risk constitutes the main reason why we have abandoned the routine practice of removing indirect hernia sacs. Likewise, the placement of staples in or around the region of the internal inguinal ring may injure or entrap the genitofemoral nerve. Such injuries usually result in transient or even permanent numbness or pain in the scrotum or labia.

Femoral nerve

Despite the fact that femoral nerve injury has not been observed in our series, it is important to discuss this particular serious complication. The femoral nerve may be injured laparoscopically as it courses beneath the iliopubic tract, lateral to the iliac artery. This type of injury is invariably due to wayward dissection or staple placement lateral to the internal inguinal ring and posterior to the iliopubic tract. Such injuries may lead to a variety of neuropathies of the lower extremity and may even necessitate re-exploration to remove staples or sutures. This particular complication should be totally preventable if the surgeon avoid dissecting or stapling posterior to the iliopubic tract, lateral to the internal inguinal ring.

Urinary bladder injury

Injuries to the urinary bladder have been described during various types of inguinal hernia repairs and, because of its preperitoneal location, this structure may also be injured during a laparoscopic repair. Large direct hernias, femoral hernias, and even some indirect hernias may have portions of the bladder 'sliding' into them, making up a portion of their wall[2]. The presence of a bladder diverticulum may also predispose the patient to bladder injury, since these areas of the wall are quite thin and are thus more easily penetrated than the normal, muscular bladder wall. Generally, bladder injuries occur during sharp dissection along the medial portion of the inguinal floor. If blunt dissection is employed during the laparoscopic dissection of the inguinal floor, injuries to the bladder are less likely to occur. Also, the routine use of an indwelling urinary catheter will keep the bladder completely decompressed, helping to prevent this complication.

An injury to the urinary bladder occurred in one patient undergoing the repair of what proved to be a right femoral hernia. An ill-advised attempt to remove the hernia sac was the mechanism of injury. The sac contained an unsuspected bladder diverticulum which was transected with the electrocautery. This problem was immediately recognized and successfully repaired laparoscopically. The subsequent recovery was uneventful.

Small bowel obstruction

The incidence of bowel obstruction following laparoscopic hernia repair is unknown, and will likely require many years to determine accurately. However, it would seem reasonable to assume that the risk of obstruction secondary to adhesions is probably quite low, due to the fact that significant adhesions are not a frequent consequence of other laparoscopic procedures. Surgeons who have had occasion to reoperate on patients following laparoscopic surgery uniformly report minimal to no peritoneal adhesions at the sites of trocar placement. This is most likely due to the lack of manipulation and trauma to the serous membrane of the visceral peritoneum. An undisturbed serosal surface has little potential for adhesion formation.

On the other hand, early postoperative bowel obstruction may occur following laparoscopic hernia repair if the peritoneum is not closed completely. One such case was encountered following a transperitoneal repair. Significant gaps existed in the peritoneal closure, which had been performed with staples. The patient presented back to hospital two days after surgery, with obvious signs and symptoms of a small bowel obstruction. Plain film radiographs of the abdomen demonstrated a considerable distance separating the staples in the fascia from those used to close the peritoneum. At the time of laparoscopic exploration the preperitoneal space contained approximately 90 cm (3 feet) of incarcerated small intestine. The obstruction was relieved laparoscopically by reducing the herniated bowel and completely closing the peritoneum with a continuous running suture. The patient recovered without further incident.

Bowel obstructions, such as the one described here, are best prevented by the careful and complete approximation of the peritoneal edges following the repair. When approximating the edges of the peritoneum with staples or clips, they should be no more than 1 cm apart, with no visible gaps in the final closure. If possible, the edges of the peritoneum should actually be overlapped rather than simply approximated. Our preferred method for closing the peritoneum and thus preventing the problem of bowel obstruction, is a running, locked suture using an absorbable material.

Recurrence of the hernia

As with any technique for repairing inguinal hernia, the actual incidence of recurrence tends to be related not only to the specific technique but also to the experience of the surgeon and the length of follow-up. Thus far, recurrences have been unusual following laparoscopic hernia repairs that employ a stapled mesh technique, but the length of follow-up remains relatively short. Generally, recurrences can be attributed to either inadequate fixation or inadequate mesh size. As each of the various techniques for laparoscopic hernia repair has evolved, the size of the prosthetic mesh has gradually increased to ensure that it adequately overlaps the surrounding normal tissues.

The single recurrence in our series of 250 repairs was due to inadequate dissection and repair of the direct space during the repair of an obvious indirect hernia. The patient presented 13 months after the initial procedure with a recurrent hernia. This ultimately proved to be a direct defect in the medial aspect of the inguinal floor. This area had not been completely covered by the original mesh prosthesis. The subsequent repair was also performed laparoscopically using the same method, but a much larger piece of mesh was used. The possibility of an open conventional repair was discussed with the patient preoperatively, and it was agreed that there would be no hesitation in converting to such an approach if the laparoscopic dissection proved too difficult.

When approaching a recurrent hernia, it should be remembered that the mesh from the previous repair makes the secondary dissection considerably more difficult and treacherous. This second dissection offers a greater potential for injury to surrounding structures, especially the major vessels in the area. During the repair of our single recurrence, no attempt was made to remove the old mesh, or to identify the iliac vein. Instead, the new sheet of mesh was simply laid over the entire floor followed by staple fixation to the surrounding structures and to the original mesh. The procedure was successfully completed laparoscopically and the patient remains without further recurrence five months later.

Other types of complications

In general discussions of laparoscopic hernia repair, concern has been expressed regarding the potential for other specific complication[3]. To date there have been no infections of any kind in our series and there have been no problems relative to testicular ischaemia. There were two patients who developed seromas in the inguinal floor, both of which resolved spontaneously. Two additional patients developed symptomatic hydroceles of the cord. These fluid collections, occurring within the remnants of indirect hernia sacs, were treated with periodic aspiration until they eventually failed to reaccumulate. Total resolution required three aspirations in one case and four in the other.

Conclusion

Several different laparoscopic techniques are currently in use for the repair of inguinal hernias. While the results from these procedures have been very promising, the surgeon should recognize the risks that are inherent to these operations. These techniques can be performed safely only when the surgeon has a clear understanding of the anatomy of the inguinal region as seen from the inside. Whatever laparoscopic approach is used, it must include cautious dissection and adherence to basic surgical principles. As with any operative procedure, the risk should diminish for each individual surgeon as experience is gained, and it is in everyone's best to share our experiences, both good and bad.

References

1. Wantz GE. Complications of inguinal hernial repair. *Surg Clin North Am* 1984; 64: 287–97.
2. Nyhus LM. Complications of hernial repair. In Artz CP, Hardy JD, eds. *Management of surgical complications*, 3rd ed. Philadelphia: JB Lippincott, 1975: 659–71.
3. Phillips E, Carroll B. Laparoscopic inguinal hernia repair. *Gastroint Endosc Clin North Am* 1993; 3: 297–307.

82

Complications and Recurrences Associated with Laparoscopic Repair of Groin Hernias: a Multi-institutional Retrospective Analysis

CIHAT TETIK, MAURICE E ARREGUI, DANIEL CASTRO, CHAD J DAVIS, JEAN L DULUCQ, ROBERT J FITZGIBBONS Jr, MORRIS E FRANKLIN, JOEL C HAMMOND, J BARRY MCKERNAN, R DAVID ROSIN, LEONARD S SCHULTZ AND FREDERICK K TOY

Hernia repair is the second most frequent procedure (after cholecystectomy) performed by the general surgeon[1]. In the USA 500 000–700 000 hernia repairs are performed each year[2,3]. Although the laparoscopic technique is a new approach to groin hernia, it is becoming more widely accepted as an alternative to traditional open techniques. The purpose of this chapter is to make a preliminary assessment of this new approach by reviewing its complications and recurrences.

Materials and methods

A questionnaire was sent to the contributing surgeons, who represented eight hospitals throughout Europe and the USA. This questionnaire was created to analyse complications and recurrences associated with laparoscopic herniorrhaphy. The study period covered over three years, from December 1989 to April 1993. A total of 1514 hernias were repaired in 1288 patients. There were 119 (7.9%) bilateral hernias and 192 (12.7%) recurrent hernias. The types of hernia are listed in Table 82.1, and the procedures used to repair them are given in Table 82.2.

Results

Eighteen intraoperative and 188 postoperative complications were seen. The total complication rate was 13.6% in 1514 hernia repairs.

Table 82.1: Types of hernias

Indirect hernias	860
Direct hernias	560
Pantaloon hernias	43
Femoral hernias	37
Obturator hernias	6
Not specified	8
Total	1514

Table 82.2: Types of repairs

Transabdominal preperitoneal mesh technique (TAPP)	553
Total extraperitoneal mesh technique (TEP)	457
Intraperitoneal onlay mesh technique (IPOM)	320
Ring closure technique	102
Plug and patch technique	82
Total	1514

Table 82.3: Intraoperative complications of laparoscopic herniorrhaphy techniques

Technique	*Related to hernia repair*	*Related to laparoscopic technique*	*Related to anaesthesia*	*Total*	*%*
Ring closure	0	1	0	1	1.0
Plug and patch	0	0	0	0	0.0
Intraperitoneal onlay mesh	2	1	0	3	0.9
Transabdominal preperitoneal mesh	1	3	1	5	0.9
Total extraperitoneal mesh	0	9	0	9	1.9
Totals	3	14	1	18	1.2

Table 82.4: Postoperative complications of laparoscopic herniorrhaphy techniques

Technique	*Local*	*Neurological*	*Testicular*	*Urinary*	*Mesh*	*Misc.*	*Total*	*%*
Ring closure	0	0	0	0	0	0	0	0
Plug and patch	0	0	1	0	6	4	11	13.4
IPOM	18	15	0	4	1	2	40	12.5
TAPP	21	7	11	12	3	2	56	10.1
TEP	56	3	11	7	0	4	81	17.7
Totals	95	25	23	23	10	12	188	12.4

Fourteen intraoperative complications were related to laparoscopic technique. These included one colon injury, a needle lost in the abdominal wall, a bleeding port site and open conversions. The open conversions were mostly in connection with early surgical experience and equipment problems. Three intraoperative complications were related to the actual hernia repair. These included injuries of the bladder, spermatic artery and epigastric artery. One complication was related to anaesthesia: the patient had bronchospasm and cardiac dysrhythmia upon induction. The procedure was cancelled.

By specific laparoscopic technique, there was one (1.0%) technique-related intraoperative complication out of 102 ring closures. It involved a bleeding port site. There were no intraoperative complications during the plug and patch technique. Three (0.9%) intraoperative complications occurred during IPOM, five (0.9%) during TAPP and nine (1.9%) during TEP (Table 82.3).

The rate of conversion to an open procedure was 0.8%. Of procedures converted to open technique eight were in connection with early experience, one was due to vascular injury (epigastric artery), one a broken stapler, one additional equipment problem and one bladder injury. An elderly patient with a large sliding hernia developed bladder injury during intraperitoneal onlay mesh repair.

Ninety-five local, 25 neurological 23 testicular, 23 urinary, 10 mesh and 12 miscellaneous postoperative complications were noted (Table 82.4). The majority of local complications were inguinal canal (36 cases) and trocar site haematoma/seroma (27 cases) and subcutaneous emphysema

(15 cases). Other local complications were hydrocele (five cases), wound infection (five cases), inguinal pain (four cases) and scrotal haematoma (three cases). These local complications were seen most commonly after total extraperitoneal mesh technique. No postoperative complications were reported after the 102 ring closures.

The most common neurological complication was lateral femoral cutaneous nerve pain. In addition, nerve pain from the genitofemoral nerve and the intermediate cutaneous branch of the femoral nerve occurred. Two of the neurological complications required repeat laparoscopy and staple removal.

Testicular complications included testicular pain in 20 cases, two cases of epidydymitis and one of orchitis. No testicular atrophy was noted in any patients. Most were transient, testicular pain lasting two to three weeks. Urinary retention (after 20 procedures) was the most common urinary complication. Other urinary complications included urinary tract infection and haematuria.

Six mesh complications such as palpable mesh and migration of mesh were seen after the plug and patch technique. There was only one infected mesh; this occurred with the IPOM technique.

There were three small bowel obstructions associated with adhesion formation. Two obstructions were between staples used to close the peritoneum, and one was at a trocar site. All of the small bowel obstructions were associated with the plug and patch technique. All required reoperation. Other miscellaneous complications included seven postoperative non-neurological pains, one osteitis pubis and one haemorrhage at a trocar site. Osteitis pubis was seen after the IPOM technique.

One mortality was noted in the postoperative period, secondary to disseminated histoplasmosis. The patient died 23 days after TEP. This death was not related to the hernia repair.

A total of 34 (2.2%) recurrences occurred after 1514 hernia repairs. A breakdown by technique used is given in Table 82.5.

Table 82.5: The rate of recurrences with laparoscopic herniorrhaphy techniques

Type of repair	*Number*	*Rate* (%)
Ring closure	3	3
Plug and patch	18	22
IPOM	7	2.2
TAPP	4	0.7
TEP	2	0.4
Total	34	2.2

Discussion

This retrospective analysis is based on a questionnaire designed to analyse more than the more serious intraoperative and postoperative complications usually reported in most hernia series (Figure 82.1). Minor complications such as asymptomatic haematomas, transient testicular or neurological pain, and so on are reported to attempt to analyse factors related to patient comfort as well as potentially serious problems associated with laparoscopic hernia repair. Because this technique continues to evolve and modifications are constantly being made, it is difficult to know at this early stage what the ultimate role, complications and recurrences of laparoscopic hernia repair will be.

Some of the notable findings in this study which have not been discussed in other publications dealing with complications include the unexpectedly high numbers of haematomas found with the TAPP and TEP repairs. This is undoubtedly related to the more extensive dissections required as well as the fact that the hernia sacs or spaces remain everted and any serous weeping or bleeding will manifest as an external haematoma. With direct hernias we now invert the sac and anchor it to Cooper's ligament, which has eliminated the problem. Indirect hernias remain a problem. Removal of the sac does not eliminate the space.

LAPAROSCOPIC HERNIA SURVEY OF COMPLICATIONS

Investigator name .... Date ....
Street .... Ph. no. .... Fax no. ....
City .... State ..... Country ....

Type of repair ❑ Ring closure ❑ Plug and patch technique ❑ Total extraperitoneal mesh
Describe technique ❑ Intraperitoneal mesh ❑ Transabdominal preperitoneal mesh ❑ Other...

....
....
....
....
....
....
....

Date this study period began .... No. of patients having open repairs ....
Date this study period ended .... No. of patients having lap repairs ....
No. of patients operated on .... No. lap hernias repaired with this technique ....

Please indicate the number of each type of hernia repaired

Direct inguinal hernias .... Femoral hernias ....
Indirect inguinal hernias .... No. recurrent hernias repaired ....
Other hernias (specify) .... Bilateral hernias ....

COMPLICATIONS *(PLEASE EXPLAIN MANAGEMENT OF EACH COMPLICATION)*

INTRAOPERATIVE

Total no. intraoperative complications ....
List no. and type comp. related to hernia repair ....
....
List no. and type comp. related to lap technique ....
....
Please list no. and type anesthetic complication ....
....
Conversion to open and reason ....
....

POSTOPERATIVE

Total no. postoperative complications ....

LOCAL COMPLICATIONS

Severe sub cutaneous emphysema ....
Hematoma/seroma trocar site ....
Hematoma/seroma inguinal canal ....
Hematoma/seroma scrotum ....
Hydrocele ....
Wound infection ....

URINARY COMPLICATIONS

Urinary retention ....
Urinary tract infection ....

Signature ______________________________

Figure 82.1 Questionnaire used for gathering prospective data on complications and recurrences.

LAPAROSCOPIC HERNIA SURVEY OF COMPLICATIONS

NEUROLOGIC COMPLICATIONS

Lateral femoral cutaneous nerve entrapment ....

Genitofemoral nerve entrapment ....

Other nerve entrapment (please indicate) ....

TESTICULAR COMPLICATIONS

Testicular pain ....

Testicular atrophy ....

Eipididymitis ....

MESH COMPLICATIONS

Infected mesh ....

Palpable mesh ....

Migration of mesh ....

MISCELLANEOUS COMPLICATIONS

Osteitis pubis ....

Pain from staples ....

Small bowel obstruction ....

Other complications list no. and type ....

TOTAL COMPLICATIONS

Total intra and post op comps. ....

RECURRENCES

No. of recurrences .... please indicate reasons for recurrence

....

....

Describe management of recurrences

....

....

....

....

....

MORTALITY

Mortality related to surgery ❍ yes ❍ no Mortality related to surgery (please explain)

....

....

Mortality unrelated to surgery ❍ yes ❍ no Mortality unrelated to surgery (please explain)

....

....

FOLLOW UP DATA

Length of follow up (mos) – range .... Length of follow up (mos) average ....

Investigator wishes to be acknowleged ❍ yes ❍ no

Investigator wishes to be anonymous ❍ yes ❍ no

Allows unrestricted use of information ❍ yes ❍ no

Signature ____________________

Figure 82.1 *continued*

The other notable finding is the testicular pain associated with these repairs. Although transient, the discomfort to the patient can be significant. The mechanism is uncertain. These problems and others will probably diminish with increasing experience and refining of technique. These two techniques are the currently more widely used and to date have the lowest recurrence rate which seems to be related to complete coverage of the inguinofemoral area with a large mesh and fixation of that mesh. Also noteworthy is that 12.7% of the hernias repaired were recurrent in this study. This suggests a higher recurrence rate than usually reported with traditional approaches.

Conclusion

This study supports the conclusion that laparoscopic repair of groin hernia can be performed safely. Complications, mostly minor, are a result of early development of technique and learning curve. As with open surgery, we must not forget that the successful repair of groin hernias is associated with the experience of the surgeon and perfection of the individual technique. This preliminary report suggests that the recurrence rate is less with large anchored mesh placed by TEP or TAPP technique than with the plug and patch technique[4–9].

References

1. Schneidman DS, ed. *Socio-Economic Factbook for Surgery* 1993. Chicago: American College of Surgeons, 1993; 37–54.
2. Condon RE, Nyhus LM. Complications of groin hernia. In: Nyhus LM, Condon RE. eds. *Hernia*, 3rd ed. Philadelphia: JB Lippincott: 1989: 253–64.
3. Rutkow IR, Robbins A. Demographic, classificatory, and socioeconomic aspects of hernia repair in the United States. *Surg Clin North Am* 1993; 73: 413–26.
4. Braeuer HL. A new method of transabdominal endoscopic repair of inguinal and femoral hernias. In: *1993 Scientific Session and Postgraduate Course*. 31 March – 3 April 1993, Phoenix, Arizona.
5. Fitzgibbons Jr R, Annibali R, Litke B, *et al.* A multicentered clinical trial on laparoscopic inguinal hernia repair. In: *1993 Scientific Session and Postgraduate Course*. 31 March – 3 April 1993, Phoenix, Arizona.
6. MacFadyen BV. Complications of laparoscopic inguinal herniorrhaphy. Presented at *Hernia '93: Advances or Controversies* symposium, 24–27 May 1993, Indianapolis, Indiana.
7. Newman L, Eubanks S, Lucas G, Mason E, Duncan T. Laparoscopic herniorrhaphy via the transperitoneal anatomic approach – a review of our first 151 repairs. In: *1993 Scientific Session and Postgraduate Course*. 31 March – 3 April 1993, Phoenix, Arizona.
8. Phillips EH, Carroll B, Fallas M, *et al.* Reasons for recurrence following laparoscopic hernioplasty. Presented at *Hernia '93: Advances or Controversies* symposium, 24–27 Mary 1993. Indianapolis, Indiana.
9. Theobald DR, Mack P, Kee SG, Wong WK, Ooi PJ. Laparoscopic inguinal herniorrhaphy with preperitoneal tension-free polypropylene mesh repair. In: *1993 Scientific Session and Postgraduate Course*. 31 March – 3 April, 1993, Phoenix, Arizona.

83

Two-phase *In vivo* Comparison Study of Adhesion Formation of the Gore-Tex Soft Tissue Patch, Marlex Mesh and Surgipro using a Rabbit Model

KARL A LEBLANC

Much controversy surrounds many aspects of laparoscopic hernia repair, including which prosthetic material is most appropriate for this type of surgery. In an attempt to address this issue, a comparison study was performed in the rabbit model to evaluate the suitability of prosthetic materials for use in laparoscopic hernia repair. Biological response was compared – with specific emphasis on the adhesion indices – using implants of three commonly used materials in inguinal and ventral hernia repair: monofilament woven polypropylene mesh (Marlex), multifilament knitted polypropylene mesh (Surgipro) and 1-mm-thick expanded polytetrafluoroethylene (ePTFE) sheeting material (Gore-Tex Soft Tissue Patch). The study was conducted in two phases. The first compared Marlex and Gore-Tex and the second compared Surgipro and Gore-Tex.

Materials and methods

The study comprised two groups of 36 adult New Zealand white rabbits. Each of the 72 animals received two 3.75 cm discs of Marlex and Gore-Tex or Surgipro and Gore-Tex, implanted intra-abdominally through an incision in the linea alba, directly adjacent to the viscera. Implants were randomized into left or right, and each animal served as its own control. Implants were sized to correspond proportionately to the average sized implant used in humans.

After the procedures, the animals had free access to standard laboratory food and water. Observations of the animals' conditions were recorded weekly by a veterinarian or animal technician.

The rabbits were sacrificed at 7, 14 and 90 days (three rabbits each at 7 and 14 days and 30 rabbits each at 90 days) and specimens were retrieved for gross and histological analysis. Each disc was removed along with 2 cm of surrounding tissue and placed in 10% buffered, neutral formalin for histological analysis. If adhesions to the materials were present, they were transected, leaving any attached tissue intact.

Adhesions were scored grossly according to a modified Diamond scale[1], which evaluates both the extent and the tenacity of the adhesions. Scoring for extent of adhesions ranged from 0 (no adhesions) to 4 (adhesions to > 75% of the implant). Scoring for tenacity included: 1 (adhesions easily separable – fibrinous), 2 (adhesions separable by blunt dissection) and 3 (adhesions require sharp dissection – fibrous).

Gore-Tex Soft Tissue Patch is a registered trademark of W.L. Gore & Associates Inc.
Marlex is a registered trademark licensed to C.R. Bard Inc.
Surgipro Mesh is a registered trademark of U.S. Surgical Corp.

For histological analysis, each specimen was embedded in paraffin, sectioned and stained with haematoxylin and eosin and Milligan's trichrome to evaluate tissue response, cellular migration and collagen deposition into the interstices and around the materials (incorporation), and inflammation.

Results

Cross observations

After seven days, 83% of both of the mesh material showed adhesions (100% of the Marlex and 75% of the Surgipro specimens) compared with 16% of the Gore-Tex. The adhesion score for the meshes was 0.57 for the Marlex and 0.42 for the Surgipro compared with 0.09 for the Gore-Tex. Results at 14 days did not change appreciably for the meshes, 100% of the Marlex and 66% of the Surgipro specimens showing adhesions (adhesion scores 0.67 and 0.33, respectively). The Gore-Tex implants showed an increase in the number of adhesions (42% compared with 16% at seven days), although the adhesion score still remained low (0.2). At 90 days, 58.6% of the Marlex mesh specimens

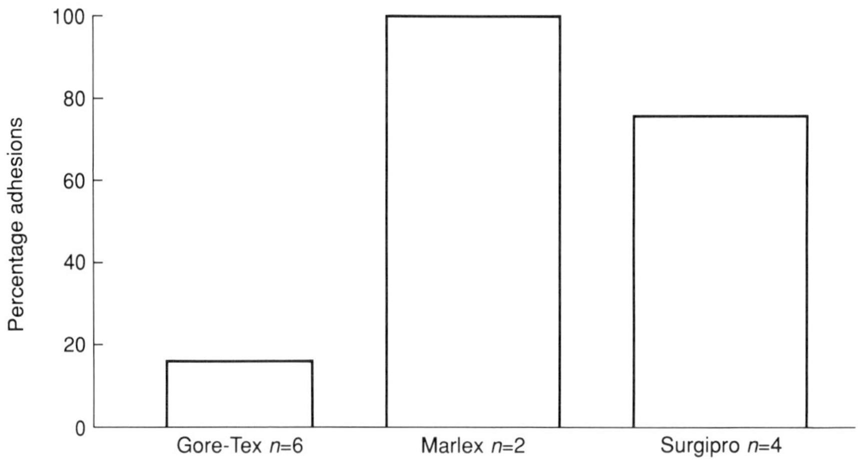

Figure 83.1: Adhesion data for the three types of implant material seven days after the procedure.

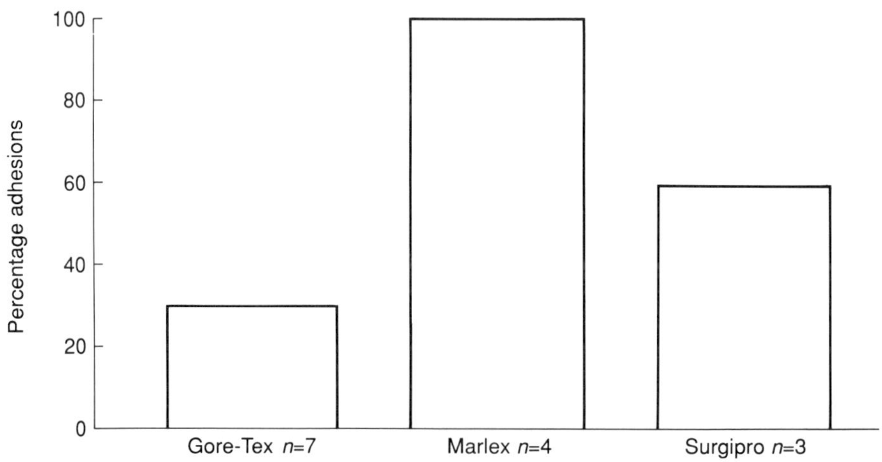

Figure 83.2: Adhesion data for the three types of implant material 14 days after the procedure.

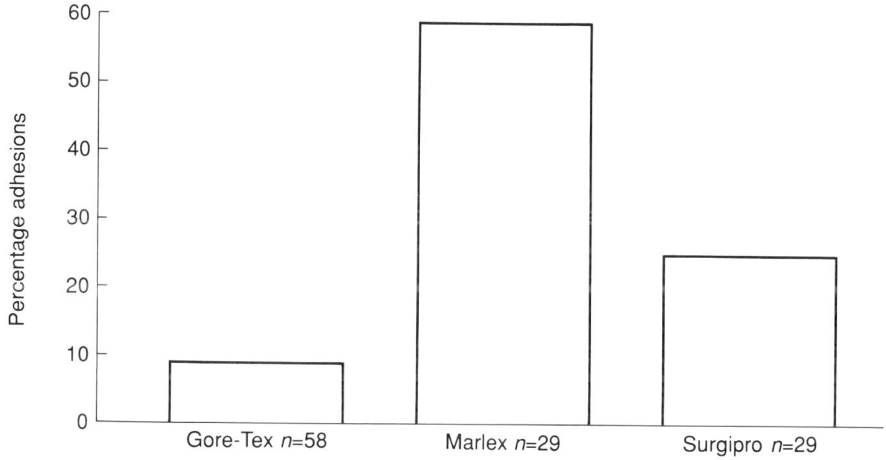

Figure 83.3: Adhesion data for the three types of implant material 90 days after the procedure.

Table 83.1: Number of adhesions at 90 days

Material	*Large bowel*	*Small bowel*	*Caecum and appendix*	*Omentum*
Gore-Tex Soft Tissue Patch	3	1	0	1
Marlex mesh	12	4	1	6
Surgipro mesh	3	1	2	2

and 27.5% of the Surgipro specimens showed adhesions compared with 8.6% of the Gore-Tex implants. Adhesion scores were 0.3 and 0.11 for the Marlex and Surgipro, respectively, with 0.04 for the Gore-Tex.

Figures 83.1–83.3 indicate the individual adhesion data for each material at each time period. Large and small bowel, caecum, appendix and omentum were adherent to the mesh specimens. The large and small bowel were usually firmly adherent and, in some cases, the serosal surface was in direct contact with the surface of the meshes. In general, the Surgipro had fewer adhesions ($p = 0.01$) than the Marlex ($p = 0.0001$), possibly because it is less stiff and coarse than the Marlex.

The Gore-Tex had fewer adhesions when compared with the meshes. Some specimens had small or large bowel loosely adherent by thin, tendinous bands. The majority of the other adhesions to the Gore-Tex patches were to the suture line or edge of the patch only (Table 83.1).

Histological observations

At seven days the Gore-Tex had a continuous lining of neomesothelialization with cellular migration into the interstices by mainly histiocytes and a few fibroblasts. At 14 days, collagen deposition into the interstices was observed, providing firm anchorage of the Gore-Tex. Collagen deposition increased with time, and by 90 days there was greater cellular ingrowth and collagen deposition into the interstices of the patch, with no evidence of encapsulation. Inflammation was not observed, although occasional foreign body giant cells were seen at the patch/tissue interface.

Both mesh materials had a tissue response typical of rough-surfaced materials. The Marlex mesh showed concentric alignment of collagen fibres around individual mesh filaments, which increased with time until a dense, hypertrophic scar was observed at 90 days. Remesothelialization was patchy owing to the presence of the scar tissue. The Surgipro mesh also showed dense, unorganized collagen fibres with irregular neomesothelialization. Inflammation was evident in both meshes, with hypercellularity around the mesh filaments that persisted at 90 days. Numerous foreign body giant cells and histiocytes were presented at seven days, in addition to lymphocytes and plasma cells at 90 days. None of the mesh samples completely reperitonealized at any time point in the study.

Conclusions

In the intra-abdominal position, the Gore-Tex had fewer adhesions than the two mesh materials. Although the Surgipro had more adhesions and more tenacious adhesions than the Gore-Tex, it exhibited fewer adhesions than the Marlex.

Histologically, the Gore-Tex showed a more normal healing response, with good ingrowth and reperitonealization and minor inflammatory response. The mesh materials exhibited a marked inflammatory response throughout the study, indicating abnormal healing. The type of response seen with the mesh materials leads to hypertrophic scar formation and calcification, which ultimately results in contraction of the scar[2] and distortion of the stiff mesh, increasing the risk of fistula formation.

Clearly, mesh materials should be used with caution in the intra-abdominal position, and may only be suitable for preperitoneal approaches to laparoscopic hernia repair. However, because the peritoneum may tear or otherwise be incompletely closed during laparoscopic hernia repair, mesh materials may still present problems.

The intraperitoneal approach to laparoscopic hernia repair takes less time to complete compared with preperitoneal repairs, and avoids many of the complexities, pitfalls and potential complications of preperitoneal approaches. If the surgeon elects to perform an intraperitoneal repair, Gore-Tex should be the surgeon's prosthetic material of choice. This study suggests that mesh materials are contraindicated for intraperitoneal placement.

References

1. Diamond MP, Linsky CB, Cunningham T, Constantine B, diZerega GS, DeCherney AH. A model for sidewall adhesions in the rabbit: reduction by an absorbable barrier. *Microsurgery* 1987; 8: 197–200.

2. Skalli O, Gabbiani G. The biology of the myofibroblast relationship to wound contraction and fibrocontractive diseases. In Henson C, ed. *The Molecular and Cellular Biology of Wound Repair.* New York: Plenum Press, 1988.

84

Prosthetic Biomaterials in Hernia Repair

ARNOLD S SEID

Although the modern era of hernia repair began more than a century ago, controversies continue about the optimal surgical technique. Recent published reports of herniorrhaphies in which mesh was not used are disappointing: re-recurrences for recurrent hernias are as high as 33% and recurrences of incisional hernias of 30% have been reported[1–4]. However, the better results reported in series in which mesh was used suggests that these prosthetic devices produce a lower incidence of recurrent hernia[5–13]. A recent editorial advocating the use of prosthetic materials for inguinal herniorrhaphy concludes that the use of endogenous tissue is physiologically naïve and structurally destructive whereas the use of a prosthetic tension-free repair is mechanically reasonable, structurally sound, and elegantly simple[14].

Despite numerous studies confirming the advantages of biomaterials in hernia repair, some bias against their use persists because of concern about rejection, infection and recurrence. Although prosthetic mesh is clearly valuable in reducing recurrences, the question remains whether there are valid contraindications to the use of a foreign material in the body, such as rejection and infection. Additionally, questions remain about which prosthetic material in a given clinical situation is most efficacious. It is the intent of the author to review the pertinent literature to answer these questions as they pertain to the repair of inguinal and incisional hernias.

Historical background

The Greeks were the first to use foreign materials to treat hernias. Around the beginning of the Common Era, a physician (probably Heliodorus) used cellulose from either the cotton or flax plant in an incision to attempt scarification of the defect[15]. For the next 1900 years, hernia treatment involved the use of trusses or cautery to produce cicatrization. The development of anaesthesia and antisepsis in the 19th century inaugurated the modern era of hernia surgery. In the 1880s, Billroth prophetically postulated the use of biomaterials to repair the weakened endogenous fascia[14]. In 1900, two reports from Germany described the first use of prosthetic material when Witzel and Goepel employed silver mesh to repair hernia defects. However, the material ultimately fragmented and proved to be unsatisfactory[16,17].

In 1951, Koontz reported the use of a tantalum mesh[18]. Subsequently, tantalum and stainless steel were both used, but they, too, failed due to fragmentation and severe inflammatory reaction[19,20]. Later, Koontz and Usher evaluated the organic polymers orlon, teflon (PTFE), dacron, and polyethelene[18,21]. In 1962, polypropylene mesh (PPM) was first used for hernia repair[22].

Initial use of teflon was disappointing, but the results improved with the introduction of microporous expanded-weave (ePTFE). In 1985, Wool used this material for a hernia repair[23].

Currently in the United States, the prosthetic materials used most extensively in inguinal and incisional hernia repairs are PPM and ePTFE.

Properties of biomaterials

A material that is to be used for long term implantation into the body to reinforce a fascial defect must have certain physical, mechanical and biocompatible properties. In 1973, Williams reviewed extensively the mechanical and physical properties of biomaterials, and in the 1950s, Cumberland and Scales identified the biocompatibility considerations[24,25,26]. Their work remains crucial to understanding the problem.

The mechanical characteristics that must be considered have been ably described by Williams, and it is beyond the scope of this chapter to detail them fully[26]. The prosthetic device must be able to withstand, over decades, the great and repeated stresses of bodily movement and changes in intraperitoneal pressure. Therefore, it must meet stringent criteria identified by Williams such as tensile strength, shear strain, elasticity, brittleness, ductility, hardness, and degree of creep and fatigue.

The physical characteristics of materials include the optical, magnetic, electrical, ratioactive and radiolucent properties. Optimally, a prosthetic patch used in herniorrhaphy would be radiolucent to avoid subsequent diagnostic imaging problems. Also, the prosthesis should be non-magnetic to preclude difficulties with MRI imaging. Optically, lucent prosthesis would be desirable for laparoscopic repair. It would allow the surgeon to visualize structures when affixing the prosthesis and thereby avoid injuring structures that otherwise would be obscured by the patch.

In the 1950s, Cumberland and Scales defined the important criteria in determining biocompatibility of bioprostheses[24,25]. These criteria remain relevant today. The material:

1 should not be physically modified by tissue fluids

2 should be chemically inert

3 should not excite an inflammatory or foreign body reaction

4 should be non-carcinogenic

5 should not produce allergy or hypersensitivity

6 should be capable of resisting mechanical strains

7 should be capable of being fabricated in form required

8 should be capable of being sterilized.

To date, PPM and ePTFE seem to best meet these demanding mechanical, physical, and biocompatible criteria, and thus are most extensively utilized. Only recently has it been suggested that these foreign materials evoke an inflammatory response. The long term clinical significance of these findings are the subject of ongoing research.

Animal studies

Despite basic similarities in these eight areas between PPM and ePTFE, major questions remain concerning the tissue response to the two meshes. Brown addressed the question of adhesion formation using a standard classification for adhesions to the mesh[27]. A hernial defect was surgically created in guinea pigs and repaired with PPM or ePTFE. At autopsy, the degree of adhesions was compared. A significant difference between the two materials was noted, with greater adhesions in the PPM ($p < 0.05$). Law performed a similar study in Sprague-Dawley rats and also found significantly greater adhesions to PPM than to ePTFE at 1, 2, 4 and 3 weeks ($p < 0.05$)[4,28]. However, at 22 weeks, this difference declined, and failed to reach statistical significance. Murphy used a similar model in a rat study, using an adhesion scale of 0–4[29]. At 107–140 days, the adhesion index in the ePTFE group was 1.37 compared to 2.62 in the PPM group ($p < .005$). Additionally, in this study Murphy compared the breakaway strength of tissue prosthetic patches on a tensionometer, and found the PPM stronger (3.02 kg/cm) than the ePTFE (2.67 kg/cm). However, the difference was not statistically significant. Brown also found in a comparison study complicated by *Staph aureus* that with or without antibiotics, significantly fewer organisms ($p < 0.05$) adhered to the ePTFE than to the PPM[27].

Mora's studies provided insight into the aetiology of infection of prosthetic mesh used in the repair of ventral hernia[30]. Sterile and endotoxin free biomaterials (Dacron velour, woven Dacron and Biomer polyurethane) were implanted subcutaneously and intraperitoneally in mice. The subcutaneous materials remained sterile. All of the intraperitoneal prostheses became colonized with enteric bacteria. The data suggests that intraperitoneal sterile reactive stimuli can produce bacterial translocation to the dense prostheses directly through the intact normal bowel wall.

Although PPM and ePTFE are generally believed to evoke little or no inflammatory response, recent work by Kossovsky undermines this presumption[31]. He injected dispersed particulate PTFE subcutaneously into dogs, mice and rabbits. Upon histologic examination of the injection sites, he found persistent chronic inflammatory reaction with progressive growth of the involved tissue volume. In addition to giant cells and macrophages, lymphocytes became apparent at three months and constituted up to 40% of the cellular infiltrate by one year. Plasma cells were also noted at the one year period in the rabbit model. Delaney implanted PPM to repair hernias in dogs and found that the mesh caused continued reaction with cellularity in the form of lymphocytes, mast cells and 2+ vascularity at four months[32]. At this time, the immunological significance of this data is unclear.

Clinical summary

Numerous clinical studies have attested to the efficacy and safety of both PPM and ePTFE in the repair of inguinal hernia[5,6,8,9,24,33]. In a combined series, Shulman reported the use of PPM in primary hernia repair with a recurrence rate of 0.2% with no evidence of mesh rejection in 3019 cases[13]. In smaller series, similar results were reported for ePTFE by Lablanc and Pailler, and Berliner[10,12].

However, the use of prosthetic materials in large abdominal wall defects is more problematic. In these cases, the potential complications of prosthetic meshes are well documented. PPM has been associated with mesh extrusion, enteric fistula, and erosion into intra-abdominal organs whereas ePTFE has been used in the repairs of large abdominal wall defects with no cases of extrusion, bowel obstructions or fistulas[34,35,36].

Conclusion

A 30 year experience with PPM and an eight year experience with ePTFE have shown that these materials are important adjuncts for successful hernia repairs. The question of which material, in what type of hernia and how and where the prosthetic material should be placed is not yet entirely resolved.

Both materials have satisfactory physical and mechanical properties and are essentially biocompatible. In inguinal herniorrhaphy, the incidence of complications associated with the prosthesis is low. Therefore, handling characteristics, the 'feel' of the material, and surgeons' preference seem to be decisive in the choice of materials. In congenital or Nyhus I hernias, simple ligation of the sac and a reconstruction of the internal ring may be a sufficient repair, thereby avoiding the minimal risks associated with prosthetic mesh. However, in cases of fascial defects with one problem of collangenolysis or a recurrent hernia, the use of either mesh offers superior results. In conventional inguinal herniorrhaphy, there seems little to differentiate between the PPM and the ePTFE. For laparoscopic repair of inguinal hernia, the physical and mechanical properties of PPM are superior to ePTFE. The PPM has more memory and more readily assumes a flat planar configuration after passing through the trocar, whereas the ePTFE is limp and difficult to manipulate laparoscopically.

In addition, the ePTFE is opaque and the surgeon's inability to see through the mesh makes the staple affixation more difficult. The history of serious complications associated with intraperitoneal mesh would suggest that in any laparoscopic hernia repair the mesh should be placed preperitoneally and that the intraperitoneal placement of prosthetic material in a routine inguinal hernia repair is contraindicated.

In the repair of large abdominal wall defects, the complicating factor is that the mesh often cannot be kept isolated from the intraperitoneal structures, specifically, bowel. Mora has shown that intraperitoneal placement of prosthetic mesh can lead to translocation of bacteria across the intact bowel wall and contaminate the mesh[30]. Preliminary data indicate the ePTFE is less likely to cause adhesions and erode into bowel than PPM. This suggests that if possible, the mesh should be kept from contact with the bowel by interposition of omentum or closure of the peritoneum. If this is not possible, the ePTFE is preferred over PPM.

The recent questions about the long-term safety of silicone gel-filled breast implants should serve as a warning that every bioprosthetic implant, designed to last decades, requires continued close scrutiny[37]. Kossovsky cautions that we must 'take the position that biomaterials can behave like any other immunogenic substance. If we would just stop fighting that and accept the hypothesis, then many clinical observations make sense, and a whole host of clinical questions come to mind. As long as there is denial of this basic hypothesis, then the science can't be advanced[38]'.

Summary

The prosthetic biomaterials have been shown to offer major advantages in the repair of inguinal and incisional hernias. They appear to be safe and efficacious with a low recurrence rate, minimal infection and no evidence of rejection. Nonetheless, a review of the literature indicates that continuous clinical scrutiny is necessary to further define the optimal means and indications for using these materials in order to avoid the adverse reactions they can evoke.

References

1. Ijzermans J, DeWilt H, Hop WOJ, Jeekel H. Recurrent inguinal hernia treated by classical hernioplasty. *Arch Surg*, 1991; **126**: 1097–100.
2. Schaap, HM, van de Pavoordt HDWM, Bast TJ. The preperitoneal approach in the repair of recurrent inguinal hernias. *Surg Gynecol Obstet*, 1992; **174**: 460–4.
3. Langer S, Christiansen J. Long-term results after incisional hernia repair. *Acta Chir Scand*, 1985; **151**: 217–19.
4. Larson GM, Harrower HW. Plastic mesh repair of incisional hernia. *Am J Surg*, 1978; **135**: 559–63.
5. Barnes JP. Inguinal hernia repair with routine use of marlex mesh. *Surg Gynecol Obstet*, 1987; **165**: 33–7.
6. Bauer JJ, Salky BA, Gelernt IM, Kree I. Repair of large abdominal wall defects with expanded polytetrafluoroethylene (PTFE). *Ann Surg*, 1987; **206**: 765–9.
7. Berliner SD. Clinical experience with an inlay expanded polytetrafluoroethylene soft tissue patch as an adjunct in inguinal hernia repair. *Surg Gynecol Obstet*, 1993; **176**: 323–6.
8. DeBord JR, Wyffels PL, Marshall JS, Miller G, Marshall WH. Repair of large central incisional hernias with expanded polytetrafluoroethylene prosthetic patches. *Postgrad Gen Surg*, 1992; **4**: 156–60.
9. Deysine M. Hernia repair with expanded polytetrafluoroethylene. *Amer J Surg*, 1992; 422–4.
10. LeBlanc KA, Booth WV. Repair of primary and secondary inguinal hernias using an expanded polytetrafluoroethylene patch. *Contemp Surg*, 1992; **41**.

11. Martin RE, Shureih S, Classen JN. Polypropylene mesh in 450 hernia repairs: evaluation of wound infections. *Contemp Surg*, 1982; **20**.

12. Pailler JL, Baranger B, Darrieus H, Schill H, Neveux Y. Clinical analysis of expanded PTFE in the treatment of recurrent and complex groin hernias. *Postgrad Gen Surg*, 1992; 168–70.

13. Shulman AG, Amid PK, Lichtenstein IL. The safety of mesh repair for primary inguinal hernias: results of 3,019 operations from five diverse surgical sources. *Am Surg*, 1992; **58**: 255–7.

14. Read RC. The development of inguinal herniorrhaphy. *Surg Clin North Am*, 1984; **64**: 185–96.

15. Carlson RI. The historical development of the surgical treatment of inguinal hernia. *Surgery*, 1956; **39**: 1031–46.

16. Goepel R. Uber die Verschliessung von Bruchpforten durch Einheilung seflochtener fertiger Silberdrahtnetze. *Verhandlungen der Deutschen Gesellschaft fur Chirurgie*, 1900; **29**: 174–7.

17. Witzel O. Ueber den Verschluss von Bauchwunden und Bruchpforten durch versenkte Silberdrahtnetze. *Zentralblatt fur Chirurgie*, 1900; **27**: 257–60.

18. Koontz AR, Kimberly RC. Further experimental work on prostheses for hernia repair. *Surg Gynecol Obstet*, 1959; **109**: 321–7.

19. Burton CC. Fascia lata, cutis, and tantalum grafts in repair of massive abdominal incisional hernias. *Surg Gynecol Obstet*, 1959; **109**: 621–8.

20. Peacock Jr, EE. Here we are: behind again! *Amer J Surg*, 1989; **157** (editorial): 187.

21. Usher FC, Wallace SA. Tissue reaction to plastics: a comparison of nylon, orlon, dacron, teflon and Marlex. *Arch Surg*, 1958; **76**: 997–9.

22. Usher FC. Hernia repair with Marlex mesh. *In*: Nyhus LM, Condon RE, eds. *Hernia*. 2nd ed. Philadelphia, Pa: JB Lippincott Company, 1978; 561–71.

23. Wool NL, Straus AK, Roseman DL. Clinical experience with Gore-Tex soft tissue patch in hernia repair: a preliminary report. *Proc Inst Med Chao*, 1985; **41**: 358–62.

24. Cumberland VH. A preliminary report on the use of prefabricated nylon weave in the repair of ventral hernia. *Med J Aust*, 1952; **1**: 143–4.

25. Scales JT. Discussion on metals and synthetic materials in relation to soft tissues: tissue reaction to synthetic materials. *Proc R Soc Med*, 1953; **46**: 647–52.

26. Williams DF. The mechanical and physical properties of materials. *In*: Williams DF, Roaf R, eds. *Implants in surgery*. Philadelphia, Pa: WB Saunders Company, 1973; 65–136.

27. Brown GL, Richardson JD, Malangoni MA, Tobin GR, Ackerman D, Polk Jr HC. Comparison of prosthetic materials for abdominal wall reconstruction in the presence of contamination and infection. *Ann Surg*, 1985; **201**: 705–11.

28. Law NW. A comparison of polypropylene mesh, expanded polytetrafluoroethylene patch and polyglycolic acid mesh for the repair of experimental abdominal wall defects. *Acta Chir Scand*, 1990; **156**: 759–62.

29. Murphy JL, Freeman JB, Dionne PG. Comparison of Marlex and Gore-Tex to repair abdominal wall defects in the rat. *Can J Surg*, 1989; **32**: 244–7.

30. Mora EM, Cardona MA, Simmons RL. Enteric bacteria and ingested inert particles translocate to intraperitoneal prosthetic materials. *Arch Surg*, 1991; **126**: 157–63.

31. Kossovsky N, Millett D, Juma S, Little N, Briggs PC, Raz S, Berg E. In vivo characterization of the inflammatory properties of poly(tetrafluoroethylene) particulates. *J Biomed Mater Res*, 1991; **25**: 1287–301.

32. Delany HM, Li J, Kim ES. Extent of peritoneal adhesions and local tissue reaction in response to absorbable vs. nonabsorbable mesh. *Contemp Surg*, 1992; **40**: 29–35.

33. Lichtenstein IL, Shulman AG, Amid PK, Montllor MM. The tension-free hernioplasty. *Amer J Surg*, 1989; **157**: 188–93.

34. Kaufman Z, Engelberg M, Zager M. Fecal fistula: A late complication of marlex mesh repair. *Dis Colon Rectum*, 1981; **24**: 543–4.

35. Schneider R, Herrington JL Jr, Granada AM. Marlex mesh in repair of a diaphragmatic defect later eroding into the distal esophagus and stomach. *Am Surg*, 1979; **45**: 337–9.

36. Voyles C, Richardson JD, Bland KI, *et al.* Emergency abdominal wall reconstruction with polypropylene mesh. Short-term benefits versus long-term complications. *Ann Surg*, 1981; **194**: 219–23.

37. Press RI, Peebles CL, Kumagi Y, Ochs RL, Tan EM. Antinuclear autoantibodies in women with silicone breast implants. *Lancet*, 1992; **340**: 1304–7.

38. Randall T. Antibodies to silicone detected in patients with severe inflammatory reactions. *JAMA*, 1992; **268**: 1821–2.

Law NW, Ellis H. Adhesion formation and peritoneal healing on prosthetic materials. *Clin Mater*, 1988; **3**: 95–101.

Nyhus LM, Pollak R, Bompeck TC, Donahue PE. The preperitoneal approach and prosthetic buttress repair for recurrent hernia: the evolution of a technique. *Ann Surg*, 1988; **208**: 733–7.

85

A Simple Stapling Technique for the Prosthetic Repair of Massive Incisional Hernias

PARVIZ K AMID, ALEX G SHULMAN AND IRVING L LICHTENSTEIN

Unacceptable recurrence rates, as high as 46%, have been reported following simple closure of large incisional hernias without utilization of biomaterials[1]. Use of prosthetic mesh, however, has improved the results, with recurrence rates of zero[2] to 11%[3], depending on the technique used. The preperitoneal prosthetic repair, described by Stoppa, has been employed successfully in Europe for many years[4,5], and has proved superior to other mesh repair techniques by American authors as well[6]. Taking advantage of new instrumentation technology for endoscopic surgery, this chapter introduces a simplified version of a previously described approach that has proved successful for many years[4–6]. The procedure is easier, faster and safer, and achieves a better cosmetic result than its predecessor. The instrument used is the Endo-Hernia stapler. This stapler, originally designed for endoscopic hernia repair, can be angulated at its tip.

In the preperitoneal approach, intra-abdominal pressure, the same force that caused the hernia, keeps the prosthesis in place and prevents recurrence. The edges of the mesh, however, should be anchored to the posterior abdominal wall to prevent wrinkling or folding until incorporation takes place. In Stoppa's procedure, this is accomplished by making multiple stab wounds on the skin around the surgical incision in order to pull the anchoring sutures of the mesh through the entire thickness of the abdominal wall. This can result in more postoperative pain, formation of haematoma and infection. It also causes multiple unsightly skin retractions (Figure 85.1).

Operative technique

The hernia sac is simply inverted into the abdomen by imbricating sutures or, if necessary, preserved in order to facilitate complete peritoneal closure. With multiloculated hernias, the septa are released in order to create one combined sac. Below the arcuate line of Douglas, the peritoneum is separated from the posterior abdominal wall for a distance of 6–8 cm beyond the edges of the defect for placement of the mesh. Above this line, if the peritoneum cannot be separated from the posterior aspect of the posterior rectus sheath, the mesh can be inserted between the rectus muscles and the anterior aspect of the posterior sheath.

The rectus muscles are reached by incising the rectus sheath. If feasible, it is preferred to incise the posterior rectus sheath because this facilitates the subsequent closure of the linea alba by preserving all the anterior rectus sheath[7]. The rectus muscles are then dissected from their posterior sheaths to a point beyond the lateral border of the muscles.

In most instances, the peritoneal cavity is not entered, resulting in a smoother postoperative course. If the peritoneum is opened, either inadvertently or intentionally, it must be closed in order to provide a physical barrier between the intestines and the mesh. This will prevent intestinal

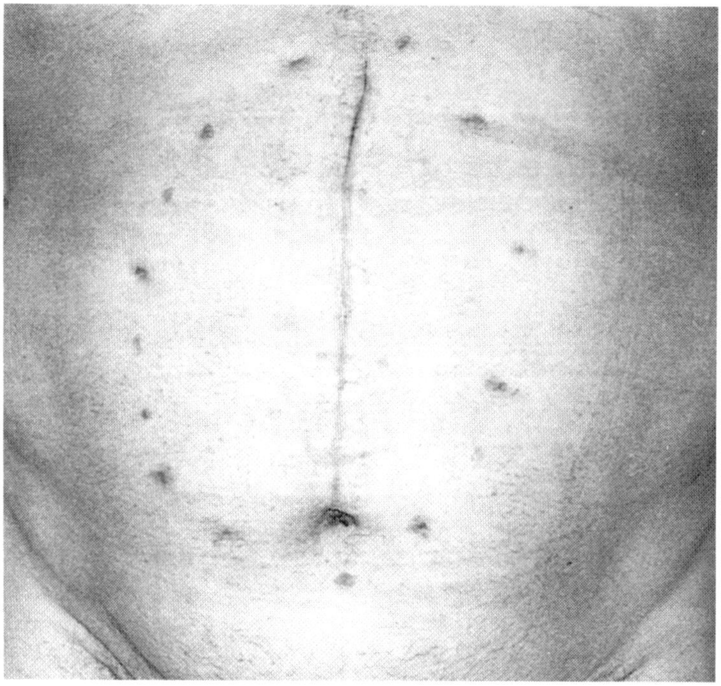

Figure 85.1: Postoperative scars of suture technique.

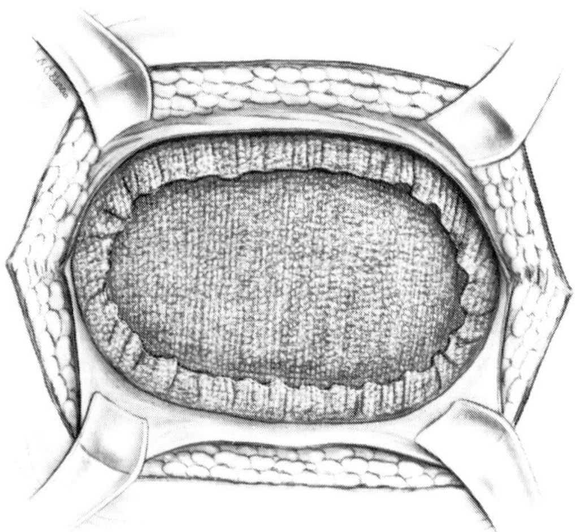

Figure 85.2: The extra mesh in the preperitoneal space is allowed to fold upon itself.

adhesions and biomaterial-related intestinal fistulae. At times, a lack of adequate peritoneal tissue due to previous multiple operations or peritonitis may make this impossible. In such instances, closure may be achieved by taking advantage of the preserved hernia sac or by borrowing tissue from the omentum. A new generation of prostheses with the selective property of incorporation with the abdominal wall, but without adherence to the intestines, is under study and may resolve this problem in the near future.

A sheet of Marlex mesh, slightly larger than needed, is used. Marlex is the preferred choice of biomaterial because its slight roughness stimulates fibroplasia and its monofilamented fibres do not promote or harbour infection. The mesh is then spread over the peritoneum. The extra mesh is allowed to fold upon itself (Figure 85.2). The tip of the Endo-Hernia stapler with a 45° upward angulation is placed into the fold of the mesh using the right hand (Figure 85.3).

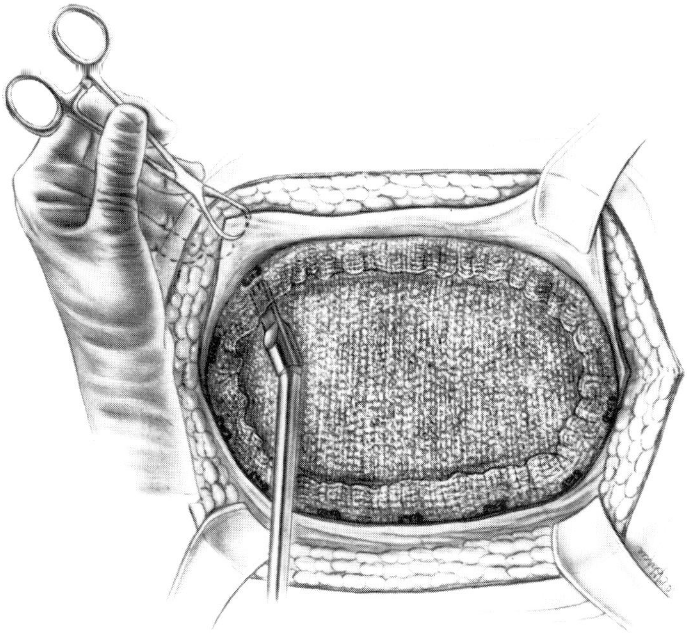

Figure 85.3: The tip of the stapler with 45-degree upward angulation is placed into the fold of the mesh.

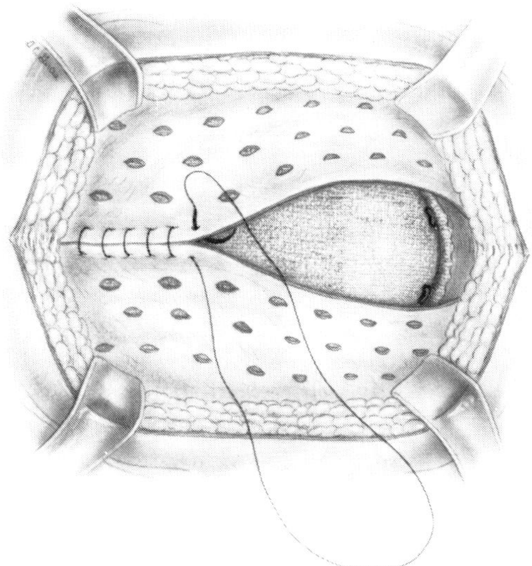

Figure 85.4: Closure of the linea alba facilitated by multiple buttonholes[7].

The left hand is used to pull the edge of the fascia upward with a clamp while simultaneously pressing against the skin from the outside to facilitate the stapling. Alternatively, the tip of the stapler can be placed in the surgeon's left hand and guided into the fold of the mesh. While the left hand is pushing the tip upward, the stapler is fired by the right hand.

Staples are placed lateral to the lateral edge of the rectus muscle, along the linea semilunaris, 3–4 cm apart. In the upper abdomen, this results in fixation of the prosthesis to the rectus sheath and restoration of some of the lost respiratory functions of the abdominal belt muscles[8]. Excess mesh is then trimmed away. The advantages of using this instrument include a considerable saving of time when compared with the suturing technique. Furthermore, as the stapler is inserted into the fold of the mesh, it helps to straighten the mesh. Upward angulation of the stapler, which is pointing away from the peritoneum, prevents injury to the underlying peritoneum and the intestines.

To exploit the intra-abdominal pressure for holding the mesh in place, the anterior rectus sheath must be closed. If this is not possible without wrinkling the mesh, closure can be facilitated by making multiple buttonholes on the anterior rectus sheath (Figure 85.4).

The surgical field should be drained, using closed suction drain placed over the mesh, and intraoperative antibiotics should be given intravenously. A postoperative low-power radiograph of the abdomen, showing the individual staples, provides a useful baseline for future follow-up.

Results

Since 1988, we have used the preperitoneal prosthetic repair in 54 patients. The stapling technique was employed for the last 25 patients. There have been no recurrences to date. This stapling technique can also be used in bilateral (Stoppa)[9] or unilateral (Wantz)[10] preperitoneal inguinal hernioplasty when these procedures are indicated.

Summary

A total of 54 large incisional hernias were successfully repaired by employing preperitoneal insertion of a large sheet of Marlex mesh. In 25 patients, the mesh was fixed in place using a simple stapling technique. The procedure exploits intra-abdominal pressure, the same force that caused the hernia, to prevent reherniation. The margins of the mesh, however, need fixation to the posterior abdominal wall to prevent folding until host tissue infiltration occurs. Fixation of mesh by this stapling technique simplifies the procedure. It is faster, easier and safer, and achieves a more acceptable cosmetic result.

References

1. George CD, Ellis H. The results of incisional hernia repair: a twelve year review. *Ann R Coll Surg Engl* 1986; **68**: 185–93.
2. Usher FC. The repair of incisional and inguinal hernias. *Surg Gynecol Obstet* 1970; 525–30.
3. Larson GM, Harrower HW. Plastic mesh repair of incisional hernias. *Am J Surg* 1978; **135**: 559–63.
4. Rives J. In collaboration with Pire JC, Flament JB, Palot JP. Major incisional hernias. In: Chevrel JP, ed. *Surgery of the Abdominal Wall.* New York: Springer-Verlag, 1987: 116–44.
5. Stoppa RE. The treatment of complicated groin and incisional hernias. *World J Surg* 1989; **13**: 545–54.
6. Wantz G. *Atlas of Hernia Surgery*. New York: Raven Press, 1991: 179–216.
7. Wantz GE. Incisional hernioplasty with Mersilene. *Surg Gynecol Obstet* 1991; **172**: 129–37.
8. Stoppa RE, Moungar F, Verhaeghe P. Surgical treatment of median supraumbilical eventrations. *J Chir (Paris)* 1992; **129**: 335–43.
9. Stoppa RE, Rives JL, Warlaumont CR, *et al.* The use of Dacron in the repair of hernias of the groin. *Surg Clin North Am* 1984; **64**: 269–85.
10. Wantz GE. Giant prosthetic reinforcement of the visceral sac for management of hernias of the groin at high risk for recurrence. *Surg Gynecol Obstet* 1989; **169**: 408–17.

86

Laparoscopic Ventral Herniorrhaphy using an Intraperitoneal Onlay Patch of Expanded Polytetrafluoroethylene

KARL A LEBLANC, WILLIAM V BOOTH AND ALBERT T SPAW

Laparoscopic surgery may prove the best method of managing ventral hernias, especially recurrent incisional hernias, obviating the need for large incisions into compromised fascia, requiring minimal dissection and producing less postoperative pain and morbidity. Most often, these procedures can be performed on an outpatient basis.

The use of a prosthetic reinforcing patch is an essential part of this surgery. The material selected must not promote the formation of dense or prolific adhesions because the patch is placed intraperitoneally, in direct contact with the abdominal viscera. Adhesions to viscera have been implicated in the formation of bowel fistulas[1–3]. We use a 1 mm-thick expanded polytetrafluoroethylene (ePTFE) patch (Gore-Tex Soft Tissue Patch) because of its extreme inertness, low foreign-body response and minimal to no adhesion formation.

This chapter reports the results of 34 laparoscopic ventral herniorrhaphies using an intraperitoneal onlay patch (IPOP) in 29 patients.

Operative technique

Twenty-nine patients ranging in age from 19 to 88 years underwent 34 laparoscopic IPOP ventral herniorrhaphies. Twenty-four were incisional, six were umbilical and four were epigastric hernias. Six were incarcerated. Ten patients were obese, two had pulmonary disease and three had heart disease. There were 14 concomitant laparoscopic procedures, including two cholecystectomies, one inguinal hernia repair, one small bowel obstruction and ten other fascial defects. Hernias ranged in size from 2 to 25 cm; the largest was about 16 × 35 cm.

All operations were performed under general anaesthesia administered via tracheal intubation, and most patients received nasogastric tubes and Foley catheters.

The abdomen was usually entered through an upper or lower midline incision, and a 10 mm trocar was inserted through which a CO_2 pneumoperitoneum was established. Additional trocars were then placed. The number and placement of trocars varied according to the location of the hernia and patient habitus, but generally two additional 10 mm trocars were placed laterally. Larger hernias generally required more trocars. We used 0°, 30° or 45° scopes, although we found that the 30° scope provided the best visualization of the defect.

The fascial margins of the defect were differentiated using enterolysis. Sharp dissection was sometimes necessary to remove omental adhesions. The ePTFE patch was sized to overlap the

Gore-Tex Soft Tissue Patch and Gore-Tex Suture are registered trademarks of W.L. Gore & Associates, Inc., Flagstaff, AZ.

margins of the defect by at least 1.5–2 cm on each side. (Through experience, we have found that it is better to make the patch larger than smaller. In one case two 15 × 20 cm patches were stapled together, to cover the defect of 16 × 35 cm.) The patch was then rolled, inserted through a trocar, unrolled and stapled in place over the defect. Usually, one edge of the patch was held in place by the assistant surgeon and the surgeon as the edge was stapled. The patch was then pulled up and the opposite edge was stapled, causing the patch to cover the initial row of staples. The remaining two edges were then stapled, completing the repair. (Approximately 25 staples were used in all.)

Average time in surgery was 45 minutes (range: 20–180 minutes).

Results

The patients were generally sent home within 23 hours of surgery, except for one patient with a small bowel obstruction who required a hospital stay and two patients with heart disease who were kept overnight for observation. All patients tolerated the procedure well.

Patients were restricted from heavy lifting for one month and other activities were limited only by their individual pain tolerance. Patients were prescribed hydrocodone 7.5 mg tablets for postoperative pain. All patients appeared to have markedly reduced pain (this was especially evident in those patients with recurrent hernias) when compared with open repair, and returned to full activity within a few days to a few weeks.

There were two complications. One patient developed an infected seroma overlying the repair about one week postoperatively. We removed the ePTFE patch via an open technique to avoid compromising the patient's status. The wound was closed primarily without a prosthesis and the patient has experienced no further problems. Another patient experienced postoperative pain and requested that the prosthesis be removed. An open technique used to remove the patch revealed no apparent source of the pain. The hernia was repaired at that time using conventional techniques with an ePTFE patch and the patient has experienced no further problems.

Four patients experienced temporary idiopathic induration at the site of the defects. These indurated areas resolved spontaneously within two months, with no complications or further sequelae.

Average follow-up is 8.64 months (longest follow-up: 14 months).

Conclusions

Laparoscopic IPOP ventral herniorrhaphy clearly decreases postoperative morbidity and pain, and lowers medical costs as a result of shorter hospital stays. Follow up will be necessary to determine if it provides acceptable complication and recurrence rates in the long term.

Laparoscopic IPOP ventral herniorrhaphy is indicated for epigastric, lower abdominal, incisional and recurrent hernias. It should not be performed on a pregnant patient. The surgeon should have adequate equipment to perform the procedure, including two large monitors to provide the surgeon and the assistant surgeon with a clear view of the operative field.

The preferred scope and optimum placement must be learned through trial and error. We have found the 30° scope to be the most useful, although we have sometimes needed the 0° and 45° scopes. The scope should be placed in the midline if possible, and we have found that, for optimum visualization, it should be placed slightly lower or higher than expected. At least two other trocars are needed, depending on the size and location of the defect.

Through experience, we have found that fixed-head staplers give the best, most consistent results (articulating-head staplers do not seem to work as well and misfire more frequently).

In the beginning of the series, we chose not to repair very large defects laparoscopically. We now repair the larger defects using laparoscopic techniques, although we generally prefer the open technique if the combined length of the trocar incisions would exceed the length of the laparotomy. Defects with extensive, dense adhesions may, ultimately, be easier to repair using open techniques.

It is extremely important to select a prosthetic material that will not evoke a dense fibrotic response, because the patch is placed intraperitoneally, in direct contact with abdominal viscera. Therefore, the polypropylene meshes are probably unsuitable for this technique. As stated, we use the ePTFE patch specifically because it is inert and supports good tissue ingrowth for a strong repair, without forming adhesions. Because we have been using ePTFE in open repairs for years without experiencing any problems, we feel that we can recommend it in this procedure with a very high degree of confidence.

Laparoscopic IPOP repair of ventral hernias is promising, providing immediate relief of symptoms with greatly decreased morbidity and reduced costs. Continued follow-up is necessary to determine long-term results.

References

1. Bauer JJ, Salky BA, Gelernt IM, Kreel I. Repair of large abdominal wall defects with expanded polytetrafluoroethylene (PTFE). *Ann Surg* 1987; **206**: 765–9.

2. DeBord JR, Wyffels PL, Marshall JS, Miller G, Marshall WH. Repair of large ventral incisional hernias with expanded polytetrafluoroethylene prosthetic patches. *Postgrad Gen Surg* 1992; **4**: 156–60.

3. Deysine M. Hernia repair with expanded polytetrafluoroethylene. *Am J Surg* 1992; **163**: 422–4.

Index